PHARMACOLOGY AND NUTRITIONAL INTERVENTION IN THE TREATMENT OF DISEASE

Edited by **Faik Atroshi**

Pharmacology and Nutritional Intervention in the Treatment of Disease
http://dx.doi.org/10.5772/57023
Edited by Faik Atroshi

Contributors

Tuomas Westermarck, Faik Atroshi, Markku Partinen, Vincent Gallicchio, Erland Johansson, Jerzy Professor Majkowski , Md, PhD, Anatoly Skalny, Mohamed Abdulla, Somdet Srichairatanakool, Maija L Castrén, Shirley Ekvall, Sangeeta Shukla, Elżbieta Płonka-Półtorak, Pekka Kaipainen, Markus Kaski, Ruhi Cakir, Tuomo Maatta, Tuula Tervo-Määttä, Anja Taanila, Maati Iivanainen, Suthat Fucharoen, Margarita G. Skalnaya

Published by InTech

Janeza Trdine 9, 51000 Rijeka, Croatia

Publishing Process Manager Iva Lipovic
Technical Editor InTech DTP team
Cover InTech Design team

First published May, 2014
Printed in Croatia

Additional hard copies can be obtained from orders@intechopen.com

Pharmacology and Nutritional Intervention in the Treatment of Disease, Edited by Faik Atroshi
p. cm.
ISBN 978-953-51-1383-6

For EU product safety concerns:
IN TECH d.o.o., Prolaz Marije Krucifikse Kozulić 3, 51000 Rijeka, Croatia,
info@intechopen.com or visit our website at intechopen.com.

Meet the editor

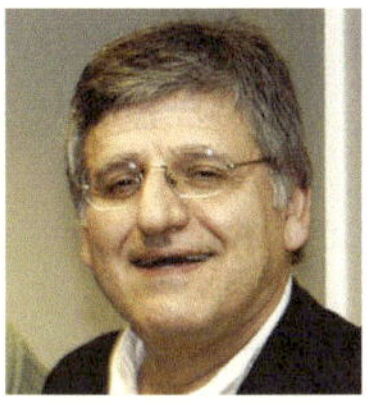

Faik Atroshi, MScBM, Licentiate, PhD clinical biomarkers, Docent, senior researcher in pharmacology and toxicology, Adjunct professor in clinical genetics and clinical nutrition, visiting professors at different international universities; Dip Genetic engineering; Dip Molecular genetics; Dip Analytical clinical pharmacology; Director, education & research satellite centre in trace elements for UNESCO; President of the Global Society for Nutrition, Environment and Health (GSNEH.com); Vice president of the Finnish society for biological medicine, chief editor of International Journal of Trends in Medicine. Research interests and publications are in the field of biomedicine and health; Free radicals and inflammation, oxidative stress and diseases, antioxidants and DNA repair.

Contents

Preface

Pharmacology and Nutritional Intervention in the Treatment of Disease covers topics of fundamental importance in biomedicine, basic principles of nutrition and pharmacology, health and disease research, as well as in basic biological research. While pharmacology is the science of drug action on biological systems, the nutritional aspect deals with general nutrition concepts with a focus on health promotion and therapeutic nutrition.

Food and nutrition play an intimate and inextricable role in all aspects of drug metabolism, comprising, among others, safety and effectiveness. The importance of food and nutrition in the bioavailability of drugs, and vice versa, has been an area of historical interest. In spite of many synthetic compounds, the most efficient drugs available are directly or indirectly related to the plant kingdom. Many plant extracts have been shown to possess pharmacological actions. There is also accumulating evidence that the pharmacological actions, i.e. drug metabolism, distribution and effectiveness, depend on the nutritional status of a person. Natural products are a constant source of potentially active compounds for the treatment of various disorders. Natural products have, however, been largely replaced by synthetic drugs during the last century. However, the adverse side-effects and poor tolerability of many of these drugs have led to the investigation of the efficacy of dietary therapies for several disorders. For example, there is a body of evidence suggesting that metabolism-based therapy could often be considered as the initial treatment plan for patients with specific epilepsy syndromes.

Nutrient-based or natural therapies are gaining popularity for many reasons. People are becoming aware of health-related information and are ready to consider disease prevention and treatments that are less intrusive than conventional allopathic medicine. Natural alternative treatments can provide an opportunity to treat a condition with a first round protocol that is less harmful for natural cell chemistry than the treatment with hard-core synthetic pharmacology. The alternative treatments are based on natural pharmacological activity as well as on cofactor activity that acts as a passive building block. Furthermore, complementary treatments have become popular because nutrigenomic science has helped us to learn more about the natural pharmacology of these remedies. This insight has allowed us to determine the activity of these natural biomedical treatments in relation to that of pharmaceutical drugs; providing reliable science-based information for safe alternative natural choices that can be applied as a first round treatment with reduced risk for side-effects. Nutrigenomic science has also allowed veterinary and human health care professionals to apply confidently complementary medicine to treat patients with natural and conventional drugs in powerful synergy. Many herbal, vitamin, antioxidant and mineral compounds have pharmacological activity similar to that of drugs and are thus able to synergize the effects of a drug leading to lower doses of the drug required for successful treatment. The synergizing effect of some of these nutrient-based compounds is due to them acting through different pathways than the drug. However, many natural compounds (both nutritional and pharmacological) can interfere with or even elevate drug activity, ranging from absorption and transport to liver metabolism and cellular activity. These interactions may change the expected pharmacology of a drug and cause unexpected side-effects.

The unique contributions of individual vitamins and trace elements and their prevalence and distribution in foods provide an ever-expanding field of research which was born on the observations made by the two-time Nobel laureate Linus Carl Pauling (1901–1994). His scientific interest shifted to orthomolecular medicine and his findings on megavitamin therapy, dietary supplements and vitamin C are well known. Furthermore, Abram Hoffer (1917–2009) supported Pauling's conclusion that clinical application of therapeutic doses of specific B vitamins such as niacin and pyridoxine can be successfully used for the management of certain forms of schizophrenia.

Drugs and nutrients are not only involved in the same processes, their availability and function are also intimately and inextricably entwined. The body's ability to process foreign substances depends on metabolic systems that rely on essential nutrients (vitamins, minerals, fatty acids, and so forth) obtained through diet. This book contains a review of what is known about the general relationships between nutrition and pharmacology, as well as issues specific to disease therapies. The importance of food and nutrition for the bioavailability of drugs, and vice versa, has been an area of historical interest. However, much has been learned about the importance of nutritional status for drug metabolism, distribution and effectiveness. The issues related to traditional therapies are highlighted as an area of clinical concern and one in need of further research. Additional attention is focused on the impact of individual micronutrients on drug pharmacokinetics and pharmacodynamics. We have to look more carefully at potential drug-nutrient interactions in the clinical setting and to ask the correct questions, particularly in settings in which poor nutrition might be anticipated. To support our ability to do that, we need to delineate more clearly the role of nutrients in pharmacology beyond just bioavailability.

Faik Atroshi, PhD
Pharmacology & Toxicology,
University of Helsinki,
Finland

Chapter 1

Epilepsy Treatment and Nutritional Intervention

Jerzy Majkowski

Additional information is available at the end of the chapter

http://dx.doi.org/10.5772/57484

1. Introduction

1.1. Epilepsy

Epilepsy is the most common chronic brain condition with epileptiform neuronal discharges, characterized by recurrent unproved seizures with at least two and at least 24 hrs apart. Epileptiform patterns in electroencephalogram (EEG) should confirm the diagnosis. It is the most expensive chronic neurological brain disorder in Europe (Andlin-Sobocki et al. 2005; Majkowski and Majkowska-Zwolińska, 2010). According to the World Health Organisation and the World Bank, the costs of epilepsy constitutes 0.5% of all diseases (Leonardi and Ustrun, 2002).

The incidence of epilepsy in the whole population is estimated as about 50-60 cases per 100.000 persons per year, and it is aged depending. In elderly, above 65 yrs old, it is increasing and about 80 yrs old is about 200 cases /100.000/year and in young preschool age children 100-150 / 100.000/year (Forsgeren, 2004). Worldwide prevalence of epilepsy is about 1% (in whole world about 50 millions of persons). However, according to Poter (1988), 45 to 100 million people worldwide were estimated to have epilepsy. Prevalence, like incidence, is age related; in age above 70 yrs it is highest (about 2%), and a little lower in infants. Extremes of life in humans are associated with increased incidence of epilepsy and increased susceptibility to oxygen stress in the developing immature brain (Lafemina et al., 2006) and in aged animals (Liang and Patel, 2004; Avramovic et al., 2012). It is an open question if there is a causal relation between these two events.

Occurrence of the first seizure, at any age, does not necessary mean epilepsy and a need for antiepileptic drug (AED) administration. It may be symptomatic and diagnostic procedure should be implemented to exclude or confirm an etiological cause. In the whole life of a person, from birth to death, at least one epileptic seizure may occur – including febrile convulsions – in about 8% of otherwise healthy population. In about one of them epilepsy will develop.

Once diagnosis of epilepsy, as defined, is established AED treatment should be started, and in majority of seizure free patients should be continued for several years after the last seizure. In at least 1/3 of epileptic patients with pharmaco-resistant epilepsy, their seizures tend to recur despite of using more than one AED. This group of patients may require life long administration of AEDs. However, a patient's drug resistancy does not imply that the patient will never become seizure-free on further adjustment of AED therapy or other treatment intervention (Kwan et al., 2010; Fröscher, 2012). Introduction of so called new generation of AEDs, while substantially better tolerated, as far as adverse events are concerned, did not make breakthrough in control of pharmaco-resistant form of epilepsy.

All AEDs, with various mechanisms of actions, can to some extent control frequency and severity of epileptic seizures, but not to prevent epileptogenesis (will be discussed in some detail later in this text) which may start after any kind of inborn or acquired brain pathology. However, AEDs may to some extent prevent secondarily cortical epileptization due to epileptic seizures and epileptiform patterns in EEG by reducing or inhibiting occurrence of seizures and/or epileptiform discharges and their spreading to various parts or whole brain structures. On the other hand some AEDs can produce oxygen stress.

In patients with AED therapy resistance, other treatment e.g. neurosurgery may be beneficial in the patients with epileptogenic focus which is precisely localized and is not in eloquent cortical areas. Vagus nerve stimulation is used in addition to AEDs in patients if their seizures are not adequately controlled and there is no possibility to perform neurosurgery (e.g. diffuse brain pathology). Ketogenic diet (KD) may be helpful in some infants and young children with severe epilepsy. Protective modulation of oxidative stress and mitochondrial function by the KD was recently reviewed (Milder and Patel, 2012). The authors highlighted potential mechanism of the KD which can ultimately result in increased production of anti-oxidants and detoxification enzymes with the protective effects of the KD. The diet in Wistar rats revealed an increase in anti-oxidant activity in hippocampus (glutathione peroxidase (GSH-Px) about 4 times) and no changes in lipoperoxidation levels (Ziegler et al., 2003). Cerebral cortex was not affected by the KD, and in cerebellum was a decrease in anti-oxidant capacity. The authors conclude that KD might contribute to protect the hippocampus from neurodegenerative sequelae of seizures. Using organotypic hippocampal slice cultures, it was shown that ketone bodies abolished hippocampal network hyperexcitability following metabolic insult (hypoxia) (Samoilova et al., 2010). The study demonstrated a direct link between metabolic resistance and better control of excessive synchronous abnormal electrical activity. Chronic in vitro ketosis has neuroprotective but not anticonvulsant activity.

However, both methods neurosurgery and KD – are used in rather small percentage of drug resistant epilepsy patients. There is a number of intervention procedures which are at experimental level, still.

In short, currently, AED administration in great majority of patients is the most successfully used symptomatic treatment of seizures but not epilepsy itself. However, long-term treatment, in particular, when polytherapy is used, may result in adverse events including cognitive function impairments, and in turn in decrease the patients' quality of life. Thus, continuous search and trials are needed to find compounds of antiepileptogenesis prevention, to improve seizure control and prevent adverse events, in particular, long term ones affecting cognitive functions. Ideas of various brain disorders, including epilepsy, are teleologicaly explicitly associated with the oxygen toxicity paradigm (Atroshi et al., 2007). Consequently, anti-oxidant interventions are logical procedure with a hope for better health care for these groups of patients. Rational for use of these essential compounds to stay healthy is that they cannot be synthesized in human body. Thus, anti-oxidant supplements could have a potential role in preventing diseases. However, in a normal diet, in high-income countries, sufficient amounts of anti-oxidants may be provided Despite of that more than one third of adults regularly take anti-oxidant supplements (Bjelakovic et al., 2013). The authors assessed whether different doses of beta-carotene, vitamin A and vitamin E affect mortality in primary or secondary prevention randomized clinical trials low risk of bias (53 trials, 241,883 persons aged 18-103 years, 44% women). The study was based on Cochrane systematic review analyzing beneficial and harmful effect of the anti-oxidant supplements in adult. Meta-regression analysis showed that the dose of vitamin A was significantly positively associated with all cause mortality. Vitamin A in a dose above recommended daily allowance (RDA) (>800 μg) did not significantly influence mortality. Beta-carotene in dose above 9.6 mg, and vitamin E in dose above the RDA (>15 mg) significantly increased mortality.

1.2. Oxygen stress

Within the last three decades interest in oxygen stress and its role in the development of oxygen pathology has been considerably increasing and the importance of this phenomenon – increasingly recognized not only in the brain disorders e.g. epilepsy (Azam et al., 2012), headache (Vurucu et al., 2013) but also in other organ function e.g. heart, vascular disorders, diabetes, nasal polyps (Bozkus et al., 2013; Büyükkaya et al., 2013; Chalghoum et al., 2012; Kim et al., 2013; Madmani et al., 2013). Moreover, for the first time the pathophysiological consequences of L-ferritin deficiency in a human helped to define the concept for new disease entity – halmarked by idiopatic generalized seizures and atypical restless leg syndrome – in 23 yrs old female (Cozzi et al., 2013). The syndrome was accompanied with diminished levels of cytosolic catalase, superoxide dismutase (SOD) 1 protein levels, enhanced reactive oxygen species (ROS) production and higher level of oxidized proteins.

Oxygen stress means that the production of free radicals and ROS has exceded physiological the anti-oxidant defence mechanism capacity (Sies, 1985; Mahle and Desgupta, 1997). In Bartosz (2006) opinion, oxygen stress research may be the key to better understanding of certain biochemical, physiological and pathological aspects of living organisms and suggests that such understanding could be applied in clinical practice. Free radicals, the product of oxygen stress, may play an important role as physiological markers which control cell process signals. However, when produced in excess, or when anti-oxidant defense system is not efficient, the free radicals may lead to cell damage. Under physiologic circumstances, the brain has sufficient anti-oxidant defense mechanisms, including GSH-Px which converts potentially harmful H_2O_2 to oxygen and water at the expense of reduced glutathione (GSH) (Wang et al., 2003).

Excessive free radical production is related to various physiological and pathological states, including aging, epileptic seizures or the use of xenobiotics, including fat-soluble drugs (Nikietic et al., 1995; Martinez-Bellesteros et al., 2004; Patel, 2004); this also applies to old and to some new AEDs (Hamed and Abdellah, 2004; Kaipainen et al., 2004; Sobaniec et al., 2006; Atroshi et al, 2007; Avcicek and Iscan, 2007; Płonka-Półtorak et al., 2011). A number of non-specific factors as well as dietary habits affect the state of anti-oxidants in the healthy elderly (Anlasik at al., 2005). This suggests that at the current level of understanding, oxidation and anti-oxidation processes are rather ubiquitous and hence non-specific for particular disorder.

In epilepsy, when the number of free radicals in the brain neurons increases, this interferes with respiratory chain in the mitochondria, destabilizes the lysosomal membranes, and lowers the convulsion threshold (Tayarani et al., 1987; Frantseva et al., 1998; Frantseva et al., 2000; Patel 2002; Waldbaum and Patel, 2010a). Neuronal firing associated with prolonged epileptic discharges and seizures may lead to a number of neurochemical changes and cascades of events at the cellular and molecular level. This in turn, results in mitochondrial dysfunction, increased ROS and nitric oxide (NO) which precede neuronal degeneration and death with possible subsequent epileptogenesis and cortical epileptization – secondary epileptogenesis – which may result in cognitive function impairments and with chronic intractable epilepsy.

Experimental data indicate that NO may be involved in various way in pathophysiology of epileptic seizures. One of interesting mechanism was suggested by Cupello et al. (1997). The authors studied the effects of NO donors and L-arginine (NO precursor) on the up-take of GABA in synaptosomes of the rat brain. They found that NO decreases synaptosomal GABA up-take and it could result in a reduced availability of GABA at the synapses – leading to an increase of neuronal firing.

Mitochondria are emerging as key participants in cell death because their association with an over-growing list o apoptosis-related problems (Chang, 2010). Peroxydation of neuronal membranes modifies their electrophysiological properties and leads to abnormal bioelectric discharges of neurones. Among diseases involving dysfunction in the mitochondrial structures, epilepsy is prominent; it is a sign of energetic anomalies in ATP synthesis due to ADP phosphorylation (Patel, 2002). Mitochondria have important vital functions such as energy production, cellular harm control, neurotransmitter synthesis and free radical production. It is still not clear which of these functions is affected in epileptic seizures (Rowley and Patel, 2013).

Bilateral intracerebra-venticular infusion of all-homocysteic acid in immature rats, resulting in seizures, demonstrated that the marked decrease (approximately 60%) of mitochondrial complex I activity persisted during up to 5 weeks of survival following these seizures (Folbergova et al., 2010). This period of survival corresponds the development of spontaneous seizures (epileptogenesis) in this model. The authors assumed that the persisting inhibition of mitochondrial complex I may lead to the enhanced production of ROS and/or nitrogen species. In this way may contribute not only to neural injury in this model of seizures but also to epileptogenesis.

An increase in spontaneous and evoked epileptic seizures in a subgroup of mice with partial inherent mitochondrial manganese superoxide dismutnase (MnSOD or SOD2) deficit and lipophylic metalloporphyrin catalytic anti-oxidant was reported (Liang and Patel, 2004; Liang et al., 2012). This effect correlated with chronic mitochondrial oxygen stress (aconitase enzyme deactivation) and reduced oxygen use. According to the authors, oxygen stress caused by free radical peroxides increases seizure susceptibility in this subgroup of mice. This susceptibility increases with age (corresponding to high incidence of epilepsy in elderly) and also with increased environmental stimulation and use of stimulants. It is interesting and worthwile to emphesize that **oxygen stress and mitochondrial dysfunction may both cause and be caused by epileptic attacks** (Heinemann et al., 2002; Patel, 2004; Sullivan et al., 2004; Waldbaum and Patel, 2010b). At present, an increasing attention is paid to the possible interaction between oxidative stress, resulting in disturbance of physiological signaling roles of calcium and free radicals in neurones, and mitochondrial dysfunction, cell damage and epilepsy (Martinc et al., 2012)

According to Dubenko and Litovchenko (2002), application of energy metabolism activators improves the clinical and electroencephalographic course of epilepsy. This has been demonstrated experimentally by positive histological changes. According to these authors, this treatment prevents neuronal harm and development of encephalopathy with its cognitive function impairments. Relation between epileptiform discharges and serious cognitive function impairments was shown in kindling animal model of epilepsy (Majkowski, 1981, 1990) and in young children without seizures but with continous spike and wave during sleep – so called electrical status epilepticus described by S.A. Tussinari (Patry et al., 1971). Thus, it was also shown that **not only epileptic seizures but also EEG discharges may cause complex metabolic neuronal lesions and oxidant/anti-oxidant disequilibrium** (Freitas et al., 2004; Ilhan et al., 2005a; Sok et al., 2006; Barros et al., 2007).

A number of experimental studies on animal models and humans have shown that all old and some new AEDs can also produce free radicals and significantly increase the peroxidation of neuronal membrane lipids and reduce the protective effects of anti-oxidants. These changes may lead to increased seizure and idiosyncratic drug effect frequency (Kurekci et al., 1995; Sudha et al., 2001; Hung-Ming et al., 2002; Hamed and Abdellach, 2009; Hamed et al., 2009; Dostalek et al., 2007).

Oxidation stress and resistance to AED effects triggers adaptive mechanisms i.e. production of endogenous anti-oxidants scavengers, which prevent the harmful effects of oxidation (Kawakami et al., 2006). These authors studied NO and endogenous anti-oxidant GSH scavengers, GSH-Px, complete (T) and superoxide dismutase (T-SOD), Mn –SOD and catalase in cerebrospinal fluid of children with various neurological disorders. All the anti-oxidant parameters were highest in children with bacterial meningitis compared with other groups. In the group of epilepsy NO, GSH and GSH-Px were higher than in the group with aseptic meningitis and the control group. In the authors' opinion oxygen stress may be related to seizure pathology and its reduction may lead to better prognosis for the course of epilepsy. Akarsu et al. (2007) came to similar conclusions. The authors studied the state of oxidation in 21 children with febrile convulsion and 21 children without febrile convulsions, assessing the level of arginase and catalase in their red blood cells, malondialdehyde (MDA) – an indicator of lipid peroxidation and NO in the plasma and cerebrospinal fluid. The control group consisted of 41 children divided into two subgroups: 1-with fever without convulsions and 2 – without fever and without convulsions. Both fever and convulsions had a significant effect on the oxidation mechanisms. Febrile and afebrile convulsions differed in their generation of oxygen stress. According to the authors, in afebrile convulsion higher levels of oxygen stress might affect prognosis adversely. This is interpreted in terms of fever as a protective factor preventing neuronal lesion during convulsions. Recently, relation between febrile convulsion and oxygen stress was studied in 32 pediatric patients who within the preceding 8 hrs had experienced respiratory tract infection and had been diagnosed with simple febrile convulsions (Abuhandan et al., 2013). Total oxidant level (TOL) and total anti-oxidant level (TAL) were measured 8 hrs after seizure. The TOL and oxidative stress index were found to be significantly high ($p<0.01$ and $p<0.01$, respectively), and TAL was significantly lower ($p< 0.03$) compared to control group 30 healthy children. The authors conclude that increased oxidative stress may increase the risk of occurrence febrile seizures.

Since oxygen stress worsen the course of epilepsy, consistently with those observations, use of anticonvulsants in conventional epilepsy therapy and hence attenuation of oxygen stress could have a positive effect on the course of epilepsy (Costello and Delanty, 2004). Many authors share this opinion. However, these results are not used to inform and guide everyday epilepsy medication.

1.3. Objective

The chapter is intended to present and discuss current state of knowledge in various animal experimental models of seizures and human epilepsy research related to epileptogenesis and complex interaction between epilepsy, AEDs, and oxygen stress. The effects of various nutritional factors which restore balance in the oxidant/anti-oxidant system, and prevent epileptic attacks and AEDs from causing brain neuronal damages in experimental and human epilepsies will be up-dated.

1.4. Search method

A literature review was conduced to November 2013. The following search terms were used: oxygen stress, oxidants and antioxidants, animal seizure models, epilepsy and AEDs. It was searched data bases PubMed-line, the Cochrane Epilepsy Group's Specialized Register, indexed and non-indexed citation and relevant papers related to beneficial of antioxidants, and possible harmful effects AEDs and epileptic seizures in animal models and in epileptic patients.

2. Research review and discussion

2.1. Epileptogenesis

Epileptogenesis is the main challenge for contemporary epileptology, still. Any nonspecific brain damage may result in process of epileptogenesis which leads to seizure occurrence and eventually to chronic epilepsy. Brain damage may be followed by immediate (with latency seconds to 1 hr) and/or early (minutes to 1 week) seizure and late (week to dozen of years) recurring seizures. Possible pathomechanism of these seizures, triggering factors, risk factors for development of epilepsy, onset after brain damage, age depending, type of clinical course of seizures, and responsiveness to AEDs are different in these groups (Majkowski, 1990).

Epileptogenic process can be arbitrarily divided into two – overlapping to some extent – stages: cascade of biochemical processes followed by better known electrophysiological stage which precedes epilepsy occurrence. Brain damage initiates a series of non-specific, complex biochemical changes at the neural, synaptic and molecular levels. Among these biochemical changes, oxygen stress resulting in disequilibrium between oxidants and antio-xidants has been postulated in pathogenesis of seizures by many authors (Ueda et al., 1998; Jacobson et al., 1999; Dal-Pizzol et al., 2000, Patel, 2002). Role of oxygen stress has been shown and discussed in experimental animal model of epileptic seizures (Mori et al., 1990; Dakin and Weaver, 1993; de la Pena and Porta-Etessam, 1998; Majkowski, 2007; Rowley and Patel, 2013; Ryan et al., 2012). The latter provided evidence for the occurrence of specific and irreversible oxidative modification of an important mitochondrial enzyme of a protein complex I. The complex is critical for cellular bioenergetics during the process of epileptogenesis. Mechanism of epileptogenesis is not known. However, data from animal models and from patients with temporal lobe epilepsy suggest that steady-state mitochondrial ROS and resulting oxidative damage of neurons occurs during different phases of epileptogenesis (Rowley and Patel, 2013). Epileptogenic substances produce, before seizure occurrence, an increase of free radicals, lipid peroxidation and decrease of GSH-Px – the most important anti-oxidant in brain. Lipid peroxidase correlates with an increase of seizure susceptibility. In turn, occurs dysfunction of the mitochondria, neuronal membrane permeability, disturbance of the balance between excessive neuronal activation and inhibition of neuronal transmission which may be due to an increase of glutaminergic or decrease of gabaergic transmitters (Murashima et al., 2005; Narkilati and Pitkanen 2005; Lasoń, 2006). These biochemical changes decrease seizure threshold and lead to epileptic neuronal discharges which may initiate kindling process (electro-epileptogenesis) leading to epileptic attacks (Tayarani et al., 1987; Majkowski, 1993; Frantseva et al., 1998; Frantseva et al., 2000; Liang and Patel, 2004; Waldbaum and Patel; 2010a). These biochemical study, indicating formation of specific protein in process of epileptogenesis, corresponds well with long-lasting synaptic plasticity which is seen in brain modification of sensory evoked potentials and epileptiform potentials development during kindling process of epileptogenesis (Majkowski and Kwast, 1981; Majkowski, 1989). Electrical kindling with its gradual development of epileptiform discharges is the most elegant model of chronic epilepsy which allows to study electrophysiological stage of epileptogenesis. Kindling phenomenon – produced by weak repeated electrical stimulation – described by Goddard et al., (1969), is characterized by widespread and long-lasting neuronal plasticity changes which can be seen in modification of behavior (seizure) and sensory evoked potential changes expressing long-lasting synaptic modification (Majkowski, 1989; 1993). This evoked potentals' modification is of the same kind as during learning processes (Majkowski and Kwast, 1981), what suggests new protein formation in the neurons is involved in epileptogenesis (Hyden, 1980).

It seems that oxygen stress may play essential role in the earliest biochemical stage of epileptogenesis – understood as formation of epileptogenic focus resulting in focal onset seizures. However, antiepileptogenic effects of various anti-oxidants used in different animal acute models of seizures is equivocal; the same anti-oxidant, and its dose, may have different effect in different models. Prevention or inhibition of epileptogenesis in different animal models, at best, shows delayed seizure occurrence in some seizure models (Zhao et at., 2006) and in some animals (Mori et al., 1990; Willmore et al., 1986; Suzer et al., 2000) but not prevention of epileptogenesis. A delay in seizure occurrence is understood as antiepileptogenic effects. In fact, it is not antiepileptogenic but anti-ictal effect. AEDs which increase seizure threshold, in the animal models and humans, may delay the first seizure occurrence e.g. in prevention of epileptogenesis of posttraumatic epilepsy, but not have antiepileptogenic effect. This delayed or diminished severity of seizures due to anticovulsants or anti-oxidants is also seen in chronic animal model of epilepsy (like kindling) with developed epileptiform neuronal discharges. This misunderstanding was shown in elegant hippocampal slice cultures as a model of traumatic brain injury, during acute and chronic (8 weeks) electrical recordings (Berdichevsky et al., 2011) Characteristic evolution of spontaneous epileptiform discharges, interictal spikes, seizure activity and electrical status epileptious was recorded. Peak cell death occurred immediately following slicing, and later secondary peak was associated with the peak of seizure-like activity. The secondary peak in neural death was abolished by either blockade of glutaminergic transmission by kynurenic acid or by elimination of ictal activity and status epilepticus by PHT. Withdrawal of these inhibitors was followed by spontaneous seizure activity recurrence. PHT anticonvulsant and neuroprotective effect disapeared after four weeks of continous administration. These interesting results show that AED may prevent seizures but not epileptogenesis. The authors conclude that in this vitro model secondary neuronal death is correlated with ictal but not interictal electrical activity.

Epilepsies in humans and in animal models of seizures or epilepsy are extremely heterogenous in their etiology, pathomechanisms and diversity of their behavioural menifestations. This heterogeneity corresponds to diversities of results in using anti-oxidants, various seizure models and animals. At present, there are no well documented – on evidence base medicine – studies with anti-oxidants in prophylaxis of epileptogenesis. The same may be said about AEDs (Beghi, 2003). The prophylactic use of AEDs should be short lasting and may be effective in immediate and early seizures. Recently, prophylatic effect for post-craniotomy seizures in patients without epilepsy was reported (Pulman et al., 2013). The authors reviewed the relevant literature and found that there is little evidence to suggest that PHT, CBZ, PB, VPA or ZNS administered prophylactically is effective or not effective.

The well documented beneficial effects of anti-oxidants are related to diminishing neurodegeneration produced by induced seizures and epileptic discharges. However, research on the role of oxygen stress opens a new chapter in epileptology with a hope of prevention biochemical processes leading to epileptiform neuronal discharges, epileptogenesis and cognitive function impairments in epileptic patients.

2.2. Preventing oxygen stress due to epileptic seizures in animal models

Research on animal experimental models (and clinical observation) has shown that epileptic seizures lead to a number of harmful activities in the brain: disturbed blood circulation, increased cerebrospinal fluid pressure, brain oedema, hypoxia, all of which lead to the sudden reduction of energy carriers (ADP, ATP, phosphocreatinine) and neuronal pH reduction. During seizures, arachidonic acid is released in the postsynaptic membranes. This has an activating effect on the presynaptic neuronal endings and leads to increased glutamate release. Arachidonic acid also increases the production of free oxygen radicals, leading to increased lipid peroxidation. These in turn may activate phospholipase C and then lead to the release of arachidonic acid from the cellular membranes, setting a vicious circle in motion (Bartosz, 2006).

2.2.1. DL-homocysteic acid-induced seizures in immature rats

Homocysteine (Hcy) is an exscitatory amino acid which markedly enhances the vulnerability of neuronal cells to excitatory and oxidative injury. Recently, it has been shown that oxidative stress, occurring in the brain of immature 12-day-old rats during and following the seizures, induced by *DL-homocysteic acid,* is apparently due to the increased free radicals production (SOD, CuZn SOD, MnSOD and GPX) and the limited anti-oxidant defense (catalase activity decrease). The pronounced and selective upregulation of SOD2 (MnSOD) indicates to increased ROS in the mitochondrial matrix. This may be associated with inhibiton of respiratory chain complex I (Folbergrová et al., 2013). The authors suggest that in addition to AED, substances with anti-oxidant properties might provide beneficial effects in treatment of epilepsy in children. Protective role of astrocytes in neuronal survival in response to the damage induced by Hcy was studied (Loureiro et al., 2010). The authors found that the cytoskeleton of cortical astrocytes (but not of neurons in culture) is a target to Hcy and effects are mediated by redox signaling. Astrocytes were able to respond to Hcy reorganizing their cytoskeleton, surviving and protecting neurons from Hcy damage.

2.2.2. Lithium-pilocarpine (Li-PIL) model of seizures

The modulatory effect of *dexamethasone (DEX)* using 5, 10, 20 mg/kg body mass of male Wistar rats was studied in Li-PIL epilepsy model (Al-Shorbagy et al., 2012). The authors found that effective anticonvulsant activity was only observed with 10 mg DEX/kg which reduced seizure production and incidence, as well as neuronal cell loss in the CA3 region of the hippocampus. It was associated with enhancements in the anti-oxidant system and interleukin as well as suppression of altered inflammatory markers. Dose 20 mg/kg DEX showed a tendency to shorten seizure latency, and neither affected seizure incidences nor CA3 neuronal loss. There was a lack of protection at 5 mg DEX/kg. The study indicates that there is an optimal dose of DEX for preventing the induction of seizures

2.2.3. The pentylenetetrazol seizure model (PTZ) and anti-oxidants

Astragalus mongholicus. The root extract of Astragalus mongholicus (AM), a traditional medicinal herbas, has powerful anticonvulsant effects in the mouse PTZ-induced seizure model (Aldarmaa et al., 2010). Moreover, this effect was associated with an inhibition of PTZ-induced increase of lipid and protein peroxidation and ROS. The authors suggest that anticonvulsant effect of AM may be mediated by its protective actions against oxidative damage and amelioration of mitochondrial dysfunction.

Erdosteine. Prior administration of erdosteine (mucoliticum), which acts as an antioxidant, attenuated OS and delayed onset of PTZ-induced seizures in mice ($p<0.05$) (Ilhan et al., 2005b). The erdosteine pretreated mice had lower levels of MDA and xanthine oxidase (oxidisers) and a higher level of SOD than control animals ($p<0.001$). Thus, administration of erdosteine reduces convulsion-induced oxygen stress and therefore may protect neurons.

Mexidol, novel original Russian synthetic anti-oxidant (2-ethylo-6-methyl-3-oxypiridine succinate) and effects of AEDs (PB, LTG, phenazepam) and alpha-tocopherol were studied in PTZ-induced seizure model in Wistar rats (Beshkatova et al., 2003). Fivefold elevation of NO production was found in the induced seizures. Also, the level of secondary products of lipid peroxydation (LPO) and thiobarbituric acid reactive substances was significantly increased in the cortex. The authors found that mexidol and PB were to be the most effective in preventing of PTZ-induced seizures among all the studied substances. The authors suppose that supression of seizure-induced NO generation and LPO increase may be involved in the mechanism of AEDs action.

Nigella sativa oil. Nigella sativa oil, a powerful antioxidant which has been used in folk medicine and the kitchen for thousands of years, prevented PTZ-induced kindling in mice much more effectively than that of valproic acid (Ilhan et al., 2005a).

Polyphenols (grape juice). Epileptic seizures and AEDs may cause oxidative damage in hepatocytes. Wistar rats received organic grap juice or conventional grape juice (rich in phenols) and saline for 17 days before PTZ-induced seizures (Rodrigues et al., 2012). The results showed that both juices conferred protection against lipid and protein oxidative damage of liver, and limited the increase in PTZ-induced NO metabolite content in liver and serum. Moreover, both juices inhibited the PTZ-induced reduction in enzymatic anti-oxidant defenses (SOD, CAT) and sulfhydryl protein in the liver and serum. These results indicate that grape juices can provide an insight into natural neuroprotective compounds and may lead to the development of new therapeutic strategies for epileptic patients (Rodrigues et al., 2012).

Polyphenols (walnut kernels). Walnuts have high concentration of phenols. Its supplementation was associated with increased seizure threshold and reduced mortality in PTZ seizure model in Wistar adult male rats (Asadi-Shekaari et al., 2012). Moreover, there was prevention of neurodegeneration. The authors suggest that this effect may be due to high concentration in walnuts of phenols, which have anticonvulsant properties. Recently, antiepileptic effects of phenols were updated by Lasoń (2013) with notion that phenols can have clinical relevance for novel approach to treatment of epilepsy.

Physical activity. It has been found that swimming training (6 weeks) protects against the increase of neural excitability and oxidative neuronal damage in PTZ-induced seizures in rats (Souza et al., 2009). EEG recordings showed that the spikes' amplitude in rats was decreased after PTZ administration in all doses following swimming.

Topiramate (TPM) and selenium. TPM and selenium had protective effects on PTZ-induced brain damage in rats by inhibiting free radical production, regulating calcium-dependent processes, and supporting the antioxidant redox system (Naziroglu et al., 2008). Recent studies indicate that selenium with/without topiramate administration in human and animals decreased seizure levels, although anti-oxidant values were increased (Naziroglu and Yürekli, 2013).

Vitamin E and selenium. Intraperitoneal administration of PTZ – an antagonist of the GABA A-receptor – induced seizures and ruptured the blood-brain barrier in rats. This has been demonstrated by means of Evans dye, used to mark the permeability of this barrier (Oztas et al., 2001). It has been suggested that free radicals are involved in the permeability of the blood-brain barrier; this permeability leads to albumin extravasation to the thalamic nuclei, brain stem, frontal cortex and occipital cortex. Animals that have been given vitamin E or selenium (Se) prior to seizure induction, had less extravasation in these structures. It has also been demonstrated that in young rats and in normotermic conditions, barrier permeability was greater in males that in females ($p<0.05$) (Oztas et al., 2007).

2.2.4. The kainic acid model (KA) and anti-oxidants

The KA model is used as a model substance in the assessment of neurotoxicity. It leads to excessive ROS production due to reduced antioxidant activity. When KA was administered to rats, lipid peroxidation of the neuronal membrane increased in proportion to seizure progression (Ueda et al., 1997). In the same model, SOD and catalase activity increased significantly on day 5 following KA administration and returned to base level three weeks later; GSH-Px activity also increased significantly on day 5 but was still high three weeks later (Bruce and Baudry, 1995). Lipid and protein peroxidation, assessed by MDA concentration, increased significantly 8 and 16 hours later, then decreased on day 2 and day 5 following KA administration. The authors attribute the rapid increase in MDA and protein peroxidation to free radicals produced in this phase of the pathological KA effect; they conclude that the changes in enzymatic scavenger activity and the reduced MDA concentration may have been caused by glia proliferation due to neuronal death.

Gastrodia elata B1 (GE). Hsieh et al. (2001) tested a traditional Chinese herb GE, used to treat epilepsy, in a controlled study using the rat KA seizure model. They found that prior administration of GE significantly reduced in vitro lipid peroxidation in the brain, an effect analogous to the effect of phenytoin (PHT) – 20 mg/kg. In the authors' opiniont GE has an antiepileptic effect and is a free radical scavenger. This antiepileptic effect may be, at least, partly attributable to the GE's vanilla component (Hsieh et al., 2000).

Melatonin. In the mouse KA model, prior or simultaneous administration of melatonin (a powerful hydroxyl radical scavenger) (20 mg/kg i.p.) had an anti-oxidising effect and prevented lipid peroxidation, cerebral mitochondria DNA damage and seizures (Mohanan and Yamamoto, 2002).

Since oxidative stress is thought to play a role in pathogenesis of hypertention and epileptogenesis, it could be used as a tool for studying co-morbidity of both conditions (Atanasova et al., 2013). The authors studied efficacy of chronic pretreatment with *melatonin,* infused via subcutaneous osmotic mini pump for 14 days, on KA-induced status epilepticus, oxidative stress and expression of heat shock protein (HSP) 72 in spontaneously hypertensive rats (SHRs) and normotensive Wistar rats. SHRs showed increase in the level of LP in frontal cortex and hippocampus and decreased cytosolic superoxide dismutase (SOD/CuZn) production in the frontal cortex compared to normotensive Wistar rats. Status epilepticus induced by KA was associated with increased LP and expression of HSP 72 in the hippocampus in the two strains, and increased SOD/CuZn production in frontal cortex of SHRs. Melatonin failed to suppress seizure incidence and intensity. However, latency was significantly increased in SHRs. Increased activity in SOD/CuZn and mitochondrial SOD Mn as well and reduced expression of HSP 72 in hippocampus was observed in Wistar rats pretreated with melatonin. **The observed strain differences in the efficacy of chronic melatonin expression before status epilepticus suggests a lack of direct link between the seizure activity and markers of oxygen stress and neurotoxicity.**

Petasites japonicum (BMP). Sok et al. (2006), studied the anticonvulsive effects of the plant grown in East Asia and used for both culinary purposes and in folk medicine. Its root extracts are still used for treating headaches and asthma. Prolonged administration of BMP, prior to KA administration, reduced mortality in mice by one half. Administration of the BMP-I subfraction reduced convulsive seizures and also significantly reduced neuronal loss in parts CA1 and CA3 of the hippocampus. The authors suggest that BMP-I is the factor responsible for prevention of oxidisation lesion in mouse brain.

SCH 58261 – a selective adenosine A(2A) receptor (A(2A)R) antagonist. KA induced seizures in young rats (21-day-old) were pretreated with SCH 58261 before (i.p.) KA administration (Bortolatto et al., 2012). It resulted in prolonged latency for the onset of the first clonic seizure and at the highest dose decreased the appearance of clonic seizures and mortality rate. The adenosine antagonist was also effective in protecting against alteration in oxidative stress parameters (ROS, CAT, GPx, and GST (glutathione S-tansferaze)) activities. Thus, SCH 58261 was protective against the induced neurotoxicity, and might represent a novel approach for the treatment of seizures.

Sesame seeds. Sesamin is a well-known antioxidant from sesame seeds and it scavenges free radicals. In KA–induced status epilepticus in mice and rats sesamin significantly decreased ROS, MDA and the mortality was decreased from 22% to 0% in rats (Hsieh et al., 2011).

Vineatrol. In the rat KA model, prior administration of vineatrol significantly reduced brain MDA levels but had no effect on the GSH levels (Gupta and Briyal, 2006). Doses exceeding 20 and 40 mg/kg lengthened the latency time to the first seizures. Additional administration of vineatrol 30 and 60 minutes after KA administration significantly reduced seizure incidence. The authors suggest that vineatrol could potentially be useful in status epilepticus.

2.2.5. The pilocarpine model of seizures, status epilepticus, oxidants and anti-oxidants

Pilocarpine, an imidasole alkaloid extracted from the leaves of the Pilocarpus jaborandi shrub, is a parasympathomimetic, a cholinergic agonist which acts similarly to acetylcholine. It is often used to evoke epileptic convulsions and status epilepticus in animal models. The mechanisms leading to seizures or status epilepticus are unknown. It is thought that oxygen stress plays an important role but it is still unknown which brain structures are more sensitive.

The pilocarpine-induced status epilepticus had differential effects on catalase level in discrete brain structures (Freitas et al., 2004; Freitas et al., 2005). The highest elevation of the enzyme level was found in the hippocampus (36%), striatum (31%) and frontal cortex (15%); no changes were found in the cerebellum. According to the authors, the endogenous increase in catalase activity, responsible for removal of free oxygen radicals which are produced during convulsions, may be an auto-regulatory compensating defence mechanism which counteracts the negative effects of oxygen stress in the status epilepticus. In this model of epilepsy, results show that oxidative stress, lipid peroxidation and nitric oxide could be responsible for neuronal damage in the hippocampus (Freitas, 2009).Other researchers have come to similar conclusions (Kawakami et al., 2006; Tejada et al., 2007). The later authors investigated pilocarpine-evoked status epilepticus and found that MDA levels increased significantly in the brain cortex (64%), suggesting oxygen injury. They found a simultaneous increase in the anti-oxidising activity of catalase enzymes (28%), GSH-Px (28%) and SOD (21%). On the other hand, vitamin E concentration in the cerebral cortex was reduced (15%) due to increased lipid peroxydation following pilocarpine administration. The amount of lipid peroxydation product in cortical neurons of the cerebral hemispheres decreased by 30% at the peak of convulsions observed 10-15 min. after i.p. picrotoxin injection. In neuroglial cells of control animals the intensity of lipid peroxydation was 1.7-2.0 times lower (Flerov et al., 2004).

Apocynin. In pilocarpine-induced status epilepticus in rats, ROS generation was increased in CA1, CA3 and dentate gyrus of dorsal hippocampus (Pestana et al., 2010). The authors found that administration of apocynin (NADPH oxidase inhibitor) for 7 days prior to pilocarpine-induced status epilepticus had protective activity: ROS production and neurodegeneration in the studied structures were decreased by an average of 20% and 61%, respectively.

Lipoic acid. In pilocarpine-induced seizures in rats there was significant increase in lipid peroxidation, nitrite level and GPx, however, no alterations were found in SOD and catalase activities (Militão et al., 2010). Administration of lipoic acid significantly reduced the lipid peroxidation level and nitrite content, and increased the SOD, catalase and GPx activities in striatum after seizures. The study supports hypothesis that brain damage induced by the oxidative process plays a crucial role in seizures pathogenic consequences, and a protective effect could be achieved using lipoic acid.

Vitamin C. In the same model in rats, prior administration of vitamin C (250 mg/kg i.p.) reduced the negative effects of oxygen stress and neuronal lesion (Santos et al., 2008). The latency time to convulsion onset following pilocarpine administration was longer and mortality in the status epilepticus was reduced compared with the group which did not receive vitamin C or received physiological saline. This study also found that in the group which only received vitamin C the level of lipid peroxidation was lower than in the group which a) received pilocarpine and b) received pilocarpine and vitamin C. In all the experimental groups, catalase activity in the hippocampus increased compared with the control group which only received physiological saline. In the authors' opinion, the neuroprotective function of vitamin C in adult rats may be due to reduced lipid peroxidation and increased catalase activity following convulsions and status epilepticus.

Vitamin E and status epilepticus. Barros et al. (2007) applied the same model and found that administration of vitamin E (200 mg/kg i.p.) 30 minutes prior to the administration of pilocarpine (400 mg/kg s.c.) leads to increased (214%) catalase activity in the hippocampus compared with rats which were only given policarpine (67%) or physiological saline. The authors conclude that increased catalase activity may be responsible for the regulation of free radicals evoked by the status epilepticus.

In pilocarpine-induced status epilepticus in rats autophagy – a process of bulk degeneration of cellular constituents through autophagosome-lysosomal pathways was studied (Cao et al., 2009). Status epilepticus induces an excess production of ROS resulting in an increase of autophagy which was a partially inhibited by pretreatment with vitamin E. The strong protective effect of vitamin E could be achieved in the same pilocarpine seizure model (Tome et al., 2010) The authors confirmed that oxidative stress occurs in rat hippocampus resulting in the brain damage and this plays a crucial role in seizure pathogenic consequences.

2.2.6. The audiogenic seizure model

Melatonin and valproic acid. Prolonged melatonin administration in rats congenitally predisposed to audiogenic convulsions (the Krushinsky-Molodkina model) had no effect on seizures evoked by a 20 times more powerful auditory stimulus (Savina et al., 2006). VPA administration significantly reduced convulsions but VPA and melatonin combination had a significantly larger anti-seizure effect: it lengthened latency time and reduced seizure severity. However, combined treatment led to much more rapid onset of myoclonia than in groups receiving either VPA or melatonin.

3. Oxygen stress and AEDs in animal models

3.1. Acetazolamide (AZM)

AZM or saline was given i.p. to Spragué Dawley rats before exposing to *hyperbaric oxygen model* – the pressure of 6 ATA of pure oxygen (Huang et al., 2004). There was a significant difference in the latency of hyperbaric oxygen-induced convulsions between AZM (200 mg/kg and 20 mg/kg) groups and saline controls ($p < 0.01$) and there was no significant difference between AZM (2 mg/kg) and saline group ($p > 0.05$). GSH-Px and MDA was increased in homogenized cortex, hippocampus and striatum in different ways and depending on the time of exposure to AZM. The results, according to the authors, suggest that AZM, which dilates the brain arteriolae, increases the supply of the oxygen breaking into the brain structures and aggravates the oxidation with its consequences.

3.2. Carbamazepine

Short term CBZ administration to roinbout trout and a low level of oxidative stress could induce adaptive responses of antioxidant enzymes, however, long-term exposure to CBZ could lead to serious oxidative damage of *fish brain* (Li et al., 2010).

3.3. Lamotrigine

LTG does not lead to detectable increases in lipid peroxidation in rats in vivo (Lu and Uetrecht, 2007). The anti-epileptic effectiveness of LTG in the *partial complex epilepsy model* (stimulation of the dentate gyrus) in rats was in reverse proportion to the level of nitric oxide (Sardo and Ferraro, 2007).

3.4. Levetiracetam

LEV (2000 mg/kg i.p.) administered prior to *pilocarpine administration* (400 mg/kg s.c.) in mice prevented lipid peroxidation increase in the hippocampus (but did not increase nitrate level or reduce catalase activity in the hippocampus or cortical glutathione) (Oliveira et al., 2007). Perhaps the anti-oxidising, neuroprotective effect of LEV and the consequent reduction of oxygen stress can be attributed to a different mechanism than the one which is active in the case of other AEDs.

3.5. Phenobarbital (PB)

Male Sprague – Dawley rats were pretreated with PB – a well known cytochrome P450 inducer (Dostalek et al., 2007). The markers of in vivo oxygen stress were influenced by PB resulting in significantly increased malondialdehyde, H_2O_2 generation and NADPH oxidation in vitro and significantly enhanced formation in vivo in liver and plasma.

3.6. Phenytoin (PHT)

PHT is known to produce ROS, which are involved in mechanism of the PHT-evoked teratogenesis and developmental toxicity. PHT initiates the oxidation damage to proteins and fats in the *maternal and embryonic liver tissue* organelle in murine rodents (Mahle and Dasgupta, 1997).

Gallagher and Sheehy (2010) used *cultured human prenatal liver slices* to study the effects of the human teratogen PHT on cell toxicity. Their findings in a relevant human model system are supportive of a protective role of GSH and alpha class glutathione S – transferases izoenzymes A1 against PHT toxicity and teratogenesis.

Using mutant catalase deficient mice and transgenic mice expressing human catalase, Abramov and Wells (2011) investigated protective importance of *embryonic catalase* against endogenous ROS and the ROS-imitating teratogen PHT in embryo culture. They provided evidence that the low level of embryonic catalase protects from developmental and xenobiotic-enhanced oxygen stress and that embryonic variations of this enzyme affect development.

3.7. Topiramate

TPM with its many mechanisms of action has undoubted effectiveness in the treatment of epilepsy in children. However, TPM administered to rat stomach for 3 months may lead to such adverse effects as toxic liver dysfunction (Huang et al., 2007). In a study of young rats it was found that small doses of TPM (40 mg/kg a day) may reduce total antioxidant capacity in the organism and lead to minor liver pathology. Large doses of TPM (80 mg/kg a day) or a combination of TPM (40 mg/kg) and VPA (300 mg/kg a day) significantly increased the risk of such adverse effects. GSH levels in the liver were significantly lower in the group taking large doses of TPM and the TPM+VPA group compared with the group taking small doses of TPM and the control group which was only given distilled water. Histopathological examination also revealed disseminated punctual necrosis, and as well lipid and degenerative changes in some hepatocytes.

TPM (40 and 80 mg/kg i.p.) had no effect on either rats' KA-induced status epilepticus or mortality but larger doses significantly reduced KA-produced lipid peroxidation (Kubera et al., 2004).

Treatment of diabetic mice with TPM, a potent mitochondrial carbonic anhydrazes (CA) inhibitor, prevented the oxidative stress caused by diabetes (Price et al., 2012). The authors studied the effects of pharmacological inhibition of mitochondrial CA activity on *streptozotocin induced-oxidative stress* and pericytes loss in the mouse brain. Pericytes are in immediate contact with endothelial cells and are vital for blood-brain barier integrity. These results provide for the first time evidence that inhibition of mitochondrial CA activity reduces diabetes-reduced oxidative stress in the mouse brain and rescuses cerebral policytes dropout. Mitochondrial CA may provide a new therapeutic targed for oxidative stress related impairments of the brain.

Anti-oxidant activity of TPM was shown also in vitro study (Cardenas-Rodrigues et al., 2013a). The results show that TPM displays scavenging capacity of superoxide, hydroxyl radical, hypochlorus acid, hydrogen peroxide, signled oxygen but not to peroxynitrite. Although TPM was less efficient than *nordihydroguaiaretic acid, dimethylthiourea, ascorbic acid, sodium pyruvate and glutathione* in its scavenging capacity. The authors conclude that anti-oxidant properties of TPM could explain it's the neuroprotective effect.

3.8. Valproic acid

In model of rat *cortical cell culture*, VPA was found to protect against the negative effects of oxygen stress (Wang et al., 2003). Administration of VPA for 7 days prevented lipid and protein oxidization anomalies and accumulation of free radicals. Short-term administration of VPA affects one or more of the neuroprotective processes.

Several mechanisms were suggested for VPA hepatotoxicity, however, most of them are associated with oxygen stress resulting in mitochondrial dysfunction. Rat liver mitochondria were obtained by differential ultra centrifugation and then incubated with different concentration of VPA (25-200μM) (Jafarian et al., 2013). The results showed that VPA could induce oxidative stress via rising in mitochondrial ROS, lipid peroxidation, mitochondrial membrane potential collapse, mitochondrial swelling and release of Cytochrome C. The authors found that these effects were well inhibited by pretreatment of isolated mitochondria with *cyclosporin A* and *butylated hydroxytoluene.* The data show that VPA exerts mitochondrial toxicity by impairing mitochondrial functions leading to oxidative stress and Cytochrome C expulsion which starts cell death signaling (Jafarian et al., 2013).

3.9. Zonisamide (ZNS)

The major mechanisms of antiepileptic ZNS are inhibition of voltage-gated Na(+) channel, T-type voltage sensitive Ca(2+)channel, Ca(2+) relasing system and neuronal depolarization-induced glutamate release, and increased release of inhibitory neurotransmitters.

In the KA convulsion model in rats, pretreatment with ZNS led to increased anti-oxidant level in the hippocampus (Ueda et al., 2005). The study was performed in freely moving rats using in vivo microanalysis and electron paramagenetic resonance spectroscopy. In the authors' opinion, ZNS has neuroprotective properties against free radicals.

Neuroprotective properties of ZNS also have been shown *in iron-induced epileptogenic foci* in the rat brain (Komatsu et al., 2000). The authors found that the level of 8-hydroxy-2. deoksy-guanosine (8-OHdG), which is used as a marker for oxidative DNA damage, increased 15 min after ferric chloride solution injections reaching maximum after 30 min. ZNS prevented the increase of the 8-OHdG within 30 min after iron solution injection. This effect may be due to the ZNS antioxidant activity and might be interesting to use it in prevention of posttraumatic epilepsy development due to blood extravasation and epileptogenic affect of free ferrum.

3.10. Old and new AEDs

Pavone and Cardile (2003) studied effects of AEDs on oxygen stress in an *astrocyte culture from rats.* Selected list of studied variables includes: lactate dehydrogenase (LDH) and glutamine synthtase (GS) levels, ROS production, lipid peroxidation and DNA fragmentation. Drugs such as CBZ, TPM and OXC caused oxygen stress whatever their dose. Gabapentin (GBP), LEV, LTG, tiagabine (TGB) and ZNS on the other hand, caused no significant metabolic changes in large or small doses. Cortical astrocytes seem to tolerate this latter group of AEDs better than the former ones.

Animal models of seizures, in particular, epilepsy and oxidative processes are useful for developing antiepileptic drugs (Majkowski et al., 2011; Rowles and Olsen, 2012). However, one of the main problems in transferring animal-based data to humans is to define effectiveness of a dose.

4. Aging and anti-oxidants of omega-3 fatty acid

Omaga-3 fatty acids supplementation was added to standard laboratory food for 6 weeks to aged 24 months old Wistar rats (Avramovic et al., 2012). The results showed befeneficial effects of omega-3 fatty acid on the brain cortex with increased SOD activity and decreased lipid peroxidation in contrast to the control grup. The changes in oxidative/antioxidative balance are due to effects of eicosapentanoic acid (EPA) and decosahexanoic (DHA) on lipids and enzyme of anti-oxidative system. Aging as a biophysiological process could be influeced by EPA and DHA.

5. Course of seizures and oxygen stress

An interesting effect of *prolonged seizures* (PS) versus *repeated-seizures* (RS) in one day old chicken *in pilocarpine-induced status epilepticus* has been reported (Tsai et al., 2010). In the PS group excessive levels of ROS and MDA, and lower activities of SOD and catalase were found when compared to the RS group ($p< 0.05$). This was associated with neuronal death in the PS group ($p < 0.01$). ROS, mitochondrial dysfunction and DNA damage played important roles in pathophysiology of the immature brain to PS-induced damage. The authors suggest that replenishment of SOD and catalase activities might be useful in protecting neurons against seizure-induced damage.

6. Sleep deprivation and oxygen stress

It is well known that *sleep deprivation* in epileptic patients may provoke seizures. The mechanism underlying this relation is unknown. Hirotsu et al. (2013) investigated changes in gene expression related to reactive oxygen species and NO production in the frontal cortex of a rodent model of temporal lobe epilepsy (PILO) in rats with *pilocarpine-induced status epilepticus* after paradoxidal sleep deprivation (PSD 24h) and total sleep deprivation (TSD 6h). The data show that PILO rats had increased NOX-2 expression and decreased SOD expression independent of sleep. Higher NOX-2 expression was observed only in PILO rats subjected to the control condition and TSD 6h. CAT expression in the frontal cortex of PILO rats submitted to PSD 24 h was reduced compared to that of PILO rats that were not sleep-deprived. In the authors opinion, the molecular changes in the frontal cortex following sleep deprivation suggest a machanism via oxidative stress.

7. Oxygen stress and AEDs in human epilepsy

AEDs have various and equivocal effects on the oxidization processes (Hamed and Abdellach, 2004; Hamed et al., 2004; Devi et al., 2008; Ounjaijean et al., 2011; Rowles and Olsen, 2012; Azam et al., 2012; Naziroglu and Yürekli, 2013;Rodriguez et al., 2013). Generally, epilepsy and prolonged AED treatment (CBZ, PHT and VPA) results in increased Zn, Ca, Na, MDA and GSH-Px. Usually, anti-oxidant trace elements' levels such as Se, Cu, Zn, Mg, and total antioxidant capacity and ceruloplasmine are low in the blood of epileptic patients. New AEDs are more prone to restore anti-oxidant system in brain. In untreated patients with epilepsy, uric acid (a powerful free oxygen radical scavenger) was elevated but the total anti-oxidant capacity in the serum was reduced, suggesting that different anti-oxidants have different activities in this epileptic group. It was found that some nutrients may have a positive effect on the reduction of seizure frequency and may improve cognitive functioning in patients with epilepsy (vitamin B_1, B_6, vitamin E, Mg, Mn, taurine, glycine, omega-3 fatty acids). In order to prevent the negative effects of AEDs, prophylactic or therapeutic replenishment of folic acid, vitamin B6, vitamin D, and L-carnitine may be advisable. In some cases melatonin may reduce seizure frequency. However, supplementation can very seldom substitute AEDs completely (Gaby, 2007). Casuistic reports may be observed e.g. in pyridoxine (vitamin B6) deficiency seizures, usually, in neonates and infants.

7.1. Carbamazepine

It has been shown CBZ-induced toxic effects in erythrocytes in epilepsy treated patients (Ficcara et al, 2013). However, some beneficial effects of CBZ has been evident as an increased release of ATP and NO derived metabolites from erythrocytes to lumen, leading to an increased NO pool in the vasculature.

7.2. Oxcarbazepine

Bolayir et al. (2004) studied the effect of OXC on anti-oxidative processes in 13 adult patients with epilepsy prior to monotherapy and after 1 year of OXC monotherapy; 15 healthy controls were included in the study. Lipid peroxidation activity, SOD, GSH-Px and catalase in the red blood cells were measured. The patients had significant differences in level of GSH-Px and SOD after 1 year of treatment compared with pre-treatment levels. MDA level was also significantly different compared with the control group and the pre-treatment assessment. These findings suggest that the anti-oxidation systems in patients treated with OXC were negatively affected after 1 year of treatment.

7.3. Phenytoin

Mahle and Dasgupta (1997) found a significant increase in blood serum concentration of lipid hydroperoxydase in PHT monotherapy compared with the control group. Total blood serum anti-oxidant capacity was lower in patients than in healthy controls. These authors found a weak correlation between lipid hydroperoxidase concentration, triglyceridemia and cholesterol levels in the serum of patients with epilepsy.

The negative consequences of oxygen stress in serum were significantly larger in women with epilepsy treated with PHT monotherapy (N=20), than in healthy women (N=20) and women with untreated epilepsy (N=12) (Liu et al., 1997). For PHT treated epileptic woman, the MDA serum level was significantly increased ($p< 0.05$), and GSH level – significantly decreased ($p< 0.005$). This was not observed in untreated epilepsy and in healthy control women. The abnormal metabolism of S-Cu, CuZn-SOD, and GSH was highly involved in the PHT-mediated toxicity. According to the authors, addition of glutathione to PHT treatment – resulting in modification of the activity of CuZn-SOD enzymes and reduction of copper absorption during pregnancy, may prevent the incidence of the foetal phenytoin syndrome.

7.4. Phenytoin and carbamazepine

Comparative studies of the effects of PHT and CBZ monotherapies found a significant increase in the blood serum level of MDA and CuZn-SOD, and a significant reduction of glutathione in a patients treated with PHT compared with a healthy control group and a group with untreated epilepsy (Liu et al., 1998). No differences were found for CBZ except for a slight increase in CuZn-SOD activity. All in all, CBZ caused fewer interferences with antioxidant activity, lipid peroxidation and the level of trace elements (Cu, Zn).

7.5. Topiramate and Selenium

Neuroprotective effects of TPM and Se deficiency play a important role in pathophysiology of seizures in epileptic patients. Demirci et al., (2013) studied effect of Se and TPM in neural PC 12 cell by evaluating Ca(2+) mobilization, lipid peroxidation and anticonvulsant levels. The results showed that Se induced protective effects on oxidative stress in PC12 cells by modulating cytosolic Ca(2+) influx and anti-oxidant levels. TPM modulated also lipid peroxidation and glutathione and vitamin C concentrations in the cell system.

7.6. Valproic acid

VPA is frequently used in epileptic patients, mainly, in young children. In some forms of idiopathic epilepsy (myoclonic and absences) is the most effective drug, however, its use is limited due to adverse events related to dose and duration of treatment. Recently, Zhang et al. (2011) studied the VPA influence on neutrophils' oxidative metabolism and oxidant status. The study were performed on 26 newly diagnosed epileptic children with idiopathic epilepsy and 30 healthy children were included as control group. The authors performed the study before, after 6 and 12 months of VPA treatment. MDA, superoxide dismutase, catalase and glutathione peroxidase were measured in plasma. The results showed that VPA may activate neutrophils and cause oxidative stress, moreover, prolonged treatment may aggravate it. Multiple regression analysis showed that the time of treatment and the activation rates of neutrophils were indicator which has positive correlation with the levels of plasma MDA and that SOD activities were inversely correlated with MDA levels.

VPA can sometimes be related to allergic idiosyncratic hepatopathy, a rare condition but more frequent in children under 2 years of age taking more than one AED. The mechanism of toxic hepatopathy is unknown but it has been suggested that it is caused by oxygen stress which leads to excessive ROS production and reduction of total anti-oxidant capacity (Chang and Abbott, 2006; Sabayan et al., 2007). Therefore, specifics which reduce oxygen stress may protect against toxic hepatopathy in patients taking VPA. Sabayan et al. (2007) have hypothesized that garlic (allium) preparations may prevent this liver damage by removing free radicals and preventing the reduction of glutathione activity which accompanies treatment with VPA.

VPA used in monotherapy for 60 days in 50 children with epilepsy (mean age 8.5 ± 3.6 years) led to liver dysfunction and free radicals which seems to produce DNA oxidation injury in the liver cells not excluding neurons (Schulpis et al., 2006). The general oxidation state, measured by the level of 8-OHdG, depended on the VPA dose. A linear relation was found between VPA serum level and degree of lipid peroxidation. In a group of children with a mean VPA concentration of 114 ± 9.7 µg/ml, peroxidation was significantly higher than in a control group of children with a mean VPA concentration of 81.0 ± 8 µg/ml. Free radicals caused DNA oxygen injury due to significant increase in the serum level of 8-OHdG. In the authors' opinions, 8-OHdG may be a good biological indicator of increased risk of VPA-related cell degeneration.

Other authors have also found a linear relation between lipid peroxidation and VPA levels in the plasma of patients with epilepsy (Martinez-Ballesteros et al., 2004). They measured lipid peroxidation spectrofluorometrically, before and after Fenton reaction evocation, in 76 patients and 4 healthy controls. Interestingly, lipid peroxidation was higher in patients with partial epilepsy than in patients with generalized epilepsy, and higher in women than in men. *The same sex-related differences in oxygen stress effects were found in PHT-treated epilepsy (Liu et al., 1997), in hyppocampal slices in patients (Li et al., 2005), in the mouse PTZ-seizure model (Oztas et al., 2007). In PTZ-seizure model in Wistar rats, seizure were more severe in females; moreover pretreatment by a nitric oxide syntase (NOS) inhibitor N-omega-nitro-L-arginine-methylester, completely prevented seizures in male rats, whereus increased severity frequency and duration in female rats, on the other hand, pretreatment by NO precursor sodium-nitroprusside increased seizure severity in male, and decreased in females (Uzum et al., 2005).*

The alteration of iron homeostasis and oxygen stress in 24 young adult epileptic patients treated with VPA monotherapy revealed a significant decrease of serum anti-oxidant levels while anti-oxidant enzyme activities increased (Ounjaijean et al., 2011). An interesting association was found between the daily dose of VPA and the concentration of non-transferrin bound iron (NTBI) (p=0.009), MDA (p=0.022) and Zn (p=0.009). Thus, the study has shown that VPA treatment in epilepsy patients contributes to the metabolism of iron, leading to the formation of NTBI and increase of oxidative stress. The alteration of iron homeostasis and oxygen stress product were not observed in the control group comprising of 24 sex and age-matched healthy volunteers.

In a recent study, Plonka-Półtorak et al. (2011) found that in long-term VPA monotherapy in adult young epileptic patients (and 21 healthy controls) frequency of seizures and duration of VPA therapy (7-14 years) were associated with changes of oxidative/antioxidative balance. The activity of erythrocyte SOD was higher in patients treated for a longer period (7-14 years) in comparison to controls (p=0.001) and patients with a short period of time ($p < 0.001$). Patients with uncontrolled epilepsy exhibited higher serum Zn than seizure-free patients (p=0.041). The most relevant parameters for anti-oxidative defence mechanism were plasma SOD, ferric reducing ability of plasma, uric acid and Zn.

It is interesting that commonly reported VPA oxidative stress effect occurs in overweight children (Verrotti et al., 2008). The study was performed on 31 epileptic children before and after 1 year of therapy with VPA. The control group consisted of 31 sex-, age-and BMI-matched healthy controls. In the authors' opinion, increase in the levels of oxidant markers (MDA) ($p < 0.001$) and lower level of antioxidant (vit. E, $p< 0.001$), probably caused by obesity, might contribute to endothelial dysfunction and arteriosclerosis in later life.

Very interesting effect of the mood stabilizing VPA on decrease of ROS in schizophrenic patient was reported (Paulsen Bda et al., 2012). Studies on schizophrenia have shown altered cell respiration and oxidative stress response, however this knowledge is acquired mainly from postmortem brain analyses or from nonneuronal cells. The authors reported very interesting results that neural cells – derived from induced pluripotent stem cell generated from skin fibroblasts of a schizopherenic patient – presented a twofold increase in extra-mitochondrial oxygen consumption as well as ROS elevated levels compared to controls. The difference *in ROS levels was reverted by the mood stabilizer valproic acid.*

7.7. Valproic acid and carbamazepine

A comparative study of the effect of two-year VPA and CBZ monotherapies on changes in the antioxidant system in children with epilepsy found significant differences in the effects of both AEDs (Yuksel et al., 2001). The levels of GSH, GSH-Px, red blood cell SOD and serum lipid peroxidation were measured. They studied two groups: 1) 25 healthy children and 2) 27 children with epilepsy untreated prior to the study onset, 14 of whom were treated with VPA and 13 with CBZ. Treatment lasted for 2 years. Laboratory tests were conducted in treatment months 13 and 24. The anti-oxidant systems in children taking VPA for 2 years were more altered than the anti-oxidant systems of children taking CBZ.

Another comparative study of CBZ and VPA in children found no differences in the serum concentrations of Cu, Zn, Mn, Se and Mg (Kurekci et al., 1995). The only difference was found for GSH-Px activity which was significantly higher in the VPA group. No differences were found in SOD levels.

7.8. Valproic acid, carbamazepine and phenobarbital

A more recent comparative study yielded slightly different results of the effect of VPA, CBZ and PB monotherapies on the oxidation and anti-oxidation systems in 122 children – including healthy controls, untreated epileptic patients and epileptic patients treated with VPA, PHT, PB (Avcicek and Iscan, 2007). The authors found that the level of total anti-oxidant capacity in serum was significantly reduced in the group with untreated epilepsy compared with the healthy group. Level of peroxidation was significantly elevated in both the untreated group with epilepsy and the CBZ treatment group compared with healthy controls. The pattern of results was similar for the children treated with PB and the control group. According to the authors, children with epilepsy are at risk of oxygen stress due to seizures and AEDs. Their oxidation and anti-oxidation processes are unbalanced. VPA restores this balance more effectively than CBZ or PB.

8. Preventing oxygen stress in human AED treated epilepsy

8.1. Melatonin

Numerous studies of melatonin conducted over the last 30 years have confirmed that this neurohormone is susceptible to circadian rhythms, has anti-oxidant properties and modulates immunological activity (Harderland et al., 2006). Melatonin affects the blood platelets and prolongs their life. It is transported by the platelets to all the body tissues. Thanks to its lipophilic function, it crosses the cell membranes easily, regulates blood-tissue exchange and interacts with the endothelial cells. Platelets can behave like mobile and wandering serotonergic and/or melatonergic elements, comparable with cerebral neurotransmitter release (Di Bella and Gualano, 2006). Melatonin is a free radical scavenger devoided of pro-oxidative activity (Tan et al., 2002) and therefore it reduces oxygen stress and prevents excessive excitotoxic effects arousal from injured neurones in various animal and human models.

In epilepsy patients melatonin is reduced compared with controls and is increased threefold following seizures (Bazil et al., 2000) Single evening dose of 5-10 mg melantion can exert a positive effect on the frequency of epileptic seizures in children with sleep disturbances (Fauteck et al., 1999).

The neuroprotective effect of melatonin has been confirmed in a randomized, double blind trial of children with epilepsy receiving VPA monotherapy (Gupta et al., 2004). The authors administered VPA+melatonin to 15 children and VPA+placebo to 14 children for 14 days. Post-test glutathione reductase (GSSG-Rd) levels were significantly higher ($p=0.05$) in the VPA +melatonin group and the percentile difference in the values of this enzyme was also significant ($p=0.005$). Thus, melatonin possesses anti-oxidant, antiexcitotoxic and free radical scavenging properties in the central nervous system.

Gupta et al. (2006) found that CBZ or VPA administered in monotherapy to 22 children with epilepsy had differential effects on melatonin serum levels. In both groups the endogenous and exogenous melatonin was measured 30 minutes after administration. The serum median level of melatonin was higher in the CBZ group 165 pg/ml (range 50-350) than in the VPA group, it was 78 pg/ml (range 13-260). In the authors' opinion these range differences in level of melatonin could be attributed to the different effects of these two AEDs, additive increase in ROS due to disease combined with CBZ, or possibly to differences in melatonin kinetics in conditions of oxidative stress.

8.2. Selenium

The neuroprotective effect of selenium in epilepsy is related to selenoproteins which are antioxidants (Atroshi et al., 2007; Naziroglu, 2009). Selenium insufficiency has been found in young children with severe mental retardation and drug-resistant epilepsy (Ramaekers et al., 1994). Oral administration of selenium (3-5 μg/kg m.c.) reduced seizure frequency, improved EEG recordings and normalized liver activity.

In another study, serum level of selenium in 30 patients with intractable epilepsy was also lower (66.88 ng/ml ± 17.58) than in healthy controls matched for age, socio-economic status and place of residence (85.93 ng/ml ± 13.93) ($p<0.05$) (Ashrafi et al., 2007). However, low selenium levels in serum did not correlate with the measured risk factors for drug-resistant epilepsy: with age of onset, infant seizures, neurological disorder or etiology of epilepsy.

It is suggested that blood GSH-Px activities could be a reliable indicator of selenium deficiency in patients with epilepsy (Naziroglu, 2009).

8.3. Plants

Assuming that AEDs can trigger free radical production and lipid peroxidation, Hung-Ming et al. (2002) studied TW970, a modified version of the Chinese herbal specific chaihu-longu-muli-tang which has antiepileptic and antioxidant properties. The TW 970 was administered for 4 months to 3 groups of adults: 1) 20 patients with drug-resistant epilepsy (at least 4 seizures a month); 2) 20 patients with mild epilepsy (fewer than 4 seizures a month), and 3) a control group of 20 healthy adults matched for age. The patients were tested prior to the introduction of TW970 and four months after introduction. In the resistant group, seizure frequency dropped from 13.4 ± 3.4 to 10.7 ± 2.5 a month but the difference was not significant ($p=0.084$). Prior to TW970 introduction, the resistant epilepsy group had significantly higher lipid peroxidation, increased MDA and CuZn-SOD activity, including reduced GSH, compared with the healthy control group. After 4 months of TW970 treatment, levels of MDA and CuZn-SOD normalized in the resistant epilepsy group whereas no significant changes in parameters were found in the mild epilepsy group, either prior to or following TW970 therapy. The authors suggest that TW970 may reduce seizure frequency in resistant epilepsy and that anti-oxidants may be responsible for this effect.

Japanise kampo (TJ-960) traditional herbal medicine was used for treatment of epilepsy (Hamada et al., 1993). The authors identified baicalein as one of the several components the most potent scavenger for radicals in $FeCl_3$-induced epilepsy model in rats. It is suggested that baicalein action is based upon radical quenching and anti-oxidant effects.

Many Native American plants are valued by local medical practitioners for their positive effects on health and a number of diseases, including epilepsy. *Celastrus paniculatus L.* (CP), *Picrorhiza kurroa (PK)* and *Withania somnifera L. (WS)* were investigated for their free radical scavenging capacity (Russo et al., 2001). It has been observed that methanolic extracts of these plants are dose-dependent free radical scavengers, and that they prevent DNA injury due to oxygen stress. PK extract had a more powerful effect than CP or WS. These favourable biological properties, reported in clinical and animal studies, have been attributed, at least in part, to their anti-stress, immune-modulating, anti-inflammatory and anti-aging effects. A similar anti-oxidant effect was observed using another plant in Ayurvedic medicine, *Bacopa monniera L.* (BM), which has free radical scavenging capacity (Russo et al., 2003).

8.4. Nootropics and anti-oxidants

It was reported that nootropics (phenotropil) and antioxidants (mexidol) potentiate AEDs in posttraumatic epilepsy treatment (Savenkov et al., 2013).The authors observed in 75 patients significant reduction of epileptic seizure frequency, decrease of epileptic changes in the EEG, improvement of cognitive function and quality of life. Coherent indicators of slow wave-activity were observed after treatment. The authors recommended to use mexidol and phenotropil with AEDs for complex treatment of posttraumatic epilepsy.

When interpreting clinically, these and the highlighted earlier results, one needs to be careful because the relationships in disease as heterogeneous as epilepsy are complex and multifactorial. Moreover, the results, usually are not conducted according to rules of evidence based medicine.

9. Drug-resistant epilepsy and polytherapy

Drug-resistant seizures force physicians to use polytherapy with various AEDs. Polytherapy increases the production of free radicals and disturbs mineral balance to a greater extent than monotherapy, leading to increased oxygen stress. Both, increased free radical production and inhibition of the enzymes which remove scavengers, lead to adverse reactions and aggravation of the morbid process (Maertens et al., 1995; Hamed et al., 2004).

Patients with chronic epilepsy and long-term AED therapy are at greater risk of atherosclerotic changes in the arteries through complex molecular mechanisms that promote atherogenesis (Hamed and Nabeshima, 2005). Metabolic dysfunctions in these patients have been attributed to altered homocysteine, lipid and lipoprotein metabolism and uric acid.

In relevant study, relationship between the carotid artery intima-media thickness (CA-IMT) and lipid profile (MDA, oxidised LDL, total anti-oxidant capacity, GSH-Px and uric acid) were assessed in 225 adult patients with epilepsy (and 60 control subjects) (Hamed et al., 2007). Compared to the control group, the CA-IMT of treated and untreated patients common carotid artery, bifurcation area and internal carotid arteries were significantly thickened in 51.1%, 73.3% and 43.6% of patients, respectively. The study supports the opinion that in patients with epilepsy, various risk factors and CA-IMT become worse, which could be attributed to epilepsy itself and/or AEDs. According to the authors, these dysfunctions are indications for routine anti-oxidant multivitamin supplementation (folic acid, vitamins B12, B6, C, E, and beta-carotene). The protective, anti-atheromatic effect of vitamins is based on their anti-oxidant and anti-inflammatory properties. Tupeev et al. (1993) found a positive effect of prolonged vitamin E treatment (600 mg/day) in patients with generalized seizures: seizure frequency was reduced, EEG improved and anti-oxidant activity increased.

In other research highlighted earlier, increased lipid hydroperoxidase concentrations were weakly correlated with the risk factors for vascular changes (triglyceridemia, cholesterolemia) (Mahle and Dasgupta, 1997).

10. The effects of surgery on oxygen stress in AED-resistant temporal lobe epilepsy

López et al. (2007) studied the activity of anti-oxidant enzymes (SOD, catalase and GSH-Px) and markers of oxygen stress induced molecular neuronal injury (MDA and ROS) before and at various times after epileptic focus resection in 9 therapy resistant patients; a control group consisted of 32 healthy individuals. All the studied variables normalized postoperatively except SOD activity.

Several earlier interesting observations seem to be related to these findings to a certain extent. Turkdogan et al. (2002) found that increased lipid peroxidation in plasma may be causally related to the presence of abnormal structural changes as assessed by brain magnetic resonance (MR), rather, than to the treatment of epilepsy with focal or generalized epileptic discharges in the EEG, duration of epilepsy, or seizure frequency (more or fewer than 1 seizure a month). The authors found an increase in plasma lipid peroxidation in 52 children with epilepsy, treated with one or more AEDs and abnormal brain MR, compared with 16 healthy children (the difference was significant, $p<0.05$). No significant differences in anti-oxidant enzymes were found in either group. Patients with well-controlled seizures and children with drug-resistant seizures but normal MRs had a higher SOD activity than children in the control group ($p<0.05$). GSH-Px (an antioxidant) activity was not significantly different in the children with epilepsy compared to the control group.

This interesting and heterogeneous picture of enzymatic activity in children with epilepsy and control children suggests that the relationship between various laboratory tests and numerous variables associated with the heterogeneity and treatment of epilepsy are very complex. Although the authors took seizure frequency into consideration, they did not state when blood tests were undertaken relative to seizure occurrence or to an imminent seizure, nor do they report EEG epileptic activity prior to the blood test. This makes it very difficult to monitor the causal relationships between the results of the various tests and their epileptic correlates.

Study of oxygen stress markers in the neocortex of drug-resistant epilepsy patients submitted to epilepsy surgery, supported human findings being in agreement with those found in animal models (Rumia et al., 2013). The concurrent increase in catalase ($p<0.01$) and decrease in GPx ($p<0.05$) together with unchanged SOD levels, suggests catalase as the main anti-oxidant enzyme in human epileptic cortex. The substantial increase in the levels of oxidants – 0_2 (-) and 8-oxo-dG in epileptic patients – in comparison with non-epileptic cortex samples – supports a connection between chronic seizures and ROS-mediated neuronal damage.

11. Conclusions

1. It seems that oxygen stress and its products may play an essential role in earliest stage of epileptogenesis. However, antioxidants as well as antiepiletic drugs do not prevent epileptogenesis. In seizure or epilepsy animal models, at best, both antioxidants or antepileptic drugs can delay the first seizure occurrence and diminish seizures' severity.

2. Research on animal models and patients with epilepsy suggests that epileptic seizures, epileptiform discharges and some AEDs (especially polytherapy) may produce oxygen stress and have a negative effect on the oxidation – anti-oxidation balance.

3. AEDs and the drug dosages have differential effects on oxygen stress. In epileptic patients (and in animal models of seizures) CBZ, OXC, PB, PHT and VPA produce oxygen stress. In experimental models of seizures, the majority of new generation AEDs has no or minor effects on oxygen stress; usually they have a more favourable effect on the oxidation and

http://dx.doi.org/10.5772/57484

anti-oxidation enzyme balance, trace elements and electrolytic homeostasis than the odler AEDs.

4. Neuroprotectors (trace elements, vitamins and other antioxidants) help to reduce seizure-induced oxygen stress and therefore it is suggested that they should supplement AED treatment. It may be expected that the long-term AED adverse events will be diminished by combination of AED with antioxidants. However, one of the main problems is to find appropriate effective dose and kind of antioxidants restoring equilibrium between oxidative and anti-oxidative processes.

5. Since some AEDs, seizures and epileptiform discharges can lead to oxidation – anti-oxidation imbalance, it seems reasonable to develop new strategies that diminish negative effects of oxygen stress properties in current epilepsy treatment. New AED synthesis, without oxidative effects, would provide better quality of epilepsy medication.

6. Further studies of oxygen stress effects are needed to understand better the mechanisms of protective effects of anti-oxidants.

7. Research on the role of oxygen stress opens a new chapter in epileptology with a hope of prevention of biochemical proceses leading to epileptogenesis, better seizure control and diminish cognitive function impaiment.

Author details

Jerzy Majkowski*

Address all correspondence to: fundacja@epilepsy.pl

Epilepsy Diagnostic and Therapeutic Center, Foundation of Epileptology, Warsaw, Poland

The authors have no conflict of interest to disclose.

References

[1] Abramov J.P., Wells P.G.: *Embryoprotective role of endogenous catalase in acatalasemic and human catalase-expressing mouse embryos exposed in culture to developmental and phenytoin-enhanced oxidative stress.* Toxicol. Sci., 2011, 120: 428-438.

[2] Abuhandan M., Calik M., Taskin A., Yetkin I., Selek S., Iscan A.: *The oxidative and antioxidative status of simple febrile seizure patients.* J. Pak. Med. Assoc., 2013, 63: 594-7.

[3] Akarsu S., Yilmaz S., Ozan S., Kurt A., Benzer F., Gurgoze M.K.: *Effects of febrile seizures on oxidant state in children.* Pediatr. Neurol., 2007, 36: 307-311.

[4] Aldarmaa J., Liu Z., Long J., Mo X., Ma J., Liu J.: *Anti-convulsant effect and mechanism of Astragalus mongholicus extract in vitro and in vivo: protection against oxidative damage and mitochondrial dysfunction.* Neurochem. Res., 2010, 35: 33-41.

[5] Al-Shorbagy M.Y., El Sayeh B.M., Abdallah D.M.: *Diverse effects of variant doses of dexamethasone in lithium-pilocarpine induced seizures in rats.* Can. J. Physiol. Pharmacol., 2012, 90:13-21.

[6] Andlin-Sobocki P., Jönss B., Wittchen H.-U., Olesen J.: Cost of disorders of the brain in Europe. Eur. J. Neurol., 2005, 12 (supl. 1): 1-27.

[7] Anlasik T., Sies H., Griffiths H.R. Mecocci P., Stahl W., Polidori M.C.: *Dietary habits are major determinants of the plasma antioxidant status in healthy elderly subject.* Br. J. Nutr., 2005, 94: 639-642.

[8] Asadi-Shekaari M., Kalantaripour T.P., Nejad F.A., Namazian E., Eslami A.:*The anticonvulsant and neuroprotective effects of walnuts on the neurons of rat brain cortex.* Avicenna J. Med. Biotechnol., 2012, 4: 155-8.

[9] Ashrafi M.R., Shabanian R., Abbaskhanian A., Nasirian A., Ghofrani M., Mohammadi M. et al.: *Selenium and intractable epilepsy: is there any correlation?* Pediatr. Neurol., 2007, 36: 25-29.

[10] Atanasova M., Petkova Z., Pechlivanova D., Dragomirova P., Blazhev A., Tchekalarova J.: *Strain-dependent effects of long-term treatment with melatonin on kainic acid-induced status epilepticus, oxidative stress and the expression of heat shock proteins*. Pharmacol. Biochem. Behav., 2013, 111: 44-50.

[11] Atroshi F., Erkki A., Westermarck T.: *The role of selenium in epilepsy and other neurological disorders*. Epileptologia, 2007, 15: 211-224.

[12] Avcicek A., Iscan A.: *The effects of carbamazepine, valproic acid and phenobarbital on the oxidative balance in epileptic children*. Eur. Neurol., 2007, 57: 65-69.

[13] Avramovic N., Dragutinovic V., Krstic D., Colovic M., Trbovic A., de Luka S. Et al.: *The effects of omega 3 fatty acid supplementation on brain tissue oxidative status in aged wistar rats*. Hippokratia, 2012, 16: 241-245.

[14] Azam F., Prasad M.V, Thangavel N.: *Targeting oxidative stress component in the therapeutics of epilepsy*. Curr. Top. Med. Chem., 2012;.12: 994-1007.

[15] Barros D.O., Xavier S.M., Barbosa C.O., Silva R.F., Freitas R.L., Maia F.D. et al.: *Effects of the vitamin E in catalase activities in hippocampus after status epilepticus induced by pilocarpine in Wistar rats*. Neurosci. Lett., 2007, 416: 227-230.

[16] Bartosz G.: *Druga twarz tlenu. (Other face of oxygen)*. Wyd. Nauk. PWN, 3rd edition, Warszawa, 2006.

[17] Bazil C.W., Short D., Crispin D., Zheng W.: *Patients with intractable epilepsy have low melatonin, which increases following seizures.* Neurology, 2000, 55: 1746-1748.

[18] Beghi E.: Overview of studies to prevent posttraumatic epilepsy. Epilepsia, 2003, 44 (Suppl. 10): 21-26.

[19] Berdichevsky Y., Dzhala V., Mail M., Staley K.J.: *Interictal spikes, seizure and ictal cell death are not necessary for post-traumatic epileptogenesis in vitro.* Neurobiol. Dis., 2012, 45: 774-785.

[20] Beshkatova V., Narkewich V., Vitskova B., Vanin A.: *The influence of anticonvulsant and antioxidant drugs on nitric oxide level and lipid peroxidation in the rat brain during penthylenetetrazole-induced epileptiform model seizures.* Prog. Neuropsychopharmacol. Biol. Psychiatry., 2003, 27: 487-492.

[21] Bjelakovic G., Nikolova D., Gluud C.: *Meta-regression analyses, meta-analyses, and trial sequential analyses of the effects of supplementation with Beta-carotene, vitamin A, and vitamin E singly or in different combinations on all-cause mortality: do we have evidence for lack of harm?* PLoS One, 2013, 8:e74558.

[22] Bolayir E., Celik K., Tas A., Topaktas S., Bakir S.: *The effects of oxcarbazepine on oxidative stress in epileptic patients.* Methods Find. Exp. Clin. Pharmacol., 2004, 26: 345-348.

[23] Bortolatto C.F., Jesse C.R., Wilhelm E.A., Nogueira C.W.: *Selective blockade of A(2A) receptor protects against neurotoxicity induced by kainic acid in young rats.* Fundam. Clin. Pharmacol., 2012, 26: 495-502.

[24] Bozkus F., San I., Ulas T., Iynen I., Yesilova Y., Guler Y., Aksoy N.: *Evaluation of total oxidative stress parameters in patients with nasal polyps.* Acta Otorhinolaryngol. Ital., 2013, 33: 248-253.

[25] Bruce A.J., Baudry M.: *Oxygen free radicals in rat limbic structures after kainate-induced seizures.* Free Radic. Biol. Med., 1995, 18: 993-1002.

[26] Büyükkaya E., Evliyaoğlu O., Islamoğlu Y., Cil H., Karakaş M.F., Burak Akçay A. et al.: *The relationship between coenzyme Q10 and severity of coronary artery disease.* Med. Glas. (Zenica), 2013, 10: 229-233.

[27] Cao L., Xu J., Lin Y., Zhao X., Liu X., Chi Z.: *Autophagy is upregulated in rats with status epilepticus and partly inhibited by vitamin E.* Biochem. Biophys. Res. Commun., 2009, 379: 949-953.

[28] Cárdenas-Rodríguez N., Coballase-Urrutia E., Huerta-Gertrudis B., García-Cruz M.E., Pedraza-Chaverri J., Coria-Jiménez R. et al.: *Antioxidant activity of topiramate: an antiepileptic agent.* Neurol. Sci., 2013a, 34: 741-747.

[29] Chalghoum A., Noichri Y., Mohamed M.H., Dandana A., Baudin B., Ferchichi S., Miled A.: *The pro-oxidant effect of angiotensin-1 converting enzyme in Tunisian patients with coronary heart disease.* Acta Biomed., 2012, 83: 202-207.

[30] Chang T.K., Abbott F.S.: *Oxidative stress as a mechanism of valproic acid-associated hepatoxicity.* Drug Metab. Rev., 2006, 38: 627-639.

[31] Chang J.C., Kou S.J, Lin W.T., Liu C.S.: *Regulatory role of mitochondria in oxidative stress and atherosclerosis.* World J. Cardiol., 2010, 2:150-159.

[32] Chuang Y.C.: *Mitochondrial dysfunction and oxidative stress in seizure-induced neuronal cell death. Acta Neurol. Taiwan,* 2010, 19 :3-15.

[33] Costello D.J., Delanty N.: *Oxidative injury in epilepsy: potential for antioxidant therapy.* Expert. Rev. Neurother., 2004, 4: 541-553.

[34] Cozzi A., Santambrogio P., Privitera D., Broccoli V., Rotundo L.I., Garavaglia B. et al.: *Human L-ferritin deficiency is characterized by idiopathic generalized seizures and atypical restless leg syndrome.* J. Exp. Med., 2013, 210: 1779-1791.

[35] Cupello A., Mainardi P., Robello M., Thellung S.: Effect of oxide donors on GABA uptake by rat brain synaptosomes. Neurochem. Res., 1997, 22: 1517-1521.

[36] Dakin K.A., Weaver D.F.: *Mechanisms of posttraumatic seizures: a quantum pharmacological analysis of the molecular properties of an epileptogenic focus following iron-induced membrane peroxidation.* Seizure, 1993, 2: 21-33.

[37] Dal-Pizzol F., Klamt F., Vianna M.M, Schröder N., Quevedo J., Benfato M.S. et al.: *Lipid peroxidation in hippocampus early and late after status epilepticus induced by pilocarpine or kainic acid in Wistar rats.* Neurosci. Lett. 2000, 291:179-182.

[38] de la Pena P., Porta-Etessam J. *Post-traumatic epilepsy.* Rev. Neurol., 1998, 26: 256-261.

[39] Demirci S., Kutluhan S., Nazıroğlu M., Uğuz A.C., Yürekli V.A., Demirci K.: *Effects of selenium and topiramate on cytosolic Ca(2+) influx and oxidative stress in neuronal PC12 cells.* Neurochem. Res., 2013, 38: 90-97.

[40] Devi P.U. Manocha A., Vahora D.: *Seizures, antiepileptics, antioxidants and oxidative stress: an insight for researchers.* Expert Opin. Pharmacother., 2008, 9: 3169-3177.

[41] Di Bella L., Gualano L.: *Key aspects of melatonin physiology: thirty years of research.* Neuro. Endocrinol. Lett., 2006, 27: 425-432.

[42] Dostalek M., Brooks J.D., Hardy K.D., Milne G.L., Moore M.M., Sharma S. et al.: *In vivo oxidative damage in rats is associated with barbiturate response but not other cytochrome P450 inducers.* Mol. Pharmacol., 2007, 72:1419-1424.

[43] Dubenko A.E., Litovchenko T.A.: *The concept of pathogenic therapy of epilepsy with medications restoring energy metabolism.* Zh. Nevrol. Psikhiatr. Im. S. S. Korsakova, 2002, 102: 25-31.

[44] Fauteck J., Schmidt H., Lerchl A., Kurlemann G., Wittkowski W.: *Melatonin in epilepsy: first results of replacement therapy and first clinical results.* Biol. Signals. Recept., 1999, 8: 105-110.

[45] Ficarra S., Misiti F., Russo A., Carelli-Alinovi C., Bellocco E., Barreca D. et al.: *Antiepileptic carbamazepine drug treatment induces alteration of membrane in red blood cells: possible positive effects on metabolism and oxidative stress.* Biochimie, 2013, 95: 833-841.

[46] Flerov M.A., Tolstukhina T.I., Gerasimova I.A.: *Free radical lipid oxidation in brain cortex neurons and neuroglia during convulsions.* Bull. Exp. Biol. Med.: 2004, 138: 341-342.

[47] Folbergrová J., Ješina P., Nůsková H., Houštěk J.: *Antioxidant enzymes in cerebral cortex of immature rats following experimentally-induced seizures: upregulation of mitochondrial MnSOD (SOD2).* Int. J. Dev. Neurosci., 2013, 31: 123-130.

[48] Folbergrová J., Jesina P., Haugvicová R., Lisý V., Houstek J.: *Sustained deficiency of mitochondrial complex I activity during long periods of survival after seizures induced in immature rats by homocysteic acid.* Neurochem. Int., 2010, 56: 394-403.

[49] Forsgren I., Beghi E., Ekman M.: *Cost of epilepsy in Europe.* Eur. J. Neurol., 2005, 12 (Suppl. 1): 54-58.

[50] Frantseva M.V., Perez Velazquez J.L., Carlen P.L.: *Changes in membrane and synaptic properties of thalamocortical circuitry caused by hydrogen peroxide.* J. Neurophysiol., 1998, 80: 1317-1326.

[51] Frantseva M.V., Perez Velazquez J.L., Tsoraklidis G.et al.: *Oxidative stress is involved in seizure-induced neurodegeneration in the kindling model of epilepsy.* Neuroscience, 2000, 97: 431-435.

[52] Freitas R.M.: *Investigation of oxidative stress involvement in hippocampus in epilepsy model induced by pilocarpine.* Neurosci Lett., 2009, 25: 462: 225-229.

[53] Freitas R.M., Nascimento V.S., Vasconcelos S.M., Sousa F.C., Viana G.S., Fonteles M.M.: *Catalase activity in cerebellum, hippocampus, frontal cortex and striatum after status epilepticus induced by pilocarpine in Wistar rats.* Neurosci. Lett., 2004, 365: 102-105.

[54] Freitas R.M., Vasconcelos S.M., Souza F.C., Viana G.S., Fonteles M.M.: *Oxidative stress in the hippocampus after pilocarpine-induced status epilepticus in Wistar rats.* FEBS J., 2005, 272: 1307-1312.

[55] Fröscher W.: *Drug resistant epilepsy.* Epileptologia, 2012, 20: 17-23

[56] Gaby A.R.: *Natural approaches to epilepsy.* Altern. Med. Rev., 2007, 12: 9-24.

[57] Gallagher E.P., Sheehy K.M.: *Effects of phenytoin on glutathione status and oxidative stress biomarker gene mRNA levels in cultured precision human liver slices.* Toxicol. Sci., 2001 59:118-26.

[58] Goddard G.V., McIntyre D.C., Leech C.K.: *A permanent change in brain function resulting from daily electrical stimulation.* Exp. Neurol., 1969, 25: 295-330.

[59] Gupta Y.K., Briyal S.: *Protective effect of vineatrol against kainic acid induced seizures, oxidative stress and on the expression of heat shock proteins in rats.* Eur. Neuropsychopharmacol., 2006, 16: 85-91.

[60] Gupta M., Gupta Y.K., Agarwal S., Aneja S., Kohli K.: *A randomized, double-blind, placebo controlled trial of melatonin add-on therapy in epileptic children on valproate monotherapy: effect on glutathione peroxidase and glutathione reductase enzymes.* Br. J. Clin. Pharmacol., 2004, 58: 542-547.

[61] Gupta M., Kohli K., Gupta Y.K.: *Modulation of serum concentrations of melatonin by carbamazepine and valproate.* Indian. J. Physiol. Pharmacol., 2006, 50: 70-82.

[62] Hamada H., Hiramatsu M., Edamatsu R., Mori A.: *Free radical scavenging action of baicalein.* Arch. Biochem. Biophys., 1993, 306: 261-266.

[63] Hamed S.A., Abdellah M.M.: *Trace elements and electrolytes homeostasis and their relation to antioxidant enzyme cavity in brain hyperexcitability of epileptic patients.* J. Pharmacol. Sci., 2004, 96: 349-359.

[64] Hamed S.A., Abdellah M.M., El-Melegy N.: *Blood levels of trace elements, electrolytes, and oxidative stress/antioxidant systems in epileptic patients.* J. Pharmacol. Sci., 2004, 96: 465-473.

[65] Hamed S.A., Hamed E.A., Hamdy R., Nabeshima T.: *Vascular risk factors and oxidative stress as independent predictors of asymptomatic atherosclerosis in adult patients with epilepsy.* Epilepsy Res. 2007, 74:183-192.

[66] Hamed S.A., Nabeshima T.: *The high atherosclerotic risk among epileptics: the atheroprotective role of multivitamins.* J. Pharmacol. Sci., 2005, 98: 340-353.

[67] Hardeland R., Pandi-Perumal S.R., Cardinali D.P.: *Melatonin.* Int. J. Biochem. Cell. Biol., 2006, 38: 313-316.

[68] Heinemann U., Buchheim K., Gabriel S., Kann O., Kovacs R., Schuchmann S.: *Cell death and metabolic activity epileptiform discharges and status epilepticus in the hippocampus.* Prof. Brain Res., 2002, 135: 197-210.

[69] Hirotsu C., Matos G., Tufik S., Andersen M.L.: *Changes in gene expression in the frontal cortex of rats with pilocarpine-induced status epilepticus after sleep deprivation.* Epilepsy Behav., 2013, 27: 378-384.

[70] Hsieh C.L., Chang C.H., Chiang S.Y., Li T.C., Tang N.Y., Pon C.Z. et al.: *Anticonvulsive and free radical scavenging activities of vanillyl alcohol in ferric chloride-induced epileptic seizures in Sprague-Dawley rats.* Life Sci., 2000, 67: 1185-1195.

[71] Hsieh C.L., Chiang S.Y., Cheng K.S., Lin Y.H., Tang N.Y., Lee C.J. et al.: *Anticonvulsive and free radical scavenging activities of Gastrodia elata Bl. In kainic acid-treated rats.* Am. J. Chin. Med., 2001, 29: 331-341.

[72] Hsieh P.F., Hou C.W., Yao P.W., Wu S.P., Peng Y.F., Shen M.L., Lin CH, Chao Y.Y., Chang M.H., Jeng K.C.: *Sesamin ameliorates oxidative stress and mortality in kainic acid-*

induced status epilepticus by inhibition of MAPK and COX-2 activation. J. Neuroinflammation, 2011, 8: 57.

[73] Huang J.L., Ma Y.W., Lian Q.L., Xu J.P., Jiang C.L., Guo M.Z., Sun X.J.: *Effect of acetazolamide on the latency of hyperbaric oxygen-induced convulsion.* Sheng Li Xue Bao., 2004, 56: 158-162.

[74] Huang J., Ren R.N., Chen C.M., Ye L.Y.: *An experimental study on hepatotoxicity of topiramate in young rats.* Zhongguo Dang Dai Er Ke Za Zhi, 2007, 9: 54-58.

[75] Hung-Ming W., Liu C.S., Tsai J.J., Ko L.Y., Wei Y.H..: *Antioxidant and anticonvulsant effect of a modified formula of chaihu-longu-muli-tang.* Am. J. Chin. Med., 2002, 30: 339-346.

[76] Hydén H.: *The learning brain during a life cycle some biochemical and psychological aspects.* Acta. Neurol. Scand. Suppl. 1980, 80: 9-27.

[77] Iivanainen M., Gaily E., : *Uudet Epilepsialääkkeet.* Duodecim, 1995, 111: 751-758.

[78] Ilhan A., Gurel A., Armatcu F. et al.: *Antiepileptogenic and antioxidant effects of Nigella sativa oil against pentylenetetrazol-induced kindling in mice.* Neuropharmacology, 2005a, 49: 456-464.

[79] Ilhan A., Aladog M.A., Kocer A., Boluk A., Gurel A., Armutcu F.: *Erdosteine ameliorates PTZ-induced oxidative stress in mice seizure model.* Brain Res. Bull., 2005b, 65: 495-499.

[80] Jacobson S.O., Cassel G.E., Persson S.A.: *Increased levels of nitrogen oxides and lipid peroxidation in the rat brain after soman-induced seizures.* Arch. Toxicol., 1999, 73, 269-273.

[81] Jafarian I., Eskandari M.R., Mashayekhi V., Ahadpour M., Hosseini M.J.: *Toxicity of valproic acid in isolated rat liver mitochondria.* Toxicol. Mech. Methods., 2013, 23: 617-623.

[82] Kaipainen P., Atroshi F.: *Effect of Phenobarbital on liver microsmal cytochrome P-450 contents and liver reduced glutathione (GSH) level in various species.* Z. Versuchstierkunde, 1986, 28: 27-31.

[83] Kaipainen P., Westermarck T., Kaski M., Iivanainen M., Atroshi F.: *Effect of valproic acid treatment on serum lipid contents in persons with intellectual disability and epilepsy.* Intellectual Disability Research, 2004, 48: 351.

[84] Kawakami Y., Monobe M., Kuwabara K., Fujita T., Maeda M., Fujino O. et al.: *A comparative study of nitric oxide, glutathione, and glutathione peroxidase activities in cerebrospinal fluid from children with convulsive diseases/children with aseptic meningitis.* Brain Dev., 2006, 28: 243-246.

[85] Kim J.B., Hama S., Hough G., Navab M., Fogelman A.M., Maclellan W.R. et al.: *Heart failure is associated with impaired anti-inflammatory and antioxidant properties of high-density lipoproteins.* Am. J. Cardiol., 2013, 112: 1770-1777.

[86] Komatsu M., Hiramatsu M., Willmore L.J.: *Zonisamide reduces the increase in 8-hydroxy-2'-deoxyguanosine levels formed during iron-induced epileptogenesis in the brains of rats.* Epilepsia, 2000, 41: 1091-1094.

[87] Kubera M., Budziszewska B., Jaworska-Feil L. Basta-Kaim A., Leskiewicz M., Tetich M.et al.: *Effect of topiramate on the kainate-induced status epilepticus, lipid peroxidation and immunoreactivity of rats.* Pol. J. Pharmacol., 2004, 56: 553-561.

[88] Kurekci A.E., Alpay F., Tanindi S., Gokcay E., Ozcan O., Akin R. et al.: *Plasma trace element, plasma glutathione peroxidase, and superoxide dismutase levels in epileptic children receiving antiepileptic drug therapy.* Epilepsia, 1995, 36: 600-604.

[89] Kwan P., Arzimanoglou A., Berg A.T. Brodie M.J., Hauser W.A., Mathern G., et al.: *Definition of drug resistant epilepsy: Consensus proposal by the ad hoc task force of the ILAE Commission of Therapeutic Strategies.* Epilepsia, 2010, 51: 1069-1077.

[90] Lafemina M.J., Sheldon R.A., Ferriero D.M.: *Acute hypoxia-ischemia results in hydrogen peroxide accumulation in neonatal but not adult mouse brain.* Pediatr. Res., 2006, 59: 680-683.

[91] Lasoń W.: *Mechanisms of drug resistance in epilepsy.* Przegl Lek., 2006, 63: 1218-1220.

[92] Lasoń W., Leśkiewicz M.: *Effect of plant polyphenols on seizures – animal studies.* Journal of Epileptology, 2013, 21, 2: 87-95.

[93] Leonardi M., Ustrun T.B.: *The global burden of epilepsy.* Epilepsia, 2002, 43, Suppl. 6:21-25.

[94] Li H., Pin S., Zeng Z., Wang M.M. Andreasson K.A. McCullough L.D.: *Sex differences in cell death.* Ann. Neurol., 2005, 58: 317-321.

[95] Li Z.H., Zlabek V., Velisek J., Grabic R., Machova J., Randak T.: *Modulation of antioxidant defence system in brain of rainbow trout (Oncorhynchus mykiss) after chronic carbamazepine treatment.* Comp. Biochem. Physiol. C. Toxicol. Pharmacol., 2010, 51:137-141.

[96] Liang L.P., Patel M.: *Mitochondrial oxidative stress and increased seizure susceptibility in SOD2 (-/+) mice.* Free Radic. Biol. Med., 2004, 36: 542-554.

[97] Liang L.P., Waldbaum S., Rowley S., Huang T.T., Day B.J., Patel M.: Mitochondrial oxidative stress and epilepsy in SOD2 deficient mice: attenuation by a lipophilic metalloporphyrin. Neurobiol. Dis., 2012, 45: 1068-1076.

[98] Liu C.S., Wu H.M., Kao S.H., Wei Y.H.: *Phenytoin-mediated oxidative stress in serum of female epileptics: a possible pathogenesis in the fetal hydantoin syndrome.* Hum. Exp. Toxicol., 1997, 16: 177-181.

[99] Liu C.S., Wu H.M., Kao S.H., Wei Y.H.: *Serum trace elements, glutathione, cooper/zinc superoxide dismutase, and lipid peroxidation in epileptic patients with phenytoin or carbamazepine monotherapy.* Clin. Neuropharmacol., 1998, 21: 62-64.

[100] López J., González M.E., Lorigados L., Morales L., Reverón G., Bauzá J.Y.: *Oxidative stress markers in surgically treated patients with refractory epilepsy.* Clin. Biochem., 2007, 40: 292-298.

[101] Loureiro S.O., Romão L., Alves T., Fonseca A., Heimfarth L., Moura Neto V. et al.: *Homocysteine induces cytoskeletal remodeling and production of reactive oxygen species in cultured cortical astrocytes.* Brain Res., 2010, 1355: 151-164.

[102] Lu W., Uetrecht J.P.: *Possible bioactivation pathways of lamotrigine.* Drug. Metab. Dispos., 2007, 35: 1050-1056.

[103] Madmani M.E, Solaiman A.Y., Tamr Agha K., Madmani Y., Shahrour Y., Essali A, Kadro W.: *Coenzyme Q10 for heart failure.* Cochrane Database Syst. Rev., 2013, 9: CD008684.

[104] Maertens P., Dyken P., Graf W., Pippenger C., Chronister R., Shah A.: *Free radicals, anticonvulsants, and the neuronal ceroid-lipofuscinoses.* Am. J. Med. Genet., 1995, 57: 225-228.

[105] Mahle C., Dasgupta A.: *Decreased total antioxidant capacity and elevated lipid hydroperoxide concentrations in sera of epileptic patients receiving phenytoin.* Life Sci., 1997, 61: 437-443.

[106] Majkowski J.: *Brain electical stimulation: kindling and memory aspects.* Acta Neurol. Scand., 1981, 64 (Suppl. 89): 101-108.

[107] Majkowski J.: *Kindling and memory.*W: *The Clinical Relevance of Kindling,* G. Blowig and M.R. Trimble (eds.), John Wiley & Sons Ltd., 1989: 87-102.

[108] Majkowski J.: *Posttraumatic epilepsy.* In: Comprehensive Epileptology. M. Dam, L. Gram (eds). Raven Press, New York, 1990, 281-288.

[109] Majkowski J.: Kindling dall'epilessia sperimentale alla psicopatologia, Monduzzi Editore, Monduzzi Bologna, 1993.

[110] Majkowski J.: *Epileptogenesis – The role of oxygen stress.* Epileptologia, 2007, 15: 225-240.

[111] Majkowski J. and Kwast O.: *Changes in somatosensory evoked potentials during kindling: analogy to learning modifications.* Epilepsia, 1981, 22: 267-274.

[112] Majkowski J., Majkowska-Zwolińska B.: Direct and Indirect Annual Costs of Patients with Epilepsy in Poland. Prospective Multicenter Study. Epileptologia, 2010, 18:141-152.

[113] Majkowski J., Westermarck T., Atroshi F.: *Oxygen stress: epilepsy and antiepilepic drugs.* Epileptologia, 2011,19: 143-157.

[114] Martinc B., Grabnar I., Vovk T.: *The role of reactive species in epileptogenesis and influence of antiepileptic drug therapy on oxidative stress.* Curr. Neuropharmacol., 2012, 10: 328-343.

[115] Martinez-Ballesteros C., Pita-Calandre E., Sanchez-Gonzalez Y., Rodriguez-Lopez C.M., Agil A.: *Lipid peroxidation in adult epileptic patients treated with valproic acid.* Rev. Neurol., 2004, 38: 101-106.

[116] Milder J., Patel M.: *Modulation of oxidative stress and mitochondrial function by the ketogenic diet.* Epilepsy Res., 2012, 100: 295-303.

[117] Militão G.C, Ferreira P.M., de Freitas R.M.: *Effects of lipoic acid on oxidative stress in rat striatum after pilocarpine-induced seizures.* Neurochem. Int., 2010, 56:16-20.

[118] Mohanan P.V., Yamamoto H.A.: *Preventive, effect of melatonin against brain mitochondria DNA damage, lipid peroxidation and seizures induced by kainic acid.* Toxicol. Lett., 2002, 129: 99-105.

[119] Mori A., Hiramatsu M., Yokoi I., Edamatsu R.: *Biochemical pathogenesis of post-traumatic epilepsy.* Pavlov. J. Biol. Sci., 1990, 205-208.

[120] Murashima Y.L., Suzuki J., Yoshii M.: *Developmental program of epileptogenesis in the brain of EL mice.*Epilepsia, 2005, 46 Suppl 5:10-16.

[121] Narkilahti S., Pitkanen A.: *Caspase 6 expression in the rat hippocampus during epileptogenesis and epilepsy.* Neurosicience, 2005, 131: 887-897.

[122] Naziroğlu M., Kutluhan S., Yilmaz M.: *Selenium and topiramate modulates brain microsomal oxidative stress values, Ca2+-ATPase activity, and EEG records in pentylenetetrazol-induced seizures in rats.* J. Membr. Biol., 2008, 225: 39-49.

[123] Nazıroglu M.: *Role of selenium on calcium signaling and oxidative stress-induced molecular pathways in epilepsy.* Neurochem. Res., 2009, 34: 2181-2191.

[124] Nazıroğlu M., Yürekli V.A.: *Effects of antiepileptic drugs on antioxidant and oxidant molecular pathways: focus on trace elements.* Cell. Mol. Neurobiol., 2013, 33: 589-599.

[125] Niketic V., Ristic S., Saicic Z.S., Spasic M., Buzadzic B., Stojkovic M.: *Activities of antioxidant enzymes and formation of the glutathione adduct of hemoglobin (Hb ASSG) in epileptic patients with long-term antiepileptic therapy.* Farmaco., 1995, 50: 811-813.

[126] Oliveira A.A., Almeida J.P., Freitas R.M., Nascimento V.S., Aguiar L.M., Júnior H.V. et al.: *Effects of levetiracetam in lipid peroxidation level, nitrite-nitrate formation and antioxidant enzymatic activity in mice brain after pilocarpine-induced seizures.* Cell. Mol. Neurobiol., 2007, 27: 395-406.

[127] Ounjaijean S., Westermarck T., Partinen M., Plonka-Poltorak E., Kaipainen P., Kaski M. et al.: *Increase in non-transferrin bound iron and the oxidative stress status in epilepsy patients treated using valproic acid monotherapy.* Int. J. Clin. Pharmacol. Ther., 2011, 49: 268-277.

[128] Oztas B., Akgul S., Seker F.B.: *Gender difference in the influence of antioxidants on the blood-brain barrier permeability during pentylenetetrazol-induced seizures in hyperthermic rat pups.* Biol. Trace Elem. Res., 2007, 118: 77-83.

[129] Oztas B., Kilic S., Dural E., Ispir T.: *Influence of antioxidants on the blood-brain barrier permeability during epileptic seizures.* J. Neurosci. Res., 2001, 66: 674-678.

[130] Patel M.N.: *Oxidative stress, mitochondrial dysfunction, and epilepsy.* Free Radic. Res., 2002, 36: 1139-1146.

[131] Patel M.: *Mitochondrial dysfunction and oxidative stress: cause and consequence of epileptic seizures.* Free Radic. Biol. Med., 2004, 37: 1951-1962.

[132] Patry G., Lyagoubi S., Tassinari C.A.: *Subclinical electrical status epilepticus' induced by sleep in children.* Arch. Neurol., 1971, 24: 242-252.

[133] Paulsen Bda S., de Moraes Maciel R., Galina A., Souza da Silveira M., dos Santos Souza C, Drummond H. et al.: *Altered oxygen metabolism associated to neurogenesis of induced pluripotent stem cells derived from a schizophrenic patient.* Cell., Transplant. 2012; 21:1547-1559.

[134] Pavone A., Cardile V.: *An in vitro study of new antiepileptic drugs and astrocytes.* Epilepsia, 2003, 44 (supl. 10): 34-39.

[135] Pestana R.R., Kinjo E.R., Hernandes M.S., Britto L.R: *Reactive oxygen species generated by NADPH oxidase are involved in neurodegeneration in the pilocarpine model of temporal lobe epilepsy.* Neurosci. Lett., 2010, 484: 187-191.

[136] Płonka-Półtorak E., Zagrodzki P., Chłopicka J., Bartoń H., Westermarck T., Kaipainen P. et al.: *Valproic acid modulates superoxide dismutase, uric acid-independent FRAP and zinc in blood of adult epileptic patients.* Biol. Trace Elem. Res. 2011, 143: 1424-1434.

[137] Poter R.J.: *Therapy of epilepsy.* Curr. Opin. Neurol. Neurosurg., 1988, 1: 205-211.

[138] Price T.O., Eranki V., Banks W.A., Ercal N., Shah G.N.: *Topiramate treatment protects blood-brain barrier pericytes from hyperglycemia-induced oxidative damage in diabetic mice.* Endocrinology, 2012, 153: 362-372.

[139] Pulman J., Greenhalgh J., Marson A.G.: *Antiepileptic drugs as prophylaxis for post-craniotomy seizures.* Cochrane Database Syst. Rev. 2013, 2: CD007286.

[140] Ramaekers V.T., Calomme M., Vanden Berghe D., Makropoulos W.: *Selenium deficiency triggering intractable seizures.* Neuropediatrics, 1994, 25: 217-223.

[141] Rodrigues A.D., Scheffel T.B., Scola G., Dos Santos M.T., Fank B., Dani C. et al.: *Purple grape juices prevent pentylenetetrazol-induced oxidative damage in the liver and serum of Wistar rats.* Nutr. Res., 2013, 33:120-1255.

[142] Rodrigues A.D., Scheffel T.B., Scola G., Santos M.T., Fank B., de Freitas S.C. et al.: *Neuroprotective and anticonvulsant effects of organic and conventional purple grape juices*

on seizures in Wistar rats induced by pentylenetetrazole. Neurochem. Int., 2012, 60: 799-805.

[143] Rowles J., Olsen M.: *Perspectives on the development of antioxidant antiepileptogenic agents.* Mini. Rev. Med. Chem. 2012, 12: 1015-1027.

[144] Rowley S., Patel M.: *Mitochondrial involvement and oxidative stress in temporal lobe epilepsy.* Free. Radic. Biol. Med., 2013, 62:121-131.

[145] Rumià J., Marmol F., Sanchez J., Giménez-Crouseilles J., Carreño M., Bargalló N. et al.: *Oxidative stress markers in the neocortex of drug-resistant epilepsy patients submitted to epilepsy surgery.* Epilepsy Res., 2013,107: 75-81.

[146] Russo A. Izzo A.A., Borrelli F., Renis M., Vanella A.: *Free radical scavenging capacity and protective effect of Bacopa monniera L. on DNA damage.* Phytother. Res., 2003, 17: 870-875.

[147] Russo A., Izzo A.A., Cardile V., Borrelli F., Vanella A.: *Indian medicinal plants as antiradicals and DNA cleavage protectors.* Phytomedicine, 2001, 8: 125-132.

[148] Sabayan B., Foroughina F., Chohedry A.: *A postulated role of garlic organosulfur compounds in prevention of valproic acid hepatotoxicity.* Med. Hypotheses, 2007, 68: 512-514.

[149] Samoilova M., Weisspapir M., Abdelmalik P., Velumian A.A., Carlen P.L.: *Chronic in vitro ketosis is neuroprotective but not anti-convulsant.* J. Neurochem., 2010, 113: 826-835.

[150] Ryan K., Backos D.S., Reigan P., Patel M.: *Post-translational oxidative modification and inactivation of mitochondrial complex I in epileptogenesis.* J. Neurosci., 2012, 32 : 11250-11258.

[151] Santos L.F., Freitas R.L., Xavier S.M., Saldanha G.B., Freitas R.M.: *Neuroprotective actions of vitamin C related to decreased lipid peroxidation and increased catalase activity in adult rats after pilocarpine-induced seizures. Pharmacol.* Biochem. Behav., 2008, 89: 1-5.

[152] Sardo P., Ferraro G.: *Modulatory effects of nitric oxide-active drugs on the anticonvulsant activity of lamotrigine in an experimental model of partial complex epilepsy in the rat.* BMC Neurosci., 2007, 3: 8-47.

[153] Savenkov A.A., Badalian O.L., Avakian G.N.: *Nootropics and antioxidants in the complex therapy of symptomatic posttraumatic epilepsy.* Zh. Nevrol. Psikhiatr. Im. S.S. Korsakova, 2013, 113: 26-34.

[154] Savina T.A., Balashova O.A., Shchipakina T.G.: *Effect of chronic consumption of sodium valproate and melatonin on seizure activity in Krushinskii-Molodkina rats.* Bull. Exp. Med., 2006, 142: 601-604.

[155] Schulpis K.H., Lazaropoulou C., Regoutas S., Karikas G.A., Margeli A., Tsakiris S., Papassotiriou I.: *Valproic acid monotherapy induces DNA oxidative damage.* Toxicology, 2006, 217: 228-232.

[156] Sies H.: *Oxidative stress.* Academic Press, New York, 1985.

[157] Sobaniec W., Sołowiej E., Kułak W., Bockowski L., Smigielska-Kuzia J., Artemowicz B.: *Evaluation of the influence of antiepileptic therapy on antioxidant enzyme activity and lipid peroxidation in erythrocytes of children with epilepsy.* J. Child Neurol., 2006, 21: 558-562.

[158] Sok D.E., Oh S.H, Kim Y.B., Kang H.G., Kim M.R.: *Neuroprotection by extract of Petasites japonicus leaves, a traditional vegetable, against oxidative stress in brain of mice challenged with kainic acid.* Eur. J. Nutr., 2006, 45: 61-69.

[159] Souza M.A., Oliveira M.S., Furian A.F., Rambo L.M., Ribeiro L.R., Lima F.D. et al.: *Swimming training prevents pentylenetetrazol-induced inhibition of Na+, K+-ATPase activity, seizures, and oxidative stress.* Epilepsia., 2009, 50: 811-823.

[160] Sudha K., Rao A.V., Rao A.: *Oxidative stress and antioxidants in epilepsy.* Clin. Chim. Acta, 2001, 303: 19-24.

[161] Sullivan P.G., Springer J.E. Hall E.D, Scheff S.: *Mitochondrial uncoupling as a therapeutic target following neuronal injury.* J. Bioenerg. Biomembr., 2004, 36: 353-356.

[162] Suzer T., Coskun E., Demir S., Tahta K.: *Lipid peroxidation and glutathione levels after cortical injection of ferric chloride in rats: effect of trimetazidine and deferoxamine.* Res. Exp. Med. (Berl.), 2000, 199: 223-229.

[163] Tan D.X., Reiter R.J., Manchester L.C., Yan M.T, El-Sawi M., Sainz R.M. et al.: *Chemical and physical properties and potential mechanisms: melatonin as a broad spectrum antioxidant and free radical scavenger.* Curr. Top. Med. Chem. 2002, 2: 181-197.

[164] Tayarani I., Chaudiere J., Lefauconnier J.M., Bourre J.M.: *Enzymatic protection against peroxidative damage in isolated brain capillaries.* J. Neurochem., 1987, 48: 1399-1402.

[165] Tejada S., Sureda A., Roca C., Gamundí A., Esteban S.: *Antioxidant response and oxidative damage in brain cortex after high dose of pilocarpine.* Brain Res. Bull., 2007, 71: 372-375.

[166] Tomé A.R., Feng D., Freitas R.M.: *The effects of alpha-tocopherol on hippocampal oxidative stress prior to in pilocarpine-induced seizures.* Neurochem Res., 2010, 35: 580-587.

[167] Tsai H.L., Chang C.N., Chang S.J.: *The effects of pilocarpine-induced status epilepticus on oxidative stress/damage in developing animals.* Brain Dev., 2010, 32: 25-31.

[168] Tupeev I.R., Kryzhanovskii G.N., Nikushkin E.V., Bordiukov M.M., Iuzefova S.M.: *The antioxidant system in the dynamic combined treatment of epilepsy patients with traditional anticonvulsant preparations and an antioxidant-alpha-tocopherol.* Biull. Eksp. Biol. Med., 1993, 116: 362-364.

[169] Turkdogan D., Toplan S., Karakoc Y.: *Lipid peroxidation and antioxidative enzyme activities in childhood epilepsy.* J. Child., Neurol., 2002, 17: 673-676.

[170] Ueda Y., Doi T., Tokumaru J., Nakajima A., Nagatomo K.: *In vivo evaluation of the effect of zonisamide on the hippocampal redox state during kainic acid-induced seizure status in rats.* Neurochem Res., 2005, 30: 1117-1121.

[171] Ueda T., Willmore L.J., Triggs W.J.: *Amygdalar injection of FeCl3 causes spontaneous recurrent seizures.* Exp. Neurol., 1998, 153: 123-127.

[172] Ueda Y., Yokoyama H., Niwa R., Konaka R., Ohya-Nishiguchi H., Kamada H.: *Generation of lipid radicals in the hippocampal extracellular space during kainic acid-induced seizures in rats.* Epilepsy Res., 1997, 26: 329-333.

[173] Uzum G., Akgun-Dar K., Bahcekapili N., Diler A.S. Ziylan Y.Z.: *Nitric oxide involvement in seizures elicited by pentylentetraloz and sex dependence.* Int. Neurosci., 2005, 115: 1503-1514.

[174] Verrotti A., Scardapane A., Franzoni E., Manco R., Chiarelli F.: *Increased oxidative stress in epileptic children treated with valproic acid.* Epilepsy Res. 2008, 78: 171-177.

[175] Vurucu S., Karaoglu A, Paksu M.S., Yesilyurt O., Oz O., Unay B., Akin R.: *Relationship between oxidative stress and chronic daily headache in children.* Hum. Exp. Toxicol., 2013, 32:113-119.

[176] Waldbaum S., Patel M.: *Mitochondrial dysfunction and oxidative stress: a contributing link to acquired epilepsy?* J. Bioenerg. Biomembr., 2010a, 42: 449-455.

[177] Waldbaum S., Patel M.: *Mitochondria, oxidative stress, and temporal lobe epilepsy.*

[178] Epilepsy Res., 2010b, 88: 23-45.

[179] Wang J.F., Azzam J.E., Young L.T.: *Valproate inhibits oxidative damage to lipid and protein in primary cultured rat cerebrocortical cells.* Neuroscience, 2003, 116: 485-489.

[180] Willmore L.J., Triggs W.J. Gray J.D.: *The role of iron-induced hippocampal peroxidation in acute epileptogenesis.* Brain Res., 1986, 382: 422-426.

[181] Wilson J.X.: *Antioxidant defense of the brain: a role for astrocytes.* Can. J. Physiol. Pharmacol., 1997, 75: 1149-1163.

[182] Yuksel A., Cengiz M., Seven M., Ulutin T.: *Changes in the antioxidant system in epileptic children receiving antiepileptic drugs: two-year prospective studies.* J. Child Neurol., 2001, 16: 603-606.

[183] Zhang Y.J., Zhang M., Wang X.C., Yu Y.H., Jin P.J., Wang Y.: *Effects of sodium valproate on neutrophils' oxidative metabolism and oxidant status in children with idiopathic epilepsy.* Zhonghua Er Ke Za Zhi. 2011, 49: 776-781.

[184] Zhao W., Swanson S.A., Ye J., Li X., Shelton J.M., Zhang W., Thomas G.D.: *Reactive oxygen species impair sympathetic vasoregulation in skeletal muscle in angiotensin II-dependent hypertension.* Hypertension, 2006, 48: 637-643.

http://dx.doi.org/10.5772/57484

[185] Ziegler D.R., Ribeiro L.C., Hagenn M., Siqueira I.R., Araujo E., Torres I.L. et al.: *Ketogenic diet increases glutathione peroxidase activity in rat hippocampus.* Neurochem. Res., 2003, 28: 1793-1797.

Chapter 2

Use of Trace Elements and Halotherapy in the Treatment of Human Diseases

Vincent S. Gallicchio

Additional information is available at the end of the chapter

http://dx.doi.org/10.5772/58235

1. Introduction

Trace elements possess important therapeutic properties. First, binding to specific macromolecules (enzymes, nucleic acids, etc.) they influence important chemical and biological processes; second, they interact amongst themselves synergistically to amplify their individual reactions. Some trace elements are also metals. Not all metals are trace elements. Metals have been used therapeutically for hundreds of years. Use of metals in the treatment of human diseases began with discoveries with gold used initially in patients with tuberculosis followed by rheumatoid arthritis. Gold identified an immunological pathogenesis in the etiology of rheumatoid arthritis, thus metals may be efficacious in other human conditions that are immunological in etiology. The antineoplastic potential of metals was further disseminated by the development of less toxic compounds such as platinum. Third, use of metals in the treatment of human cancers has improved the therapeutic effectiveness response to this diverse group of diseases. Fourth, lithium use in clinical medicine revolutionized treating psychiatric mood disorders. Central to the biological action of lithium is its ability to influence brain and central nervous system chemistry, thereby providing spectacular results in the treatment of affective and other psychiatric mood disorders, in particular, suicide prevention. Discoveries defining alternative non-psychiatric clinical use of lithium continue to intrigue clinical medicine based upon a key discovery demonstrating lithium can effectively influence stem cells. Halotherapy is using salt compounds as initial and maintenance therapy of human respiratory aliments. Used by the Greeks and Romans, halotherapy has existed for thousand of years. It is associated with the therapeutic effectiveness attributed to spas. Today halotherapy has gained resurgence with its use as personalized medicine in the treatment of human diseases.

2. Trace elements as medicines

2.1. Role and function as medicine for the treatment of human diseases

Trace element properties are the core of their therapeutic activity based upon their activity in chemical reactions such as binding to macromolecules like enzymes and nucleic acids, inhibiting specific biological reactions, and their interactions with other elements. These general properties, specifically the binding to large molecules are far from specific, which helps explain why their use has gained interest and popularity over the years in a wide range of diseases in which trace elements have been implicated as medicine. Although trace elements as metals have been associated with human use for centuries, the scientific basis for their use as medicines in humans began with the gold compounds, initially in patients with tuberculosis and later in rheumatoid arthritis. Although other drugs have been developed to treat these infectious and inflammatory diseases, gold has retained an important position in the treatment of these diseases especially in certain cultures. Gold-induced effects on the immune system in rheumatoid arthritis are observed in conditions where autoimmune is involved. Trace element metal complexes have been used as anti-cancer therapy. They have been widely used by the development of less toxic compounds such as platinum and possibly other trace elements. Simultaneously there have been improvements in the administration of these compounds. This increases their therapeutic efficacy in the treatment of specific diseases. There are specific types of cancers that respond to trace elements. The gastrointestinal system represents another area where trace elements have a therapeutic role both in the control of intraluminal acidity and nutrient availability. The central nervous system is another area for trace element therapeutics. This involves the use of lithium. Lithium has provided significant results in the treatment of affective, bi-polar and manic disorders. More recently lithium has shown the ability to influence stem cells derived from a number of different sites in the human body. Thus, lithium may also have clinical use in human alignments or injuries such as spinal chord conditions where here-to-fore these patients were committed to a lifetime of paralysis. An example is spinal chord injuries where lithium use with stem cells can improve clinical outcomes in these patients who previously were non-treatable. With a very wide range of other conditions in which they are employed, trace element use provides a compelling illustration of the importance of trace elements in human disease.

2.2. Boron

In the periodic table boron finds its place in group 13 comprising boron, aluminum, gallium, indium, thallium, and ununtrium. Boron group elements are characterized by having three electrons in their outer energy levels (valence layers) [1]. These elements have also been referred to as icosagens and triels [2].

Boron is classified as a metalloid. Boron occurs sparsely, probably because bombardment by the subatomic particles produced from natural radioactivity disrupts its nuclei. Aluminum occurs widely on earth, and is the third most abundant element in the Earth's crust (8.3%)[3]. Gallium is abundant on earth, while Indium is the 61st most abundant element in the earth's crust. Thallium is found in moderate amounts. Ununtrium is never found in nature and therefore is termed a synthetic element.

Many of the elements found in this group have fundamental roles in biology. Boron is a trace element in humans and is also essential for some plants. Lack of boron can lead to stunted plant growth, while excess boron thus can cause harm by inhibiting growth. Aluminum has neither a biological role nor significant toxicity associated with it and is considered safe. Both indium and gallium can stimulate metabolism with gallium credited with the ability to bind to iron proteins; however, thallium is highly toxic interfering with numerous vital enzymes. When boron was used as a pesticide it contributed to these effects [4].

Boron is a very light element because of its atomic number of five. In nature it is almost never found free thus it is very low in abundance, comprising only 0.001% (10 ppm)[5] of the Earth's crust. It is known to occur in over a hundred different minerals and ores; however, the main source is borax, but it is also found in complex compounds [6]. Areas in the world that mine boron include Argentina, Bolivia, China, Peru, Turkey and the United States. Turkey is by far the most important accounting for around 70% of all boron extracted in the world. For the United States it is the state of California that engages in significant production [7].

Boron is essential for many plants. Plant cells use it for strengthening cell walls. It is classified as a trace element in humans, but there is debate over its significance in human nutrition. The chemistry of boron allows it to form carbohydrate complexes so its role in nutrition in the human body may be more important than previously thought. Boron has also been shown to replace iron in some of its functions, particularly in wound healing [8]. Aluminum has no known biological role in animals or plants. Gallium is not essential for the human body, but it does interact with iron that allows it to become bound to iron bound and transport proteins [9]. Gallium can also stimulate metabolism. Indium and its heavier complexes have no known biological role, although in small amounts like gallium, indium salts can stimulate metabolism [10].

All elements within the boron group can be toxic. Many are only toxic to plants, some only to animals with some to both. An example of boron toxicity is it harms barley in concentrations exceeding 20 mM [11]. In plants the symptoms of boron toxicity are numerous, such as: reduced cell division, decreased shoot and root growth, decreased production of leaf chlorophyll, inhibition of photosynthesis, lowering of stomata conductance, reduced proton extrusion from roots, and deposition of lignin and sub-origin [12].

In human medicine, boron is found in the form of boric acid, which is used as a topical astringent and as an ophthalmologic irrigant. Sodium borate is bacteriostatic and commonly added to cold creams, washes, and mouth rinses. Boron compounds found in over-the-counter supplements are reported to enhance mental attentiveness from studies that found alterations in the electroencephalogram in the presence of a low-boron diet. These studies reported also that there's a correlation between a low-boron diet and a decrease in mental alertness. There is no evidence however, that diet supplementations of boron compounds, above the levels derived from a normal balanced diet can enhance mental acuity or improve alertness. When sprinkled in crevices and corners, boric acid powder controls rodents and insects. Boron compounds are used to enhance the cytotoxicity associated with the use of radiation therapy.

2.3. Calcium

Calcium (Ca) with the atomic number of 20 is a soft gray alkaline earth metal that is the 5th most abundant element by mass found in the earth. Calcium is also the fifth-most-abundant dissolved ion both molarity and mass in seawater, following sodium, chloride, magnesium, and sulfate [13]. For living organisms calcium is essential, in particular where movement of the cytoplasmic calcium ion Ca^{2+}into and out of functions as a signal for many cellular processes.

Calcium salts are colorless. As with magnesium salts and other alkaline earth metal salts, calcium salts are often quite soluble in water. Notable exceptions include the hydroxides such as the sulfates, carbonates and phosphates. When in solution, the calcium ion to the human taste varies remarkably, being reported as mildly salty, sour, "mineral like" or even "soothing." It is apparent that many animals can taste, or develop a taste, for calcium, and use this sense to detect the mineral in a variety of locations and sources [14]. In human nutrition, soluble calcium salts may be added to tart juices without much effect to the average palate.

Calcium is the fifth-most-abundant element by mass in the human body, where it is a common cellular ionic messenger with many functions like enzymes. It also serves as a structural element in bone. It has a relatively high atomic number. Calcium in the skeleton causes bone to be radio-opaque. The human body's solid components following drying or burning of organics, as an example observed following cremation, contributes to about a third of the total "mineral" mass remaining in the body. Approximately one kilogram of calcium is composed in the average skeleton with the remaining mineral content being composed of mostly phosphorus and oxygen.

Calcium should be a very important component of the human diet and is a mineral necessary for life. The National Osteoporosis Foundation states that calcium should play an important role in building stronger, denser bones both early in life and in keeping bones strong and healthy later in adulthood. Approximately 99 percent of the body's calcium is stored in the bones and teeth [15]. In the body calcium has other important uses such as in exocytosis, specifically in neurotransmitter release, and muscle contraction. In the electrical system of the heart, calcium replaces sodium as the mineral that depolarizes the cell, proliferating the action potential. In cardiac muscle, sodium influx initiates an action potential, but during the efflux of potassium, the cardiac myocyte experiences calcium influx, prolonging the action potential and creating a plateau phase of dynamic equilibrium. Long-term deficiency of calcium can lead to rickets and poor blood clotting and in menopausal women it can lead to osteoporosis, where the bone deteriorates creating an increased risk of fractures. While lifelong calcium deficits can affect bone and tooth formation, over-retention causes an increase in blood calcium called hypercalcemia, impaired kidney function and decreased absorption of other minerals [16, 17]. Sources suggest there's a correlation between high calcium intake (2000 mg per day, or twice the U.S. recommended daily allowance, equivalent to six or more glasses of milk per day) and prostate cancer [18]. High calcium intakes or absorption were previously thought to contribute to the development of kidney stones; however, high calcium intake has been associated with a lower risk for kidney stones in more recent research [19-21], because Vitamin D is required to absorb calcium.

Milk and cheese as dairy products are well-known sources of calcium. Some individuals are allergic to dairy products. There are people who are lactose-intolerant leaving them unable to consume non-fermented dairy products in quantities larger than about half a liter per serving. Others, especially vegans avoid dairy products for ethical and health reasons.

Many good vegetable sources of calcium exist as in seaweeds such as kelp, wakame, and hijiki; nuts and seeds like almonds, hazelnuts, sesame, pistachios, molasses, soy beans, figs, quinoa, okra, rutabaga, broccoli, dandelion leaves, and kale. In addition, for some drinks like soymilk or orange juice, it is typical to be fortified with calcium. Numerous vegetables, notably spinach, chard, and rhubarb have high calcium content, but they may also contain varying amounts of oxalic acid that binds calcium and reduces its absorption. The same problem may to a degree affect the absorption of calcium from amaranth, collard and chicory greens. This process may also be related to the generation of calcium oxalate. An overlooked source of calcium is eggshell, which can be ground into a powder and mixed into food or a glass of water [22-24]. The calcium content of most foods can be found in the USDA National Nutrient Database [25].

Calcium supplements are used to prevent and to treat calcium deficiencies. Office of Dietary Supplements (National Institutes of Health) recommends that no more than 600 mg of supplement should be taken at a time because the percent of calcium absorbed decreases as the amount of calcium in the supplement increases [26]. It is therefore recommended to spread doses throughout the day [27]. Recommended daily calcium intake for adult's ranges from 1000 to 1300 mg [27]. Calcium supplements may have side effects such as bloating and constipation in some people. It is suggested that taking the supplements with food may aid in nullifying these side effects [27]. Vitamin D is added to some calcium supplements. Proper vitamin D status is important because vitamin D is converted to a hormone in the body, which then induces the synthesis of intestinal proteins responsible for calcium absorption [28].

A study investigating the effects of personal calcium supplement use on cardiovascular risk was reported in the Women's Health Initiative Calcium/Vitamin D Supplementation Study (WHI CaD Study) found a modestly increased risk of cardiovascular events, particularly myocardial infarction in postmenopausal women. A broad recommendation of calcium/ vitamin D supplements is therefore not warranted. In osteoporosis such studies often do not test calcium alone, but rather combinations of calcium and vitamin D. Randomized controlled clinical trials found both positive [29] and negative [30-33] effects. The different results may be explained by doses of calcium and underlying rates of calcium supplementation in the control groups [34]. A meta-analysis [35] by the international Cochrane Collaboration of two randomized controlled trials [36-37] found that calcium "might contribute to a moderate degree to the prevention of adenomatous colonic polyps. More recent studies were conflicting, and one that was positive for effect did control for a possible anti-carcinogenic effect of vitamin D, which was found to be an independent positive influence from calcium-alone on cancer risk [38].

A randomized controlled trial found that 1000 mg of elemental calcium and 400 IU of vitamin D_3 had no effect on colorectal cancer [39]. A randomized controlled trial found that 1400–1500 mg supplemental calcium and 1100 IU vitamin D_3 reduced aggregated cancers with a relative risk of 0.402 [40]. An observational cohort study found that high calcium and vitamin D intake was associated with lower risk of developing premenopausal breast cancer [41].

Compared with other metals, the calcium ion and most calcium compounds have low toxicity. This is not surprising given the very high natural abundance of calcium compounds in the environment and in organisms. Calcium poses few serious environmental problems, with kidney stones the most common side effect in clinical studies. Acute calcium poisoning is rare, and difficult to achieve unless calcium compounds are administered intravenously. For example, the oral median lethal dose (LD^{50}) for rats for calcium carbonate and calcium chloride are 6.45 [42] and 1.4 g/kg [43] respectively.

Calcium metal is hazardous because of its sometimes-violent reactions with water and acids. Calcium metal is found in some drain cleaners where it functions to generate heat and calcium hydroxide that saponifies fats and liquefies proteins, e.g., hair that block drains. When swallowed calcium metal has the same effect on the mouth, esophagus and stomach, and can be fatal [44].

Excessive consumption of calcium carbonate antacids/dietary supplements, over a period of weeks or months can cause milk-alkali syndrome with symptoms ranging from hypercalcemia to potentially fatal renal failure. What constitutes "excessive" consumption is not well known and, it is presumed, varies a great deal from person to person. Persons consuming more than 10 grams/day of $CaCO_3$ (=4 g Ca) are at risk of developing milk-alkali syndrome [45], but the condition has been reported in at least one person consuming only 2.5 grams/day of $CaCO_3$ (=1 g Ca), an amount usually considered moderate and safe [46]. Oral calcium supplements diminish the absorption of thyroxine when taken within four to six hours of each other [47]. Thus, people taking both calcium and thyroxine run the risk of inadequate thyroid hormone replacement and thence hypothyroidism if they take them simultaneously or near-simultaneously [48]. Excessive calcium supplementation can be detrimental to cardiovascular health, especially in men [49, 50].

2.4. Chromium

Trivalent chromium (Cr (III) or Cr^{3+}) occurs in trace amounts in foods and waters, and appears to be benign [51]. In contrast, hexavalent chromium (Cr (VI) or Cr^{6+}) is very toxic and mutagenic when inhaled. Cr (VI) has not been established as a carcinogen when in solution, although it may cause allergic contact dermatitis (ACD) [52].

Chromium deficiency, involving a lack of Cr (III) in the body, or perhaps some complex of it, such as glucose tolerance factor is controversial, or is at least extremely rare. Chromium has no verified biological role and has been classified by some as *not* essential for mammals [53]. However, other reviews have regarded it as an essential trace element in humans [54]. It is a reddish crystalline powder, 12.5% Cr (III) by weight, very sparingly soluble in water. Chromium deficiency has been attributed to only three people on long-term parenteral nutrition, which is when a patient is fed a liquid diet through intravenous drips for long periods of time [55].

Although no biological role for chromium has ever been demonstrated, dietary supplements for chromium include chromium (III), chromium (III) picolinate, chromium (III) polynicotinate, and related materials. The benefit of those supplements is questioned by some studies [56]. The use of chromium-containing dietary supplements is controversial, owing to the absence of any verified biological role, the expense of these supplements, and the complex effects of their use [57]. The popular dietary supplement chromium picolinate, complex generates chromosome damage in hamster cells (due to the picolinate ligand) [58]. In the United States the dietary guidelines for daily chromium uptake were lowered in 2001 from 50–200 μg for an adult to 35 μg (adult male) and to 25 μg (adult female)[59].

No comprehensive, reliable database of chromium content of food currently exists [60]. Data reported prior to 1980 is unreliable due to analytical error [56]. Chromium content of food varies widely due to differences in soil mineral content, growing season, plant cultivar, and contamination during processing. 60]. In addition, large amounts of chromium (and nickel) leech into food cooked in stainless steel [61,62].

The acute oral toxicity for chromium (VI) ranges between 50 and 150 μg/kg [61]. In the body, chromium (VI) is reduced by several mechanisms to chromium (III) already in the blood before it enters the cells. The chromium (III) is excreted from the body, whereas the chromate ion is transferred into the cell by a transport mechanism, by which also sulfate and phosphate ions enter the cell. The acute toxicity of chromium (VI) is due to its strong oxidational properties. After it reaches the blood stream, it damages the kidneys, the liver and blood cells through oxidation reactions. Hemolysis, renal and liver failure are the results of these damages. Aggressive dialysis can improve the situation [63].

The carcinogenity of chromate dust has been known for a long time. In 1890 the first publication described the elevated cancer risk of workers in a chromate dye company [64,65]. Three mechanisms have been proposed to describe the genotoxicity of chromium (VI). The first mechanism includes highly reactive hydroxyl radicals and other reactive radicals that are by products of the reduction of chromium (VI) to chromium (III). The second process includes the direct binding of chromium (V), produced by reduction in the cell, and chromium (IV) compounds to DNA. The last mechanism attributed the genotoxicity to the binding to the DNA of the end product of the chromium (III) reduction [66].

In some people chromium salts (chromates) are also the cause of allergic reactions. Chromates are often used to manufacture, amongst other things, leather products, paints, cement, mortar and anti-corrosives. Contact with products containing chromates can lead to allergic contact dermatitis and irritant dermatitis, resulting in ulceration of the skin, sometimes referred to as "chrome ulcers". This condition is often found in workers that have been exposed to strong chromate solutions in electroplating, tanning and chrome-producing manufacturers [67,68]. As chromium compounds were used in dyes and paints and leather tanning, these compounds are often found in soil and groundwater at abandoned industrial sites that now need environmental cleanup and remediation of contaminated land. Primer paint containing hexavalent chromium is still widely used for aerospace and automobile refinishing applications [69].

2.5. Copper

Copper is essential to all living organisms as a trace dietary mineral because it is a key constituent of the respiratory enzyme complex cytochrome c oxidase. In mollusks and crustacean copper is a constituent of the blood pigment hemocyanin, which is replaced by the iron-complexed hemoglobin in fish and other vertebrates. The main areas where copper is found in humans are liver, muscle and bone [70]. Copper compounds are used as bacteriostatic substances, fungicides and wood preservatives. Numerous antimicrobial efficacy studies have been conducted in the past 10 years regarding copper's efficacy to destroy a wide range of bacteria, as well as influenza A virus, adenovirus, and fungi [93].

Copper-alloy touch surfaces have natural intrinsic properties to destroy a wide range of microorganisms, *E.coli,* methicillin-resistant *Staphylococcus aureus,* influenza A virus, adenovirus, and fungi [71]. Some 355 copper alloys were proven to kill more than 99.9% of disease-causing bacteria within just two hours when cleaned regularly [72]. The U.S. Environmental Protection Agency (EPA) has approved the registrations of these copper alloys as antimicrobial materials with public health benefits [72], which allows manufacturers to legally make claims as to the positive public health benefits of products made with registered antimicrobial copper alloys. In addition, the EPA has approved a long list of antimicrobial copper products made from these alloys, such as bedrails, handrails, over-bed tables, sinks, faucets, door knobs, toilet hardware, computer keyboards, health club equipment, shopping cart handles, etc. (for a comprehensive list of products. Copper doorknobs are used by hospitals to reduce the transfer of disease and Legionnaires' disease is suppressed by copper tubing in plumbing systems [73]. Antimicrobial copper alloy products are now being installed in healthcare facilities in the U.K., Ireland, Japan, Korea, France, Denmark, and Brazil and in the subway transit system in Santiago, Chile, where copper-zinc alloy handrails will be installed in some 30 stations by 2014 [74-76].

Copper proteins have diverse roles in biological electron transport and oxygen transportation, processes that exploit the easy interconversion of Cu (I) and Cu (II) [77-79]. The biological role for copper commenced with the appearance of oxygen in earth's atmosphere [80]. The protein hemocyanin is the oxygen carrier in most mollusks and some arthropods such as the horseshoe crab (*Limulus polyphemus*) [81]. Because hemocyanin is blue, these organisms have blue blood, not the red blood found in organisms that rely on hemoglobin for this purpose. Structurally related to hemocyanin are the lactases and tyrosinases. Instead of reversibly binding oxygen, these proteins hydroxylate substrates, illustrated by their role in the formation of lacquers [79].

Copper is also a component of other proteins associated with the processing of oxygen. In cytochrome c oxidase, which is required for aerobic respiration, copper and iron cooperate in the reduction of oxygen. Copper is also found in many superoxide dismutases, proteins that catalyze the decomposition of superoxides, by converting it to oxygen and hydrogen peroxide:

$$2\,HO_2 \longrightarrow H_2O_2 + O_2 \tag{1}$$

Several copper proteins, such as the "blue copper proteins" do not interact directly with substrates hence they are not enzymes. These proteins relay electrons by the process called electron transfer [79].

Copper is an essential trace element in plants and animals, but not in some microorganisms. The human body contains copper at a level of about 1.4 to 2.1 mg per kg of body mass [82]. Stated differently, the recommended daily allowance (RDA) for copper in normal healthy adults is quoted in the range of 0.97 mg/day to 3.0 mg/day [83]. Copper is absorbed in the gut, and then transported to the liver then bound to albumin [84]. After processing in the liver, copper is distributed to other tissues in a second phase. Copper transport here involves the protein ceruloplasmin, which carries the majority of copper in blood. Ceruloplasmin also carries copper that is excreted in milk, and is particularly well absorbed as a copper source [85]. Copper in the body normally undergoes enterohepatic circulation (about 5 mg a day, vs. about 1 mg per day absorbed in the diet and excreted from the body), and the body is able to excrete some excess copper, if needed, via bile, which carries some copper out of the liver that is not then reabsorbed by the intestine [84,85].

Because of its role in facilitating iron uptake, copper deficiency can produce anemia-like symptoms, neutropenia, bone abnormalities, hypopigmentation, impaired growth, increased incidence of infections, osteoporosis, hyperthyroidism, and abnormalities in glucose and cholesterol metabolism. Conversely, Wilson's disease causes an accumulation of copper in body tissues. Severe deficiency can be found by testing for low plasma or serum copper levels, low ceruloplasmin, and low red blood cell superoxide dismutase levels; these are not sensitive to marginal copper status. The cytochrome c oxidase activity of leucocytes and platelets has been stated as another factor in deficiency, but the results have not been confirmed by replication [86].

Gram quantities of various copper salts have been taken in suicide attempts and produced acute copper toxicity in humans, possibly due to redox cycling and the generation of reactive oxygen species that damage DNA [87,88]. Corresponding amounts of copper salts (30 mg/kg) are toxic in animals [89]. A minimum dietary value for healthy growth in rabbits has been reported to be at least 3 ppm in the diet [90]. However, higher concentrations of copper (100 ppm, 200 ppm, or 500 ppm) in the diet of rabbits may favorably influence feed conversion ratio, growth rates, and carcass dressing percentages [91].

Chronic copper toxicity does not normally occur in humans because of transport systems that regulate absorption and excretion. Autosomal recessive mutations in copper transport proteins can disable these systems, leading to Wilson's disease with copper accumulation and cirrhosis of the liver in persons who have inherited two defective genes [82].

2.6. Gold

Gold is a chemical element with the symbol Au and atomic number 79. It is a dense, soft, malleable, and ductile metal with an attractive, bright yellow color and luster that is maintained without tarnishing in air or water. Chemically, gold is a transition metal and a group 11 element. It is one of the least reactive chemical elements, solid under standard conditions. The metal therefore occurs often in free elemental form, as nuggets or grains in rocks, in veins and in alluvial deposites. Less commonly, it occurs in minerals as gold compounds, such as with tellurium as calaverite, sylvanite and krennerite. Gold is perhaps the most anciently administered medicine [92] and known to the ancients [93-94] with apparent paradoxes with respect to its toxicology. This information suggests there are still serious gaps in understanding of action of gold on physiology [95].

In medieval times, gold was often seen as beneficial for the health, in the belief that something so rare and beautiful could not be anything but healthy. Even some modern esotericists and forms of alternative medicine assign metallic gold a healing power [96]. Some gold salts do have anti-inflammatory properties and are used as pharmaceuticals in the treatment of arthritis and other similar conditions. Gold-based injections have been explored as a means to help to reduce the pain and swelling of rheumatoid arthritis and tuberculosis [97]. However, only salts and radioisotopes of gold are of pharmacological value, as elemental (metallic) gold is inert to all chemicals it encounters inside the body.

Gold alloys are used in restorative dentistry, especially in tooth restorations, such as crowns and permanent bridges. The gold alloys' slight malleability facilitates the creation of a superior molar mating surface with other teeth and produces results that are generally more satisfactory than those produced by the creation of porcelain crowns. The use of gold crowns in more prominent teeth such as incisors is favored in some cultures and discouraged in others.

Colloidal gold preparations, such as the use of gold in nanoparticle suspensions in water are intensely red-colored, and can be made with tightly controlled particle sizes up to a few tens of nanometers across by reduction of gold chloride with citrate or ascorbate ions. Colloidal gold is used in research applications in medicine, biology and materials science. The technique of immunogold labeling exploits the ability of the gold particles to adsorb protein molecules onto their surfaces. Colloidal gold particles coated with specific antibodies can be used as probes for the presence and position of antigens on the surfaces of cells [98]. In ultrathin sections of tissues viewed by electron microscopy, the immunogold labels appear as extremely dense round spots at the position of the antigen [99].

Gold, or alloys of gold and palladium are applied as conductive coating to biological specimens and other non-conducting materials such as plastics and glass to be viewed in a scanning electron microscope. The coating, which is usually applied by sputtering with argon plasma, has a triple role in this application. Gold's very high electrical conductivity drains an electrical charge; therefore, its very high density provides stopping power for electrons in the electron beam, helping to limit the depth to which the electron beam penetrates the specimen. This improves definition of the position and topography of the specimen surface and increases the spatial resolution of the image. Gold also produces a high output of secondary electrons when irradiated by an electron beam, and these low-energy electrons are the most commonly used signal source in the scanning electron microscope [100]. The isotope gold-198 (half-life 2.7 days) is used in nuclear medicine, in some cancer treatments and for treating other diseases [101,102].

2.7. Iodine

Iodine and its compounds are primarily used in nutrition, and industrially in the production of acetic acid and certain polymers. Iodine's relatively high atomic number, low toxicity, and ease of attachment to organic compounds have made it a part of many X-ray contrast materials in modern medicine. Iodine has only one stable isotope. A number of iodine radioisotopes are also used in medical applications.

Iodine is found on Earth mainly as the highly water-soluble iodide ion 1-that concentrates it in oceans and brine pools. Like the other halogens, free iodine occurs mainly as a diatomic molecule I_2, and then only momentarily after being oxidized from iodide by an oxidant like free oxygen. In the universe and on Earth, iodine's high atomic number makes it a relatively rare element. However, its presence in ocean water has given it a role in biology. It is the heaviest essential element utilized widely by life in biological functions. Iodine's rarity in many soils, due to initial low abundance as a crust-element, and also leaching of soluble iodide by rainwater, has led to many deficiency problems in land animals and inland human populations. Iodine deficiency affects about two billion people and is the leading preventable cause of intellectual disabilities [103].

Iodine is required by higher animals, which use it to synthesize thyroid hormones, which contain the element. Because of this function, radioisotopes of iodine are concentrated in the thyroid gland along with nonradioactive iodine. If inhaled, the radioisotope iodine-131, which has a high fission yield, concentrates in the thyroid, but is easily remedied with non-radioactive potassium iodide treatment.

Potassium iodide has been used as an expectorant, although this use is increasingly uncommon. In medicine, potassium iodide is usually used to treat acute thyrotoxicosis, usually as a saturated solution of potassium iodide. It is also used to block uptake of iodine-131 in the thyroid gland when this isotope is used as part of radiopharmaceuticals (such as iobenguane) that are not targeted to the thyroid or thyroid-type tissues.

Iodine-131, in the chemical form of iodide is a component of nuclear fallout and a particularly dangerous one owing to the thyroid gland's propensity to concentrate ingested iodine, where it is kept for periods longer than this isotope's radiological half-life of eight days. For this reason, if people are exposed to a significant amount of environmental radioactive iodine (iodine-131 in fallout), they may be instructed to take non-radioactive potassium iodide tablets. The typical adult dose is one 130 mg tablet per 24 hours, supplying 100 mg (100,000 micrograms) iodine, as iodide ion. Typical daily dose of iodine to maintain normal health is of order 100 micrograms. By ingesting this large amount of non-radioactive iodine, radioactive iodine uptake by the thyroid gland is minimized [104].

Diatrizoic acid, an iodine-containing radio contrast agent Iodine, as an element with high electron density and atomic number absorbs X-rays well. Therefore, it may be used as a radio contrast agent by filtering out imaging X-rays weaker than 33.3 keV, where iodine's innermost electrons begin absorbing X-rays strongly due to the photoelectric effect [105.] Organic compounds of a certain type (typically iodine-substituted benzene derivatives) are thus used in medicine as X-ray radio contrast agents for intravenous injection. This is often in conjunction with advanced X-ray techniques such as angiography and CT scanning. At present, all water-soluble radio contrast agents rely on iodine.

2.8. Iron

Iron is a chemical element with the symbol Fe (from Latin: *ferrum*) and atomic number 26. It is a metal in the first transition series. It is the most common element (by mass) forming the planet Earth as a whole, forming much of Earth's outer and inner core. It is the fourth most common element in the Earth's crust. Iron's very common presence is due to its abundant production as a result of fusion in high-mass stars, where the production of nickel-56 (which decays to the most common isotope of iron) is the last nuclear fusion reaction that is exothermic. This causes radioactive nickel to become the last element to be produced before collapse of a supernova leads to the explosive events that scatter this precursor radio nucleotide of iron abundantly into space.

Iron is abundant in biology [106]. Iron-proteins are found in all living organisms, ranging from the evolutionarily primitive archaea to humans. The color of blood is due to the hemoglobin, an iron-containing protein. As illustrated by hemoglobin, iron is often bound to cofactors, e.g. in hemes. The iron-sulfur clusters are pervasive and include nitrogenase, the enzymes responsible for biological nitrogen fixation. Influential theories of evolution have invoked a role for iron sulfides in the iron-sulfur world theory.

Structure of heme, in the protein additional ligand would be attached to Fe. Iron is a necessary trace element found in nearly all-living organisms. Iron-containing enzymes and proteins, often containing heme prosthetic groups participate in many biological oxidations and in transport. Examples of proteins found in higher organisms include hemoglobin, cytochrome and catalase [107]. Iron is pervasive, but particularly rich sources of dietary iron include red meat, lentils, beans, poultry, fish, leaf vegetables, watercress, tofu, chickpeas, black-eyed peas, blackstrap molasses, fortified bread, and fortified breakfast cereals. Iron in low amounts is found in molasses, teff and farina. Iron in meat (heme iron) is more easily absorbed than iron in vegetables [108]. Although some studies suggest that heme/hemoglobin from red meat has effects that may increase the likelihood of colorectal cancer [109,110]. There is still some controversy [111] and even a few studies suggesting that there is not enough evidence to support such claims [112].

Iron provided by dietary supplements is often found as iron (II) fumarate, although iron sulfate is cheaper and is absorbed equally well. Elemental iron, or reduced iron, despite being absorbed at only one third to two thirds the efficiency (relative to iron sulfate) [113] is often added to foods such as breakfast cereals or enriched wheat flour. Iron is most available to the body when chelated to amino acids [114] and is also available for use as a common iron supplement. Often the amino acid chosen for this purpose is the cheapest and most common amino acid, glycine, leading to "iron glycinate" supplements [115]. The Recommended Dietary

Allowance (RDA) for iron varies considerably based on age, gender, and source of dietary iron (heme-based iron has higher bioavailability) [116]. Infants may require iron supplements if they are bottle-fed cow's milk [117]. Blood donors and pregnant women are at special risk of low iron levels and are often advised to supplement their iron intake [118]. Iron acquisition poses a problem for aerobic organisms, because ferric iron is poorly soluble near neutral pH. Thus, bacteria have evolved high-affinity sequestering agents called siderophores [119-121].

After uptake, in cells, iron storage is carefully regulated as "free" as iron ions do not exist as free. A major component of this regulation is the protein transferrin, which binds iron ions absorbed from the duodenum and carries it in the blood to cells [122]. In animals, plants, and fungi, iron is often the metal ion incorporated into the heme complex. Heme is an essential component of cytochrome proteins, which mediate redox reactions, and of oxygen carrier proteins such as hemoglobin, myoglobin, and leg hemoglobin.

Inorganic iron contributes to redox reactions in the iron-sulfur clusters of many enzymes, such as nitrogenase involved in the synthesis of ammonia from nitrogen and hydrogen and hydrogenate. Non-heme iron proteins include the enzymes methane monooxygenase oxidizes methane to methanol, ribonucleotide reductase, reduces ribose to deoxyribose in DNA synthesis, hemerythrins involved in oxygen transport and fixation in marine invertebrates, and purple acid phosphatase hydrolysis of phosphate esters. Iron distribution is heavily regulated in mammals, partly because iron ions have a high potential for biological toxicity [123].

Iron uptake is tightly regulated by the human body, which has no regulated physiological means of excreting iron. Only small amounts of iron are lost daily due to mucosal and skin epithelial cell sloughing, so control of iron levels is mostly by regulating uptake [124]. Regulation of iron uptake is impaired in some people as a result of a genetic defect that maps to the HLA-H gene region on chromosome 6. In these people, excessive iron intake can result in iron overload disorders, such as hemochromatosis. Many people have a genetic susceptibility to iron overload without realizing it or being aware of a family history of the problem. For this reason, it is advised that people do not take iron supplements unless they suffer from iron deficiency and have consulted a doctor. Hemochromatosis is estimated to cause disease in between 0.3 and 0.8% of Caucasians [125]. MRI finds that iron accumulates in the hippocampus of the brains of those with Alzheimer's disease and in the substantia nigra of those with Parkinson disease [126].

Large amounts of ingested iron can cause excessive levels of iron in the blood. High blood levels of free ferrous iron react with peroxides to produce free radicals, which are highly reactive and can damage DNA, proteins, lipids, and other cellular components. Thus, iron toxicity occurs when there is free iron in the cell, which generally occurs when iron levels exceed the capacity of transferrin to bind the iron. Damage to the cells of the gastrointestinal tract can also prevent them from regulating iron absorption leading to further increases in blood levels. Iron typically damages cells in the heart, liver, and elsewhere, which can cause significant adverse effects, including coma, metabolic coma, metabolic acidosis, shock, liver failure, coagulopathy, adult respiratory distress syndrome, long-term organ damage, and even death [127]. Humans experience iron toxicity above 20 milligrams of iron for every kilogram of mass, and 60 milligrams per kilogram is considered a lethal dose [128]. Overconsumption of iron, often the result of children eating large quantities of ferrous sulfate tablets intended for adult consumption, is one of the most common toxicological causes of death in children under six [128]. The Dietary Reference Intake (DRI) lists the Tolerable Upper Intake Level (UL) for adults as 45 mg/day. For children under fourteen years old the UL is 40 mg/day. The medical management of iron toxicity is complicated and can include use of a specific chelating agent called deferoxamine to bind and expel excess iron from the body [127,129].

2.9. Lithium

Lithium (from Greek *lithos* 'stone') is a chemical element with symbol Li and atomic number 3. It is a soft, silver-white metal belonging to the alkali metal group of chemical elements. Under standard conditions it is the lightest metal and the least dense solid element. Like all alkali metals, lithium is highly reactive and flammable. For this reason, it is typically stored in mineral oil. When cut open, lithium exhibits a metallic luster, but contact with moist air corrodes the surface quickly to a dull silvery gray, then black tarnish. Because of its high reactivity lithium never occurs freely in nature, and instead, only appears in compounds, which are usually ionic. Lithium occurs in a number of pegmatite minerals, but due to its solubility as an ion is present in ocean water and is commonly obtained from brines and clay. On a commercial scale, lithium is isolated electrolytically from a mixture of lithium chloride and potassium chloride. Lithium and its compounds have several industrial applications, including heat-resistant glass and ceramics, high strength-to-weight alloys used in aircraft, lithium batteries and lithium-ion batteries. These uses consume more than half of lithium production.

Trace amounts of lithium are present in all organisms. The element serves no apparent vital biological function, since animals and plants survive in good health without it; however, its central role in reproduction has been documented [130]. In the absence of lithium when tested in a number of vertebrate species (fowl, cows and goats) showed an increase in spontaneous abortions amongst these species. In humans lithium administered as any of several lithium salts has proved to be useful as a mood-stabilizing drug in the treatment of bipolar disorder due to neurological effects of the ion in the human body [131].

Lithium is found in trace amount in numerous plants, plankton, and invertebrates, at concentrations of 69 to 5,760 parts per billion (ppb). In vertebrates the concentration is slightly lower, and nearly all vertebrate tissue and body fluids have been found to contain lithium ranging from 21 to 763 ppb [132]. Marine organisms tend to bioaccumulate lithium more than terrestrial ones [133]. It is not known whether lithium has a physiological role in any of these organisms [132], but nutritional studies in mammals have indicated its importance to health, leading to a suggestion that it be classed as an essential trace element with an RDA of 1 mg/day [134]. Observational studies in Japan, reported in 2011, suggested that naturally occurring lithium in drinking water might increase human lifespan [135].

Lithium is useful in the treatment of bipolar disorder [136]. Lithium salts may also be helpful for related diagnoses, such as schizoaffective disorder and cyclic major depression. The active part of these salts is the lithium ion Li^+[137]. They may increase the risk of developing Ebstein's cardiac anomaly in infants born to women who take lithium during the first trimester of pregnancy [135]. The most exciting results for lithium are its reported non-psychiatric medical effects that are centered on the ion's ability to influence the proliferation of stem cells first identified from hematopoietic tissues [138, 139]. This effect has now been demonstrated to also take place in the regeneration of neurological tissues, thus the use of lithium to treat spinal chord injuries through a mechanism that involves enhancing stem cell regeneration of damaged neurons is very exciting.

2.10. Magnesium

Magnesium is a chemical element with the symbol Mg and atomic number 12. Its common oxidation number is+2. It is an alkaline earth metal and the eighth most abundant element in the Earth's crust and ninth in the known universe as a whole [140]. Magnesium is the fourth most common element in the Earth as a whole (behind iron, oxygen and silicon), making up 13% of the planet's mass and a large fraction of the planet's mantle. The relative abundance of magnesium is related to the fact that it easily builds up in supernova stars from a sequential addition of three helium nuclei to carbon (which in turn is made from three helium nuclei). Due to magnesium ion's high solubility in water, it is the third most abundant element dissolved in seawater [141]. Magnesium is produced in stars larger than 3 solar masses by fusing helium and neon in the alpha process at temperatures above 600 megakelvins.

The free element (metal) is not found naturally on Earth, as it is highly reactive. Once produced, it is coated in a thin layer of oxide, which partly masks this reactivity. The free metal burns with a characteristic brilliant white light, making it a useful ingredient in flares. The metal is now mainly obtained by electrolysis of magnesium salts obtained from brine. Commercially, the chief use for the metal is as an alloying agent to make aluminum-magnesium alloys, sometimes called magnalium or magnelium. Since magnesium is less dense than aluminum these alloys are prized for their relative lightness and strength.

In human physiology, magnesium is the eleventh most abundant element by mass in the human body. Its ions are essential to all living cells, where they play a major role in manipulating important biological polyphosphate compounds like ATP, DNA, and RNA. Hundreds of enzymes thus require magnesium ions to function. Magnesium compounds are used medicinally as common laxatives, and antacids, e.g., milk of magnesia, and in a number of situations where stabilization of abnormal nerve excitation and blood vessel spasm is required (e.g., to treat eclampsia). Magnesium ions are sour to the taste, and in low concentrations they help to impart a natural tartness to fresh mineral waters.

Pharmaceutical preparations of magnesium are used to treat magnesium deficiency and hypomagnesemia, as well as eclampsia [142]. Usually in lower dosages, magnesium is commonly included in dietary mineral preparations, including many multivitamin preparations.

Sorted by type of magnesium salt, biological applications of magnesium include:

- Magnesium sulfate, as the heptahydrate called Epsom salts, is used as bath salts, as a laxative, and as a highly soluble fertilizer [143].

- Magnesium hydroxide, suspended in water, is used in milk of magnesia antacids and laxatives.
- Magnesium chloride, oxide, gluconate, malate, orotate, glycinate and citrate are all used as oral magnesium supplements. Some have claimed that oral magnesium supplements are therapeutic for Restless Leg Syndrome (RLS) in some individuals [144].
- Magnesium borate, magnesium salicylate, and magnesium sulfate are used as antiseptics.
- Magnesium bromide is used as a mild sedative (this action is due to the bromide, not the magnesium).
- Magnesium stearate is a slightly flammable white powder with lubricating properties. In pharmaceutical technology, it is used in the manufacturing of numerous kinds of tablets to prevent the tablets from sticking to the equipment during the tablet compression process (i.e., when the tablet's substance is pressed into tablet form).

Magnesium carbonate powder is used by athletes such as gymnasts, weightlifters and climbers to eliminate moisture and improves the grip on gymnastic apparatus, and lifting and climbing rocks.

Because of the important interaction between phosphate and magnesium ions, magnesium ions are essential to the basic nucleic acid chemistry of life, and thus are essential to all cells of all known living organisms. Over 300 enzymes require the presence of magnesium ions for their catalytic action, including *all* enzymes utilizing or synthesizing ATP, or those that use other nucleotides to synthesize DNA and RNA. ATP exists in cells normally as a chelate of ATP and a magnesium ion.

Plants have an additional use for magnesium in that chlorophylls are magnesium-centered porphyrins. Magnesium deficiency in plants causes late-season yellowing between leaf veins, especially in older leaves, and can be corrected by applying Epsom salts, which is rapidly leached, or else crushed dolomitic limestone to the soil.

Magnesium is a vital component of a healthy human diet. Human magnesium deficiency (including conditions that show few overt symptoms is relatively rare [145], although only 32% of people in the United States meet the RDA-DRI; [146] low levels of magnesium in the body has been associated with the development of a number of human illnesses such as asthma, diabetes, and osteoporosis [147]. Taken in the proper amount magnesium plays a role in preventing both stroke and heart attack. The symptoms of people with fibromyalgia, migraines, and girls going through their premenstrual syndrome are less severe and magnesium can shorten the length of the migraine symptoms [148,149].

Adult human bodies contain about 24 grams of magnesium, with 60% in the skeleton, 39% intracellular (20% in skeletal muscle), and 1% extracellular [150]. Serum levels are typically 0.7–1.0 mmol/L or 1.8–2.4 mEq/L. Serum magnesium levels may appear normal even in cases of underlying intracellular deficiency, although no known mechanism maintains a homeostatic level in the blood other than renal excretion of high blood levels. Intracellular magnesium is correlated with intracellular potassium. Magnesium is absorbed in the gastrointestinal tract, with more absorbed when status is lower. Magnesium competes with calcium in the human body [151]. In this way it actually keeps calcium in check. However, this can cause a calcium deficiency if calcium levels are already low [152]. Low and high protein intake inhibit magnesium absorption, and other factors such as phosphate, phytate, and fat affect absorption. Absorbed dietary magnesium is largely excreted through the urine, although most magnesium "administered orally" is excreted through the feces [153]. Magnesium status may be assessed roughly through serum and erythrocyte Mg concentrations and urinary and fecal excretion, but intravenous magnesium loading tests are likely the most accurate and practical in most people [154]. In these tests, magnesium is injected intravenously; retention of 20% or more indicates deficiency [155]. Other nutrient deficiencies are identified through biomarkers, but none are established for magnesium [156].

The UK recommended daily values for magnesium is 300 mg for men and 270 mg for women [157.] Spices, nuts, cereals, coffee, cocoa, tea, and vegetables are rich sources of magnesium [158]. Green leafy vegetables such as spinach are also rich in magnesium as they contain chlorophyll. Observations of reduced dietary magnesium intake in modern Western countries compared to earlier generations may be related to food refining and modern fertilizers that contain no magnesium [153].

Numerous pharmaceutical preparations of magnesium, as well as magnesium dietary supplements are available. Magnesium oxide, one of the most common forms in magnesium dietary supplements because it has high magnesium content per weight, has been reported the least bioavailable [159,160]. Magnesium citrate has been reported as more bioavailable than oxide or amino acid chelate forms [161].

Excess magnesium in the blood is freely filtered at the kidneys, and for this reason it is difficult to overdose on magnesium from dietary sources alone [148]. With supplements, overdose is possible, particularly in people with poor renal function; occasionally, with use of high cathartic doses of magnesium salts, severe hypermagnesemia has been reported to occur even without renal dysfunction [162]. Alcoholism can produce a magnesium deficiency, which is easily reversed by oral or parenteral administration, depending on the degree of deficiency [163]. Magnesium concentrations in plasma or serum may be measured to monitor for efficacy and safety in those receiving the drug therapeutically, to confirm the diagnosis in potential poisoning victims or to assist in the forensic investigation in a case of fatal over dosage. The newborn children of mothers who received parenteral magnesium sulfate during labor may exhibit toxicity at serum magnesium levels that were considered appropriate for the mothers [164].

There has been some speculation that magnesium deficiency can lead to depression. Cerebral spinal fluid (CSF) magnesium has been found low in treatment-resistant suicidal depression and in patients that have attempted suicide. Brain magnesium has been found low amounts using phosphorus nuclear magnetic resonance spectroscopy, an accurate means for measuring brain magnesium. Blood and cerebral spinal fluid (CSF) magnesium does not appear well correlated with major depression [165]. Magnesium chloride in relatively small doses was found as effective in the treatment of depressed elderly type 2 diabetics with hypomagnesemia as imipramine 50 mg daily [166].

Results from a meta-analysis of randomized clinical trials demonstrated that magnesium supplementation lowers high blood pressure in a dose dependent manner [167]. Low serum magnesium levels are associated with metabolic syndrome, diabetes mellitus type 2 and hypertension [168]. Low serum magnesium levels have been associated with a higher risk of developing metabolic syndrome [169]. Magnesium therapy is recommended by the 2006 Guidelines for Management of Patients With Ventricular Arrhythmias and the Prevention of Sudden Cardiac Death for patients with ventricular arrhythmia associated with torsade de pointes that present with long QT syndrome as well as for the treatment of patients with digoxin intoxication-induced arrhythmias [170]. Magnesium is also the drug of choice in the management of pre-eclampsia and eclampsia [171].

Besides its therapeutic role, magnesium has an additional beneficial effect on calcification. Patients with chronic kidney disease have a high prevalence of vascular calcification, and cardiovascular disease is the leading cause of death in this population. Several *in vitro* and animal studies point towards a protective role of magnesium through multiple molecular mechanisms. Magnesium is a natural calcium antagonist and both human and animal studies have shown that low circulating magnesium levels are associated with vascular calcification [172]. Results from an observational study conducted in the general Japanese population demonstrated that lower serum magnesium levels were significantly and independently associated with a greater average intima-media thickness and the risk of at least two carotid plaques [173]. Magnesium supplementation might be useful in reducing the progression of atherosclerosis in chronic dialysis patients [174]. Low serum magnesium may be an independent risk factor for death in patients with chronic kidney disease [175] and patients with mildly elevated serum magnesium levels could have a survival advantage over those with lower magnesium levels [176].

Since the kidneys are responsible for the excretion of magnesium, anyone with a heart or kidney disorder should not take any extra magnesium except under their doctor's supervision. It is very rare to overdose on magnesium from food [152]; however people who ingest large amounts of milk of magnesia (as a laxative or antacid), Epsom Salts (as a laxative or tonic), or magnesium supplements may overdose, especially if they suffer from kidney problems. Too much magnesium can cause several serious health problems, including nausea, vomiting, severely lowered blood pressure, confusion, slowed heart rate, respiratory paralysis, deficiencies of other minerals, coma, cardiac arrhythmia, cardiac arrest, and death. At very high doses, it can even be fatal [152]. However the most common side effects of magnesium toxicity are stomach upset and diarrhea [36].

2.11. Manganese

Manganese is a chemical element designated by the symbol Mn. It has the atomic number 25. It is found as a free element in nature often in combination with iron and in many minerals. Manganese is a metal with important industrial metal alloy uses, particularly in stainless steels. In biology, manganese (II) ions function as cofactors for a large variety of enzymes with many functions [177]. Manganese enzymes are particularly essential in detoxification of superoxide free radicals in organisms that must deal with elemental oxygen. Manganese also functions in the oxygen-evolving complex of photosynthetic plants. The element is a required trace mineral for all known living organisms. In larger amounts, and apparently with far greater activity by inhalation, it can cause a poisoning syndrome in mammals, with neurological damage, which is sometimes irreversible.

Manganese is an essential trace nutrient in all known forms of life [178]. The classes of enzymes that have manganese cofactors are very broad, and include oxidoreductases, transferases, hydrolases, lyases, isomerases, ligases, lectins, and integrins. Reverse transcriptase found in many retroviruses contains manganese. The best-known manganese-containing polypeptides may be arginase, the diphtheria toxin and Mn-containing superoxide dismutase [179].

Mn-(super oxide dismutase (SOD) is the type of SOD present in eukaryotic mitochondria, and also in most bacteria (this fact is in keeping with the bacterial-origin theory of mitochondria). The Mn-SOD enzyme is probably one of the most ancient, for nearly all organisms living in the presence of oxygen use it to deal with the toxic effects of superoxide, formed from the 1-electron reduction of oxygen. Exceptions include a few kinds of bacteria, and related lactobacilli, which use a different nonenzymatic mechanism, involving manganese (Mn^{2+}) ions complexed with polyphosphate directly for this task, indicating how this function possibly evolved in aerobic life.

The human body contains about 12 mg of manganese, which is stored mainly in the bones; in the tissue, it is mostly concentrated in the liver and kidneys [20]. In the human brain, the manganese is bound to manganese metalloproteins, most notably glutamine synthetase in astrocytes [180]. Manganese is also important in photosynthetic oxygen evolution in chloroplasts in plants. The oxygen-evolving complex (OEC) is a part of photosystem II contained in the thylakoid membranes of chloroplasts; it is responsible for the terminal photo oxidation of water during the light reactions of photosynthesis, and has a metalloenzyme core containing four atoms of manganese [181]. For this reason, most broad-spectrum plant fertilizers contain manganese.

Manganese compounds are less toxic than those of other widespread metals, such as nickel and copper [182]. However, exposure to manganese dusts and fumes should not exceed the ceiling value of 5 mg/m^3 even for short periods because of its toxicity level [183]. Manganese poisoning has been linked to impaired motor skills and cognitive disorders [184-186]. In 2005, a study suggested a possible link between manganese inhalation and central nervous system toxicity in rats [187]. The Occupational Safety and Health Administration in the United States regulates exposure to manganese [188]. Generally, exposure to ambient Mn air concentrations in excess of 5 μg Mn/m3 can lead to Mn-induced symptoms. Increased ferroportin protein expression in human embryonic kidney (HEK293) cells is associated with decreased intracellular Mn concentration and attenuated cytotoxicity, characterized by the reversal of Mn-reduced glutamate uptake and diminished lactate leakage [189].

Waterborne manganese has a greater bioavailability than dietary manganese. According to results from a 2010 study [190] higher levels of exposure to manganese in drinking water levels are associated with increased intellectual impairment and reduced intelligence quotients in school-age children. It is hypothesized that long-term exposure to the naturally occurring manganese in shower water puts up to 8.7 million Americans at risk [191-193]. Manganese overexposure is most frequently associated with manganism, a rare neurological disorder associated with excessive manganese ingestion or inhalation. Historically, persons employed in the production or processing of manganese alloys [194,195] have been at risk for developing manganism; however, current health and safety regulations protect workers in developed nations [158]. The disorder was first described in 1837 by British academic John Couper in two patients who were manganese grinders [196].

Manganism is a biphasic disorder. In its early stages, an intoxicated person may experience depression, mood swings, compulsive behaviors, and psychosis. Early neurological symptoms give way to late-stage manganism, which resembles Parkinson's disease. Symptoms include weakness, monotone and slowed speech, an expressionless face, tremor, forward-leaning gait, inability to walk backwards without falling, rigidity, and general problems with dexterity, gait and balance [197,198]. Unlike Parkinson's disease, manganism is not associated with loss of smell and patients are typically unresponsive to treatment with L-DOAP [195]. Symptoms of late-stage manganism become more severe over time even if the source of exposure is removed and brain manganese levels return to normal [197].

Several recent studies attempt to examine the effects of chronic low-dose manganese overexposure on development in children. The earliest study of this kind was conducted in the Chinese province of Shanxi. Drinking water there had been contaminated through improper sewage irrigation and contained 240–350 μg Mn/L. Although WMn concentrations at or below 300 μg Mn/L are considered safe by the US EPA and 400 μg Mn/L are considered safe by the World Health Organization, the 92 children sampled (between 11 and 13 years of age) from this province displayed lower performance on tests of manual dexterity and rapidity, short-term memory, and visual identification when compared to children from an uncontaminated area. More recently, a study of 10-year-old children in Bangladesh showed a relationship between WMn concentration in well water and diminished IQ scores. A third study conducted in Quebec examined school children between the ages of 6 and 15 living in homes that received water from a well containing 610 μg Mn/L; controls lived in homes that received water from a 160 μg Mn/L well. Children in the experimental group showed increased hyperactive and oppositional behaviors [192].

Chronic low-dose manganese intoxication is strongly implicated in a number of neurodegenerative disorders, including Alzheimer's disease, Parkinson's disease, and amyotrophic lateral sclerosis. It may also play a role in the development of multiple sclerosis, restless leg syndrome, and Huntington's disease. A protein called DMT1 is the major transporter involved in manganese absorption from the intestine, and may be the major transporter of manganese across the blood-brain barrier. DMT1 also transports inhaled manganese across the nasal epithelium. The putative mechanism of action is that manganese overexposure and/or dysregulation lead to oxidative stress, mitochondrial dysfunction, glutamate-mediated excitoxicity, and aggregation of proteins.

2.12. Platinum

Platinum is a chemical element with the chemical symbol Pt and an atomic number of 78. Its name is derived from the Spanish term *platina,* which is literally translated into "little silver" [198,199]. It is a dense, malleable, ductile, precious, gray-white transition metal. Platinum is used in catalytic converters, laboratory equipment, electrical contacts and electrodes, platinum resistance thermometers, dentistry equipment, and jewelry. Because only a few hundred tons are produced annually, it is a scarce material, and is highly valuable and is a major precious metal commodity. Being a heavy metal, it leads to health issues upon exposure to its salts, but due to its corrosion resistance, it is not as toxic as some metals [200]. Compounds containing platinum, most notably cisplatin, are applied in chemotherapy against certain types of cancer [201].

In the laboratory, platinum wire is used for electrodes; platinum pans and supports are used in thermo gravimetric analysis because of the stringent requirements of chemical inertness upon heating to high temperatures (~1000 °C). Platinum is used as an alloying agent for various metal products, including fine wires, noncorrosive laboratory containers, medical instruments, dental prostheses, electrical contacts, and thermocouples. Platinum-cobalt, an alloy of roughly three parts platinum and one part cobalt, is used to make relatively strong permanent magnets [202, 203]. Platinum-based anodes are used in ships, pipelines, and steel piers [204]. According to the Centers for Disease Control and Prevention, short-term exposure to platinum salts may cause irritation of the eyes, nose, and throat, and long-term exposure may cause both respiratory and skin allergies. The current OSHA standard is 2 micrograms per cubic meter of air averaged over an 8-hour work shift [205].

Platinum-based antineoplastic agents are used in chemotherapy, and show good activity against some tumors. As platinum is a catalyst in the manufacture of the silicone rubber and gel components of several types of medical implants (breast implants, joint replacement prosthetics, artificial lumbar discs, vascular access ports, etc.), the possibility platinum could enter the body and cause adverse effects have merited study. The Food and Drug Administration and other institutions have reviewed the issue and found no evidence to suggest toxicity *in vivo* [206,207].

2.13. Potassium

Potassium is a chemical element with symbol K (from Neo-Latin *kalium*) and atomic number 19. Elemental potassium is a soft silvery-white alkali metal that oxidizes rapidly in air and is very reactive with water, generating sufficient heat to ignite the hydrogen emitted in the reaction and burning with a lilac flame.

Potassium ions are necessary for the function of all living cells. Potassium ion diffusion is a key mechanism in nerve transmission, and potassium depletion in animals, including humans, results in various cardiac dysfunctions. Potassium accumulates in plant cells, and thus fresh fruits and vegetables are a good dietary source of it. Conversely, most plants except specialist halophytes are intolerant of salt, and sodium is present in them only in low concentrations. This resulted in potassium first being isolated from potash, the ashes of plants, giving the element its name. For the same reason, heavy crop production rapidly depletes soils of potassium, and agricultural fertilizers consume 95% of global potassium chemical production [208].

Potassium is the eighth or ninth most common element by mass (0.2%) in the human body, so that a 60 kg adult contains a total of about 120 g of potassium [209]. The body has about as much potassium as sulfur and chlorine, and only the major minerals calcium and phosphorus are more abundant [210].

Potassium cations are important in neuron (brain and nerve) function, and in influencing osmotic balance between cells and the interstitial fluid, with their distribution mediated in all animals (but not in all plants) by the so-called Na+/K+ATPase pump [211]. This ion pump uses ATP to pump three sodium ions out of the cell and two potassium ions into the cell, thus creating an electrochemical gradient over the cell membrane. In addition, the highly selective potassium ion channels (which are tetramers) are crucial for the hyperpolarization, in for example neurons, after an action potential is fired. The most recently resolved potassium ion channel is KirBac3.1, which gives a total of five potassium ion channels (KcsA, KirBac1.1, KirBac3.1, KvAP, and MthK) with a determined structure [212]. All five are from prokaryotic species.

Potassium can be detected by taste because it triggers three of the five types of taste sensations, according to concentration. Dilute solutions of potassium ions taste sweet, allowing moderate concentrations in milk and juices, while higher concentrations become increasingly bitter/alkaline, and finally also salty to the taste. The combined bitterness and saltiness of high-potassium solutions makes high-dose potassium supplementation by liquid drinks a palatability challenge [213,214]. Potassium is also important in preventing muscle contraction and the sending of all nerve impulses in animals through action potentials. By nature of their electrostatic and chemical properties, K^+ions are larger than Na^+ions, and ion channels and pumps in cell membranes can distinguish between the two types of ions, actively pumping or passively allowing one of the two ions to pass, while blocking the other [215]. A shortage of potassium in body fluids may cause a potentially fatal condition known as hypokalemia, typically resulting from vomiting, diarrhea, and/or increased diuresis [216]. Deficiency symptoms include muscle weakness, paralytic ileus, ECG abnormalities, decreased reflex response and in severe cases respiratory paralysis, alkalosis and cardiac arrhythmia [217].

Potassium is an essential macro mineral in human nutrition; it is the major cation (positive ion) inside animal cells, and it is thus important in maintaining fluid and electrolyte balance in the body. Sodium makes up most of the cations of blood plasma at a reference range of about 145 mmol/L (3.345 g)(1 mmol/L=1mEq/L), and potassium makes up most of the cell fluid cations at about 150 mmol/L (4.8 g). Plasma is filtered through the glomerulus of the kidneys in enormous amounts, about 180 liters per day [218]. Thus 602 g of sodium and 33 g of potassium are filtered each day. All but the 1–10 g of sodium and the 1–4 g of potassium likely to be in the diet must be reabsorbed. Sodium must be reabsorbed in such a way as to keep the blood volume exactly right and the osmotic pressure correct; potassium must be reabsorbed in such a way as to keep serum concentration as close as possible to 4.8 mmol/L (about 0.190 g/L) [219]. Sodium pumps in the kidneys must always operate to conserve sodium. Potassium must sometimes be conserved also, but, as the amount of potassium in the blood plasma is very small and the pool of potassium in the cells is about thirty times as large, the situation is not so critical for potassium. Since potassium is moved passively [220,221] in counter flow to sodium in response to an apparent (but not actual) Donnan equilibrium [222] the urine can never sink below the concentration of potassium in serum except sometimes by actively excreting water at the end of the processing. Potassium is secreted twice and reabsorbed three times before the urine reaches the collecting tubules [223]. At that point, it usually has about the same potassium concentration as plasma. At the end of the processing, potassium is secreted one more time if the serum levels are too high. If potassium were removed from the diet, there would remain a minimum obligatory kidney excretion of about 200 mg per day when the serum declines to 3.0–3.5 mmol/L in about one week [224] and can never be cut off completely, resulting in hypokalemia and even death [225].

The potassium moves passively through pores in the cell membrane. When ions move through pumps there is a gate in the pumps on either side of the cell membrane and only one gate can be open at once. As a result, approximately 100 ions are forced through per second. Pores have only one gate, and there is only one kind of ion that can stream through, at 10 million to 100 million ions per second [226]. The pores require calcium in order to open [225] although it is thought that the calcium works in reverse by blocking at least one of the pores [228]. Carbonyl groups inside the pore on the amino acids mimic the water hydration that takes place in water solution [229] by the nature of the electrostatic charges on four carbonyl groups inside the pore [230].

A potassium intake sufficient to support life can in general be guaranteed by eating a variety of foods. Clear cases of potassium deficiency (as defined by symptoms, signs and a below-normal blood level of the element) are rare in healthy individuals. Foods rich in potassium include parsley, dried apricots, dried milk, chocolate, various nuts (especially almonds and pistachios), potatoes, bamboo shoots, bananas, avocados, soybeans, and bran, although it is also present in sufficient quantities in most fruits, vegetables, meat and fish [231].

Epidemiological studies and studies in animals subject to hypertension indicate that diets high in potassium can reduce the risk of hypertension and possibly stroke (by a mechanism independent of blood pressure), and a potassium deficiency combined with an inadequate thiamine intake has produced heart disease in rats [232]. There is some debate regarding the optimal amount of dietary potassium. For example, the 2004 guidelines of the Institute of Medicine specify a DRI of 4,700 mg of potassium (100 mEq), though most Americans consume only half that amount per day, which would make them formally deficient as regards this particular recommendation [233, 234]. Likewise, in the European Union, in particular in Germany and Italy, insufficient potassium intake is somewhat common [235]. Italian researchers reported in a 2011 meta-analysis that a 1.64 g higher daily intake of potassium was associated with a 21% lower risk of stroke [234].

Supplements of potassium in medicine are most widely used in conjunction with loop diuretics and thiazides, classes of diuretics that rid the body of sodium and water, but have the side effect of also causing potassium loss in urine. A variety of medical and non-medical supplements are available. Potassium salts such as potassium chloride may be dissolved in water, but the salty/bitter taste of high concentrations of potassium ion make palatable high concentration liquid supplements difficult to formulate [234]. Typical medical supplemental doses range from 10 mmol (400 mg, about equal to a cup of milk or 6 US flu oz (180 ml) of orange juice) to 20 mmol (800 mg) per dose. Potassium salts are also available in tablets or capsules, which for therapeutic purposes are formulated to allow potassium to leach slowly out of a matrix, as very high concentrations of potassium ion (which might occur next to a solid tablet of potassium chloride) can kill tissue, and cause injury to the gastric or intestinal mucosa. For this reason, law in the US to only 99 mg of potassium limits non-prescription supplement potassium pills.

Individuals suffering from kidney diseases may experience adverse health effects from consuming large quantities of dietary potassium. End stage renal failure patients undergoing therapy by renal dialysis must observe strict dietary limits on potassium intake, as the kidneys control potassium excretion, and buildup of blood concentrations of potassium (hyperkalemia) may trigger fatal cardiac arrhythmia.

2.14. Selenium

Selenium is a chemical element with symbol Se and atomic number 34. It is a nonmetal with properties that are intermediate between those of its periodic table column-adjacent chalcogen elements sulfur and tellurium. It rarely occurs in its elemental state in nature, or as pure ore compounds. Jons Jacob Berselius, who noted the similarity of the new element to the previously known tellurium, discovered selenium in 1817.

Selenium salts are toxic in large amounts, but trace amounts are necessary for cellular function in many organisms, including all animals. Selenium is a component of the antioxidant enzymes glutathione peroxidase and thioredoxin reductase (which indirectly reduce certain oxidized molecules in animals and some plants). It is also found in three deiodinase enzymes, which convert one thyroid hormone to another. Selenium requirements in plants differ by species, with some plants requiring relatively large amounts, and others apparently requiring none [237].

Although it is toxic in large doses, selenium is an essential micronutrient for animals. In plants, it occurs as a bystander mineral, sometimes in toxic proportions in forage (some plants may accumulate selenium as a defense against being eaten by animals, but other plants such as locoweed require selenium, and their growth indicates the presence of selenium in soil) [237]. Selenium is a component of the unusual amino acids selenocysteine and selenomethionine. In humans, selenium is a trace element nutrient that functions as cofactor for reduction of antioxidant enzymes, such as glutathione peroxidases [238] and certain forms of thioredoxin reductase found in animals and some plants (this enzyme occurs in all living organisms, but not all forms of it in plants require selenium).

The glutathione peroxidase family of enzymes (GSH-Px) catalyzes certain reactions that remove reactive oxygen species such as hydrogen peroxide and organic hydroperoxides.

$$2\,GSH + H_2O_2 \text{----} GSH\text{-}Px \longrightarrow GSSG + 2\,H_2O \tag{2}$$

Selenium also plays a role in the functioning of the thyroid gland and in every cell that uses thyroid hormone, by participating as a cofactor for the three of the four known types of thyroid hormone deiodinases, which activate and then deactivate various thyroid hormones and their metabolites: the iodothyronine deiodinases are the subfamily of deiodinase enzymes that use selenium as the otherwise rare amino acid selenocysteine. Only the deiodinase iodotyrosine, which works on the last breakdown products of thyroid hormone, does not use selenium [239].

Selenium may inhibit Hashimoto's disease, in which the bodies own thyroid cells are attacked as alien. A reduction of 21% in antibodies was reported with the dietary intake of 0.2 mg of selenium [240]. Increased dietary selenium intakes reduce the effects of mercury toxicity [241] and it is now recognized that the molecular mechanism of mercury toxicity involves irreversible inhibition of selenoenzymes that are required to prevent and reverse oxidative damage in brain and endocrine tissues [242,243]. Dietary selenium comes from nuts, cereals, meat, mushrooms, fish, and eggs. Brazil nuts are the richest ordinary dietary source (though this is soil-dependent, since the Brazil nut does not require high levels of the element for its own needs). In descending order of concentration, high levels are also found in kidney, tuna, crab, and lobster [244,245].

The human body's content of selenium is believed to be in the 13–20 milligram range [246]. The substance loosely called selenium sulfide (approximate formula SeS_2) is the active ingredient in some anti-dandruff shampoos [247]. The selenium compound kills the scalp fungus Malassezia, which causes shedding of dry skin fragments. The ingredient is also used in body lotions to treat Tinea versicolor due to infection by a different species of *Malassezia* fungus [248].

Selenium may be measured in blood, plasma, serum or urine to monitor excessive environmental or occupational exposure, confirm a diagnosis of poisoning in hospitalized victims or to assist in a forensic investigation in a case of fatal over dosage. Some analytical techniques are capable of distinguishing organic from inorganic forms of the element. Both organic and inorganic forms of selenium are largely converted to monosaccharide conjugates (selenosugars) in the body prior to being eliminated in the urine. Cancer patients receiving daily oral doses of selenothionine may achieve very high plasma and urine selenium concentrations [249]. Selenium deficiency is rare in healthy, well-nourished individuals. It can occur in patients with severely compromised intestinal function, those undergoing total parenteral nutrition, and [250] in those of advanced age (over 90). Also, people dependent on food grown from selenium-deficient soil are at risk. Although New Zealand has low levels of selenium in its soil, adverse health effects have not been detected [251]. Selenium deficiency as defined by low (<60% of normal) selenoenzyme activity levels in brain and endocrine tissues only occurs when a low selenium status is linked with an additional stress, such as high exposures to mercury [252] or as a result of increased oxidant stress due to vitamin E deficiency [253].

There are interactions between selenium and other nutrients, such as iodine and vitamin E. The effect of selenium deficiency on health remains uncertain, particularly in relation to

Kashin-Beck disease [254]. Also, there are interactions between selenium and other minerals, such as zinc and copper, it seems that high does of Se supplement to pregnant animal might disturb the Zn:Cu ratio which, in turn, leads to Zn reduction. It can be concluded that the Zn status should be monitored when high dose of Se is supplemented to pregnant animal. Further studies needs to be done with higher levels of Se supplement to confirm these interactions [255].

In some regions (e.g. various regions within North America) where low available selenium levels in soil lead to low concentrations in dry matter of plants, Se deficiency in some animal species may occur unless dietary (or injected) selenium supplementation is done [256]. Ruminants are particularly susceptible. In general, absorption of dietary selenium is lower in ruminants than in non-ruminants, and is lower from forages than from grain [257] Ruminants grazing certain forages, e.g. some white clover varieties containing cyanogenic glycosides, may have higher selenium requirements, [258] presumably because of cyanide from the aglycone released by glucosidase activity in the rumen [258] and inactivation of glutathione peroxidases due to absorbed cyanide's effect on the glutathione moiety [260]. Neonate ruminants at risk of WMD (white muscle disease) may be administered both selenium and vitamin E by injection; some of the WMD myopathies respond only to selenium, some only to vitamin E, and some to either [261]. A number of correlative epidemiological studies have implicated selenium deficiency (as measured by blood levels) in a number of serious or chronic diseases, such as cancer [259], diabetes [262], HIV/ AIDS [263] and tuberculosis. In addition, selenium supplementation has been found to be a chemopreventive for some types of cancer in some types of rodents. However, in randomized, blinded, controlled prospective trials in humans, selenium supplementation has not succeeded in reducing the incidence of any disease, nor has a meta-analysis of such selenium supplementation studies detected a decrease in overall mortality [264].

2.15. Sodium

Sodium is a chemical element with the symbol Na (from Latin: *natrium*) and atomic number 11. It is a soft, silvery-white, highly reactive metal and is a member of the alkali metals; its only stable isotope is ^{23}Na. The free metal does not occur in nature, but instead must be prepared from its compounds; was first isolated by Humphry Davy in 1807 by the electrolysis of sodium hydroxide. Sodium is the sixth most abundant element in the Earth's crust, and exists in numerous minerals such as feldspars and rock salt. Many salts of sodium are highly water-soluble, and their sodium has been leached by the action of water so that chloride and sodium (NaCl) are the most common dissolved elements by weight in the Earth's bodies of oceanic water.

In humans, sodium is an essential nutrient that regulates blood volume, blood pressure, osmotic equilibrium and pH; the minimum physiological requirement for sodium is 500 milligrams per day [265]. Sodium chloride is the principal source of sodium in the diet, and is used as seasoning and preservative, such as for pickling and jerky; most of it comes from processed foods [266]. The DRI for sodium is 2.3 grams per day [266], but on average people in the United States consume 3.4 grams per day [267], the minimum amount that promotes hypertension [268]; this in turn causes 7.6 million premature deaths worldwide [269].

The renin-angiotensin system regulates the amount of fluids and sodium in the body. Reduction of blood pressure and sodium concentration in the kidney results in the production of renin, which in turn produces aldosterone and angiotensin, retaining sodium in the urine. Because of the increase in sodium concentration, the production of renin decreases, and the sodium concentration returns to normal [270]. Sodium is also important in neuron function and osmoregulation between cells and the extracellular fluid, their distribution mediated in all animals by Na+/K+-ATPase [271]; hence, sodium is the most prominent cation in extracellular fluid [272].

In C4 plants, sodium is a micronutrient that aids in metabolism, specifically in regeneration of phosphoenolpyruvate and synthesis of chlorophyll [273]. In others, it substitutes for potassium in several roles, such as maintaining turgor pressure and aiding in the opening and closing of stomata [274]. Excess sodium in the soil limits the uptake of water due to decreased water potential, which may result in wilting; similar concentrations in the cytoplasm can lead to enzyme inhibition, which in turn causes necrosis and chlorosis [275]. To avoid these problems, plants developed mechanisms that limit sodium uptake by roots, store them in cell vacuoles, and control them over long distances [276]; excess sodium may also be stored in old plant tissue, limiting the damage to new growth.

2.16. Zinc

Zinc, in commerce also spelter, is a metallic chemical element; it has the symbol Zn and atomic number 30. It is the first element of group 12 of the periodic table. Zinc is, in some respects, chemically similar to magnesium, because its ion is of similar size and its only common oxidation state is+2. Zinc is the 24th most abundant element in the Earth's crust and has five stable isotopes. The most common zinc ore is sphalerite (zinc blende), a zinc sulfide mineral. The largest mineable amounts are found in Australia, Asia, and the United States. Zinc production includes froth flotation of the ore, roasting, and final extraction using electricity.

Zinc is an essential mineral of "exceptional biologic and public health importance" [277]. Zinc deficiency affects about two billion people in the developing world and is associated with many diseases [278]. In children it causes growth retardation, delayed sexual maturation, infection susceptibility, and diarrhea, contributing to the death of about 800,000 children worldwide per year [277]. Enzymes with a zinc atom in the reactive center are widespread in biochemistry, such as alcohol dehydrogenase in humans [279]. Consumption of excess zinc can cause ataxia, lethargy and copper deficiency.

Zinc is included in most single tablet over-the-counter daily vitamin and mineral supplements [280]. Preparations include zinc oxide, zinc acetate, and zinc gluconate [281]. It is believed to possess antioxidant properties, which may protect against accelerated aging of the skin and muscles of the body; studies differ as to its effectiveness [282]. Zinc also helps speed up the healing process after an injury [281]. It is also suspected of being beneficial to the body's immune system. Indeed, zinc deficiency may have effects on virtually all parts of the human immune system [282]. The efficacy of zinc compounds when used to reduce the duration or severity of cold symptoms is controversial [283]. A 2011 systemic review concludes that supplementation yields a mild decrease in duration and severity of cold symptoms [284].

Optimum dosing and formulation have not been determined. The studies included in the 2011 review used a variety of forms and doses of zinc, including zinc gluconate or zinc acetate lozenges and zinc sulfate syrup. The doses ranged from 30 to 160 milligrams per day. The researchers noted the following: *"Given the variability in the populations studied (no studies from low-or middle-income countries), dose, formulation and duration of zinc used in the included studies, more research is needed to address these variabilities and determine the optimal duration of treatment as well as the dosage and formulations of zinc that will produce clinical benefits without increasing adverse effects, before making a general recommendation for zinc in treatment of the common cold."*

Zinc serves as a simple, inexpensive, and critical tool for treating diarrheal episodes among children in the developing world. Zinc becomes depleted in the body during diarrhea, but recent studies suggest that replenishing zinc with a 10-to 14-day course of treatment can reduce the duration and severity of diarrheal episodes and may also prevent future episodes for up to three months [285]. The Age-Related Eye Disease Study determined that zinc could be part of an effective treatment for age-related macular degeneration [286]. Zinc supplementation is an effective treatment for acrodermatitis enteropathica, a genetic disorder affecting zinc absorption that was previously fatal to babies born with it [287]. Gastroenteritis is strongly attenuated by ingestion of zinc, and this effect could be due to direct antimicrobial action of the zinc ions in the gastrointestinal tract, or to the absorption of the zinc and re-release from immune cells (all granulocytes secrete zinc), or both [288,289]. In 2011, researchers at John Jay College of Criminal Justice reported that dietary zinc supplements could mask the presence of drugs in urine. Similar claims have been made in web forums on that topic [289].

Although not yet tested as a therapy in humans, a growing body of evidence indicates that zinc may preferentially kill prostate cancer cells. Because zinc naturally homes to the prostate and because the prostate is accessible with relatively non-invasive procedures, its potential as a chemotherapeutic agent in this type of cancer has shown promise [290]. However, other studies have demonstrated that chronic use of zinc supplements in excess of the recommended dosage may actually increase the chance of developing prostate cancer, also likely due to the natural buildup of this heavy metal in the prostate [291]. Topical zinc preparations include those used on the skin, often in the form of zinc oxide. Zinc preparations can protect against sunburn in the summer and windburn in the winter [292]. Applied thinly to a baby's diaper area (perineum) with each diaper change, it can protect against diaper rash [292]. Zinc lactate is used in toothpaste to prevent halitosis [138]. Zinc pyrithione is widely applied in shampoos because of its anti-dandruff function [293]. Zinc ions are effective antimicrobial agents even at low concentrations [294].

Zinc is an essential trace element, necessary for plants [295], animals [296], and microorganisms [297]. Zinc is found in nearly 100 specific enzymes [298], serves as structural ions in transcription factors and is stored and transferred in metallothioneins [299]. It is "typically the second most abundant transition metal in organisms" after iron and it is the only metal that appears in all enzyme classes [295]. In proteins, Zn ions are often coordinated to the amino acid side chains of aspartic acid, glutamic acid, cysteine and histidine. The theoretical and computational description of this zinc binding in proteins (as well as that of other transition metals) is difficult [300]. There are 2-4 grams of zinc [301] distributed throughout the human body. Most zinc is in the brain, muscle, bones, kidney, and liver, with the highest concentrations in the prostate and parts of the eye [302]. Semen is particularly rich in zinc, which is a key factor in prostate gland function and reproductive organ growth [303].

In humans, zinc plays "ubiquitous biological roles"[275.] It interacts with a wide range of organic ligands [275], and has roles in the metabolism of RNA and DNA, signal transduction, and gene expression. It also regulates apoptosis. A 2006 study estimated that about 10% of human proteins (2800) potentially bind zinc, in addition to hundreds which transport and traffic zinc; a similar *in silico* study in the plant *Arabidopsis thaliana* found 2367 zinc-related proteins [293].

In the brain, zinc is stored in specific synaptic vesicles by glutamatergic neurons [304] and can modulate brain excitability [305]. It plays a key role in synaptic plasticity and so in learning [159]. However, it has been called the brain's dark horse [306] since it also can be a neurotoxin, suggesting zinc homeostasis plays a critical role in normal functioning of the brain and central nervous system [307]. Zinc deficiency is usually due to insufficient dietary intake, but can be associated with malabsorption, acrodermatitis enteropathica, chronic liver disease, chronic renal disease, sickle cell disease, diabetes, malignancy, and other chronic illnesses [4]. Symptoms of mild zinc deficiency are diverse [308]. Clinical outcomes include depressed growth, diarrhea, impotence and delayed sexual maturation, alopecia, eye and skin lesions, impaired appetite, altered cognition, impaired host defense properties, defects in carbohydrate utilization, and reproductive teratogenesis [305]. Mild zinc deficiency depresses immunity [306], although excessive zinc does also [299]. Animals with a diet deficient in zinc require twice as much food in order to attain the same weight gain as animals given sufficient zinc [309]. Groups at risk for zinc deficiency include the elderly, children in developing countries, and those with renal insufficiency. The zinc chelator phytate, found in seeds and cereal bran, can contribute to zinc malabsorption [278].

Despite some concerns [310], western vegetarians and vegans have not been found to suffer from overt zinc deficiencies any more than meat-eaters [311]. Major plant sources of zinc include cooked dried beans, sea vegetables, fortified cereals, soy foods, nuts, peas, and seeds [306]. However, phytates in many whole-grains and fiber in many foods may interfere with zinc absorption and marginal zinc intake has poorly understood effects. There is some evidence to suggest that more than the US RDA (15 mg) of zinc daily may be needed in those whose diet is high in phytates, such as some vegetarians [308]. These considerations must be balanced against the fact that there is a paucity of adequate zinc biomarkers, and the most widely used indicator, plasma zinc, has poor sensitivity and specificity [312]. Diagnosing zinc deficiency is a persistent challenge [277].

Nearly two billion people in the developing world are deficient in zinc [278]. In children it causes an increase in infection and diarrhea, contributing to the death of about 800,000 children worldwide per year [275]. The World Health Organization advocates zinc supplementation for severe malnutrition and diarrhea [313]. Zinc supplements help prevent disease and reduce mortality, especially among children with low birth weight or stunted growth [313]. However, zinc supplements should not be administered alone, since many in the developing world have several deficiencies, and zinc interacts with other micronutrients [314].

3. Halotherapy

Salt therapy, halotherapy or speleotherapy [315] is the use of salt mines, caves or other forms of exposure to salt air in the belief that this confers a health benefit. These natural deposits of mineral halite are derived from evaporated ancient lakes and seas. The unrefined rock salt, primarily sodium chloride, also includes varying concentrations of other mineral salts such as calcium and magnesium, manganese and sulfates, which have additional therapeutic properties depending on the source [316]. The special characteristics of the microclimate of a salt mine include stable air temperature, humidity and lack of airborne pollutants such as pollens, and are unique to each mine. At depth the air pressure is also significantly higher than above ground, which has been found to benefit sufferers of respiratory diseases in studies conducted at the Dead Sea, which is below sea level.

There are records of improvements in the breathing of miners in Roman and medieval times. Dr. Felix Boczkowski, a physician at the Polish salt mine at Wieliczka wrote in 1843 that the miners there did not suffer from lung diseases and his successor set up a spa based upon these observations [317]. Modern use of this therapy started in Germany when Dr. Karl Hermann Spannagel [318] noticed improvement in the health of his patients after they hid in the Kluterthöhle karst cave to escape heavy bombing. It is now practiced in places such as Bystrianska in Slovakia [319] Wieliczka in Poland [320], Solotvyno in Ukraine [320] and many other East European countries [321].

Halogenerators are used to simulate the salted atmosphere of salt mines. These highly developed machines crush rock salt into dry micrometer sized particles, ionize the particles, and release them into the air. Salt particles of sizes 0.1-2.5 micrometers are able to escape the natural defenses of the upper airways and travel deep into the lung to the level of the alveoli. Typically used in a small room with floors and walls lined with rock salt, known as artificial salt room.

Salt lamps are another method of salt therapy. A large crystal of natural salt is hollowed out and heated with a tealight or lightbulb. The crystals give off an attractive glow in various colors of pink, orange, red or purple according to the minerals present.

Special home saline therapy devices were developed with the scope of making salt therapy easily available at home, replicating the seashore or speleotherapy aerosol. Hand-held devices and ultrasonic salinizer, use rock salt to create the microscopic breathable particles of salt. The hand-held salt inhaler uses dry rock salt and can deliver the salt aerosol by breathing through the mouth and exhaling through the nose, offering 1–2 hours daily exposure. The ultrasonic salinizer uses saline solution [322] made with natural rock salt, to create the salt aerosol. These salt particles are released into the indoor air and freely breathed during the night, offering 7–8 hours daily exposure, especially for chronic respiratory diseases [323]. Breathing an aerosol of hypertonic salt water (3-7% NaCl) has been found effective as a treatment for the heavy build up of mucus typical of cystic fibrosis [323]. The benefits of this treatment were first noticed by sufferers in Australia who were exposed to the natural aerosol of ocean salt spray [323].

The use of saline solution delivered by a nebulizer to treat bronchiolitis in children has also been systematically reviewed. The conclusion was current evidence suggests nebulized 3% saline may significantly reduce the length of hospital stay and improve the clinical severity score in infants with acute viral bronchiolitis [323].

Author details

Vincent S. Gallicchio

Departments of Biological Sciences and Public Health Sciences, College of Agriculture, Forestry and Life Science and College of Health and Human Development, USA

References

[1] Kotz J., Treicher P., and Townsend J.R. editors. Chemistry and Chemical Reactivity. Belmont, USA; Thomson Books; p. 351; 2009.

[2] Earths, Metals, Aluminum. Scribd. March, 2013.

[3] Soviet Aluminum from Clay. The New Scientist 1960;191,89.

[4] Dobbs M., editor. Clinical Neurotoxicology: Syndromes, Substances, and Environments, Philadelphia, PA, USA; p. 276-278; 2009.

[5] Kotz J., Treicher P., and Townsend J.R. editors. Chemistry and Chemical Reactivity. Belmont, USA; Thomson Books; p. 979; 2009

[6] Klein C., Hurlburt C., Jr., editors. Manual of Minerology, 20th ed., Wiley, Philadelphia, PA, USA, p. 343-347, 1985.

[7] Zbayolu, G.; Poslu, K. Mining and Processing of Borates in Turkey. Mineral Processing and Extractive Metallurgy Review 9 (1–4) 245–254; 1992.

[8] Crichton, R. R., Biological Inorganic Chemistry: An Introduction. UK. p. 9; 2008.

[9] Krebs R. E., The History and Use of Our Earth's Chemical Elements: A Reference Guide. Greenwood Press. p. 176; 2006.

[10] Fangsen X. Advances in Plant and Animal Boron Nutrition. Dordrecht, Netherlands: Springer. p. 84; 2007.

[11] Lovatt C.J., Bates L.M. Early effects of excess boron on photosynthesis and growth. Journal of Experimental Botany 1984;35 (3) 297–305.

[12] Dickson A.G., Goyet, C. Handbook of method for the analysis of the various parameters of the carbon dioxide system in seawater, version 2. ORNL/CDIAC; 1994:74.

[13] Tordoff M.G. Calcium: Taste, Intake, and Appetite. Physiological Reviews 2001:81(4): 1567–97.

[14] Dietary Supplement Fact Sheet: Calcium. Office of Dietary Supplements, NIH. Retrieved 31 March 2011.

[15] Standing Committee on the Scientific Evaluation of Dietary Reference Intakes, Food and Nutrition Board, Institute of Medicine. Dietary Reference Intakes for Calcium, Phosphorus, Magnesium, Vitamin D and fluoride. 1997. Washington DC: The National Academies Press.

[16] Committee to Review Dietary Reference Intakes for Vitamin D and Calcium; Institute of Medicine. A. Catharine Ross, Christine L. Taylor, Ann L. Yaktine, Heather B. Del Valle, ed. 2011, Dietary Reference Intakes for Calcium and Vitamin D.

[17] Giovannucci E, Rimm EB, Wolk A, *et al.* Calcium and fructose intake in relation to risk of prostate cancer. Cancer Research 1998;38(3) 442–7.

[18] Curhan G.C., Willett W.C., Rimm E.B., Stampfer M.J. A prospective study of dietary calcium and other nutrients and the risk of symptomatic kidney stones. The New England Journal of Medicine 1993;328(12) 833–8.

[19] Bihl G., Meyers A. Recurrent renal stone disease-advances in pathogenesis and clinical management. Lancet 2001;358(9282) 651–6.

[20] Hall W.D., Pettinger M., Oberman A. Risk factors for kidney stones in older women in the Southern United States. Am J Med Sci 2001;322(1)12–8.

[21] Schaafsma A., Beelen, G.M. Eggshell powder, a comparable or better source of calcium than purified calcium carbonate: piglet studies. Journal of the Science of Food and Agriculture 1999;79(12) 1596-0.

[22] Schaafsma, A., van Doormaal, J.J., Muskiet, F.A., Hofstede, G.J., Pakan, I., van der Veer E. Positive effects of a chicken eggshell powder-enriched vitamin-mineral supplement on femoral neck bone mineral density in healthy late post-menopausal Dutch women. Br. J. Nutr. 2002;87(3) 267–75.

[23] Rovenský, J., Stancíková, M., Masaryk, P., Svík, K., Istok, R. Eggshell calcium in the prevention and treatment of osteoporosis. Int J Clin Pharmacol Res 2003;23(2–3) 83–92.

[24] USDA Nationals Nutrient Database

[25] Standing Committee on the Scientific Evaluation of Dietary Reference Intakes, Food and Nutrition Board, Institute of Medicine. Dietary Reference Intakes for Calcium, Phosphorus, Magnesium, Vitamin D and fluoride. 1997. Washington DC: The National Academies Press.

[26] Committee to Review Dietary Reference Intakes for Vitamin D and Calcium; Institute of Medicine. A.C. Ross, C. L., Taylor., A.L. Yaktine., H.B. Del Valle., ed. Dietary Ref-

erence Intakes for Calcium and Vitamin D. 2001. Washington DC: The National Academies Press.

[27] Giovannucci E., Rimm E.B., Wolk A., *et al.* Calcium and fructose intake in relation to risk of prostate cancer. Cancer Research 1998;58(3): 442–7.

[28] Dawson-Hughes B., Harris S.S., Krall E.A., Dallal G.E. Effect of calcium and vitamin D supplementation on bone density in men and women 65 years of age or older. N. Engl. J. Med. 1997;337(10): 670–6.

[29] Jackson R.D., LaCroix A.Z., Gass M. Calcium plus vitamin D supplementation and the risk of fractures. N. Engl. J. Med. 2006;354(7): 669–83.

[30] Grant A.M., Avenell A., Campbell M.K. Oral vitamin D3 and calcium for secondary prevention of low-trauma fractures in elderly people (Randomised Evaluation of Calcium Or vitamin D, RECORD): a randomised placebo-controlled trial. Lancet 2005;365(9471): 1621–8.

[31] Porthouse J., Cockayne S., King C. Randomised controlled trial of calcium and supplementation with cholecalciferol (vitamin D3) for prevention of fractures in primary care. BMJ 2005;330(7498): 1003-6..

[32] Prince R.L., Devine A., Dhaliwal S.S., Dick I.M. (2006). Effects of calcium supplementation on clinical fracture and bone structure: results of a 5-year, double blind, placebo-controlled trial in elderly women. Arch. Intern. Med. 2006;166(8): 869–75.

[33] Fletcher R.H. Calcium plus Vitamin D plus did not prevent hip fracture or colorectal cancer in postmenopausal woman. ACP J. Club 2006;145(1): 4–5.

[34] Weingarten M.A., Zalmanovici A., Yaphe J. Dietary calcium supplementation for preventing colorectal cancer and adenomatous polyps. In Weingarten, M. A.. Dietary calcium supplementation for preventing colorectal cancer, adenomatous polyps and calcium metabolisism disorder. Cochrane database of systematic reviews (Online) (3): CD003548.

[35] Baron J.A., Beach M., Mandel J.S. (1999). Calcium supplements for the prevention of colorectal adenomas. Calcium Polyp Prevention Study Group. N. Engl. J. Med. 1999;340(2): 101–7.

[36] Bonithon-Kopp C., Kronborg O., Giacosa A., Räth U., Faivre J. Calcium and fibre supplementation in prevention of colorectal adenoma recurrence: a randomised intervention trial. European Cancer Prevention Organisation Study Group. Lancet 2000;356(9238): 1300–6.

[37] Lappe J.M., Travers-Gustafson D., Davies K.M., Recker R.R., Heaney R.P. (2007). Vitamin D and calcium supplementation reduces cancer risk: results of a randomized trial. American Journal of Clinical Nutrition 2007;85(6): 1586–91.

[38] Wactawski-Wende J., Kotchen J.M., Anderson G.L Calcium plus vitamin D supplementation and the risk of colorectal cancer. N. Engl. J. Med. 2006;354(7): 684–96.

[39] Lappe J.M., Travers-Gustafson D., Davies K.M., Recker R.R., Heaney R.P. Vitamin D and calcium supplementation reduces cancer risk: results of a randomized trial. Am. J. Clin. Nutr. 2007;85(6): 1586–91.

[40] Lin J., Manson J.E., Lee I.M., Cook N.R., Buring J.E., Zhang S.M. Intakes of calcium and vitamin D and breast cancer risk in women. *Arch. Intern. Med.* 2007;167(10): 1050–9.

[41] Lewis R. J. Sax's Dangerous Properties of Industrial Materials (9 ed.). New York, NY: Van Nostrand Reinhold; 1996. p. 635.

[42] ITII. Toxic and Hazardous Industrial Chemicals Safety Manual. Tokyo, Japan: The International Technical Information Institute. 1988. p. 101

[43] Rumack B.H.. POISINDEX. Information System Micromedex, Inc., Englewood, CO; CCIS Volume 143. Hall A.H., Rumack B.H. (Eds), 2010.

[44] Beall D.P., Henslee H.B., Webb H.R., Scofield R.H. Milk-alkali syndrome: a historical review and description of the modern version of the syndrome. Am. J. Med. Sci. 2006;331(5): 233–42

[45] Picolos M.K., Orlander P.R. Calcium carbonate toxicity: The updated milk-alkali syndrome; report of 3 cases and review of the literature. Endocrine Practice 2005;4(11): 272–80.

[46] Singh, N., Singh P., Hershman J. (2000). Effect of calcium carbonate on the absorption of levothyroxine. JAMA: the Journal of the American Medical Association. 2000;283(21): 2822–2825.

[47] Harding, A. Calcium May Help with Weight Loss. http://www.rxalternativemedicine.com/headline-news.asp (accessed 10 July 2013).

[48] Michaëlsson K., Melhus H., Warensjö-Lemming E., Wolk A., Byberg L, Long term calcium intake and rates of all cause and cardiovascular mortality: community based prospective longitudinal cohort study. BMJ 2013;346:f228.

[49] Xiao Q., Murphy R.A., Houston D.K., Harris T.B., Chow W.H., Park Y. (2013). Dietary and supplemental calcium intake and cardiovascular disease mortality: the National Institutes of Health-AARP diet and health study. JAMA Internal Medicine. 2013;173(8): 639–646.

[50] Mertz W. Chromium in Human Nutrition: A Review. Journal of Nutrition 1993;123 (4): 626–33.

[51] ToxFAQs:Chromium. Agency for Toxic Substances & Disease Registry. Centers for Disease Control and Prevention. 2001 (accessed July 20, 2013).

[52] Bona K. R., Love S., Rhodes N. R., McAdory D., Sinha S. H., Kern N., Kent J., Strickland J., Wilson A., Beaird J., Ramage J., Rasco J.F., Vincent J. B. Chromium is not an essential trace element for mammals: Effects of a "low-chromium" diet. JBIC Journal of Biological Inorganic Chemistry 2011;16(3): 381-85.

[53] Anderson R. A. Chromium as an Essential Nutrient for Humans. Regulatory Toxicology and Pharmacology 1997;26(1 Pt 2): S35–S41.

[54] Moukarzel A. Chromium in parenteral nutrition: too little or too much? Gastroenterology 2009;137(5 Suppl): S18–S28.

[55] Vincent J. B. Chromium: Celebrating 50 years as an essential element? Dalton Transactions 2010;39(16): 3787–94.

[56] Cronin J. R. The Chromium Controversy. Alternative and Complementary Therapies 2004;10(1): 39–42.

[57] Stearns D.M. Chromium (III) picolinate produces chromosome damage in Chinese hamster ovary cells. FASEB J. 1995;9(15):1643–8.

[58] Vincent J. B. Recent advances in the nutritional biochemistry of trivalent chromium. Proceedings of the Nutrition Society 2007;63(1): 41–47.

[59] Thor M.Y., Harnack L., King D., Jasthi B., Pettit J. Evaluation of the comprehensiveness and reliability of the chromium composition of foods in the literature. J Food Compost Anal 2011;24(8): 1147–1152.

[60] Kamerud K.L., Hobbie K.A., Anderson K.A. Stainless Steel Leaches Nickel and Chromium into Foods During Cooking. J Agric Food Chem. 2013:61(39): 9495-501

[61] Flint G.N., Packirisamy S. Purity of food cooked in stainless steel utensils. Food Addit Contam 1997;14(2): 115–26.

[62] Dayan A.D., Paine A. J. Mechanisms of chromium toxicity, carcinogenicity and allergenicity: Review of the literature from 1985 to 2000. Human & Experimental Toxicology 2001;20(9): 439–451.

[63] Newman D. A case of adeno-carcinoma of the left inferior turbinated body, and perforation of thenasal septum, in the person of a worker in chrome pigments. Glasgow Medical Journal 1990;33: 469–70.

[64] Langard S. One Hundred Years of Chromium and Cancer: A Review of Epidemiological Evidence and Selected Case Reports. American Journal of Industrial Medicine 1990;17(2): 189–214.

[65] Cohen M. D., Kargacin B., Klein C. B., Costa M. Mechanisms of chromium carcinogenicity and toxicity. Critical Reviews in Toxicology 1993;23(3): 255–81.

[66] Chrome Contact Allergy. DermNet NZ. http://dermnetnz.org/dermatitis/chrome-allergy.html (accessed 13 December 2013).

[67] Basketter D., Horev L., Slodovnik D., Merimes S., Trattner A., Ingber A. Investigation of the threshold for allergic reactivity to chromium. Contact Dermatitis 2000;44(2): 70–4.

[68] Baselt R. C. (2008). Disposition of Toxic Drugs and Chemicals in Man (8th ed.). Foster City: Biomedical Publications. 2008, pp. 305–307.

[69] Johnson M.D., Larry E., ed. Copper. Merck Manual Home Health Handbook. 2008, Merck Sharp & Dohme Corp., a subsidiary of Merck & Co., Inc., http://www.merckmanuals.com/404.html (accessed 12 December 2013).

[70] Copper Touch Surfaces. http://www.coppertouchsurfaces.org/antimicrobial/bacteria/index.html (accessed 12 December 2013.

[71] EPA registers copper-containing alloy products. May 2008. http://www.epa.gov/pesticides/factsheets/copper-alloy-products.htm (accessed 12 December 2013.

[72] Biurrun A., Caballero L., Pelaz C., León E., Gago A. Treatment of a Legionella pneumophila-Colonized Water Distribution System Using Copper-Silver Ionization and Continuous Chlorination. Infection Control and Hospital Epidemiology 1999;20(6): 426–428.

[73] Chilean subway protected with Antimicrobial Copper-Rail News. Rail.co. http://www.rail.com (accessed 12 December 2013)

[74] Codelco to provide antimicrobial copper for new metro lines (Chile). Construpages.com.ve. http://www.construpages.com.ve/nl/noticia_nl.php?

[75] PR 811 Chilean Subway Installs Antimicrobial copper (pdf). Antimicrobialcopper.com

[76] Vest K.E., Hashemi H.F., Cobine P.A. Chapter 13 The Copper Metallome in Eukaryotic Cells. In: Banci L. (Ed.). Metallomics and the Cell. Metal Ions in Life Sciences 2013;12. Springer.

[77] Vest K.E., Hashemi H. F., Cobine P. A. Chapter 12 The Copper Metallome in Prokaryotic Cells. In: Banci L. (Ed.). Metallomics and the Cell. Metal Ions in Life Sciences 2013;12. Springer.

[78] Lippard S.J., Berg J. Principles of bioinorganic chemistry. University Science Books: Mill Valley, CA; 1994.

[79] Decker H., Terwilliger N. COPs and Robbers: Putative evolution of copper oxygen-binding proteins. Journal of Experimental Biology 2000, 203(Pt 12): 1777–1782.

[80] *Horseshoe crab*. University of Delaware.

[81] Copper. In: Recommended Dietary Allowances. Washington, D.C.: National Research Council, Food Nutrition Board, NRC/NAS. 1980. pp. 151–154.

[82] http://www.copper.org/consumers/health/cu_health_uk.html

[83] Copper sulfate. http://pmep.cce.cornell.edu/profiles/extoxnet/carbaryl-dicrotophos/copper-sulfate-ext.html (accessed 18 December 2013)

[84] Adelstein S.J., Vallee B.L. (1961). Copper metabolism in man. New England Journal of Medicine 1961;265(18): 892–97.

[85] Bonham, M. The immune system as a physiological indicator of marginal copper status? British Journal of Nutrition 2002;87(5): 393–403.

[86] Li Y., Trush M., Yager J. DNA damage caused by reactive oxygen species originating from a copper-dependent oxidation of the 2-hydroxy catechol of estradiol. *Carcinogenesis* 1994;15(7): 1421–27.

[87] Gordon S., John M. Endothelial cell injury due to copper-catalyzed hydrogen peroxide generation from homocysteine

[88] Pesticide Information Profile for Copper Sulfate. Cornell University

[89] Hunt C.E., Carlton W.W. Cardiovascular Lesions Associated with Experimental Copper Deficiency in the Rabbit. Journal of Nutrition 1965;87(4): 385–94.

[90] Ayyat M.S., Marai I.F.M., Alazab A.M. Copper-Protein Nutrition of New Zealand White Rabbits under Egyptian Conditions. *World Rabbit Science* 1995;3: 113–18.

[91] Kean W.F., Kean I.R.L. Clinical pharmacology of gold. Inflammopharmacology 2008;16(3): 112–25.

[92] Moir, D.M. (1831). Outlines of the ancient history of medicine. (accessed 12 December 2013) http://www.books.google.com

[93] Mortier T. An experimental study on the preparation of gold nanoparticles and their properties, PhD thesis, University of Leuven, May 2006.

[94] Merchant, B. Gold, the Noble Metal and the Paradoxes of its Toxicology. Biologicals 1998;26(1): 49–59.

[95] The healing power of precious metals.

[96] Messori L, Marcon G. "Gold Complexes in the treatment of Rheumatoid Arthritis". In Sigel, Astrid. *Metal ions and their complexes in medication*. CRC Press. 2004, pp. 280–301.

[97] Faulk, W.P., Taylor G.M. An immunocolloid method for the electron microscope. Immunochemistry 1971;8(11): 1081–3.

[98] Roth J., Bendayan M., Orci L. "FITC-protein A-gold complex for light and electron microscopic immunocytochemistry". *The journal of histochemistry and cytochemistry: official journal of the Histochemistry Society* 1980;28(1): 55–7.

[99] Bozzola J.J., Russell L.D. *Electron microscopy: principles and techniques for biologists*. Jones & Bartlett Learning. 1999, p. 65.

[100] Nanoscience and Nanotechnology in Nanomedicine: Hybrid Nanoparticles in Imaging and Therapy for Prostate Cancer. Radiopharmaceutical Sciences Institute, University of Missouri-Columbia.

[101] Hainfeld J.F., Dilmanian F., Avraham S., Daniel N., Smilowitz H.M. (2008). Radiotherapy enhancement with gold nanoparticles". *Journal of Pharmacy and Pharmacology* 2008;60(8): 977–85.

[102] McNeil D.G., Jr. In Raising the World's I.Q., the Secret's in the Salt. New York Times, 2006 (accessed 2 December 2013) http://www.nytimes.com/2006/12/16/health/16iodine.html?fta=y&_r=0

[103] U.S. Centers for Disease Control "CDC Radiation Emergencies", U.S. Centers for Disease Control, U.S. Centers for Disease Control, October 11, 2006 (accessed 3 November 2013) http://www.bt.cdc.gov/radiation/ki.asp

[104] Lancaster J.L. Chapter 4: Physical Determinants of Contrast, in Physics of Medical X-Ray Imaging. The University of Texas Health Science Center. (accessed 7 November 2013) http://ric.uthscsa.edu/personalpages/lancaster/DI-II_Chapters/DI_chap4.pdf [

[105] Dlouhy A.C., Outten C.E. Chapter 8, The Iron Metallome in Eukaryotic Organisms. In Banci, Lucia (Ed.). Metallomics and the Cell. Metal Ions in Life Sciences 2013;12. Springer.

[106] Lippard S.J., Berg J.M. Principles of Bioinorganic Chemistry. Mill Valley: University Science Books, 1994.

[107] Food Standards Agency-Eat Well, Be Well-Iron Deficiency. Food Standards Agency – Eat well, be well – Iron deficiency. Eatwell.gov.uk (accessed 8 October 2013). http://www.nhs.uk/conditions/Food-poisoning/Pages/Introduction.aspx

[108] Sesink A.L. Red meat and colon cancer: the cytotoxic and hyperproliferative effects of dietary heme. *Cancer Research* 1999;59(22): 5704–9.

[109] Glei M., Klenow S., Sauer J., Wegewitz U., Richter K., Pool-Zobel B.L. Hemoglobin and hemin induce DNA damage in human colon tumor cells HT29 clone 19A and in primary human colonocytes. Mutat. Res. 2006;594(1–2): 162–171.

[110] Sandhu M.S., White I.R., McPherson K. Systemic Review of the Prospective Cohort Studies on Meat Consumption and Colorectal Cancer Risk: A Meta-Analytical Approach. Cancer Epidemiology, Biomarkers & Prevention 2001;10(5): 439–46.

[111] Eating Red Meat Will Not Increase Colorectal Cancer Risk, Study Suggests. ScienceDaily. (accessed 6 November 2013) http://www.sciencedaily.com/releases/2007/06/070611113729.htm

[112] Hoppe M., Hulthén L., Hallberg L. The relative bioavailability in humans of elemental iron powders for use in food fortification. European Journal of Nutrition 2005; 45(1): 37–44.

[113] Pineda O., Ashmead H.D. Effectiveness of treatment of iron-deficiency anemia in infants and young children with ferrous bis-glycinate chelate". *Nutrition* 2001;17(5): 381–4.

[114] Ashmead H. Conversations on Chelation and Mineral Nutrition. Keats Publishing. 1989

[115] Dietary Reference Intakes: Elements (PDF). The National Academies. 2001. (accessed 5 October 2013) http://www.iom.edu

[116] Iron Deficiency Anemia. MediResource. (accessed 12 October 2013) http://bodyandhealth.canada.com/condition_info_details.asp?disease_id=274

[117] Milman N. Serum ferritin in Danes: studies of iron status from infancy to old age, during blood donation and pregnancy. International Journal of Hematology 1996;63(2): 103–35.

[118] Neilands J.B. Siderophores: structures and function of microbial iron transport compounds. *The Journal of Biological Chemistry* 1995;270(45): 26723–6.

[119] Neilands J.B. Microbial Iron Compounds. Annual Review of Biochemistry 1981;50:715–31.

[120] Boukhalfa H., Crumbliss A.L. Chemical aspects of siderophore mediated iron transport. BioMetals 2002;15(4): 325–39.

[121] Rouault T.A. How Mammals Acquire and Distribute Iron Needed for Oxygen-Based Metabolism. PLoS Biology 2003;1(1): e9.

[122] Nanami M., Ookawara T., Otaki Y., Ito K., Moriguchi R., Miyagawa K., Hasuike Y., Izumi M., Eguchi H., Suzuki K., Nakanishi T. Tumor necrosis factor-a-induced iron sequestration and oxidative stress in human endothelial cells. Arteriosclerosis, thrombosis, and vascular biology 2005;25(12): 2495–2501.

[123] Ramzi S.C., Vinay K., Tucker C., Stanley L.R. Robbins pathologic basis of disease. Saunders. 1999

[124] Durupt S., Durieu I., Nové-Josserand R., Bencharif L., Rousset H., Vital D.D. Hereditary hemochromatosis. Rev Med Interne 2000;21(11): 961–71.

[125] Brar S., Henderson D., Schenck J., Zimmerman E.A. Iron accumulation in the substantia nigra of patients with Alzheimer's disease and Parkinsonism. Archives of Neurology 2009;66(3): 371–4.

[126] Cheney K., Gumbiner C., Benson B., Tenenbein M. (1995). Survival after a severe iron poisoning treated with intermittent infusions of deferoxamine. J Toxicol Clin Toxicol 1995;33(1): 61–6.

[127] Toxicity, Iron (Medscape) (accessed 3 October 2013) http://emedicine.medscape.com/article/815213-overview [

[128] Tenenbein M. Benefits of parenteral deferoxamine for acute iron poisoning. *J Toxicol Clin Toxicol* 1996;34(5): 485–489.

[129] Some Facts About Lithium. ENC Laboratories. (accessed 7 October 2013) http://www.enclabs.com/lithium.html

[130] Anke M., Arnhold W., Groppel B., Krause U. The Biological Importance of Lithium. In Lithium in Biology and Medicine: New Applications and Developments. Eds. G.N. Schrauzer and K.F. Klippel, VCH, Weiheim, 1990, p.147.

[131] Schrauzer G.N., Klippel K.F. Lithum in Biology and Medicine: New Applications and Developments. VCH, Weiheim, 1990, p. 1-209.

[132] Chassard-Bouchaud C., Galle P., Escaig F., Miyawaki M. Bioaccumulation of lithium by marine organisms in European, American, and Asian coastal zones: microanalytic study using secondary ion emission. Comptes rendus de l'Academie des sciences. Serie III, Sciences de la vie 1984;299(18): 719–24.

[133] Schrauzer G.N. Lithium: Occurrence, dietary intakes, nutritional essentiality. Journal of the American College of Nutrition 2002,21(1): 14–21.

[134] Zarse K., Terao T., Tian J., Iwata N., Ishii N., Ristow M. (2011). Low-dose lithium uptake promotes longevity in humans and metazoans. European Journal of Nutrition 2011;50(5): 387–9.

[135] Kean,S. The Disappearing Spoon. 2011. (accessed 3 November 2013) http://www.theguardian.com/science/2011/nov/10/disappearing-spoon-sam-kean-review

[136] Yacobi S., Ornoy A. Is lithium a real teratogen? What can we conclude from the prospective versus retrospective studies? A review. Isr J Psychiatry Relat Sci 2008;45(2): 95–106.

[137] Gallicchio V.S., Chen M.G. Modulation of murine pluripotential stem cell proliferation *in vivo* with lithium carbonate. Blood 1980;56(6): 1150-52.

[138] Gallicchio VS. Lithium and the Blood. V.S. Gallicchio (ed.), Kargar. 1991, p. 1-150.

[139] *Abundance and form of the most abundant elements in Earth's continental crust*. (accessed 2 November 2013) http://www.gly.uga.edu/railsback/Fundamentals/ElementalAbundanceTableP.pdf

[140] Housecroft C.E., Sharpe A.G. Inorganic Chemistry (3rd ed.). 2008. Prentice Hall. p. 305–6.

[141] Ash R. The Top 10 of Everything 2006: The Ultimate Book of Lists. Dk Pub. 2006 (accessed 2 October 2013) http://www.plymouthlibrary.org/faqelements

[142] Anthoni F.J. The Chemical composition of seawater. 2006 (accessed 2 October 2013) http://www.seafriends.org.nz/oceano/seawater.htm

[143] Euser A.G., Cipolla M. J. Magnesium Sulfate for the Treatment of Eclampsia: A Brief Review. Stroke 2009;40(4): 1169–1175.

[144] Gowariker V., Krishnamurthy V.P., Gowariker S., Dhanorkar M., Paranjape K. The Fertilizer Encyclopedia, p. 224. 2009 p. 224. 2009. (accessed 3 October 2013) http://books.google.com/books?id=GP1caeWDUWkC&pg=PA224#v=onepage&q&f=false

[145] NYU Langone Medical Center. Restless Lee Syndrome. Med.nyu.edu (accessed 4 October 2013) http://www.med.nyu.edu/content?ChunkIID=21806

[146] Magnesium. Ods.od.nih.gov. 2009 (accessed 4 November 2013) http://ods.od.nih.gov/factsheets/Magnesium-HealthProfessional/

[147] Lack of Energy? Maybe It's Your Magnesium Level. United States Department of Agriculture. 2004. (accessed 4 October 2013) http://www.ars.usda.gov/is/AR/archive/may04/energy0504.htm?pf=1

[148] University of Maryland Medical Center. Magnesium. 2013 (accessed 3 November 2013) http://umm.edu/health/medical/altmed/supplement/magnesium

[149] University of Maryland. Magnesium. 2013. (accessed 7 May 2013) http://umm.edu/health/medical/altmed/supplement/magnesium

[150] Larsson S.C., Virtanen M.J., Mars M., Männistö S., Pietinen P., Albanes D., Virtamo J. "Magnesium, calcium, potassium, and sodium intakes and risk of stroke in male smokers". Arch. Intern. Med. 2008;168(5): 459–65.

[151] Dietary Supplemental Fact Sheet-Magnesium. US National Institute of Health. 2013 (accessed 2 October 2013) http://ods.od.nih.gov/factsheets/Magnesium-HealthProfessional/

[152] Magnesium. University of Maryland Medical Center". 2013 (accessed 3 November 2013) http://umm.edu/health/medical/altmed/supplement/magnesium.

[153] Wester P.O. Magnesium. Am. J. Clin. Nutr. 1987;45 5 Suppl): 1305–12.

[154] Arnaud M.J. Update on the assessment of magnesium status". Br. J. Nutr. 2008;99 Suppl 3: S24–36.

[155] Rob P.M., Dick K., Bley N., Seyfert T., Brinckmann C., Höllriegel V., Friedrich H.J., Dibbelt L., Seelig M.S. (1999). Can one really measure magnesium deficiency using the short-term magnesium loading test? J. Intern. Med. 1999;246(4): 373–378.

[156] Franz K.B. A functional biological marker is needed for diagnosing magnesium deficiency. J Am Coll Nutr 2004;23(6): 738S–41S.

[157] Vitamins and minerals-others-NHS Choices. Nhs.uk. 2012 (accessed 9 October 2013) http://www.nhs.uk/Conditions/vitamins-minerals/Pages/Other-vitamins-minerals.aspx

[158] Dietary Supplement Fact Sheet: Magnesium. Office of Dietary Supplements. 2012 (accessed 3 October 2013) http://ods.od.nih.gov/factsheets/Magnesium-HealthProfessional/

[159] Firoz M, Graber M. Bioavailability of US commercial magnesium preparations. *Magnes Res* 2001;14(4): 257–62.

[160] Lindberg J.S., Zobitz M.M., Poindexter J.R., Pak C.Y. Magnesium bioavailability from magnesium citrate and magnesium oxide. J Am Coll Nutr 1990:9(1): 48–55.

[161] Walker A.F., Marakis G., Christie S., Byng M. Magnes Res 2003;16(3): 183–91.

[162] Kontani M., Hara A., Ohta S., Ikeda T. Hypermagnesemia induced by massive cathartic ingestion in an elderly woman without pre-existing renal dysfunction. Intern. Med. 2005;44(5): 448–452.

[163] Giannini, A. J. Drugs of Abuse (Second ed.). Los Angeles: Physicians Management Information Co. 1997.

[164] Baselt R., Disposition of Toxic Drugs and Chemicals in Man, 8th edition, Biomedical Publications, Foster City, CA, 2008.

[165] Eby G. 3rd., Eby K.L Magnesium for treatment-resistant depression: a review and hypothesis. Medical hypotheses 2010;74(4): 649–660.

[166] Barragán-Rodríguez L., Rodríguez-Morán M., Guerrero-Romero F. Efficacy and safety of oral magnesium supplementation in the treatment of depression in the elderly with type 2 diabetes: a randomized, equivalent trial. Magnesium research: official organ of the International Society for the Development of Research on Magnesium 2008;21(4): 218–23.

[167] Jee S.H., Miller E.R. 3rd., Guallar E., Singh V.K., Appel L.J., Klag M.J. The effect of magnesium supplementation on blood pressure: a meta-analysis of randomized clinical trials. Am J Hypertens 2002;15(8): 691–696.

[168] Geiger H., Wanner C. Magnesium in Disease. Clin Kidney *J* 2012;5 (Suppl 1): i25–i38.

[169] Guerrero-Romero F., Rodriguez-Moran M. Low serum magnesium levels and metabolic syndrome. Acta Diabetol 2002;39(4): 209–213.

[170] Zipes D.P., Camm A.J., Borggrefe M. et al. (2012). ACC/AHA/ESC 2006 Guidelines for Management of Patients with Ventricular Arrhythmias and the Prevention of Sudden Cardiac Death: a report of the American College of Cardiology / American Heart Association Task Force and the European Society of Cardiology Committee for Practice Guidelines (writing committee to develop Guidelines for Management of Patients with Ventricular Arrhythmias and the Prevention of Sudden Cardiac Death): developed in collaboration with the European Heart Rhythm Association and the Heart Rhythm Society. *Circulation* 2012;114(10): e385–e484.

[171] James M.F. Magnesium in obstetrics. Best Pract Res Clin Obstet Gynaecol. 2010;24(3): 327–337.

[172] Hashimoto T., Hara A., Ohkubo T., Kikuya M., Shintani Y., Metoki H., Inoue R., Asayama K., Kanno A., Nakashita M., Terata S., Obara T., Hirose T., Hoshi H., Totsune K, Satoh H, Imai Y (2010). "Serum magnesium, ambulatory blood pressure, and carotid artery alteration: the Ohasama study". *Am J Hypertens* 2010;23(12): 1292–1298.

[173] Massy Z.A., Drüeke T.B. Magnesium and outcomes in patients with chronic kidney disease: focus on vascular calcification, atherosclerosis, and survival. Clin Kidney J 2012;5 (Suppl 1): i52–i61.

[174] Turgut F., Kanbay M., Metin M.R., Uz E., Akcay A., Covic A. Magnesium supplementation helps to improve carotid intima media thickness in patients on hemodialysis. Int Urol Nephrol 2008;40(4): 1075–1082.

[175] Passlick-Deetjen J., Wang W. et al. Magnesium and mortality risk in hemodialysis patients. European Renal Association (ERA) and European Dialysis and Transplant Association (EDTA 2010), XLVII Congress, 25–28 June, Munich, Germany. Oral presentation.

[176] Shimura E., Okuno S., Yamakawa T., Inaba M., Nishizawa Y. Serum magnesium concentration is a significant predictor of mortality in maintenance hemodialysis patients. Magnes Res 2007;20(4): 237–244.

[177] Science Safety: Chapter 8. Government of Manitoba, 2007. (accessed 2 October 2013) http://www.edu.gov.mb.ca

[178] Roth, J., Ponzoni S., Aschner M. Chapter 6 Manganese Homeostasis and Transport. In Banci, Lucia (Ed.). *Metallomics and the Cell.* Metal Ions in Life Sciences 2013;12. Springer.

[179] Emsley J. Manganese. Nature's Building Blocks: An A-Z Guide to the Elements. Oxford, UK: Oxford University Press. 2001. p. 249–53, 2001.

[180] Law N., Caudle M., Pecoraro V. Manganese Redox Enzymes and Model Systems: Properties, Structures, and Reactivity. Advances in Inorganic Chemistry 1998;46. p. 305.

[181] Takeda, A. Manganese action in brain function. Brain Research Reviews 2003;41(1): 79–87.

[182] Dismukes G.C., Willigen R. T. van. Manganese: The Oxygen-Evolving Complex & Models. "Manganese: The Oxygen-Evolving Complex & Models". Encyclopedia of Inorganic Chemistry, 2006.

[183] Hasan H. Manganese. The Rosen Publishing Group. p. 31., 2008.

[184] Manganese Chemical Background. Metcalf Institute for Marine and Environmental Reporting University of Rhode Island, 2006.

[185] Risk Assessment Information System Toxicity Summary for Manganese. Oak Ridge National Laboratory. 2008.

[186] Ong K.L., Tan T.H., Cheung W.L. Potassium permanganate poisoning – a rare cause of fatal self poisoning. Emergency Medicine Journal 1997;14: 43–5.

[187] Young R., Critchley J.A., Young K.K., Freebairn R.C., Reynolds A.P., Lolin Y.I. Fatal acute hepatorenal failure following potassium permanganate ingestion. Human & Experimental Toxicology 1996;15(3): 259–61.

[188] Elsner R.J.F., Spangler J.G. Neurotoxicity of inhaled manganese: Public health danger in the shower? Medical Hypotheses 2005;65(3): 607–616.

[189] Safety and Health Topics: Manganese Compounds (as Mn). (accessed 2 October 2013) http://www.osha.gov

[190] Yin Z., Jiang H., Lee E.S., Ni M., Erikson K.M., Milatovic D., Bowman A.B., Aschner M. Ferroprotein is a manganese-responsive protein that decreases manganese cytotoxicity and accumulation. Journal of Neurochemistry 2010;112(5): 1190–8.

[191] Bouchard M.F., Sébastien S., Benoit B., Melissa L., Marie-Ève B., Thérèse B., Elyse L., David C. B., Donna M. Intellectual Impairment Impairment in School-Age in School-Age Children. Environmental Health Perspectives 2010;119(1): 138–143.

[192] Finley, J.W., Davis, C.D. (1999). Manganese deficiency and toxicity: Are high or low dietary amounts of manganese cause for concern? BioFactors 1999;10(1): 15–24.

[193] Barceloux D., Barceloux D. Manganese. Clinical Toxicology 1999;37(2): 293.

[194] Baselt R. Disposition of Toxic Drugs and Chemicals in Man, 8th edition, Biomedical Publications, Foster City, CA, 2008, pp. 883–86.

[195] Normandin L., Hazell A.S. Manganese neurotoxicity: an update of pathophysiologic mechanisms. Metabolic Brain Disease 2002;17(4): 375–87.

[196] Couper J. On the effects of black oxide of manganese when inhaled into the lungs. *Br. Ann. Med. Pharm. Vital. Stat. Gen. Sci.* 1837;1: 41–2.

[197] Cersosimo M.G., Koller W.C. The diagnosis of manganese-induced parkinsonism. NeuroToxicology 2007;27(3): 340–46.

[198] Platinum (pt). Encyclopædia Britannica Online. Encyclopædia Britannica Inc., 2012. (accessed 24 October 2013) http://www.britannica.com

[199] Harper, Douglas. "platinum". Online Etymology Dictionary. (accessed 26 October 2013) http://www.on_line_etymology_dictionary [

[200] Lagowski J.J., ed. Chemistry Foundations and Applications 3. Thomson Gale. 2004. pp. 267–68.

[201] Wheate N.J., Walker S., Craig G.E., Oun R. The status of platinum anticancer drugs in the clinic and in clinical trials. Dalton transactions (Cambridge, England : 2003), 2010;39(35): 8113–27.

[202] Krebs R.E. Platinum. *The History and Use of our Earth's Chemical Elements*. Greenwood Press. 1998. p. 124–27.

[203] CRC contributors. Platinum. In Lide, David R. *CRC Handbook of Chemistry and Physics* 4. New York: CRC Press. 2007-2008. p. 26.

[204] Occupational Health Guideline for Soluble Platinum Salts (as Platinum). Centers for Disease Control and Prevention. (accessed 9 October 2013) http://www.cdc.gov/niosh/docs

[205] Occupational Health Guideline for Soluble Platinum Salts (as Platinum). (accessed 23 October 2013) http://www. cdc.gov/niosh/docs/81-123

[206] FDA Backgrounder on Platinum in Silicone Breast Implants. U.S. Food and Drug Administration. Archived from the original on 2008. (accessed 24 October 2013) http://www.fda.gov/cdrh/breastimplants/platinum.html

[207] Brook M. Platinum in silicone breast implants. Biomaterials 2006;27(17): 3274–86.

[208] Haynes W.M., ed. CRC Handbook of Chemistry and Physics (92nd ed.). 2011 CRC Press. p. 4.122.

[209] Abdel-Wahab M., Youssef S., Aly A., el-Fiki S., el-Enany N., Abbas M. A simple calibration of a whole-body counter for the measurement of total body potassium in humans. International Journal of Radiation Applications and Instrumentation. Part A. Applied Radiation and Isotopes 1992;43(10): 1285–89.

[210] Chang R. Chemistry. McGraw-Hill Higher Education. 2007. p. 52.

[211] Campbell N. Biology. Menlo Park, California: Benjamin/Cummings Pub. Co. 1987. p. 795.

[212] Hellgren M, Sandberg L., Edholm O. A comparison between two prokaryotic potassium channels (K_{ir}Bac1.1 and KcsA) in a molecular dynamics (MD) simulation study. Biophysical Chemistry 2006;120(1): 1–9.

[213] Institute of Medicine (U.S.). Committee on Optimization of Nutrient Composition of Military Rations for Short-Term, High-Stress Situations; Institute of Medicine (U.S.). Committee on Military Nutrition Research. Nutrient Composition of Rations for Short-Term, High-Intensity Combat Operations. National Academies Press. 2006. p. 287.

[214] Shallenberger R.S. Taste Chemistry. Springer. 1993. p. 120.

[215] Lockless S.W., Zhou M., MacKinnon R. Structural and thermodynamic properties of selective ion binding in a K+channel. PLoS Biol 2007;5(5): e121.

[216] Slonim A.D., Pollack M.M. Potassium. Pediatric critical care medicine. Lippincott Williams & Wilkins. 2006. p. 812.

[217] Visveswaran K. (2009). Hypokalemia. Essentials of Nephrology (2nd ed.). BI Publications. 2009; p. 257.

[218] Potts W.T.W., Parry G. *Osmotic and ionic regulation in animals*. Pergamon Press. 1964.

[219] Lans H.S., Stein I. F., Meyer K.A. (1952). The relation of serum potassium to erythrocyte potassium in normal subjects and patients with potassium deficiency. American Journal of Medical Science 1952;223(1): 65–74.

[220] Bennett C.M., Brenner B.M., Berliner R.W. Micropuncture study of nephron function in the rhesus monkey. Journal of Clinical Investigation 1968;47 (1): 203–216.

[221] Solomon A.K. Pumps in the living cell. Scientific American 1962;207(2): 100–8.

[222] Kernan R.P. Cell potassium (Transport in the life sciences). New York: Wiley. 1980. p. 40-8.

[223] Squires R.D., Huth E.J. Experimental potassium depletion in normal human subjects. I. Relation of ionic intakes to the renal conservation of potassium. Journal of Clinical Investigation 1959;38(7): 1134–48.

[224] Fiebach N.H., Barker L.R., Burton J.R., Zieve P.D. Principles of Ambulatory Medicine. Lippincott Williams & Wilkins. 2007. p. 748–50.

[225] Gadsby D.C. Ion transport: spot the difference. Nature 2004;427(6977): 795–97.

[226] Jiang Y., Lee A., Chen J., Cadene M., Chait B.T., MacKinnon R. Crystal structure and mechanism of a calcium-gated potassium channel. Nature 2002;417 6888): 515–22.

[227] Shi N., Ye S., Alam A., Chen L., Jiang Y. Atomic structure of a Na^+-and K^+-conducting channel. Nature 2006;440(7083): 570–74.

[228] Zhou Y., Morais-Cabral J.H., Kaufman A., MacKinnon R. Chemistry of ion coordination and hydration revealed by a K^+channel-Fab complex at 2.0 A resolution. Nature 2001;414(6859): 43–8.

[229] Noskov S.Y., Bernèche S., Roux B. Control of ion selectivity in potassium channels by electrostatic and dynamic properties of carbonyl ligands. Nature 2004;431(7010): 830–834.

[230] Potassium Food Charts. Asia Pacific Journal of Clinical Nutrition. (accessed 25 October 2013). http://www.apjcn.nhri.org.tw/server/info

[231] Folis R.H.Myocardial Necrosis in Rats on a Potassium Low Diet Prevented by Thiamine Deficiency. Bull. Johns-Hopkins Hospital 1942;71: 235.

[232] DRI, Dietary Reference Intakes for Water, Potassium, Sodium, Chloride, and Sulfate. Washington, D.C.: National Academies Press. 2001. (accessed 24 October 2013) http://www.nap.edu/openbook.php?isbn=0309091691

[233] Grim C.E., Luft F.C., Miller J.Z., Meneely G.R., Battarbee H.D., Hames C.G., Dahl L.K. Racial differences in blood pressure in Evans County, Georgia: relationship to sodium and potassium intake and plasma renin activity. Journal of Chronicle Diseases 1980;33(2): 87–94.

[234] Karger S. Energy and nutrient intake in the European Union. Annals of Nutrition and Metabolism 2004;48 2 (suppl): 1–16.

[235] D'Elia L., Barba G., Cappuccio F., Strazzullo P. Potassium Intake, Stroke, and Cardiovascular Disease: A Meta-Analysis of Prospective Studies. The Journal of the American College of Cardiology 2011;57(10): 1210–19.

[236] Ruyle G. Poisonous Plants on Arizona Rangelands. (2009). The University of Arizona. (accessed 30 October 2013) http://www.cals.arizona/edu/arec/pubs

[237] Linus Pauling Institute at Oregon State University. (accessed 2 November 2013) http://www.lpi.oregonstate.edu/infocenter/minerals/selenium

[238] "Selenium". Linus Pauling Institute at Oregon State University. (accessed 2 November 2013) http://www.lpi.oregonstate.edu/infocenter/minerals/selenium

[239] Mazokopakis E.E., Papadakis J.A., Papadomanolaki M.G., Batistakis A.G., Giannakopoulos T.G., Protopapadakis E.E., Ganotakis E.S. Effects of 12 months treatment with L-selenomethionine on serum anti-TPO Levels in Patients with Hashimoto's thyroiditis. Thyroid: official journal of the American Thyroid Association 2007;17(7): 609–12.

[240] Ralston N.V., Ralston C.R., Blackwell J.L. 3rd., Raymond L.J. Dietary and tissue selenium in relation to methylmercury toxicity. Neurotoxicology 2008;29 (5): 802–11.

[241] Ralston N.V.C., Raymond L.J. Dietary selenium's protective effects against methylmercury toxicity. Toxicology 2010;278(1): 112–123.

[242] Carvalho C.M.L., Chew H.S.I.,; Hashemy J., Lu A., Holmgren A. Inhibition of the human thioredoxin system: A molecular mechanism of mercury toxicity. Journal of Biological Chemistry 2008;283(18): 11913–11923.

[243] Gladyshev V.N., Hatfield D.L. Selenocysteine-containing proteins in mammals. Journal of Biomedical Science 1999;6(3): 151–160.

[244] Stadtman T.C. Selenocysteine. Annual Review of Biochemistry 1996;65: 83–100.

[245] Schroeder H.A., Frost D.V., Balassa J.J. Essential trace metals in man: Selenium. Journal of chronic diseases 1970;23(4): 227–43.

[246] Selenium (IV) Sulfide. Pharmacy Codes. (accessed 23 November 2013) http://www.pharmacycode.com/selenium_sulfide.html

[247] Selenium sulfide. DermNetzNZ. 2009 (accessed 23 November 2013) http://www.dermnetnz.org/treatments/selenium.html

[248] Baselt R. Disposition of Toxic Drugs and Chemicals in Man (8 ed.). Foster City, CA: Biomedical Publications. 2008. p. 1416–20.

[249] Brain P., Cousens R. Weed Research. Weed Research 1989;29(2): 93–6.

[250] Ravaglia G., Forti P., Maioli F., Bastagli L., Facchini A., Mariani E., Savarino., Sassi S., Cucinotta D., Lenaz G. Effect of micronutrient status on natural killer cell immune function in healthy free-living subjects aged >=90y1. American Journal of Clinical Nutrition 2000;71 (2): 590–598.

[251] MedSafe Editorial Team. Selenium. (2009) Prescriber Update Articles. New Zealand Medicines and Medical Devices Safety Authority.. (accessed 24 November 2013) http://www.medsafe.govt.nz/profs/puarticles/sel.htm

[252] Ralston N.V.C., Raymond L.J. Dietary selenium's protective effects against methylmercury toxicity. *Toxicology* 2010;278(1): 112–123.

[253] Mann J., Truswell A.S. *Essentials of Human Nutrition* (2nd ed.). Oxford University Press. 2002.

[254] Moreno-Reyes R., Mathieu F., Boelaert M., Begaux F., Suetens C., Rivera M.T., Nève J., Perlmutter N., Vanderpas J. Selenium and iodine supplementation of rural Tibetan children affected by Kashin-Beck osteoarthropathy. American Journal of Clinical Nutrition 2003;78(1): 137–144.

[255] Kachuee R., Moeini M., Suori M. The effect of dietary organic and inorganic selenium supllmentation on serum Se, Cu, Fe and Zn status during the late in Merghoz goats and their kids. Small Ruminant Research 2013;110(1). pp. 20–7.

[256] National Research Council, Subcommittee on Sheep Nutrition. Nutrient requirements of sheep. 6th ed., National Academy Press, Washington, 1985.

[257] National Research Council, Committee on Nutrient Requirements of Small Ruminants. Nutrient requirements of small ruminants. National Academies Press, Washington. 2007.

[258] Coop I.E., Blakely R.L. The metabolism and toxicity of cyanides and cyanogenic glycosides in sheep. N. Z. J. Sci. Technol. 1949;30: 277–91.

[259] Kraus R.J., Prohaska J.R., Ganther H.E. (1980). "Oxidized forms of ovine erythrocyte glutathione peroxidase. Cyanide inhibition of 4-glutathione:4-selenoenzyme". Biochem. Biophys. Acta 1980;615(1): 19–26.

[260] Kahn C.M., (ed.). Merck veterinary manual. 9th ed. Merck & Co., Inc., 2005. Whitehouse Station.

[261] Ip C. Lessons learned from basic research in selenium and cancer prevention. The Journal of Nutrition. 1998;128(11): 1845–54.

[262] Rayman M.P. The importance of selenium to human health. The Lancet 2000;356(9225): 233–41.

[263] Bjelakovic G., Nikolova D., Gluud L.L., Simonetti R.G., Gluud C. Antioxidant supplements for prevention of mortality in healthy participants and patients with various diseases. In Bjelakovic G.. Cochrane database of systematic reviews (Online) 2012;3: CD007176. http://summaries.cochrane.org/CD007176/antioxidant-supplements-for-prevention-of-mortality-in-healthy-participants-and-patients-with-various-diseases

[264] Sodium and Potassium Quick Health Facts. *health.ltgovernors.com*. (accessed 30 November 2013) http://www.health.itgovernors.com

[265] Dietary Reference Intakes: Water, Potassium, Sodium, Chloride, Sulfate. Food and Nutrition Board, Institute of Medicine, United States National Academies. (2004). (accessed 30 November 2013) http://www.iom.edu/reports/2004.

[266] U.S. Department of Agriculture; U.S. Department of Health and Human Services (2010) Dietary Guidelines for Americans.. (accessed 30 November 2013) http://www.usda.gov/human

[267] Geleijnse J.M., Kok F.J., Grobbee D.E.(2004). Impact of dietary and lifestyle factors on the prevalence of hypertension in Western populations. European Journal of Public Health 2004;14(3): 235–39.

[268] Lawes C.M., Vander Hoorn S., Rodgers A. International Society of Hypertension (2008). Global burden of blood-pressure-related disease, 2001. Lancet 371 (9623): 1513–18.

[269] McGuire M., Beerman K.A. Nutritional Sciences: From Fundamentals to Food. Cengage Learning. p. 546. 2011.

[270] Campbell N. Biology. Benjamin/Cummings. 1987. p. 795.

[271] Srilakshmi B. Nutrition Science (2nd ed.). New Age International. 2006. p. 318. (accessed 30 November 2013) http://www.books.google.com

[272] Kering M.K. (2008). "Manganese Nutrition and Photosynthesis in NAD-malic enzyme C4 plants Ph.D. dissertation". University of Missouri-Columbia. 2008. (accessed 30 November 2013) http://www.mospace.umsystem.edu/xmlui/bitstream/handle/10355/7201

[273] Subbarao G.V., Ito O., Berry W.L., Wheeler R.M. Sodium—A Functional Plant Nutrient. Critical Reviews in Plant Sciences 2003;22(5): 391–416.

[274] Zhu J.K. Plant salt tolerance. Trends in Plant Science. 2001;6(2): 66–71.

[275] Plants and salt ion toxicity. Plant Biology. (accessed 30 November 2013). http://www.plant-biology.com/salt-ion-toxicity.php

[276] Angelici R.J. Synthesis and Technique in Inorganic Chemistry. Mill Valley, CA: University Science Books. 1999.

[277] Zinc. (accessed 30 November 2013) http://www.infinityfoundation.com/mandala/t_est/t_es_agraw_zinc_frameset.htm

[278] Zinc. (accessed 30 November 2013) http://www.ancient-asia-journal.com/article/view/aa.

[279] Hambidge K.M., Krebs N.F. Zinc deficiency: a special challenge. J. Nutr. 2007;137(4): 1101–5.

[280] Walker J.C.F. Primary Wood Processing: Principles and Practice. Springer. 2006. p. 317.

[281] ZDDP Engine Oil-The Zinc Factor. Mustang Monthly. (accessed 30 November 2013) http://www.mustangmonthly.com/techarticles

[282] DiSilvestro R.A. Handbook of Minerals as Nutritional Supplements. CRC Press. 2004. p. 135, 155.

[283] Milbury P.E., Richer A.C. Understanding the Antioxidant Controversy: Scrutinizing the "fountain of Youth". Greenwood Publishing Group. 2008. p. 99.

[284] Keen C.L., Gershwin M.E. Zinc deficiency and immune function. Annual review of nutrition 1990;10: 415–31.

[285] Bhutta Z.A., Bird S.M., Black R.E., Brown K.H., Gardner J.M., Hidayat A., Khatun F., Martorell R. (2000). Therapeutic effects of oral zinc in acute and persistent diarrhea in children in developing countries: pooled analysis of randomized controlled trials. The American journal of clinical nutrition 2000;72(6): 1516–22.

[286] Age-Related Eye Disease Study Research Group (2001). A Randomized, Placebo, Placebo-Controlled, Clinical Trial of High-Dose Supplementation with Vitamins C and E, Beta Carotene, and Zinc for Age-Related Macular Degeneration and Vision Loss: AREDS Report No. 8. Arch Ophthalmology 2001;119(10): 1417–36.

[287] Bodsworth C.The Extraction and Refining of Metals. CRC Press. 1994. p. 148.

[288] Valko M., Morris H., Cronin M.T.D. Metals, Toxicity and Oxidative Stress. Current Medicinal Chemistry. 2005;12 (10): 1161–208.

[289] Venkatratnam A., Nathan L. Zinc Reduces the Detection of Cocaine, Methamphetamine, and THC by ELISA Urine Testing. Journal of Analytical Toxicology 2011;35(6): 333–40.

[290] Shah M., Christopher K., Nathan H., Lents M.K. Hoyer, Nimah J., Claudette K., Baldassare J.J. Direct intra-tumoral injection of zinc-acetate halts tumor growth in a xenograft model of prostate cancer. Journal of Experimental and Clinical Cancer Research 2005;28(84): 84.

[291] Leitzmann M.F., Stampfer M.J., Wu K., Colditz G.A., Willett W.C., Giovannucci E.L. Zinc Supplement Use and Risk of Prostate Cancer. JNCI Journal of the National Cancer Institute 2003;95(13):1004.

[292] World's Oldest Pills Treated Sore Eyes World's oldest pills treated sore eyes". *New Scientist*. 7 January 2013. (accessed 5 December 2013) http://www.newsscientist.com/article/dn23049-worlds-oldest-pills-treated-sore-eyes.html

[293] Eby G. Zinc lozenges: cold cure or candy? Solution chemistry determinations. *Bioscience Reports* 2004;24(1): 23.

[294] Eby G. (2010). Zinc lozenges as cure for the common cold-a review and hypothesis. Medical Hypotheses 2010;74(3): 482.

[295] Gupta C.K., Mukherjee T.K. Hydrometallurgy in Extraction Processes. CRC Press. 1990. p. 62.

[296] Frankland-Duppa Reaction. 2012. (accessed 2 December 2013). http://www.drugfuture.com/organicamereactions/onr144.tm

[297] Kim J.G., Walsh P.J. From Aryl Bromides to Enantioenriched Benzylic Alcohols in a Single Flask: Catalytic Asymmetric Arylation of Aldehydes". Angewandte Chemie International Edition 2006;45 25): 4175.

[298] Wapnir, Raul A. (1990). Protein Nutrition and Mineral Absorption. Boca Raton, Florida: CRC Press. ISBN 0-8493-5227-4.

[299] Prasad A.S. Zinc in Human Health: Effect of Zinc on Immune Cells. *Mol. Med.* 2008;14(5–6): 353–7.

[300] Sugarman B. Zinc and infection. *Review of Infectious Diseases* 1983;5(1): 137–47.

[301] NRC 2000, p. 443 (accessed 3 December 2013) http://www.epa.gov/ncer/publications/workshop/pdf/howarth.

[302] Cotton 1999, pp. 625–629 (accessed 3 December 2013) http://.www.ag.arizona.edu/pubs/crops/az1170/az11706a

[303] Brandt E.G., Hellgren M., Brinck T., Bergman T., Edholm O. Molecular dynamics study of zinc binding to cysteines in a peptide mimic of the alcohol dehydrogenase structural zinc site. Phys. Chem. Chem. Phys. 2009;11(6): 975–83.

[304] Rink L. Gabriel P. Zinc and the immune system. Proc Nutr Soc 2000;59(4): 541–52.

[305] National Agricultural Library. Nal.usda.gov. 2011. (accessed 3 November 2013). http://www.nal.usda.gov/

[306] Wapnir R. A. Protein Nutrition and Mineral Absorption. Boca Raton, Florida: 1990. CRC Press.

[307] Gadallah M.A.A. Effects of indole-3-acetic acid and zinc on the growth, osmotic potential and soluble carbon and nitrogen components of soybean plants growing under water deficit. Journal of Arid Environments 2000;44(4): 451.

[308] Zinc-Summary. Dietary Reference Intakes for Vitamin A, Vitamin K, Arsenic, Boron, Chromium, Copper, Iodine, Iron, Manganese, Molybdenum, Nickel, Silicon, Vanadium, and Zinc (2001). Institute of Medicine, Food and Nutrition Board. (accessed 3 November 2013). http://www.books.nap.edu/openbook.php

[309] Blew J.O. Wood Preservatives. Department of Agriculture, Forest Service, Forest Products Laboratory. 1953. (accessed 3 November 2013) http://www.ir.library/oregonstate.edu/xmlui/bitstream/handle/1957/816

[310] Rosado J.L. Zinc and copper: proposed fortification levels and recommended zinc compounds. Journal of Nutrition. 2003;133(9): 2985S–9S.

[311] Hotz C., DeHaene J., Woodhouse L.R., Villalpando S., Rivera J.A., King J.C. Zinc absorption from zinc oxide, zinc sulfate, zinc oxide+EDTA, or sodium-zinc EDTA does not differ when added as fortificants to maize tortillas. *Journal of Nutrition* 2005;135(5): 1102–5.

[312] Barrie S.A., Wright J.V., Pizzorno J.E., Kutter E., Barron P.C. Comparative absorption of zinc picolinate, zinc citrate and zinc gluconate in humans. Agents Actions 1987;21(1–2): 223–8.

[313] DiSilvestro R.A., Swan M. Comparison of Four Commerically Available Zinc Supplements for Performance in a Zinc Tolerance Test. The FASEB Journal. 2008;22: 693.3.

[314] Ibs K.H., Rink L. Zinc-altered immune function. Journal of Nutrition 2003;133 5 Suppl 1): 1452S–6S.

[315] Parfitt T. Ukrainian salt mines reinvented as a haven for asthma sufferers. The Guardian. 2005. (accessed 4 November 2013) http://www.guardian.co.uk/world/2005/dec/03

[316] Beamon S.P., Falkenbach A., Fainburg G., Linde K. Speleotherapy for asthma. *Speleotherapy for asthma*, Cochrane Summaries, October 7, 2009. (accessed 6 November 2013) http://www.summaries.cochrane.org/cd0017471/speleotherapy-for-asthma

[317] Valjent R. Caves offer asthma relief for tourists. The Slovak Spectator 2007. (accessed 7 November 2013) http://www.spectator.sk/articles/view/27566/3

[318] Skulimowski M.M. The microclimatic effect of the subterranean chambers of the Wieliczka Salt Mine in the treatment of bronchial asthma. *Annals of Allergy* 1968;26(2): 66–9.

[319] Fawkes H. Ukrainian mine helps asthmatics. BBC. 2006. (accessed 3 November 2013) http://www.news.bbc.co.uk/1/hi/world/europe/457388.htm

[320] Simionca I., Jaroslav C., Slavic P., Hoteteu O.M.M., Enache L., Stoian G. (2012). The XIVth International Symposium of Speleotherapy. (accessed 6 November 2013) http://www.salinetherapy.com/wp-uploads/2013/03/abstracts_of_ the_xiv_th_international_symposium_of_speleotherapy_turda__rom__ania__2012

[321] Zhang L., Mendoza-Sassi R., Wainwright C.A., Klassen T.P (2008), Nebulized hypertonic saline solution for acute bronchiolitis in infants., in Zhang, Linjie, *The Cochrane Database of Systematic Reviews* (John Wiley) 2008.(4): CD006458, (accessed 7 November 2013) http://www.mrw.interscience.wiley.com/cochrane/cisysrev/articles/cd006458

[322] Wark P., McDonald V.M. Nebulised hypertonic saline for cystic fibrosis. Cochrane Database of Systematic Reviews 2009, Issue 2. Art. No.: CD001506.

[323] Elliott J. Dose of salts to ease cystic fibrosis. BBC. 2006. (accessed 7 November 2013) http://www.news.bbc.co.uk/health/4700408.htm

Chapter 3

Oxidative Stress and Dietary Interventions in Autism: Exploring the Role of Zinc, Antioxidant Enzymes and Other Micronutrients in the Neurobiology of Autism

Maija L. Castrén, Tuomas Westermarck and
Faik Atroshi

Additional information is available at the end of the chapter

http://dx.doi.org/10.5772/57512

1. Introduction

Autism Spectrum Disorders (ASD) consist of a set of complex neurodevelopmental disorders characterised by impaired communication and social behaviour, and repetitive or stereotyped pattern of behaviour. The prevalence of ASD has increased in recent decades to 0.6-1% [1-3]. Broadening of the diagnostic criteria and increased awareness of autism among parents and health professionals likely contribute to the prevalence increase. However, the reason for the increase is not completely understood. Alterations of developmental processes and gene expression profiles have been identified in ASD but neuronal mechanisms and perturbations of neuronal networks underlying the ASD phenotype are unclear. ASD varies in severity and the clinical phenotype reflects multifactorial background [4]. Co-morbidity with some genetic syndromes and autism exist [5]. Affected males outnumber females roughly 4:1 [6-8]. The family studies imply that the autism has a strong genetic basis but no single high risk genes for ASD are identified [9]. Hundreds of de novo mutations with extreme locus heterogeneity have been identified in genes encoding protein network ranked for autism candidate genes [10]. Recent studies suggest that environmental factors could play a much larger role in susceptibility to ASD than earlier expected [4]. Since the population's genetic inheritance is relatively constant over longer periods, the increased incidence rate of autism during last decades could indicate that there is an important environmental component in the etiology of autism [11].

The symptoms of ASD appear in childhood and persist throughout the person's lifetime. Since there is evidence that an initiating event for autism may appear early in intrauterine life, an early diagnosis and treatment could be possible. However, the early diagnostic uncertainties and the nature of deficits unfortunately often delay the diagnosis. Besides limited social and communication skills, behavioural and emotional symptoms, abnormal sensory responses and activity levels often seen as attention deficits are common in ASD individuals [12-14]. Intellectual disability associates often with autism (30-60%) and epilepsy is seen in about 25% of individuals diagnosed with ASD [1, 8, 15]. Many autistic children exhibit behavioural and sleep problems and aggression towards others or self as symptoms of their condition.

Unfortunately, there is no cure for autism and symptomatic treatment optimal for autistic individuals without major side effects is lacking. Improvement in patient care – both treatment and rehabilitation – directly influence the prospects of individuals with neurological disorders, including their abilities to integrate to the society and need for life-time support. Behavioural problems in ASD increase stress of people who take care of autistic children and dealing with these problems can be extremely challenging. The child's symptoms might result from an overload of demands (allergens, infectious agents, toxins, psychosocial stresses, inflammation, oxidative stress) in combination with weakness or susceptibilities, which impaired ability to respond to the demands (impaired energy production, inherited enzyme weakness, nutritional deficiencies, osteopathic disorders, sleep deficits, hormone imbalances, etc.) and increased vulnerability. There is evidence that many interrelated environmental factors may act as risk factors to development of autism [16].

2. Evidence for the role of oxidative injury in autism and the rational use of antioxidant therapy in autism

There is compelling evidence that cumulative damage by oxidative species play a role in many diseases including autism [17]. Reactive oxygen species (ROS) are unstable and aggressive molecules, which have the tendency to give their unpaired electron to other cellular molecules or snatch electrons from other molecules to attain stability [18]. ROS can be neutralized by antioxidant defence systems, including antioxidant enzymes and antioxidant compounds. Dismutation of the superoxide species, which is catalyzed by superoxide dismutases (SOD), leads to the formation of hydrogen peroxide. This can in turn be metabolized to water by catalases or peroxidases. Superoxide and hydrogen peroxide also undergo a series of iron-catalyzed reactions to yield hydroxyl free radicals (OH-). These are highly toxic themselves and can also generate more free radicals by reaction with other biomolecules, such as proteins or membrane fatty acids.

Antioxidants are compounds that reduce the production of free radicals and ameliorate the oxidative injury. In contrast to the rapid production of toxic oxygen species, the capacity of antioxidant systems, such as the enzyme SOD, catalase, glutathione (gamma-glutamylcysteinylglycine, GSH) peroxidase, and vitamins C and E, is limited, and there is a lag time in their adaptation. Dietary antioxidants and micronutrients in the diet, such as zinc, influence the development and function of immune cells, the activity of stress-related proteins and antioxidant enzymes, and help to maintain genomic integrity and stability [19, 20]. All these physiological functions occur through the action of proteins involved in the regulation of zinc homeostasis such as metallothioneins which bind zinc with high affinity but, at the same time, release free zinc ions in response to oxidative/nitrosative stress that modulates the expression of zinc-dependent genes, activates antioxidant enzymes and has impact on immune response [21]. Zinc may induce the synthesis of metallothionein that act as a scavengers of metals and free radicals [22, 23]. The release of zinc from metallothioneins represents an intracellular response to stress. Biochemical modification of stress-related proteins might represent a useful target to influence zinc homeostasis and related mechanisms in autism.

A number of studies have implicated disturbed zinc metabolism to the neurobiology of autism. Many children with ASD are shown to suffer from zinc deficiency and excess copper levels [24, 25]. Low levels of zinc during development can adversely affect learning, memory, and attention [26]. Zinc deficiency has also been shown to associate with a behavioural syndrome characterized by reduced activity levels and slower response times [27]. Zinc is an important nutrient for the immune system, and supplementation with this mineral has been shown to reduce the duration of the common cold by suppressing the viral inflammation in the respiratory tract [28-30]. Zinc deficiency can result in a weakened intestinal immune system, which makes the digestive tract more prone to infection with certain parasites [31]. It is also reported in maldigestion and/or malabsorption that often associate with autism [32, 33]. There is evidence that zinc is required for intestinal wound healing and zinc is necessary to maintain the health and integrity of epithelial cells that line the intestines.

A variety of environmental factors that affect brain development during embryonic and perinatal periods may play a part in autism. These risk factors could be influenced by genetic mutations in genes involved in the inflammatory response such as TNF-alpha and interleukin 6 (IL-6) and in the maintenance of zinc homeostasis such as metallothioneins [34]. Il-6 has been associated with neurodegenerative disorders and autism [35, 36]. In genetic studies, measurable differences associated with genes that encode enzymes and other proteins impacting the methylation cycle, the folate metabolism and the glutathione system are reported between children with autism and healthy controls [37]. In particular differences in allele frequency and/or significant gene-gene interactions for genes encoding the reduced folate carrier (RFC), transcobalamin II (TCN2), catechol-O-methyltransferase (COMT), methylenetetrahydrofolate reductase (MTHFR), and one of the glutathione transferases (GST M1) are found. These genetic results, combined with the biochemical observations of dysfunction in the methylation cycle, strongly suggest that variations in genes associated with this cycle and its related biochemistry are involved in the genetic predisposition to developing autism.

How genetic mutations contribute to autism is not clearly understood. A hypothesis for treatment of a genetic form of autism with intellectual disability and epilepsy caused by BCKDH (Branched Chain Ketoacid Dehydrogenase Kinase) mutations by dietary amino acid supplementation was recently put forward [38]. Mutations inactivating a protein called BCKD-kinase prevent the breakdown of branched-chain amino acids. Normally, the amino acids are transported across the blood-brain barrier by special transporters. Since plasma amino acids compete with each other for transportation into the brain, the brain amino acid concentration will be substantially changed by low levels of branched-chain amino acids that affect the expression of transporters. The amino acids serve as precursors for neurotransmitters like dopamine and serotonin, which play a role in mood and pleasure-seeking, and whose activities are likely associated with autism.

Recent studies have associated mitochondrial dysfunction with autism [39, 40]. Defects and malfunction observed in the mitochondria of autistic children suggest that oxidative stress in mitochondria could influence the onset of autism and explain the immunological anomalies present in autistic children. While many inherited genetic mitochondrial disorders occur in the mitochondria of all cells in the body, some are limited to specific cell sites, such as the brain cells which rely largely on mitochondria for energy [41, 42].

3. Potential targets for treatment to modulate oxidative stress status

Selenium (Se) is a micronutrient and mineral. It is a structural component and a co-factor of the antioxidant enzyme glutathione peroxidase. For this reason, supplementation with selenium can modestly increase glutathione levels in persons who are selenium deficient. Selenium has an antagonistic action on mercury and other toxic metals. No association of autism with hair concentrations of selenium was found in a recent meta-analysis [43].

Zinc (Zn) Zinc is an important cofactor for metabolism relevant to neurotransmitters, prostaglandins, and melatonin, and indirectly affects dopamine metabolism. It is necessary for 100 different metalloenzymes and metal–enzyme complexes [44], many of them in the central nervous system. It contributes to structure and function of the brain [45]. Zinc is considered to be an important mineral for children. It is suggested that infants need more zinc for growth and development than older children and that that lack of zinc early in life may be linked with the development of autism. Zinc deficiency has been implicated in hyperactivity and jitters [46]. Children with autism have been shown to have lower zinc/copper ratios than normally developing peers and disturbed zinc homeostasis is suggested as a risk factor for neurodegenerative diseases [24, 25, 47].

N-Acetyl-L-Cysteine (NAC) NAC is sulphur-containing (sulfhydryl) amino acid which is present in many proteins, and is in the same class as the amino acid methionine. NAC is a naturally occurring amino sugar and is a form of cysteine which has been demonstrated to facilitate the short term cellular detoxification of alcohol, tobacco smoke, acetaminophen poisoning and environmental pollutants in several *in vitro* studies. NAC supplementation over long periods associates with modest increases in serum glutathione, but has not proven particularly useful in the treatment of chronic, long-term intracellular glutathione deficiencies. Furthermore, therapeutic levels of NAC are relatively toxic. At therapeutic doses, oral NAC supplementation can cause significant side effects. Cerebral symptoms, nausea, blurred vision, and vomiting are associated with NAC supplementation.

Vitamin A and E Retinol, the most useful form of vitamin A, (along with retinal and retinoic acid) and vitamin E are lipid-soluble. They can build up in the body and cause toxicity in excess amounts. Vitamin A is believed to improve sensory perception, language, and attention [48].

http://dx.doi.org/10.5772/57512

Autistic children could have a vitamin A deficiency because of gastrointestinal inflammation caused by leaky gut syndrome, allergies or viral infections. Lower levels of vitamin E are reported in ASD patients than in healthy controls [49, 50].

Vitamin $B_6$and B_{12} Some forms of epilepsy are linked with deficiency of B vitamins. Lowered concentrations of B vitamins have been linked with cognitive decline and dementia in older adults. No statistically significant differences were found in plasma B_{12} levels between ASD cases and controls in meta-analysis [51]. Beneficial effects from high dose supplementation of vitamin B_6 with magnesium are shown in a subgroup of ASD individuals. Magnesium is combined to the treatment to prevent hyperactivity that can be caused by vitamin B_6 taken alone [52]. Peripheral neuropathy is a rare side effect of high dose vitamin B_6 treatment which generally disappears when supplementation is finished.

Folic acid Folic acid, the synthetic form of folate or vitamin B_9, during the first month of pregnancy may reduce child's risk of autism [53]. Folate, vitamin B_6 and vitamin B_{12} are important coenzymes of the homocysteine-degrading remethylation and transsulfuration pathways [54] and their deficiencies can lead to an elevated serum concentration of homocysteine (hyperhomocysteinemia). In addition, B vitamins play a crucial role in the reduction of oxidative stress and in the methylation of different proteins [55]. Serum and plasma levels of folic acid are not affected in children with ASD when compared with control subjects and homocysteine show no association with ASD [51].

Vitamin C Higher or not abnormal plasma levels of vitamin C have been reported in individuals with ASD when compared with controls [49, 50]. There is evidence that vitamin C brings about significant improvement in people with autism [56]. Vitamin C softens stools and can help in constipation by making the stools easier to pass.

Magnesium (Mg) Plasma magnesium levels are shown to be lower in autistic than control children [57]. Magnesium is usually combined with vitamin B_6 supplement in ASD [52]. The efficacy of this treatment in ASD remains to be verified. Magnesium has been helpful for many autistic children who suffer from constipation. Magnesium is a smooth muscle relaxant, and it helps to pass stools by promoting rhythmic contractions of the intestinal smooth muscle. High magnesium supplementation can cause diarrhea as a side effect and the dose of magnesium should be increased gradually until the desired effects are achieved.

Phenol sulfotransferase (PST) Phenol sulfotransferase is an enzyme involved in liver detoxification. Researchers have proposed that PST is compromised in autistic children. A study [58] demonstrated that the PST enzyme system was functioning at sub-optimal levels in more than half of the autistic children tested. Since the deficiency of sulfur in the bloodstream and impairment of the PST system interferes with the body's ability to process and eliminate phenols, this may explain why many children with autism are so sensitive to phenols ingested via certain foods. Low levels of plasma sulphate are reported in autistic children when compared with age-matched control children [59].

Coenzyme Q_{10} Classical mitochondrial diseases associate with a subset of autism cases. Both nuclear and mitochondrial genes can underlie mitochondrial dysfunction that is associated with autism [60]. Coenzyme Q10 administration in rats increases mitochondrial concentrations, extended survival times, and exhibited neuroprotective effects [61]. In human, coenzyme Q10 has also been shown to be beneficial in patients with mitochondrial disease [62].

Uric acid Urate is the final oxidation product of purine metabolism. A subset of autistics display higher uric acid excretion to urine than controls [63].

Amino acids There is evidence that children with ASD are likely to have abnormalities in amino acid metabolism. Gastrointestinal problems and selective eating may contribute to these changes. In several studies, an increased plasma level of glutamate that is the major excitatory neurotransmitters in the central nervous system is a consistent finding [64]. The level of glutamine and proteins that are involved in transforming glutamate to GABA, an inhibitory neurotransmitter in brain, are shown to be decreased in children with autism [65]. In addition, the levels of essential amino acids are reduced in urine of ASD individuals. Raised glutamic acid levels and reduced plasma glutamine are also found in individuals with Asperger syndrome and their siblings and parents [66].

L-Arginine Arginine is a semi-essential amino acid because the human body does not always manufacture an adequate supply. Arginine deficiency may result from digestive [67]problems or selective eating in ASD. It has been found that autistic subjects have more essential amino acid deficiencies than controls [67] and high plasma levels of arginine were reported in a recent mass spectroscopy study of high-functioning ASD males [68].

Lithium Lithium appears to be an essential mineral in small quantities for good mental health. Low levels of lithium have been reported in the hair of children with autism and their mothers when compared with not autistic children and their mothers in Arizona.

Prostaglandins (PGs) Accumulation of the very long chain fatty acids (VLCFAs) in the membrane of red cells of autistic individuals [69] indicates involvement of peroxisomal beta oxidation in the pathophysiology of ASD. Peroxisomes are cellular organelles which are important in the biotransformation of endogenous compounds in lipid metabolism, including fatty acids, steroids, and prostaglandins They are pivotal for the formation of myelin, neurotransmission, detoxification of exogenous compounds and xenobiotic [70]. Defects in peroxisomal beta oxidation [71] may link disturbances in endocrine, gastrointestinal, and immune systems as well as cytochrome P450 enzyme nitric oxide synthase (NOS) and nitric oxide formation (NO) in ASD [69]. Plasma prostaglandin E2 (PGE2) and leukotriene levels have been shown to higher in ASD than control individuals [49].

Cytokines Inflammation and immune system dysfunction are implicated in neuropsychiatric disorders such as ASD, attention deficit hyperactivity disorder, and schizophrenia. In fact, there is a significant overlap in the pathogenic factors, structural and functional abnormalities of brain, and clinical manifestations. Altered immune responses in ASD children are seen as decreased responsiveness of peripheral blood mononuclear cells to mitogen stimulation, reduced number of T lymphocytes, elevated levels of interleukin 1 receptor antagonist and elevated production of tumor necrosis factor (TNF)-α and interleukin-1β (IL-1β) by blood mononuclear cells. An emerging area of research in autism is the role of prenatal exposure to inflammatory mediators during critical developmental periods. Epidemiological data have revealed significant correlations between prenatal exposure to pathogens, including influenza,

http://dx.doi.org/10.5772/57512

and the occurrence of autism [72]. It was suggested that the cytokine interleukin-10 (IL-10) could play a key role in the mechanisms that lead to alterations in the adaptive immune response in individuals with autism [73]. Croonenberghs et al. [74] found elevated levels of interleukin-12 and gamma interferon in autistic patients. They reported that proinflammatory cytokines may induce some of the behavioral symptoms of autism, including social withdrawal, resistance to novelty and sleep disturbances.

3.1. Defects of antioxidant system in fragile X syndrome, a variant of ASD

Fragile X syndrome (FXS) is a common cause of inherited intellectual disability and the most common monogenic cause of autism [75]. Neurobehavioral symptoms of FXS include restricted repetitive and stereotyped patterns of behavior, hyperactivity, defects in sensory integration, and communication difficulties. About 30% of FXS males fulfill the standardized criteria of autism [76-78]. Improved understanding of the FXS etiology has facilitated clinical trials to identify targeted treatments with potential to reverse or improve behavioral and cognitive deficits in FXS. Studies of the animal models of FXS suggest that an imbalance in gamma-aminobutyric acid (GABA)/glutamate transmission is involved in the pathogenesis of behavioural defects.

Defects of antioxidant system is seen as altered levels of components of the glutathione system and higher levels of reactive oxygen species, nicotinamide adenine dinucleotide phosphate (NADPH)-oxidase activation, lipid peroxidation and protein oxidation are found in the murine model of FXS [79]. These findings have led to research to treat FXS individuals with anti-oxidants. High doses of alpha-tocopherol have been shown to reduce hyperactivity, anxiety, and corticosterone levels in *Fmr1* knockout mice, the mouse model for FXS [80]. Similar beneficial effects have been shown experimentally with melatonin which is a sleep hormone in addition to its effects as an anti-oxidant [81]. GABA-B was identified as a drug target in treatment of FXS and autism. Recent studies show that arbaclofen and STX209, an oral selective GABA type B (GABA-B) receptor agonist, have the potential to normalize the deficient inhibitory neurotransmission in FXS and autism [82-84]. In addition, clinical trials with metabotrobic glutamate receptor antagonists and donepezil in FXS are on-going [82]. Furthermore, beneficial effects of minocycline and lithium on the functional defects of FXS individuals remain to be properly evaluated.

3.2. Antioxidant properties of zinc

Several mechanisms can be involved in antioxidant function of zinc. First, zinc may protect protein sulfhydryl groups from oxidative modification by influencing the conformation and reducing potential of thiol groups. Since the sulfhydryl groups are required for the catalytic activities of several enzymes, zinc protects the enzyme's activity from oxidative inactivation. Second, zinc may antagonize the activity of transition metals such as iron and copper. Zago and Oteiza [85] showed that zinc may compete with copper and iron ions and prevent transition metal mediated oxidative modifications. Third mechanism for the antioxidant property of zinc is that zinc may reduce oxidative damage indirectly by modulating antioxidant defence including (a) enzymes which catalytically remove free radicals and reactive species, like superoxide dismutase, catalase, and glutathione peroxidase; (b) proteins which minimize the availability of pro-oxidants, like transferrins, ceruloplasmin and metallothioneins; (c) low-molecular-mass ROS and RNS scavengers, like glutathione, ascorbic acid, uric acid, and alpha-tocopherol.

3.2.1. *Zinc deficiency*

Inadequate zinc intake has been implicated in many diseases; however, no laboratory test can clearly distinguish zinc deficiencies [86, 87]. Most at risk of zinc deficiency are young children, teenage girls, and people over age 71. Although zinc deficiency is largely uncommon in the developed world, it has been estimated to affect about 2 billion people worldwide. Elderly people, those with lower incomes, and those with less education may be apt to consume inadequate amounts of zinc. Zinc deficiency can be caused by insufficient dietary intake of the mineral and also by some underlying conditions including malabsorption syndrome, liver and renal disease, diabetes, sickle cell disease and other chronic illnesses [88, 89]. Appropriate absorption of nutrients depends on an intact intestine and intestinal injuries can lead to zinc deficiency. This may cause appetite loss and diarrhea which speeds the downward spiral of zinc loss and tissue damage [90]. Supplementation with 12.5-50 μM zinc has been shown to enhance epithelial cell restitution, the initial step of wound healing. Zinc has been found to help healing of intestinal lesions that associate with inflammatory bowel disease that is a serious intestinal disorder.

Improved neurophysiologic performance, positive growth response, and significantly reduced mortality and morbidity with zinc supplementation have been observed in Chinese children [91]. Zinc deficient animals display an increased susceptibility to exogenous oxidative stress such as endotoxin exposure and hyperoxia [92] and zinc is thought to protect macromolecules such as proteins, lipids and DNA from oxidative damage. Mice defective in CuZnSOD develop neurological damage and cancer at an accelerated rate as they age [16]. Zinc depletion affects the expression of metallothioneins that are low-molecular-weight proteins with high cysteine content and high affinity for metal ions [93]. In addition, zinc depletion decreases α-tocopherol and ascorbate levels in liver and lung [94], but may not change α-tocopherol level in testes [95]. Moreover, plasma uric acid concentration has been shown to be elevated occasionally in zinc-deficient rats [96].

3.2.2. *The role of zinc in reversing synaptic deficits in autism*

There is evidence that zinc deficiency plays a role in autism [24] and the zinc-dependent mechanisms underlying the neurobiology of autism are under active investigation. Zinc plays important roles in nucleic acid/protein synthesis, cell replication, tissue growth and repair. Zinc finger proteins (ZNF81 and ZNF182) are the largest class of DNA binding proteins encoded in the human genome [97] and mutations involving genes encoding these proteins have been shown to associate with mental retardation [98]. Zinc is a regulator core component of the postsynaptic density (PSD), an active zone at the synapse. A low postsynaptic availability of zinc has been shown to affect the activity dependent increase of proteins of the ProSAP/Shank family which are linked to ASD [99]. Mice with acute zinc deficiency were shown to

http://dx.doi.org/10.5772/57512

display behavioural abnormalities such as over-responsivity and hyperactivity-like behaviour whereas prenatal zinc deficiency caused ASD-related behaviour such as deficits in vocalization and social behaviour. Furthermore, low zinc levels were shown to increase the incidence of seizures, hypotonia, attention deficits, and hyperactivity in patients with Phelan-McDermid syndrome, an ASD caused by haploinsufficiency of a member of ProSAP/Shank family.

In the brain, zinc is in its ionic form (Zn^{2+}) within synaptic vesicles of glutamatergic nerve terminals or bound to metalloproteins and intracellulary mobilized by oxidative stress. $Zn^{2+}$is thought to be released from the nerve terminals in an activity-dependent manner synaptically and it may be a key modulator of neuronal activity and survival. Extracellular $Zn^{2+}$is involved in the regulation of the balance of excitation and inhibition, and exogenously applied Zn^{2+}have effects on the activity of glutamate, $GABA_A$, and glycine ionotropic receptors.

Zinc homeostasis in the brain is maintained by the blood-brain and blood-cerebrospinal fluid barriers. Researchers are beginning to understand zinc's role in maintaining the structural integrity of the endothelia, which line the blood vessels, and the epithelia, which line the gastrointestinal tract. In atherosclerosis, arterial endothelial cells are destroyed by oxidating fatty acids and inflammatory immune factors. Zinc deficiency magnifies the defect. Supplementation with zinc has recently been found to protect the integrity of the blood vessel cell lining which helps maintain immune function in the elderly [100]. Within two months of zinc supplementation, resistance improves, and the chances of surviving an infection increase [101]. The critical role of zinc to immune function is consistent with its beneficial effects against infection. Supplement of zinc, as well as vitamin C, may enhance the activity of natural killer cells. Deficiencies of zinc, as well as vitamins A and D, conversely reduce natural killer cell function [102].

3.3. Copper-Zinc and Cadmium-Zinc Imbalance

Many metallic elements play an important role in the maintenance of human health and an imbalance in trace elements may be a significant factor in a wide variety of physical and psychiatric conditions. Copper and zinc are regarded as neurotransmitters and they are both found in high concentrations in the hippocampus of brain. Elevated copper and depressed zinc levels have been associated with hyperactivity, attention deficit disorders, depression, and ASD [103]. Also, many individuals with ASD or paranoid schizophrenia have elevated blood copper levels combined with other biochemical imbalances [19,20].

The actions of selenium, zinc, and copper are all intermingled in the regulation of detoxifying and antioxidant enzymes. Zinc may induce a decrease in intracellular cadmium accumulation and the sequestration of cadmium by cadmium-induced metallothionine [104]. However, the actual activity of cadmium/zinc-metallothionine-whether protective or damaging-is believed to depend on various parameters governed by the extracellular and intracellular environment [105].

3.4. Reduced glutathione

Glutathione is present in two forms in the body; in a "reduced" or an "oxidized" form. The reduced form or "L" type glutathione is the most active form and is found in healthy cells. Reduced glutathione is responsible for all vital biological activity /function of glutathione in the body. In normal healthy cells the oxidized glutathione is quickly recycled back to its active reduced state and the majority of glutathione in the body is present in its reduced form. Reduced glutathione is a tripeptide composed of the amino acids glutamine, cysteine, and glycine (gamma-glutamylcysteinylglycine, GSH).

GSH is synthesized sequentially by glutamate-cysteine ligase (GCL) and GSH synthase (GS) [106]. The cystine/glutamate antiporter controls the biosynthesis of GSH by transporting cystine, the rate-limiting precursor of GSH synthesis, into the cell in exchange for glutamate [107]. Methylmercury (MeHg) administration induces oxidative stress in cortex which could be antagonized by riluzole induced GSH synthesis through activation of glutamate transporters (GluTs) [108].

GSH is the major cellular antioxidant and plays an important role in the protection of cells against damage from free radicals and other electrophils and also influences cellular radiosensitivity, cellular response to hyperthermia, and cytotoxicity to some kinds of chemotherapeutic agents. It protects the body against the damage caused by exposure to toxins and is a powerful detoxifier of heavy metals. Early studies showed the role of GSH in inflammation [18]. GSH delivery to the central nervous system (CNS) is limited due to its poor stability and low bioavailability.

3.4.1. Application/role of reduced glutathione (GSH) in autism

The impact of glutathione in autism has been described [109]. Children with autism have been shown to have low plasma levels of metabolites in the pathway of glutathione redox metabolism [110] suggesting that children with autism have a more oxidized extracellular GSSG. If dietary GSH is insufficient, oxidative stress, toxicity and cell damage may occur to mucosal cells in the small intestine. The elimination of fat-soluble compounds, especially heavy metals like mercury and lead are dependent upon adequate levels of glutathione.

In autism the methylation cycle was found to be blocked at methionine synthase, which is the step of homocysteine methylation for formation of methionine [11, 111]. A significant decrease in the level of plasma methionine and lowering of the ratio of S-adenosylmethionine to S-adenosylhomocysteine are two effects of this blocking. The latter change results in a decreased capacity to promote methylation reactions. In addition, the flow through the transsulfuration pathway was also reduced leading to lower plasma levels of cysteine and glutathione and a lowered ratio of reduced to oxidized glutathione. The lowered ratio of reduced to oxidized glutathione reflects a state of oxidative stress [112]. The block in the methylation cycle and alterations of glutathione were found to be linked, since supplements used to restore the normal function of the methylation cycle (methylcobalamin, folinic acid and trimethylglycine) also restored the levels of reduced and oxidized glutathione [111].

3.4.2. *The role of GSH-enzymes in the metabolism of arachidonic acid*

The tissue content of GSH is normally very high, in some tissues concentration up to 5 mM is found. The function of GSH is often tissue protective, and GSH plays a central role as a cofactor in numerous enzyme reactions. GSH-peroxidase (GSH-Px) is one of the GSH-enzymes located in the circulation almost exclusively in the red cells, various GSH-transferases that have peroxidise-like activity and bind chemicals, and γ-glutamyl transferase that reflects the liver function and is involved in the transport of amino acids across the cell membrane. GSH is also consumed by some cytochromes, most notably cytochrome P-450. Several steps in the metabolism of arachidonic acid may be normally regulated by GSH-enzymes [113]. An early observation was that GSH may function as a chemical cofactor or coenzyme in the formation of some PGs, particularly PGEs [114].

The findings of several studies indicate that alterations of cellular methylation capacity, antioxidant defence, and oxidative stress contribute to the pathophysiology of autism. An imbalance in intracellular levels of GSH and GSSG could provide a biochemical explanation for multisystem issues, such as increased frequency of infections, gastrointestinal pathology, impaired detoxification and neurologic pathology, associated with both autism and glutathione depletion.

The abnormal metabolite levels in pathways of methionine, folate, and glutathione metabolism observed in autism may reflect subtle changes in gene products that regulate activity in these pathways [37, 110]. Even small variations in the gene expression and enzyme activity, when expressed chronically, could have a significant impact on downstream metabolism. Many autistic children have been shown to exhibit a threefold reduction in the ratio of "active" GSH to "inactive" glutathione (GSSSSG). Cysteine, another substance needed for GSH synthesis, was also significantly reduced, suggesting that the building blocks for GSH synthesis are insufficient in ASD [11].

3.5. Gluten vs. Glutamate (glutamic acid) vs. Glutamine

Glutamic acid is the major excitatory neurotransmitter that increases the firing of neurons in the central nervous system. It is converted into glutamine and in GABAergic neurons to GABA, an inhibitory neurotransmitter. Glutamic acid and its neurologically inactive sibling, glutamine, are amino acids. Glutamic acid is found in most foods but it is particularly abundant in gluten grains (wheat, barley, rye), soy/legumes/peanuts, dairy products, nuts, seeds, meats and the gluten-grain substitutes (quinoa, amaranth, tapioca as well as the non-gluten grains millet, flax and sorghum). Cells lining the intestinal tract convert glutamate to glutamine, which in turn is used by the villi to maintain the health and integrity. The conversion of glutamate to glutamine happens also in liver and kidneys, which is fortuitous because many food substances that are rich in glutamic acid – namely gluten grains, casein (from dairy), and soy – are three of the four food substances that damage the villi and their ability to make the conversion. Glutamine is converted to glutamate by a mitochondrial enzyme, the phosphate-activated glutaminase.

3.6. N-Acetyl-L-Cysteine and glutathione

N-Acetyl-L-Cysteine (NAC) is an antioxidant that helps increase glutathione synthesis which, in turn, helps the body defends against harmful toxins. NAC is the acetyl derivative of L-cysteine. While L-cysteine plays important metabolic roles as a key antioxidant, a glutathione precursor and a natural source of sulfur for metabolism, it is unstable and can become degraded during absorption. NAC on the other hand, is more stable than L-cysteine. Taken orally, NAC converts into L-cysteine after being absorbed, and raises blood and tissue cysteine levels.

4. Summary and conclusion

It is generally accepted that complex diseases such as autism is influenced by genetic alterations at multiple and variable sites that interact to reach a threshold of toxicity that triggers the disease expression. When expressed chronically even small variations in the gene expression and enzyme activity caused by genetic changes and environmental factors could have a significant impact on downstream metabolism leading to development of autism. A metabolic imbalance can promote chronic oxidative stress and impaired methylation capacity which results in alterations of normal developmental maturation of neurologic and immunologic systems associated with autism. The production of free radicals is critical in the regulation of many biological functions, cellular damage, and the pathogenesis of disorders affecting central nervous system. Oxidative stress is shown to play a role in many neuropsychiatric disorders, including ASD. Understanding of functional connections of autism-associated genes and the impact of environmental risk factors on cellular responses linked to ASD phenotype will allow to distinguish disease-related pathological as well as compensatory processes and to identify targets for treatment of different features associated with ASD. The human genetic heterogeneity increases the complexity of the effects of environmental factors. New biomarkers are desired to support clinical trials which are the final way to find out the efficiency of new types of interventions.

Abbreviations

ASD, autism spectrum disorders; FXS, Fragile X syndrome, GABA, gamma-aminobutyric acid; GSH, gamma-glutamylcysteinylglycine; IL-6, interleukin 6; NAC, N-Acetyl-L-Cysteine; PST, phenol sulfotransferase; ROS, reactive oxygen species; SOD, superoxide dismutases; VLCFA, very long chain fatty acids

Acknowledgements

We thank for the grants from the Academy of Finland, the Arvo and Lea Ylppö Foundation, and the Finnish Brain Research Foundation.

http://dx.doi.org/10.5772/57512

Author details

Maija L. Castrén[1,2], Tuomas Westermarck[3] and Faik Atroshi[4]

1 Institute of Biomedicine/Physiology, University of Helsinki, Helsinki, Finland

2 Division of Child Neurology, Hospital for Children and Adolescents, Helsinki University Central Hospital, Helsinki, Finland

3 Rinnekoti Foundation, Espoo, Finland

4 Department of Pharmacology and Toxicology, University of Helsinki, Finland

References

[1] Kim YS, Leventhal BL, Koh YJ, Fombonne E, Laska E, Lim EC, Cheon KA, Kim SJ, Kim YK, Lee H, Song DH, Grinker RR. Prevalence of autism spectrum disorders in a total population sample. Am J Psychiatry. 2011;168:904-12.

[2] Gillberg C. On the relationship between epidemiological and clinical samples. J Autism Dev Disord. 1984;14:214-7.

[3] Nygren G, Cederlund M, Sandberg E, Gillstedt F, Arvidsson, T, Carina Gillberg, I, Westman Andersson G, Gillberg C. The prevalence of autism spectrum disorders in toddlers: A population study of 2-year-old swedish children. J Autism Dev Disord. 2012;42:1491-7.

[4] Hallmayer J, Cleveland S, Torres A, Phillips J, Cohen B, Torigoe T, Miller J, Fedele A, Collins J, Smith K, Lotspeich L, Croen LA, Ozonoff S, Lajonchere C, Grether JK, Risch N. Genetic heritability and shared environmental factors among twin pairs with autism. Arch Gen Psychiatry. 2011;68:1095-102.

[5] Moss J, Howlin P. Autism spectrum disorders in genetic syndromes: implications for diagnosis, intervention and understanding the wider autism spectrum disorder population. J Intellect Disabil Res. 2009;53:852-73.

[6] Fombonne E. Epidemiological surveys of autism and other pervasive developmental disorders: an update. J Autism Dev Disord. 2003;33:365-82.

[7] Fombonne E, Du Mazaubrun C, Cans C, Grandjean H. Autism and associated medical disorders in a French epidemiological survey. J Am Acad Child Adolesc Psychiatry. 1997;36:1561-9.

[8] Mattila M, Kielinen M, Linna SL, Jussila K, Ebeling H, Bloigu R, Joseph RM, Moilanen I. Autism spectrum disorders according to DSM-IV-TR and compared with

DSM-V Draft criteria: an epidemiological study. J Am Acad Child Adolesc Psych 2011;50:583-92.

[9] Folstein S, Rosen-Sheidley B. Genetics of autism: complex aetiology for a heterogeneous disorder. Nat Rev Genet. 2001;2:943-55.

[10] O'Roak B, Vives L, Girirajan S, Karakoc E, Krumm N, Coe BP, Levy R, Ko A, Lee C, Smith JD, Turner EH, Stanaway IB, Vernot B, Malig M, Baker C, Reilly B, Akey JM, Borenstein E, Rieder MJ, Nickerson DA, Bernier R, Shendure J, Eichler EE. Sporadic autism exomes reveal a highly interconnected protein network of de novo mutations. Nature. 2012;485:246-50.

[11] James S, Melnyk S, Jernigan S, Cleves MA, Halsted CH, Wong DH, Cutler P, Bock K, Boris M, Bradstreet JJ, Baker SM, Gaylor DW. Metabolic endophenotype and related genotypes are associated with oxidative stress in children with autism. Am J Med Genet B Neuropsychiatr Genet. 2006;141B:947-56.

[12] Hughes J. Update on autism: A review of 1300 reports published in 2008. Epilepsy Behavior. 2009;16:569-89.

[13] Hughes J, Melyn M. EEG and seizures in autistic children and adolescents: further findings with therapeutic implications. Clin EEG Neurosci. 2005;36:15-20.

[14] Mayes S, Calhoun SL. Symptoms of autism in young children and correspondence with the DSM. Infants Young Children. 1999;12:90-7.

[15] Tuchman R, Rapin I. Epilepsy in autism. Lancet Neurol. 2002;1:352-8.

[16] Grabrucker A. Environmental factors in autism. Front Psychiatry. 2013;3:118.

[17] Parellada M, Moreno C, Mac-Dowell K, Leza JC, Giraldez M, Bailón C, Castro C, Miranda-Azpiazu P, Fraguas D, Arango C. Plasma antioxidant capacity is reduced in Asperger syndrome. J Psychiatr Res. 2012;46:394-401.

[18] Atroshi F, Westermarck T Differences in the arterior-venous red blood cell glutathione level across the human mammary gland; Experimental data and theoretical implications. In: Rice-Evans C, editor. Free Radical Cell Damage and Disease. London: Richelieu Press; 1986. p. 295-302.

[19] Sensi S, Jeng JM. Rethinking the excitotoxic ionic milieu: the emerging role of Zn(2+) in ischemic neuronal injury. Curr Mol Med. 2004;4:87-111.

[20] Mecocci P, Polidori MC, Troiano L, Cherubini A, Cecchetti R, Pini G, Straatman M, Monti D, Stahl W, Sies H, Franceschi C, Senin U. Plasma antioxidants and longevity: a study on healthy centenarians. Free Radic Biol Med. 2000;28:1243-8.

[21] Hijova E. Metallothioneins and zinc: their functions and interactions. Bratisl Lek Listy. 2004;105:230-4.

[22] Mulder T, van der Sluys Veer A, Verspaget HW, Griffioen G, Pena AS, Janssens AR, Lamers CB. Effect of oral zinc supplementation on metallothionein and superoxide

dismutase concentrations in patients with inflammatory bowel disease. J Gastroenterol Hepatol. 1994;9:472-7.

[23] DiLeo V, D'Inca R, Barollo M, Tropea A, Fries W, Mazzon E, Irato P, Cecchetto A, Sturniolo GC. Effect of zinc supplementation on trace elements and intestinal metallothionein concentrations in experimental colitis in the rat. Dig Liver Dis. 2001;33:135-39.

[24] Yasuda H, Yoshida K, Yasuda Y, Tsutsui T. Infantile zinc deficiency: association with autism spectrum disorders. Sci Rep. 2011;1:129.

[25] Yasuda H, Yasuda Y, Tsutsui T. Estimation of autistic children by metallomics analysis. Sci Rep. 2013;3:1199.

[26] Golub M, Keen CL, Gershwin ME, Hendrickx AG. Developmental zinc deficiency and behavior. J Nutr. 1995;125(8 Suppl):2263S-71S.

[27] Golub M, Keen CL, Gershwin ME. Moderate zinc-iron deprivation influences behavior but not growth in adolescent rhesus monkeys. J Nutr. 2000;130(2S Suppl):354S-7S.

[28] Novick S, Godfrey JC, Pollack RL, Wilder HR. Zinc-induced suppression of inflammation in the respiratory tract, caused by infection with human rhinovirus and other irritants. Med Hypotheses. 1997;49:347-57.

[29] Garland M, Hagmeyer KO. The role of zinc lozenges in treatment of the common cold. Ann Pharmacother. 1998;32:63-9.

[30] Eby G, Davis DR, Halcomb WW. Reduction in duration of common colds by zinc gluconate lozenges in a double-blind study. Antimicrob Agents Chemother. 1984;25:20-4.

[31] Scott M, Koski KG. Zinc deficiency impairs immune responses against parasitic nematode infections at intestinal and systemic sites. J Nutr. 2000;130, 5S Suppl:1412S-20S.

[32] Naveh Y, Lee-Ambrose LM, Samuelson DA, Cousins RJ. Malabsorption of zinc in rats with acetic-acid induced enteritis and colitis. J Nutr. 1993;123:1389-95.

[33] Wapnir R. Zinc deficiency, malnutrition and the gastrointestinal tract. J Nutr. 2000;130(5S Suppl):1388S-92S.

[34] Cousins R. A role of zinc in the regulation of gene expression. Proc Nutr Soc. 1998;57:307-11.

[35] Morales I, Farias G, Maccioni RB. Neuroimmunomodulation in the pathogenesis of Alzheimer's disease. Neuroimmunomodulation. 2010;17:202-4.

[36] Wei H, Zou H, Sheikh AM, Malik M, Dobkin C, Brown WT, Li X. IL-6 is increased in the cerebellum of autistic brain and alters neural cell adhesion, migration and synaptic formation. J Neuroinflammation. 2011;8:52.

[37] Main P, Angley MT, Thomas P, O'Doherty CE, Fenech M. Folate and methionine metabolism in autism: a systematic review. Am J Clin Nutr. 2010;91:1598-620.

[38] Novarino G, El-Fishawy P, Kayserili H, Meguid NA, Scott EM, Schroth J, Silhavy JL, Kara, M, Khalil, RO, Ben-Omran, T, Ercan-Sencicek, AG, Hashish, AF, Sanders, SJ, Gupta AR, Hashem HS, Matern D, Gabriel S, Sweetman L, Rahimi Y, Harris RA, State MW, Gleeson JG. Mutations in BCKD-kinase lead to a potentially treatable form of autism with epilepsy. Science. 2012;338:394-7.

[39] Rossignol D, Frye RE. Mitochondrial dysfunction in autism spectrum disorders: a systematic review and meta-analysis. Mol Psychiatry. 2012;17:290-314.

[40] Giulivi C, Zhang YF, Omanska-Klusek A, Ross-Inta C, Wong S, Hertz-Picciotto I, Tassone F, Pessah IN. Mitochondrial Dysfunction in Autism. JAMA. 2010;304:2389-96.

[41] Zeviani M, Antozzi C. Defects of Mitochondrial DNA. Brain Pathol. 1992;2:121-32.

[42] Howell N. Human Mitochondrial Diseases: Answering Questions and Questioning Answers. Int Rev Cytol. 1999;186:49-116.

[43] De Palma G, Catalani S, Franco A, Brighenti M, Apostoli P. Lack of Correlation Between Metallic Elements Analyzed in Hair by ICP-MS and Autism. J Autism Dev Disord. 2012;42:342-53.

[44] Toren P, Eldar S, Sela BA, Wolmer L, Weitz R, Inbar D, Koren S, Reiss A, Weizman R, Laor N. Zinc deficiency in attention-deficit hyperactivity disorder. Biol Psychiatry. 1996;40:1308-10.

[45] Black M. Zinc deficiency and child development. Am J Clin Nutr. 1998;68(2 suppl): 464S-9S.

[46] Aggett P, Harries JT. Current status of zinc in health and disease states. Arch Dis Child. 1979;54:909-17.

[47] Szewczyk B. Zinc homeostasis and neurodegenerative disorders. Front Aging Neurosci. 2013;5:33.

[48] Megson M. Is autism a G-alpha protein defect reversible with natural vitamin A? Med Hypotheses. 2000;54:979-83.

[49] Al-Gadani Y, El-Ansary A, Attas O, Al-Ayadhi L. Metabolic biomarkers related to oxidative stress and antioxidant status in Saudi autistic children. Clin Biochem. 2009;42:10-1.

[50] Krajcovicova-Kudlackova M, Valachovicova M, Mislanova C, Hudecova Z, Sustrova M, Ostatnikova D. Plasma concentrations of selected antioxidants in autistic children and adolescents. Bratisl Lek Listy. 2009;110:247-50.

[51] Frustaci A, Neri M, Cesario A, Adams JB, Domenici E, Dalla Bernardina B, Bonassi S. Oxidative stress-related biomarkers in autism: systematic review and meta-analyses. Free Radic Biol Med. 2012;52:2128-41.

[52] Murza K, Pavelko SL, Malani MD, Nye C. Vitamin B6-magnesium treatment for autism: the current status of the research. Magnes Res. 2010;23:115-7.

[53] Berry J. Maternal prenatal folic acid supplementation is associated with a reduction in development of autistic disorder. J Pediatrics. 2013;163:302-6.

[54] Selhub J. Homocysteine metabolism. Annu Rev Nutr. 1999;19:217-46.

[55] Herrmann W, Herrmann M, Obeid R. Hyperhomocysteinaemia: a critical review of old and new aspects. Curr Drug Metab. 2007;8:17-31.

[56] Dolske M, Spollen J, McKay S, Lancashire E, Tolbert L. A preliminary trial of ascorbic acid as supplemental therapy for autism. Prog Neuropsychopharmacol Biol Psychiatry. 1993;17:765-74.

[57] Strambi M, Longini M, Hayek J, Berni S, Macucci F, Scalacci E, Vezzosi P. Magnesium profile in autism. Biol Trace Elem Res. 2006;109:97-104.

[58] Waring R, Klovrza LV. Sulphur Metabolism in Autism. J Nutr Envir Med. 2000;10:25-32.

[59] Alberti A, Pirrone P, Elia M, Waring RH, Romano C. Sulphation deficit in "low-functioning" autistic children: a pilot study. Biol Psychiatry. 1999;46:420-4.

[60] Oliveira G, Diogo L, Grazina M, Garcia P, Ataíde A, Marques C, Miguel T, Borges L, Vicente AM, Oliveira CR. Mitochondrial dysfunction in autism spectrum disorders: a population-based study. Dev Med Child Neurol. 2005;47:185-9.

[61] Matthews R, Yang L, Browne S, Baik M, Beal MF. Coenzyme Q10 administration increases brain mitochondrial concentrations and exerts neuroprotective effects. Proc Natl Acad Sci USA. 1998;95:8892-7.

[62] Sobreira C, Hirano M, Shanske S, Keller RK, Haller RG, Davidson E, Santorelli FM, Miranda AF, Bonilla E, Mojon DS, Barreira AA, King MP, DiMauro S. Mitochondrial encephalomyopathy with coenzyme Q10 deficiency. Neurology. 1997;48:1238-43.

[63] Page T, Coleman M. Purine metabolism abnormalities in a hyperuricosuric subclass of autism. Biochim Biophys Acta. 2000;1500:291-6.

[64] Ghanizadeh G. Increased glutamate and homocysteine and decreased glutamine levels in autism: A review and strategies for future studies of amino acids in autism. Dis Markers. 2013;35:281-6.

[65] Shimmura C, Suda S, Tsuchiya KJ, Hashimoto K, Ohno K, Matsuzaki H, Iwata K, Matsumoto K, Wakuda T, Kameno Y, Suzuki K, Tsujii M, Nakamura K, Takei N,

Mori N. Alteration of plasma glutamate and glutamine levels in children with high functioning autism. PLoSONE. 2011;6.

[66] Aldred S, Moore KM, Fitzgerald M, Waring RH. Plasma amino acid levels in children with autism and their families. J Autism Dev Disord. 2003;33:93-7.

[67] Arnold G, Hyman SL, Mooney RA, Kirby RS. Plasma amino acids profiles in children with autism: potential risk of nutritional deficiencies. J Autism Dev Disord. 2003;33:449-54.

[68] Kuwabara H, Yamasue H, Koike S, Inoue H, Kawakubo Y, Kuroda M, Takano Y, Iwashiro N, Natsubori T, Aoki Y, Kano Y, Kasai K. Altered Metabolites in the Plasma of Autism Spectrum Disorder: A Capillary Electrophoresis Time-of-Flight Mass Spectroscopy Study. PLoS One. 2013;8:e73814.

[69] Adams J, Audhya T, McDonough-Means S, Rubin RA, Quig D, Geis E, Gehn E, Loresto M, Mitchell J, Atwood S, Barnhouse S, Lee W. Effect of a vitamin/mineral supplement on children and adults with autism. BMC Pediatr. 2011;11:111.

[70] Kane P, Kane E. Peroxisomal disturbances in autistic spectrum disorder. J Ortho Med. 1997;12:207-18.

[71] Luers G, Beier K, Hashimoto T, Fahimi HD, Völkl A. Biogenesis of peroxisomes: sequential biosynthesis of the membrane and matrix proteins in the course of hepatic regeneration. Eur J Cell Biol. 1990;52:175-84.

[72] Moser H, Moser AB. Very long -chain fatty acids in diagnosis, pathogenesis, and therapy of peroxisomal disorders. Lipids. 1996;31:S141-5.

[73] Parker-Athill E, Tan J. Maternal immune activation and autism spectrum disorder: interleukin-6 signaling as a key mechanistic pathway. Neurosignals. 2010;18:113-28.

[74] Molloy C, Morrow A, Meinzen-Derr J, Schleifer K, Dienger K, Manning-Courtney P, Altaye M, Wills-Karp M. Elevated cytokine levels in children with autism spectrum disorder. J Neuroimmunol. 2006;172:198-205.

[75] Croonenberghs J, Bosmans E, Deboutte D, Kenis G, Maes M. Activation of the inflammatory response system in autism. Neuropsychobiology. 2002;45:1-6.

[76] Garber K, Visootsak J, Warren ST. Fragile X syndrome. Eur J Hum Genet. 2008;16:666-72.

[77] Hagerman R, Hoem G, Hagerman P. Fragile X and autism: Intertwined at the molecular level leading to targeted treatments. Molecular Autism. 2010;1(1):1-14.

[78] Brown WT, Jenkins E, Cohen IL, Fisch GS, Wolf-Schein EG, Gross A, Waterhouse L, Fein D, Mason-Brothers A, Ritvo E, et al. Fragile X and autism: a multicenter survey. Am J Med Genet. 1986;23:341-52.

[79] Hernandez RN FR, Vaurio R, Passanante NM, Thompson RE, Kaufmann WE. Autism spectrum disorder in fragile X syndrome: a longitudinal evaluation. Am J Med Genet. 2009;149A(6):1125-37.

[80] el Bekay R, Romero-Zerbo Y, Decara J, Sanchez-Salido L, Del Arco-Herrera I, Rodríguez-de Fonseca F, de Diego-Otero Y. Enhanced markers of oxidative stress, altered antioxidants and NADPH-oxidase activation in brains from Fragile X mental retardation 1-deficient mice, a pathological model for Fragile X syndrome. Eur J Neurosci. 2007;26:3169-80.

[81] de Diego-Otero Y, Romero-Zerbo Y, el Bekay R, Decara J, Sanchez L, Rodriguez-de Fonseca F, del Arco-Herrera I. Alpha-tocopherol protects against oxidative stress in the fragile X knockout mouse: an experimental therapeutic approach for the Fmr1 deficiency. Neuropsychopharmacology. 2009;34:1011-26.

[82] Romero-Zerbo Y, Decara J, el Bekay R, Sanchez-Salido L, Del Arco-Herrera I, de Fonseca FR, de Diego-Otero Y. Protective effects of melatonin against oxidative stress in Fmr1 knockout mice: a therapeutic research model for the fragile X syndrome. J Pineal Res. 2009;46:224-34.

[83] Healy A, Rush R, Ocain T. Fragile X syndrome: An update on developing treatment modalities. ACS Chem Neurosci. 2011;2:402–10.

[84] Emmitte K. Recent advances in the design and development of novel negative allosteric modulators of mGlu(5). ACS Chem Neurosci. 2011;2:411-32.

[85] Hopkins C. ACS chemical neuroscience molecule spotlight on STX209 (arbaclofen). ACS Chem Neurosci. 2011;2:381.

[86] Zago M, Oteiza PI. The antioxidant properties of zinc: interactions with iron and antioxidants. Free Radic Biol Med. 2001;15:266-74.

[87] Ma J, Betts NM. Zinc and copper intakes and their major food sources for older adults in the 1994-96 continuing survey of food intakes by individuals (CSFII). J Nutr. 2000;130:2838-43.

[88] Lowe N. In search of a reliable marker of zinc status-are we nearly there yet? Nutrition. 2005;21:883-4.

[89] Prasad A. Zinc deficiency in women, infants and children. J Am College Nutr. 1996;15:113-20.

[90] Prasad A. Discovery of human zinc deficiency: 50 years later. J Trace Elem Med Biol. 2012;26:66-9.

[91] Semrad C. Zinc and intestinal function. Curr Gastroenterol Rep. 1999;1:398-403.

[92] Sandstead H, Penland JG, Alcock NW, Dayal HH, Chen XC, Li JS, Zhao F,Yang JJ. Effects of repletion with zinc and other micronutrients on neuropsychologic performance and growth of Chinese children. Am J Clin Nutr. 1998;68:470S-5S.

[93] Sakaguchi S, Iizuka Y, Furusawa S, Ishikawa M, Satoh S, Takayanagi M. Role of Zn(2+) in oxidative stress caused by endotoxin challenge. Eur J Pharmacology. 2002;451:309-16.

[94] Tapiero H, Tew KD. Trace elements in human physiology and pathology: zinc and metallothioneins. Biomed Pharmacother. 2003;57:399-411.

[95] Taylor C, Bray TM. Increased lung copper-zinc-superoxide dismutase activity and absence of magnetic resonance imaging-detectable lung damage in copper-deficient rats exposed to hyperoxia. J Nutr. 1991;121:467-73.

[96] Oteiza P, Olin KL, Fraga CG, Keen CL. Oxidant defense systems in testes from zinc-deficient rats. Proc Soc Exp Biol Med. 1996;213:85-91.

[97] Kfoury G, Reinhold JG, Simonian SJ. Enzyme activities in tissues of zincdeficient rats. J Nutr. 1968;95:102-10.

[98] Tupler R, Perini G, Green MR. Expressing the human genome. Nature. 2001;409:832-3.

[99] Alesi V, Bertoli M, Barrano G, Torres B, Pusceddu S, Pastorino M, Perria C, Nardone AM, Novelli A, Serra G. 335.4kb microduplication in chromosome band Xp11.2p11.3 associated with developmental delay, growth retardation, autistic disorder and dysmorphic features. Gene. 2012;505:384-7.

[100] Grabrucker S, Jannetti L, Eckert M, Gaub S, Chhabra R, Pfaender S, Mangus K, Reddy PP, Rankovic V, Schmeisser MJ, Kreutz MR, Ehret G, Boeckers TM, Grabrucker AM. Zinc deficiency dysregulates the synaptic ProSAP/Shank scaffold and might contribute to autism spectrum disorders. Brain. 2013;[Epub ahead of print].

[101] Meerarani P, Ramadass P, Toborek M, Bauer HC, Bauer H, Hennig B. Zinc protects against apoptosis of endothelial cells induced by linoleic acid and tumor necrosis factor alpha. Am J Clin Nutr. 2000;71:81-7.

[102] Mocchegiani E, Muzzioli M. Therapeutic application of zinc in human immunodeficiency virus against opportunistic infections. J Nutr. 2000;130(5S Suppl):1424S-31S.

[103] Erickson K, Medina EA, Hubbard NE. Micronutrients and innate immunity. J Infect Dis. 2000;182(Suppl1):5S-10S.

[104] Barlow P, Francois PE, Goldberg IJL, Richardson I, Izmeth MGA, Kumpeson K, Sykes P. Trace metal abnormalities in long- stay hyperactive mentally handicapped children and agitated senile dements. J R Soc Med. 1986;79:581-3.

[105] Kaji T, Mishima A, Koyanagi E, Yamamoto C, Sakamoto M, Kozuka H. Possible mechanism for zinc protection against cadmium cytotoxicity in cultured vascular endothelial cells. Toxicology. 1992;76:257-70.

[106] Müller T, Schuckelt, R, Jaenicke, L. Evidence for radical species as intermediates in cadmium/zinc-metallothionein-dependent DNA damage in vitro. Environ Health Perspect. 1994;102 Suppl 3:27-9.

[107] Ramani K, Tomasi, ML, Yang, H, Ko, K, Lu, SC. Mechanism and significance of changes in glutamate-cysteine ligase expression during hepatic fibrogenes. J Biol Chem. 2012;287:36341-55.

[108] Sato H, Tamba, M, Kuriyama-Matsumura, K, Okuno, S, Bannai, S. Molecular cloning and expression of human xCT, the light chain of amino acid transport system xc-. Antioxid Redox Signal. 2000;2:665-71.

[109] Deng Y, Xu, ZF, Liu, W, Xu, B, Yang, HB, Wei, YG. Riluzole-triggered GSH synthesis via activation of glutamate transporters to antagonize methylmercury-induced oxidative stress in rat cerebral cortex. Oxid Med Cell Longev. 2012;2012:534705.

[110] Frye R, Melnyk, S, Fuchs, G, Reid, T, Jernigan, S, Pavliv, O, Hubanks, A, Gaylor, DW, Walters, L, James, SJ. Effectiveness of methylcobalamin and folinic Acid treatment on adaptive behavior in children with autistic disorder is related to glutathione redox status. Autism Res Treat. 2013;2013:609705.

[111] Rose S, Melnyk, S, Pavliv, O, Bai, S, Nick, TG, Frye, RE, James, SJ. Evidence of oxidative damage and inflammation associated with low glutathione redox status in the autism brain. Transl Psychiatry. 2012;2:e134.

[112] James S, Melnyk, SB, Jernigan, S, Janak, L, Cutler, P, Neubrander, JM. Metabolic biomarkers of increased oxidative stress and impaired methylation capacity in children with Autism. Amer J Clin Nutr. 2004;80:1611-17.

[113] Németh I, Boda, D. The ratio of oxidized/reduced glutathione as an index of oxidative stress in various experimental models of shock syndrome. Biomed Biochim Acta. 1989;48:S53-7.

[114] Rouzer C, Scott, WA, Griffith, OW, Hamill, AL, Cohn, ZA. Arachidonic acid metabolism in glutathione-deficient macrophages. Proc Natl Acad Sci USA. 1982;79:1621-5.

[115] Mimata H, Tanigawa, T, Ogata, J, Takeshita, M. Regulation of prostaglandin synthesis by reduced glutathione in urinary bladder epithelium. J Urol. 1988;139:616-20.

Chapter 4

Antioxidants as Complementary Medication in Thalassemia

Somdet Srichairatanakool and Suthat Fucharoen

Additional information is available at the end of the chapter

http://dx.doi.org/10.5772/57372

1. Introduction

Iron is an essential trace element found in all cellular forms of life and plays a crucial role in oxygen sensing and transport, electron transfer, and catalysis [1]. In ancient times, iron was used in medicine for the treatment of the following diseases; alopecia, acne, vesicular bollus, encrusting eruptions, erysipelas, paronychia, vaginal discharges, wounds, hemorrhoids, gout, tuberculosis, diarrhea, perianal fistulas, excessive lacrimation, vomiting, weakness, edema, fevers and cystitis [2]. Secondary iron overload in β-thalassemia patients is commonly caused by increased dietary iron absorption and can be a result of multiple blood transfusions [3]. Consequently, the excessive active iron catalyzes the production of a variety of reactive oxygen species (ROS), such as superoxide anions ($O_2^{\bullet -}$), hydrogen peroxide (H_2O_2) and hydroxyl radicals ($HO^{\bullet}$) via Haber-Weiss and Fenton reactions. The ROS is attributed to the function of the metal in the redox cycle and can damage many cells and tissues including the heart, liver, pancreas, erythrocytes and endocrine glands resulting in dysfunctions of the organs [4]. Hydrogen peroxide is normally applied to kill microorganisms in neutrophils; nevertheless, an excess amount can be toxic.

β-Thalassemia patients suffer from ineffective erythropoiesis and require regular blood transfusions to compensate for having chronic anemia. Transfused red blood cells (RBC) are taken up and degraded by the reticuloendothelial system (RES) or tissue macrophages, leading to a high accumulation of intracellular iron and saturation of plasma transferrin. The excess iron appears in successive forms of toxic iron as a labile iron pool (LIP), and non-transferrin bound iron (NTBI) and labile plasma iron (LPI) [5-7]. Effective iron chelators are required to remove the toxic irons in order to prevent oxidative damage in the vital organs, particularly the heart and liver. Iron chelators must be absorbed via the gastrointestinal tract into the blood circulation and target tissues readily, and show minimal side effects. They should complex directly onto the plasma iron as well as the cellular iron; afterwards, the complexes can be excreted from the body easily [8]. Serum oxidant activity in young β-thalassemia major patients with iron overload is directly correlated with the serum ceruloplasmin and copper concentrations, and with serum iron (SI) concentration and total iron-binding capacity (TIBC), but not with serum vitamin E concentration [9]. Levels of antioxidant enzymes such as superoxide dismutase (SOD), catalase (CAT) and glutathione peroxidase (GPx) were greatly elevated in the RBC of β-thalassemia minor patients to fight cellular increased oxidant and are close to normal values in the RBC of β-thalassemia major patients due to the presence of transfused normal RBC [10]. Levels of antioxidant compounds such as serum retinol (vitamin A), carotenoids, α-tocopherol (vitamin E) were decreased in β-thalassemia major patients [11, 12]. Supplements of the antioxidant vitamins can prevent some of the damage in the thalassemic RBC membrane. Thus, antioxidant therapy can be a supplemental medical regime to meliorate pathophysiological complications and improve quality of life of thalassemia patients.

2. Iron overload in thalassemia patients

2.1. Causes of iron overload

Patients with β-thalassemia have a partial or complete lack of ability to synthesize the β-chains of hemoglobin [13]. This process of β-globin chain synthesis is controlled by gene that is found to be present in Chromosome 11. There are more than 200 points of mutation and rare deletions of this gene. The production of the β-globin chain can range from near normal to completely absent, leading to varying degrees of excess α-globins in the β-globin chain production. In the β-thalassemia trait, the one gene defect is asymptomatic and results in microcytosis and mild anemia. β-thalassemia major or Cooley anemia results from either severely reduced synthesis or the absence of synthesis in both genes. If the synthesis of the beta chain is less severely reduced, the person will have beta thalassemia intermedia. These persons experience symptoms that are less severe and do not require lifelong transfusions to survive past the age of 20 years [14]. The amount of iron (20 - 30 mg) required for the daily production of 300 billion RBCs is provided mostly by the iron that is recycled by the macrophages [6]. Importantly, iron stored in the macrophages is safe and does not lead to oxidative damage [15]. Iron overload can be caused by an increase in dietary iron absorption in hereditary hemochromatosis patients [16] and by multiple blood transfusions in β-thalassemia patients. Duodenal iron absorption in normal persons is approximately 1 – 2 mg/day and balanced with iron excretion at 1 – 2 mg/day. Though thalassemia intermedia patients do not receive transfusions, abnormal iron absorption produces an increase in the body's iron burden evaluated to 2 – 5 g/year (3 - 9 mg iron/day) [17]. Regular blood transfusions (420 ml/unit of donor blood equivalent to 200 mg of iron) lead to double iron accumulation. Increased iron absorption along with multiple blood transfusions in thalassemia patients can result in hemosiderosis, oxidative stress, hypercoagulability, liver inflammation, cardiomyopathy, endocrine dysfunctions and bone deformity, of which the complications can be meliorated by many drugs and agents (Figure 1).

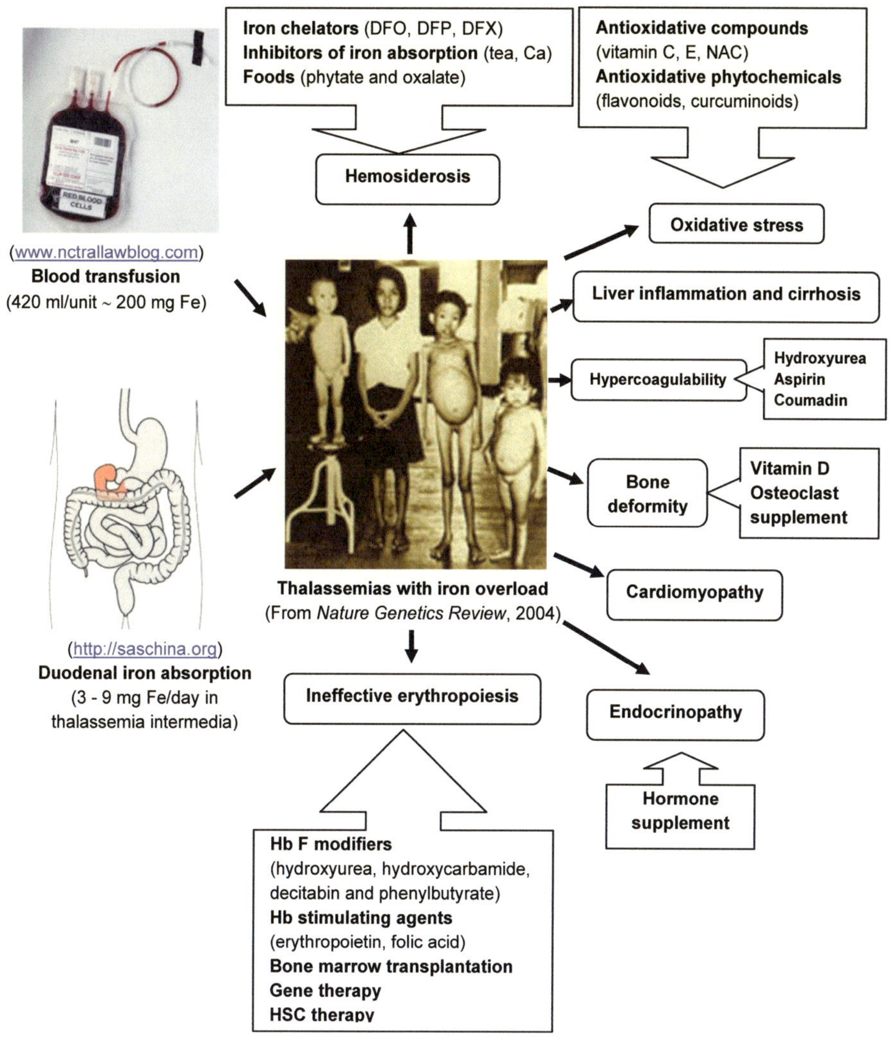

Figure 1. Complications and treatments of thalassemia patients with iron overload

Consequently, iron overload and accumulation introduces progressive damage in the liver, heart and in the endocrine glands. Plasma NTBI occurs in patients who have had multiple blood transfusions. NTBI was originally identified in reference [18] for playing a major role in the pathological conditions of iron overload. Circulating NTBI, as well as LPI, is detected whenever the capacity of transferrin to incorporate iron is derived either from the GI tract or when RES becomes a limiting factor. Both forms of toxic iron appear primarily in transfused patients where the TIBC has been surpassed [19]. Pathologically, the NTBI fraction seems to be translocated across the cell membrane irregularly, while the LPI is redox active and susceptible to chelation [20]. Chronic iron overload has been attributed to highly elevated levels of plasma iron and high accumulations of tissue iron. Excessive iron accumulation in the vital organs is the cause of various liver diseases (e.g. hepatitis, hepatic fibrosis and hepatocellular carcinoma), cardiomyopathies (e.g. cardiac arrhythmia and heart failure) and endocrine gland dysfunction (e.g. diabetes, growth retardation, hypogonardism and hypoparathyroidism) [21, 22].

2.2. Chemistry of catalytic iron

Iron acts as a cofactor within the active site of key enzymes in the biochemical pathways and as a chemical catalyst in the unique redox activity. The iron can cycle between two oxidation states, ferric ion [Fe(III) or Fe^{3+}] and ferrous ion [Fe(II) or Fe^{2+}], allowing it to act as an electron donor and acceptor [23]. The biochemical functions of iron in vital cells are dependent on its chemical properties. Limitation of iron bioavailability under aerobic conditions occurs when the Fe^{2+} is rapidly oxidized in the solution to insoluble Fe^{3+} at physiological pH [$K_{\text{free Fe(III)}} = 10^{-18}$ M] [24]. Fe(III) iron is the most stable state of the biological complexes at physiological oxygen concentrations. Many complexes of iron and biomolecules (protein or simpler molecules) are involved with reduction potential or redox potential (E_h). The E_h of complexed iron in the range of a biological oxidant is +820 mV to the reductant at −320 mV, the redox reactions are reversible whereas the reaction may be irreversible for the iron complexes when the reduction potential occurs outside this range [1].

Iron is a crucial enzyme cofactor that acts in the reduction-oxidation reaction in the metabolism in the cells. Of outstanding interest, iron deposition in the heart cells can lead to oxidative stress and cellular damage [25-27]. Heart failure is the leading cause of death among hemosiderotic β-thalassemia patients, of whom, around 60% die of this cardiac failure [28-30]. The importance of metals to both enzymatic reactions and oxidative stress makes them the key players in mitochondria. Mitochondria are the primary energy-generating organelles of the cells that produce ATP through a chain of enzymatic complexes that require cytochromes iron and sulfur-iron, and are highly sensitive to oxidative damage. Moreover, the heart is one of the most mitochondria-rich tissues in the body, making metals of particular importance to cardiac function [31]. In cardiac cells, excess iron may result in oxidative stress and an alteration of myocardial function because of the DNA damage that is caused by hydrogen peroxide through the Fenton reaction [6, 32]. Harmful effects of iron overload on the hearts of patients with β-thalassemia major can be monitored [25, 33-38] and treatment with effective iron chelators can protect these patients from cardiac arrhythmia [39, 40]. Iron catalyzes the production of ROS including $O_2^{\bullet -}$, H_2O_2 and $^{\bullet}OH$ via Haber-Weiss and Fenton reactions (Figure 2).

$$O_2^{\bullet -} + H_2O_2 \xrightarrow{\text{Fe / Cu}} HO^{\bullet} + HO^{-} + O_2 \qquad \textit{Haber-Weiss reaction}$$

$$Fe^{2+} + H_2O_2 \longrightarrow Fe^{3+} + HO^{\bullet} + HO^{-} \qquad \textit{Fenton reaction}$$

Figure 2. Hydroxyl radical formation in metals-catalyzed Haber-Weiss and Fenton reactions [41]

http://dx.doi.org/10.5772/57372

Another Fenton reagent can be hemichromes, which are a family of denatured methemoglobins [42]. Hydroxyl radicals might be most harmful to lipid, protein and DNA, which are the essential cell components (Figure 3). The •OH-induced membrane damage can be related directly to a membrane-associated Fenton reagent [43]. Oxidative cell damage has been attributed to the emergence of excessive levels of LPI that promote the production of ROS to a level that exceeds the cellular defense capacity [44].

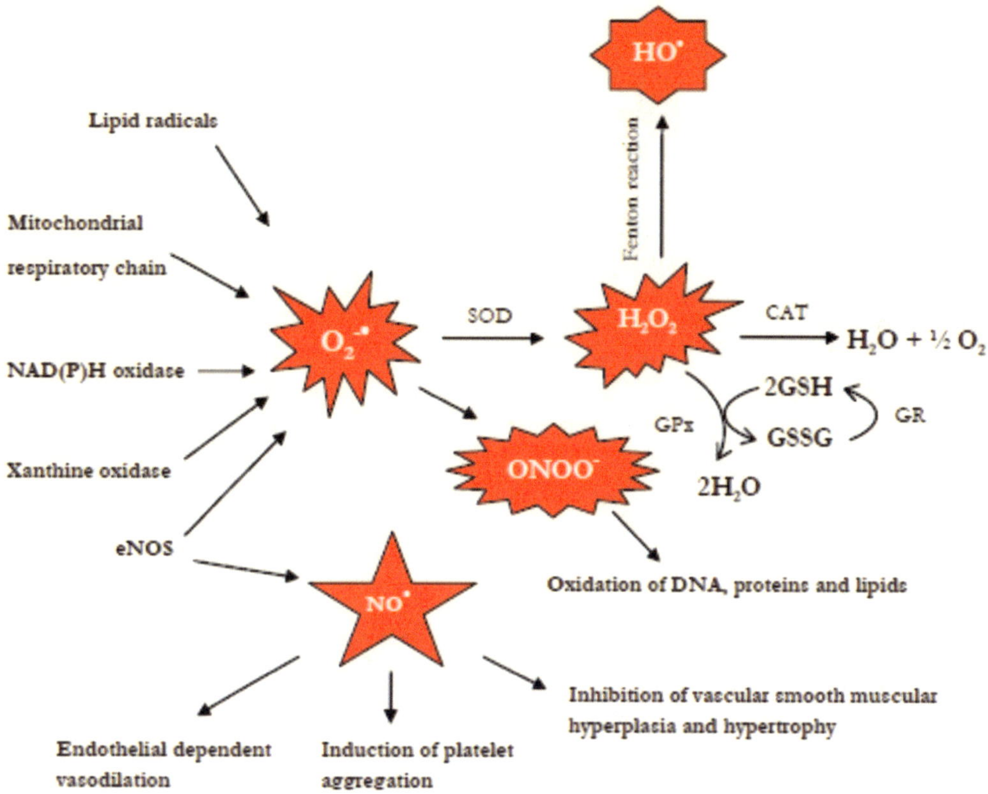

(CAT = catalase, GSH = reduced glutathione, GSSG = oxidized glutathione, SOD = siperoxide dismutase, GPx = glutathione peroxidase, GR = glutathione reductase)

Figure 3. Production and harmfulness of ROS (Reprinted with modification from [45])

In β-thalassemia major patients, an outpouring of catabolic iron overwhelms the capacity of iron-transporting protein transferrin, and generates NTBI and redox-active LPI in the plasma compartment. Cytosolic LIP has been shown to be comprised of transitory Fe (II) and Fe (III) forms which are possibly mediated by specific cellular iron reductases [20, 44]. In sub-cellular organelles, mitochondrial iron serves in the formation of protein iron-sulfur clusters and porphyrins. Additionally, endosomal iron provides the translocation of the endocytosed iron into cytosol or mitochondria, while lysosomal iron is associated with the products of iron-protein degradation [46, 47]. LIP is a source of chelatable and redox-active transient iron in the cells that serves as a crossroads of the cellular iron metabolism. The nature of the LIP has been revealed by its capacity to promote ROS generation in its "rise and fall" patterns. LIP plays a role as a self-regulatory pool that is sensed by cytosolic iron-regulatory proteins (IRP) and its feedback is regulated by an IRP-dependent expression of iron import and storage. The LIP can also be modulated by biochemical mechanism that override the IRP regulatory loops and contributes to basic cellular functions.

2.3. Oxidative stress in thalassemia patients

In one study, β-thalassemia children were found to have elevated levels of thiobarbituric acid reactive substances (TBARS), NAD(P)H oxidase (NOX) and SOD activity. Additionally, they were found to have decreased levels of CAT activity and reduced glutathione (GSH) concentration, along with unchanged GPx activity in their plasma compared to the plasma of the controls' [48]. Seminal SOD and CAT activities of homozygous β-thalassemic patients with iron overload were increased, probably due to a compensatory reaction to the persistence of high levels of ROS. Increased seminal lipid peroxidation could have contributed to the impairment of sperm motility [49]. Erythrocyte free reactive (non-heme) iron was significantly higher in β-thalassemia patients with HbE (30% >controls), which was associated with a high level of serum TBARS (86% >controls) [50]. Elevated serum ferritin showed a positive correlation with elevated levels of such liver enzymes as aspartate aminotransferase (AST), alanine aminotransferase (ALT) and alkaline phosphatase (ALP), but not γ-glutamyl transferase (GGT), confirming hepatic iron overload. Serum ferritin also showed a positive correlation with elevated levels of plasma TBARS and SOD. Plasma TBARS concentrations were increased in patients with α-thalassemia trait, and increased to the highest level in Hb H disease patient. Plasma levels of vitamin A, C, and E were significantly decreased in α- and β-thalassemia patients [51, 52]. In addition, their RBC revealed lower levels of vitamin E, GSH, CAT and SOD [51].

Isolated Hb chains can behave as pro-oxidants that can trigger oxidation of low-density lipoprotein (LDL). Importantly, the descending order of the different Hb chains to the relative oxidation of LDL protein, Apoprotein B (ApoB) and lipid parts was: α-globin chains > β-globin chains > HbA. This indicates that the extracellular globin chains may be the trigger of the lipoprotein alterations observed in β-thalassemia patients [53] and suggests that iron overload should be involved in the oxidative stress shown in the cells [54]. In comparison with apoprotein E2 (apoE2) and apoprotein E3 (apoE3) apoprotein E4 (apoE4) is considered the least efficient under conditions of oxidative stress in thalassemia patients and this imples that apoE4 is a genetic risk factor for left venticular dysfunction [55]. Mean triglyceride concentrations were not significantly different between thalassemia patients and the controls. Total cholesterol and LDL-cholesterol concentrations were found to be lower in β-thalassemia major and thalassemia intermediate patients than in the controls (p <0.001), while HDL-cholesterol concentrations were lower in thalassemia intermediate patients (p<0.03) [56]. This may account for increased erythropoiesis and cholesterol consumption in thalassemia intermediate patients, and iron overload and oxidative stress in β-thalassemia major patients. A previous

http://dx.doi.org/10.5772/57372

revision suggested that iron-induced free radical formation in thalassemia patients might lead to lipid peroxidation, LDL oxidation, stimulation of apoptosis and other damaging processes. The essence in the chelating and antioxidant treatments of thalassemia patients has to be considered within the context of free radical damage and its prevention [57].

Afanas'ev identified the major routes of superoxide damaging effects in the mitochondria. These include initiation of apoptosis through a reduction of cytochrome c, activation of uncoupled proteins by superoxide and a competition between superoxide and nitric oxide at the Complex IV site (or cytochrome oxidase). The author suggests an application of effective free radicals scavengers (rutin and flavonoids) for the treatment of thalassemic patients [58, 59]. From a comprehensive study in Indonesia, non-transfused thalassemia intermedia patients showed mild signs of oxidative stress and increased hemoglobin degradation, but revealed no significant indication of tissue or cell damage. Transfusion-dependent β-thalassemia major patients showed a highly significant decrease in antioxidants and thiols, and a tremendous iron overload along with cell damage. This situation was made even worse in long-term transfused patients [60]. ROS and lipid peroxidation were found to be higher, and GSH lower, in thalassemic RBC compared with normal RBC at the baseline as well as following the hydrogen peroxide treatment. These effects were reversed by treatment with antioxidative *N*-acetylcysteine (NAC) [61]. Platelets obtained from β-thalassemia patients contained higher ROS and lower GSH contents than those from normal donors, indicating a state of oxidative stress. Exposure of platelets to oxidants such as hydrogen peroxide and tert-butylhydroperoxide, or to the platelet activators (e.g. thrombin), ionophore (e.g. valinomycin) or phorbol myristyl acetate (PMA), stimulated the platelets' oxidative stress. Iron, hemin and thalassemic RBC also stimulated the platelets' oxidative stress. Therefore, oxidative stress of the platelets can lead to the activation of thromboembolic events [62]. Basal ROS level expressed as mean fluorescent intensity (FI) was higher in thalassemia polymorphonuclear cells (PMN) (FI = 95.6±19.8) than in normal PMN (FI = 12.7±4.5). Treatment of thalassemia PMN with PMA markedly increased the basal ROS level; in comparison, treatment with antioxidants, such as NAC, vitamins C and vitamin E, reduced their basal ROS but enhanced their PMA response. Administration of effective antioxidants may compromise their antibacterial capacity and give prophylaxis for recurrent infections [63].

DNA damage can be caused by iron-induced free radicals in thalassemia patients. Lymphocytes from a normal female did not respond to ferric chloride or hemosiderin, but did to ferrous chloride and ferrous sulphate. Comparatively, lymphocytes from an Australian patient with Hb S/β-thalassemia (double heterozygote-sickle phenotype) were more sensitive to ferrous sulphate treatment. Interestingly, desferrioxamine (DFO) and deferiprone (DFP) reduced the response [64]. Erythrocyte GPx activity was significantly lower in non-chelated β-thalassemia major patients than those chelated with either DFO or DFP [65]. β-Thalassemia major patients were deficient in vitamin A, C, D, B and folic acid [66]. Levels of ceruloplasmin concentrations and its ferroxidase activity were significantly higher in the thalassemia patients than in the healthy controls. Interestingly, the levels were significantly higher in thalassemia patients with Hp2-2 phenotype than in patients with other phenotypes, suggesting that thalassemia patients with Hp 2-2 phenotype are under greater iron-driven oxidative stress [67]. Reduction of delta-aminolevulinic acid synthase (δ-ALA) activity and an increase of peroxiredoxin-2 expression in thalassemic erythroid cells might represent two novel stress-response protective systems [68].

2.4. Iron chelation therapy

Nowadays, DFO, DFP and deferasirox (DFX) are iron chelators of choice used for the treatment of β-thalassemia patients with iron overload. Their chemical structures are shown in Figure 4 [69-72]. DFO (Desferal®) is the first drug that was introduced in the 1970s to treat iron overload. The hexadentate chelator has an extremely high affinity for iron (III) (DFO : Fe = 1:1, $K_a = 10^{29}$) and a much lower affinity for other metal ions, such as zinc, calcium and magnesium [73]. DFO is poorly absorbed from the GI tract and rapidly excreted in the urine (plasma half-life of 5 - 10 minutes), it must be therefore administered parenterally; intravenously (*iv*), intramuscularly (*im*) or subcutaneously (*sc*) [8, 74]. However, the drug exhibits side effects including an elevated body iron burden, serious neurotoxicity and abnormalities of cartilage formation [75-78]. DFP (L1 or Ferriprox®), a synthetic bidentate chelator, has been the first orally active drug available for clinical use. A previous study demonstrated DFP decreased serum ferritin and liver iron concentrations in transfusion-dependent thalassemia patients [79]. Using magnetic resonance imaging (MRI) technique, DFP was able to reduce cardiac iron overload and improve cardiac function more effectively when compared to patients treated with DFO [80]. Recently, the Government Pharmaceutical Organization (GPO) of Thailand has manufactured and launched domestically produced DFP product (GPO-L-One®) for the treatment of Thai thalassemia patients with iron overload. This will make the in-house DFP cheaper and more available than the imported DFP. However, its side effects include nausea, vomiting, gastrointestinal disturbance, leucopenia and thrombocytopenia and zinc deficiency, as they are typically observed these side effects are being evaluated in the patients [81, 82]. DFX (ICL670 or Exjade®), a tridentate oral chelator with a high affinity and specificity for iron, has been clinically used for the treatment of transfusion-dependent thalassemia patients since 2003 [83-85]. Efficacy and safety of DFX uses have previously been evaluated and reported [83, 84, 86-88]. Common side effects of DFX are abdominal symptoms (usually diarrhea), skin exanthems, elevated serum creatinine levels and renal tubular dysfunction [70].

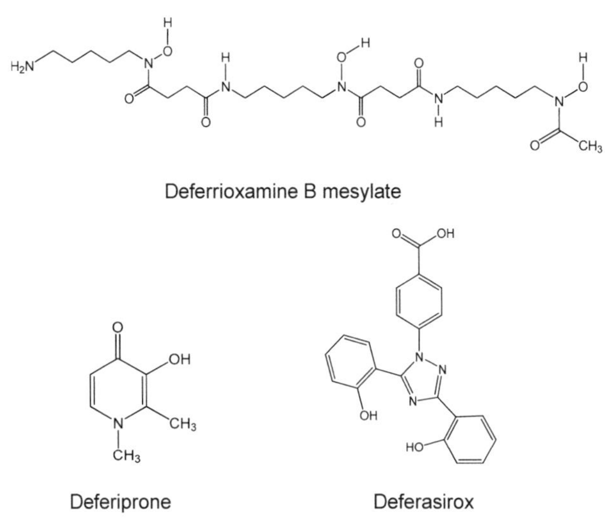

Figure 4. Chemical structures of DFO, DFP and DFX (Redrawn with modification from [89])

In the medical regimen, DFO must be subcutaneously infused in β-thalassemia patients for extensive periods in order to achieve a negative iron balance, ranging from 8 to 12 hours, five to seven times per week, and at a daily dosage of 20 to 60 mg/kg body weight [72]. The patients experienced pain and swelling at the injection site, cumulatively leading to poor patient compliance [89, 90]. DFO chelation along with DFP or DFX has been designed to improve the efficacy and to diminish the adverse effects in the treated patients [91, 92]. Ideally, the iron chelator should be orally active, cheap and highly specific for iron, but not for other metal ions, and should freely penetrate into the target tissues, so as to get the patients compliant and show minimal side effects. Chelators can act upon different iron pools, including transferrin-bound iron (TBI), NTBI and LPI in plasma compartment, and LIP in cytoplasm to form iron-chelate(s) which will then be excreted in the urine and feces [8]. Clinical efficacy of chelation therapy has been evaluated at different periods of time, generally by following up the levels of the biochemical markers, including ferritin, total iron, TIBC, transferrin saturation, NTBI and LPI in plasma with colorimetry [93, 94], and of tissue biopsied iron with pathological examination (Perl's staining), as well as in organ iron with a semi-quantum uncoupled inductive device (SQUID) and magnetic resonance imaging (MRI) techniques [95-98]. Encompassing forms of plasma NTBI are readily chelated by effective iron chelators [19]. However, the pathologically relevant fraction of NTBI is that which is seemingly translocated across cell membranes in a non-regulated manner and leads to excessive iron accumulation in the liver, heart, pancreas and endocrine organs [20]. The LPI fraction is not only an accessible diagnostic marker of iron overload and cell toxicity, but also a clinical parameter for assessing the mode and efficacy of chelation therapy.

3. Antioxidants

Antioxidants can be defined as compounds that inhibit or delay, but do not completely prevent oxidation. There are two basic categories of antioxidants, namely synthetic and natural antioxidants.

3.1. Synthetic antioxidants

Mostly, the synthetic antioxidants that are widely used are phenolic compounds; for example, butylated hydroxyanisole, butylated hydroxytoluene, tertiary-butylhydroquinone and gallic acid (GA) derivatives.

3.2. Natural antioxidants

Natural antioxidants are found to be present in many sources such as plants, fungi, microorganism and even animal tissues. Phenolic compounds are also the majority group of natural antioxidants. The three important groups of antioxidant are tocopherols, flavonoids and phenolic acid. Natural antioxidants have been widely used in complementary and alternative medicines; in comparison, the synthetic antioxidants have reported signs of toxicological evidence and caution should be imposed in their use. Most importantly, some natural antioxidants are more potent, efficiency and safer than synthetic antioxidants.

Synthetic antioxidant	Natural antioxidant
Inexpensive	Expensive
Widely applied	Use restricted to some products
Medium to high antioxidant activity	Wide-ranging antioxidant activity
Increasing safety concerns	Perceived as innocuous substances
Use banned in some cases	Increasing use and expanding application
Low water solubility	Broad range of solubility
Decreasing interest	Increasing interest

Table 1. Advantage and disadvantage of natural and synthetic antioxidants.

Advantages and disadvantages of the antioxidants are mentioned in Table 1. Most natural antioxidants are obtained in the diet from natural sources, especially from food of plant origin. Vegetables, fruits, and other foodstuffs are the best sources of these natural antioxidants. These antioxidants include vitamin C, vitamin E, carotenoids and polyphenol compounds. Antioxidants that are derived from natural sources are preferred by consumers. This is due to concerns over the toxic and carcinogenic effects of the synthetic antioxidants. Phenolic compounds include a large class of phytochemicals with interesting biological properties. Recently, the roles of these natural compounds in counteracting the negative effects of ROS/RNS and maintaining the redox homeostasis of biological fluids have been reported. Commonly, antioxidants can neutralize potentially harmful ROS in the cells before they induce lipid and proteins oxidation. Antioxidants from plants are believed to be useful in preventing aging, atherosclerosis, cancer, peptic ulcer, liver diseases and other degenerative pathologies, such as cancer, diabetes, Alzheimer's and Parkinson's diseases.

Antioxidants are any substances that significantly delay or inhibit oxidation of the oxidized substrate. These can greatly reduce the adverse damage to oxidants by crumbling or scavenging free radicals before they react with biological targets such as biomolecules, subcellular organelles, cells and tissues. The defense systems against the damage induced by ROS/reactive nitrogen species (RNS) fall into three categories: 1) preventive antioxidants that suppress free radical formation, 2) radical-scavenging antioxidants that inhibit initiation of chain reactions and intercept chain propagation and repair processes, and 3) adaptation to generate and transfer appropriate antioxidant enzymes. The hydrophilic antioxidants include vitamin C, uric acid, bilirubin, albumin, and the lipophilic antioxidants include vitamin E, ubiquinol and carotenoids. The radicals-scavenging antioxidant is described as a primary antioxidant, such as flavonoids and vitamin E (α-tocopherol), and the others that do not involve direct scavenge radical are secondary antioxidants.

4. Potential antioxidants for use in thalassemias

Oxidative stress is not only a simple imbalance between the production and scavenging of ROS, but also a dysfunction of the enzymes involved in ROS production. Dysfunction of NOX, uncoupling endothelial nitric oxide synthase (eNOS), activation of xanthine oxidase (XO) and dysfunction of the mitochondria are underlying signs of oxidative stress; therefore, NOX is one of important therapeutic targets [99]. Pharmacological agents and approaches, as shown in Figure 5, can be implemented to relieve oxidative stress by the following mechanisms.

1) Inhibition of NAD(P)H oxidase activity:

1.1) Apocynin (methoxy-substituted catechol) is a natural compound that has a structure related to vanillin and exhibits anti-inflammatory activity, blocks an assembly of $p47^{phox}$ onto membrane complex, decreases production of superoxide, enhances production of nitric oxide and disrupts active NOX complex [100].

1.2) Chimeric peptides, such as polyethylene glycol-superoxide and NOX inhibitory peptide (gp91dstat), can inhibit association of $p47^{phox}$ with $gp91^{phox}$ [101] and synthesis of Angiotensin converting enzyme II (ACE-II) a dipeptidyl carboxy-peptidase that generates the vasoconstricting peptide angiotensin II [102].

1.3) Compound S17834 (e.g. benzo(b)pyran-4-one) inhibits NOX activity and superoxide radical production and attenuates atherosclerotic lesions in apolipoprotein-E-deficient mice [103].

1.4) Statins (e.g. simvastatin) are hydroxymethylglutaryl CoA (HMG CoA) reductase inhibitor hypocholesterolemic drugs that can prevent production of hydrogen peroxide and superoxide radicals, interfere with the renin-angiotensin-aldosterone system, and inhibit NOX activation and expression [99]. Currently, Zacharski and colleagues have demonstrated that statins increased HDL/LDL ratios and reduced serum ferritin levels in subjects with advanced peripheral arterial disease. The results imply that statins may improve cardiovascular disease (CVD) outcomes, possibly by countering the pro-inflammatory effects of excess iron stores [104].

1.5) ACE-II inhibitors (e.g. captopril, enalapril and quinapril) may act as antioxidants and down-regulate the vascular NOX system. Angiotensin II, through Angiotensin I (AT1) receptor activation, can induce vasoconstriction, cell growth, actions of pro-inflammatory cytokines and profibrogenic agents, and the production of vascular ROS, such as superoxide radicals [105]. Hence, the ACE-II inhibitors would lower ROS production and prevent vascular and renal changes.

1.6) AT1 receptor antagonists (e.g. candesartan, losartan and irbesartan) reduce the expression of NOX enzyme components, resulting in lower superoxide levels and increased nitric oxide bioavailability in rat blood vessels [106].

1.7) Other blockers including calcium channel blocker (e.g. amlodipine, nifedipine and dihydropyridine), β-blocker (e.g. metoprolol, propranolol and nebivolol) and α-receptor blocker (e.g. doxazosin) can inhibit or interfere with functions of NOX activity [106, 107].

2) Vitamins and dietary antioxidants (e.g. vitamin C, vitamin E, β-carotene, polyphenols, flavonoids, olive oil and nuts) can decrease the oxidation of LDL (bad cholesterol), improve vascular endothelial functions, enhance NOS activity and attenuate NOX activity in rat aorta.

3) L-Arginine is a nitric oxide generator that can improve vascular function and regulate NOS expression and synthesis.

4) Thiol-containing compounds (e.g. α-lipoic acid and NAC) potentially inhibit LDL oxidation, decrease oxidative stress, and attenuate hypertension, insulin resistance and oxidative stress.

5) Estrogen and hormone replacement therapy can reduce the morbidity and mortality associated with CVD, lower production of superoxide radicals, up-regulate NOS gene expression, activate cyclo-oxygenase (COX) gene and reduce the production of vasoconstrictor endothelin.

6) Cu/Zn SOD (MW = 31 kD) mimetics are selective synthetic compounds; for example, M40401 (MW = 483), M40403 (MW = 501), SC-55858, that either inhibit their formation or remove superoxide anion [108].

7) Xanthine oxidase inhibitors (e.g. oxypurinol and allopurinol) improve endothelial function in hypercholesterolemic subjects, type II diabetic mellitus (DM) patients, congestive heart failure (CHF) and cigarette smokers.

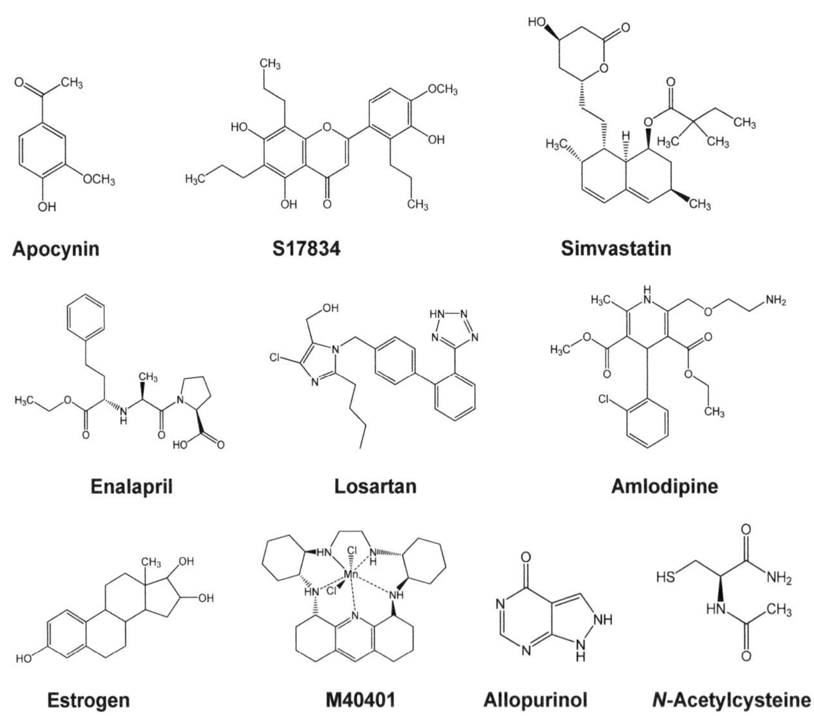

Figure 5. Drugs used for therapeutic purposes exhibits antioxidant activity

5. Benefits of antioxidants in thalassemia patients

5.1. Administration in thalassemia patients

β-Thalassemia major patients who suffered from leg ulcers and were treated with ascorbic acid (3 g/day) for eight weeks showed a high rate of either complete or partial healing [109]. Improvement of ulcer healing in β-thalassemia major patients was observed when they were orally administered with pentoxifylline (1.2 g/day) which is xanthine derivative and functions as a competitive non-selective phosphodiesterase inhibitor [110]. Plasma antioxidant enzyme activity and selenium concentration increased in subjects with the Hb Lepore trait and were found to be significantly low in those patients with the α-thalassemia trait, while erythrocyte Se content was significantly increased in α-thalassemia patients [111]. *N*-allylsecoboldine may act as an effective antioxidant and protect cells against oxidative damage in β-thalassemic red blood cells [112]. Plasma vitamin E levels were lower in β-thalassemia intermedia patients compared to the controls and these levels were positively correlated with vitamin E in the LDL [113]. Treatment of the patients with vitamin E (600 mg/day, orally) for nine months improved the antioxidant/oxidant balance in the plasma, LDL particles and red blood cells, and counteracted the lipid peroxidation processes [114].

Significant decrease of GSH and proliferation in peripheral blood mononuclear cells (PBMC) were found in β-thalassemia major patients, probably due to the abnormality of cell mediated immunity (CMI) under iron overload conditions. Treatment of the patients with silymarin, which is an extract of milk thistle seed containing anti-hepatotoxic silibinin, led to a restoration of the GSH levels and PBMC proliferation, suggesting antioxidant and immunostimulatory activities and the benefits of using flavonoids to normalize immune dysfunction in β-thalassemia major patients [115]. *In vitro* treatment of blood cells from β-thalassemia patients with *N*-acetylcysteine amide (AD4), NAC and vitamin C increased the reduced GSH content of RBC, platelets and PMN leukocytes, and reduced their ROS. Intra-peritoneal injection of AD4 to β-thalassemic mice (150 mg/kg) reduced the parameters of oxidative stress (p <0.001). These may imply the superiority of AD4, compared to NAC, in reducing oxidative stress markers in thalassemic cells, both *in vitro* and *in vivo,* and also providing a significant reduced sensitivity of thalassemic RBC to hemolysis and phagocytosis by macrophages [116]. *In vitro* treatment of blood cells from β-thalassemia patients with fermented papaya preparation (FPP) increased the GSH content in the RBC, platelets and PMN leukocytes, and reduced their ROS, membrane lipid peroxidation and phosphatidylserine (PS) externalization. Importantly, oral administration of FPP to β-thalassemia mice (50 mg/mouse/day for 3 months) and to thalassemia patients (3 g x 3 times/day for 3 months) reduced the levels of the oxidative stress parameters significantly. Suggestively, the FFP would be beneficial in reducing thalassemic RBC sensitivity to hemolysis and phagocytosis by macrophages, improving PMN ability to generate the oxidative burst and to reduce the platelet tendency to undergo activation [117].

Treatment of thalassemic RBC with erythropoietin (Epo) increased their GSH content and reduced their ROS, membrane lipid hydroperoxides, and PS exposure. Injection of Epo into heterozygous β-thalassemia mice reduced the oxidative markers. Probably, Epo might likely be an antioxidant that can alleviate symptoms of hemolytic anemia and reduced susceptibility of RBC to undergo hemolysis and phagocytosis [118]. Thalassemic lymphocytes exhibited approximately a two-fold increase in the sensitivity to treatment of food mutagen/carcinogen, 3-amino-1-methyl-5H-pyrido(4,3-b)indole (or Trp-P-2) *in vitro*. However, treatment with flavonoids (quercetin and kaempferol) reduced the responses to Trp-P-2 to untreated control levels, significantly [119]. Transfusion-dependent thalassaemia patients were vitamin E deficient (0.45±0.21 mg/dl in all patients, 0.43±0.19 mg/dl in splenectomized patients), when compared to healthy subjects (0.76±0.22 mg/dl). Replacement therapy with vitamin E is necessary to correct its low serum levels easily (0.36±0.13 mg/dl before therapy and 1.19±0.35 mg/dl after therapy) [120]. Paraoxonase (PON) and arylesterase activities were significantly lower in β-thalassemia major patients than in the control healthy subjects, whereas total oxidant status, total peroxide concentration levels, and the oxidative stress index were significantly higher in the patients than in the controls in reference [121]. In addition, the activity of prolidase, a hydrolytic enzyme involved in collagen degradation was significantly increased in β-thalassemia major patients (53.7±8.7 U/l) compared to the control group (49.2±7.2 U/l). Total oxidant status was significantly increased in the patients (5.31±3.14 mmol H_2O_2 equivalent/l) compared to the controls (3.49±2.98 μmol H_2O_2 equivalent/l). Oxidative stress index was significantly increased in the patients (3.86±3.28 arbitrary unit) compared to the controls (2.53±2.70 arbitrary unit), while antioxidant capacity expressed as TEAC (1.61±0.30 μM) in the patients' plasma and this was not significantly different from that (1.64±0.33 μM) of the controls' plasma [122]. Administration of lipophilic antioxidant vitamin E (10 mg/kg/day for 4 weeks) is beneficial in the management of transfusion-dependant β-thalassemia HbE patients [123]. A current study has demonstrated that levels of iron parameters, such as serum ferritin, NTBI and transferrin receptors, were significantly increased in β-thalassemia major and thalassemia intermedia patients, compared to the controls and in severe cases when compared to the mild cases. Levels of serum ferritin, MDA, NTBI and GSSG/GSH were significantly increased in thalassemia intermedia patients; activities of serum glutathione reductase (GR), GPx and SOD were significantly reduced in these patients; while serum ascorbic acid concentrations were mildly reduced in the patients [124]. Interestingly, DFP has been reported to be a potent pharmaceutical antioxidant [125].

Patients with Hb H disease, β-thalassemia/Hb E and β-thalassemia major had vitamin E deficiency; however, supplements of vitamin E and selenium to the patients prevented RBC oxidation and increased RBC resistance to oxidative damage [126, 127]. There were no significant differences in the mean serum vitamin A, E concentrations and the vitamin E/cholesterol ratio between pregnant women with normal hemoglobin and hemoglobinopathies (Hb E and thalassemia) [128]. Patients with β^0-thalassemia/Hb E disease with lower blood Hb concentration had significantly higher erythrocyte SOD activity and the Hb concentrations were inversely correlated with the SOD activities ($p < 0.001$) [129]. Supplementation of vitamin C plus vitamin E has greater benefits than vitamin E alone in promoting antioxidant status [130]. Administration of CoQ_{10} (100 mg/day) for six months markedly increased activities of plasma SOD, CAT and GPx, and decreased plasma MDA concentration of β-thalassemia HbE patients [131]. Increased oxidative stress in β-thalassemia/Hb E patients relates to higher levels of MDA, SOD and GPx in RBC, serum NTBI, and lower level of RBC GSH.

5.2. Intervention of antioxidants in β-knockout (BKO) thalassemia mice

Nowadays, all clinical trials in humans and animals need to be approved by highly experienced ethical committees. Accurate animal models that recapitulate the phenotype and genotype of patients with β-thalassemia would enable researchers to develop possible therapeutic approaches. In this case thalassemic mice have been developed by groups of researchers [132-135]. The Thalassemia Research Center at Mahidol University, Salaya Campus in collaboration with the Murdoch Children Research Institute Melbourne, Australia have inbred wild type (WT) C57BL/6, β-knock (BKO) thalassemia ($Hb\beta^{th-3}/Hb\beta^{+}$), β-thalasssemia/HbE ($LCR\varepsilon^{G}\gamma^{A}\gamma\delta\beta^{E}$) $Hb\beta^{+}/Hb\beta^{+}$) (HT HbE), double heterozygous ($LCR\varepsilon^{G}\gamma^{A}\gamma\delta\beta^{E}$) $Hb\beta^{+}/Hb\beta^{th-3}$) (DH) and rescued β-thalassemia Hb E ($LCR\varepsilon^{G}\gamma^{A}\gamma\delta\beta^{E}$) $Hb\beta^{0}/Hb\beta^{0}$) (rescued β/HbE) mice in order to investigate the properties of the potential antioxidants and iron-chelating agents.

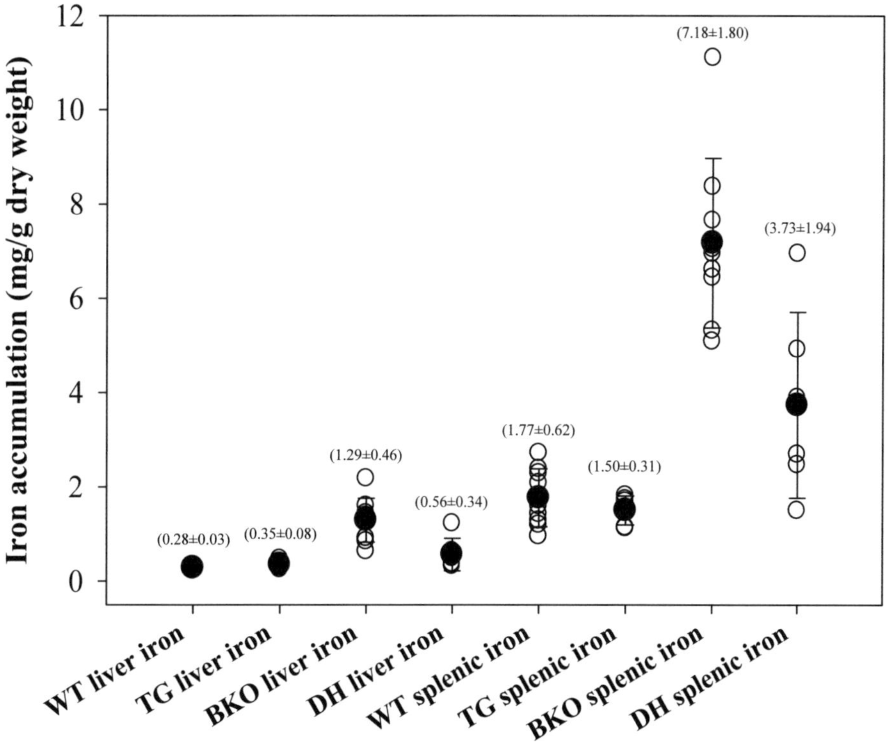

Figure 6. Iron deposition in the livers and spleens of the wild type (WT), transgenic (TG), β-knockout (BKO) thalassemia and double heterozygous (DH) thalassemia mice (S. Srichairatanakool, unpublished data)

Having measured the amounts of tissue iron of the WT and thalassemia mice, the BKO mice had the highest iron content accumulated in the livers and spleens when compared to the TG mice and WT mice, which the splenic iron content was far higher than the liver iron content (Figure 7). The results indicated that anemic conditions persisting in the BKO mice were similar to β-thalassemia intermedia and enhanced an increase of duodenal iron absorption for accelerating erythropoiesis. In our experimentations, feeding the BKO mice with a high iron diet (such as iron ferrocene) can load iron into their blood and tissue compartments, leading to iron overload and oxidative tissue damage. Their hematological parameters were determined and are illustrated in Table 2 [136]. Most importantly, the BKO thalassemia mice were found to be the most anemic when compared to the other types of thalassemia mice and their phenotype mimiced the human thalassemia intermedia patients. The mice heterozygous for deletion of the β-globin gene appear normal, but their hematologic indices show the characteristics that were typical of thalassemia intermedia. These include dramatically decreased hematocrit (Hct), hemoglobin (Hb) and red blood cell counts [136]. Bone deformities and splenic enlargement due to increased hematopoiesis [137], and iron overload in the vital organs (e.g. spleen, liver and kidneys) were also found in the heterozygous β-thalassemic mice, in reference [138].

Mice	RBC ($x10^6$ cells/μl)	Hb (g/dl)	Hct (%)	MCV (fl)	MCH (pg)	RDW (%)	Reticulocyte (%)	ROS (Mean FI)	PS cell (%)
WT	8.37±0.54	13.35±0.85	39.32±3.22	46.95±1.41	15.96±0.48	12.64±1.25	3.88±0.74	7.51±3.85	1.06±0.56
HT Hb E	7.95±0.36	12.24±0.56	35.69±1.58	44.93±0.84	15.40±0.35	14.47±0.79	4.65±0.86	3.28±0.43	0.87±0.29
BKO	5.34±0.63	7.06±0.61	22.86±2.05	43.05±2.95	13.32±1.09	23.17±2.53	29.01±5.76	170.1±24.6	3.35±0.75
DH	8.32±0.51	12.81±1.09	38.55±3.15	46.34±2.33	15.41±0.96	14.15±1.16	3.64±1.70	13.86±2.98	1.07±0.35
Rescued β/ Hb E	8.87+0.87	11.08±1.17	38.02±3.54	42.93±2.06	12.52±0.51	20.03±1.43	15.12±3.33	117.4±67.2	1.24±0.72

Abbreviations: Hb = hemoglobin, Hct = hematocrit, MCV = mean corpuscular volume, MCH = mean corpuscular hemoglobin, RDW = RBC distribution width, ROS = reactive oxygen species, PS = phosphatidylserine.

Table 2. Hematological parameters (mean±SD) of erythrocyte WT and β-thalassemia mice (Redrawn from Wannasuphaphol et al. [136]

5.2.1. *Curcuminoids*

Curcuminoids derived from *Curcuma longa* Linn. (turmeric) contained curcumin (diferuloylmethane), demethoxycurcumin (*p,p'*-dihydroxyldicinnamoylmethane), as well as *bis*-demethoxycurcumin (*p*-hydroxylcinnamoylmethane), which curcumin was found to be the most abundant and major active compound (Figure 7). Phenolic, methylene and β-diketo groups in the curcumin molecule participated in antioxidant, iron-chelating, free radical-scavenging and anti-lipid peroxidation activities.

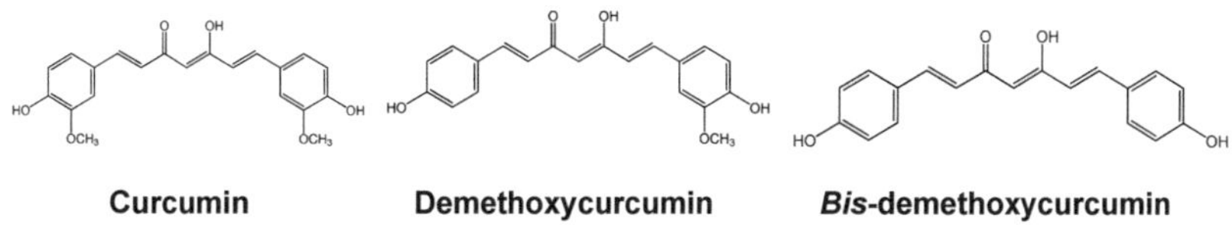

Figure 7. Chemical structures of curcumin, demethoxycurcumin and *bis*-demethoxycurcumin found in turmeric *Curcuma longa* Linn (Redrawn from http://www.molecular-cancer.com/18 September 2013)

Interestingly, curcumin can bind ferric and ferrous ions, in a concentration-dependent manner and with a molar ratio of 1:1, to form a red colored complex with a predominant peak at 500 nm. The curcumin itself chelates biological iron (e.g. plasma NTBI) and can work with DFP in lowering plasma NTBI levels more efficiently *in vitro* [139]. Curcuminoids effectively reduced levels of plasma NTBI, and liver weight index, non-heme iron, plasma and liver MDA concentrations, but increased the plasma GSH concentrations of iron-loaded BKO thalassemic mice [138]. Our results of the atomic absorption spectrometric and Perl's staining examinations demonstrated that curcumin was able to decrease the accumulation of heart iron and to depress heart rate variability of BKO mice with iron overload, suggesting the cardioprotective effect of curcumin [140]. Treatment of β-thalassemia HbE patients with curcuminoids (Thailand GPO product, 500 mg/day) for three months increased erythrocyte SOD as well as the GPx activities and GSH concentrations, and lowered levels of plasma NTBI and platelet factor-3 like activity [141, 142]. The same researcher group has been using a cocktail containing DFP, vitamin E, NAC and the curcuminoids for treatment of the thalassemia patients and expected that the treatment would improve their iron overload and oxidative stress more effectively (Kalpravidh and coworkers, personal communication). A recent study has reported that iron content of HDL-2 and HDL-3 from β-thalassemia/HbE patients was higher while the cholesterol content was lower than those levels found in the healthy subjects. Thalassemic HDL-2 and HDL-3 had increased levels of conjugated diene, lipid hydroperoxide and TBARS. The thalassemic HDL had lower peroxidase activity than the control HDL and could not protect against $CuSO_4$-induced oxidation of LDL [143].

5.2.2. Tea

Recently, the demand for green tea has increased due to current trends in human health concerns and preference. The main components found in green tea are polysaccharides, flavonoids, vitamins B, C, E, γ-aminobutyric acid, catechin compounds and fluoride. Among them, catechin compounds have been of focus for their strong antioxidant capacity. The pharmaceutical activities of the components have been studied. Tea (*Camellia sinensis*) is an excellent source of polyphenols, namely catechins, including (-)-epicatechin (EC), (-)-epicatechin 3-gallate (ECG), (-)-epigallocatechin (EGC), (-)-epigallocatechin 3-gallate (EGCG), (+)-catechin (C) and (-)-gallocatechin (GC). Among them, EGCG exerted the strongest antioxidant capacity and was found to be the most abundant, as well. It has been reported that catechins possess free radical scavenging abilities and iron chelating properties [144]. Green tea also showed a protective effect under various oxidative-related pathologic conditions.

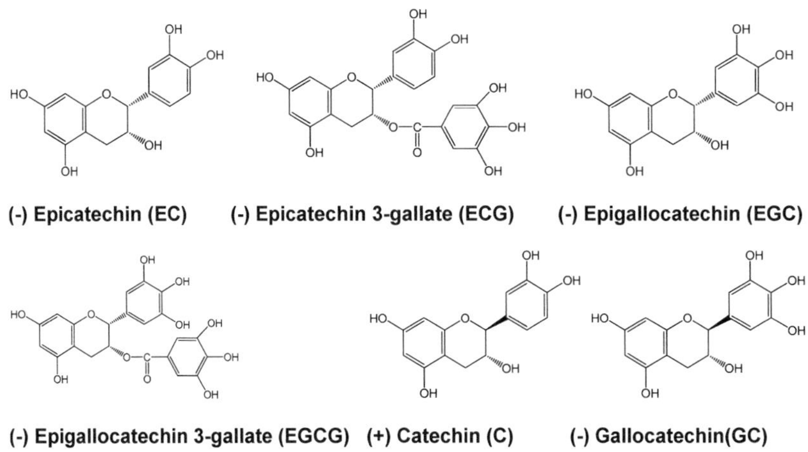

Figure 8. Chemical structures of catechins in tea (*Camellia sinensis*) (Redrawn from [145])

Drinking tea produced a 41 – 95% inhibition of dietary iron absorption in five β-thalassemia major and one β-thalassemia intermedia cases, which the iron absorption increased strikingly in the β-thalassemia intermedia cases, in references [146, 147]. Interestingly, Thai researchers have elucidated that green tea extract (GTE) and EGCG fraction were able to decrease iron (as NTBI) in plasma, eliminate plasma lipid-peroxidation product (as TBARS) and destroy the formation of erythrocyte ROS *in vitro* [144, 148] and in iron-loaded rats [149]. In addition, the GTE inhibited or delayed the deposition of hepatic iron in regularly iron-loaded BKO thalassemic mice effectively. This implies a prevention of iron-induced ROS generation and consequently liver damage and fibrosis by green tea consumption [150]. Our group has found that elevated levels of plasma NTBI and lipid peroxidation tended to be normalized in the BKO mice in response to oral therapy with GTE, while their plasma GSH concentrations were also increased by up to 2-times. The mice exhibited a decrease of the lipid peroxidation product and an improvement in the oxidant–antioxidant balance in erythrocytes. Importantly, GTE was effective in inhibiting hemolysis and thereby prolonged RBC half-life in the BKO mice (Sakaewan Ounjaijean PhD thesis. Chiang Mai University; 2011). Our current study has shown that the treatment of iron-loaded mouse hepatocytes and human hepatoma (HepG2) cells with GTE (0 – 100 mg/dl) and EGCG (0 – 200 μM) removed intracellular LIP and ROS efficiently, and relieved the mitochondrial membrane collapse, implying a hepatoprotective effect of green tea catechins in the hepatocytes with iron overload [151].

5.2.3. Mango (Mangifera indica L.)

Mangoes can be considered a good source of dietary antioxidants, such as ascorbic acid, carotenoids and phenolic compounds. *β*-carotene was found to be the most abundant carotenoid in several cultivars. The nutritional value of mango is that it is a source of vitamin C and provitamin A. Mangiferin (1,3,6,7-tetrahydroxyxanthone-2-glucopyranoside) (Figure 9) can interact with iron and other cations and also shows antioxidant activity by eliminating the superoxide radical *in vitro*, in which 100 μM of mangiferin was equivalent to the activity of 1

U/ml of SOD. This also revealed the pharmacologic effects modulating gene expression that were related to the inflammatory response [152]. Mangiferin xanthone modulates the expression of many genes critical for apoptosis regulation, viral replication, tumorigenesis, inflammation and autoimmune diseases, suggesting its possible value in the treatment of inflammatory diseases and/or cancer [153]. Vimang mango peel extract with a high mangiferin content acted as an antioxidant and complexed with Fe^{3+} efficiently, leading to protection of iron-induced oxidative liver damage and DNA fragmentation [154, 155]. Hydrolysable gallotannin present in mango kernels showed the inhibitory effects of bacterial growth, which was probably due to their iron-complexing properties [156].

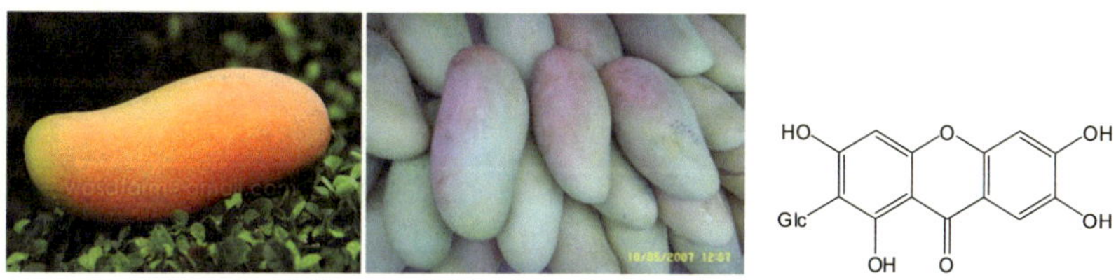

Ripe and green Mahajanaka mango

mangiferin

(www.nanagarden.com)

Figure 9. Fresh mango and chemical structure of mangiferin (Redrawn from [157])

Kaew mango peel extract can chelate both Fe^{3+} and Fe^{2+} to form the products with different predominant wavelengths, of which the binding was found to be dose-dependent and affinity-different. The green peel extract tended to exhibit stronger iron-binding abilities than the ripe peel extract and it is likely that the green peel might contain different kinds and amounts of phytochemical ingredients (Figure 10).

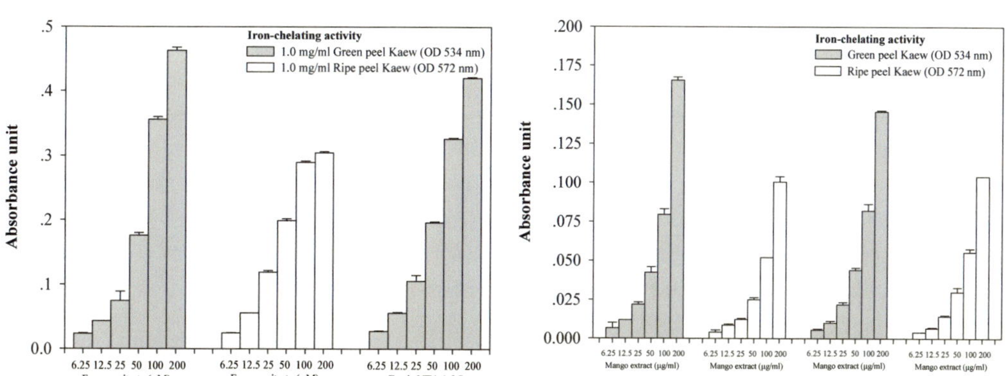

Figure 10. Iron-chelating activity of aqueous extract of Kaew mango peel (Srichairatanakool, S. unpublished data)

As shown in Table 2, the degree of antioxidant activity of the mango peel extracts were found to be Mahajanaka (ripe > green) > Chok-anan (green > ripe) > Namdocmai (green > ripe) > Kaew (ripe ~ green). The antioxidant activities were well correlated with their total phenolic contents and vitamin C concentrations. Incredibly, amounts of vitamin C in the extracts were lower than those of the total phenolic compounds. Mangiferin contents in the peel extracts were very low.

Mango/Status	Antioxidant activity (mg TEAC/g extract)	Total phenolics (mg GAE/g extract)	Vitamin C (mg/g extract)	Mangiferin (mg/g extract)
Mahajanaka/Ripe	225.6±4.4	107.6±9.6	5.49±0.23	1.49±0.25
Mahajanaka/Green	114.3±7.4	44.8±5.9	0.96±0.07	0.57±0.10
Chok-Anan/Ripe	120.1±5.4	46.0±7.0	0.75±0.08	4.62±0.37
Chok-Anan/Green	192.4±4.5	85.7±7.7	4.22±0.22	6.80±0.06
Namdocmai/Ripe	102.9±4.9	49.7±8.5	0.69±0.03	0.25±0.01
Namdocmai/Green	33.1±2.6	5.3±0.8	0.27±0.091	0.25±0.01
Kaew/Ripe	63.2±0.2	34.8±0.7	ND	0.02
Kaew/Green	65.3±0.1	55.9±0.3	ND	0.43

ND = not determined.

Table 3. Antioxidant activity, total phenolics, vitamin C and mangiferin contents (mean±SD) in aqueous extracts from ripe and green mango peels (Sricharatanakool, S. unpublished data)

5.2.4. Rice (Oryza sativa and Oryza glaberrima)

Rice is an economic cereal plant ±that is grown in many countries in Asian and Africa. Varieties of Asian rice include Thai rice (*O. sativa* cv. indica), Indonesian rice (*O. sativa* cv. javanica) and Japanese rice (*O. sativa* cv. japonica). Additionally, we have listed African rice (*O. glaberrima*). Regarding its nutritional values, rice grain contains carbohydrates (e.g. amylose and amylopectin) and rice bran is abundant in inositol, inositol hexaphosphate (or phytate), oil, ferulic acid, γ-oryzanol, phytosterol and tocotrienol. The ingredients in rice bran likely prevent carcinogenesis, hyperlipidemia, fatty liver, gallstone disease and heart diseases [158]. Red and purple rice bran possesses several fold higher hydrophilic and lipophilic anti-oxidative phenolics and flavonoids (predominantly cyanidine-3-glycoside) levels than freeze-dried blueberry and broccoli. Rice grass contains chlorophyll as a major ingredient and pheophytin (or pheo) as the second most abundant component (Figure 11). Pheophytin is synthesized in rice grass, spinach (*Spinacia oleracea*) leaves and *Michelia alba* leaves, but is not a degradation product of chlorophyll [159], and the compound reveals a level of antioxidant activity that is similar to that of ubiquinone [160].

Spinach pheophytin a (λ_{max} 409 nm) and pheophytin b (λ_{max} 435 nm) can chelate ferric ion and produce the Fe-pheophytin a complex (λ_{max} 393 nm) and Fe-pheophytin b complex (λ_{max} 421 nm) [161]. Germinating rice grain synthesizes iron-chelating compounds, deoxymugineic acid

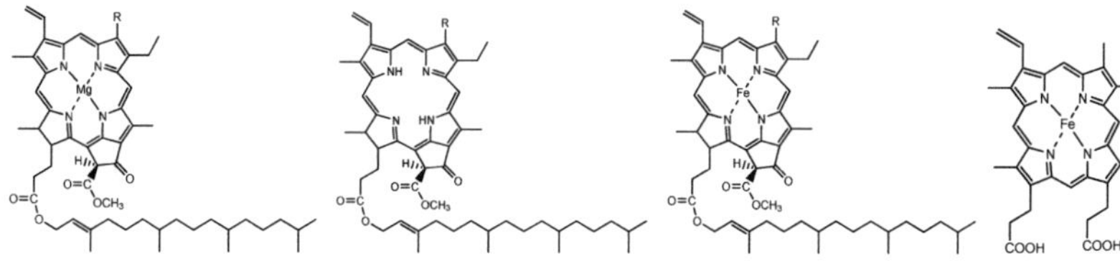

Figure 11. Chemical structures of chlorophyll, pheophytin, iron-pheophytin complex and heme [161]

and nicotinamine, and sequesters iron from the ground for their growth and development [162]. Interestingly, wheat grass (WG) juice which has been used as a general-purpose health tonic in Indian medicine and has shown at least a 25% reduction in the number of blood transfusions needed in β-thalassemia major patients [163] and also increased their blood hemoglobin levels [164]. Nonetheless, a contradictory report has shown that the oral administration of WG juice tablets for one year was not effective in reducing blood transfusions in transfusion-dependent β-thalassemia major patients [165].

Pimpilai and colleagues from Maejo University, Chiang Mai investigated the antioxidant activity of the Thai black rice grass (TBRG), Thai red rice grass (TRRG) and Thai fragrant rice grass (TFRG) extracts by using the TEAC colorimetric method and found that they exhibited antioxidant properties. The extracts dose dependently bound Fe^{3+} (ferric NTA) and Fe^{2+} (ferrous citrate) and formed the complex(s) with maximal absorption values at 393, 378 and 580 nm, respectively (personal communication). HPLC analysis showed different amounts of catechin derivatives as follows: 3.27 mg C, 4.51 mg EC and 5.19 mg EGCG in 1 g TBRG extract; 4.48 mg C, 6.22 mg EC and 5.23 mg EGCG in 1 g TRRG extract; and 5.89 mg C, 4.38 mg EC and 5.26 mg EGCG in 1 g TFRG extract. Currently, Pimpilai and Srichairatanakool have found that feeding rice grass (Sukhothai 1) extract (100 mg/kg body weight) along with a high iron diet to β-thalassemia mice for three months slightly increased their blood hemoglobin concentrations from 10.04±0.51 to 11.04±1.14 g/dl (unpublished data), while treatment with the extract (0, 50 and 100 μg/ml) decreased levels of liver MDA (153.6±44.7, 102.9±22.4 and 102.4±58.0 μg/mg tissue protein, respectively) and levels of labile iron (100±13, 120±1 and 125±5% fluorescent intensity, respectively) in iron-loaded HepG2 cell cultures. Therefore, the rice grass extracts would contain antioxidant compounds including chlorophyll, pheophytin and catechin derivatives, of which the two latter may play important roles in iron chelation and anti-lipid peroxidation to ameliorate oxidative tissue damage in the thalassemia cases with iron overload. Consequently, rice grass extracts need to be clinically studied in thalassemia patients in the near future.

6. Evaluation of oxidative stress and antioxidant status in thalassemias

Electron paramagnetic resonance (EPR) 'radical probe' was used to determine the total oxidative status in patients affected by thalassemia, and to evaluate new strategies of chelation, new chelators, or the efficacy of antioxidant formulas [166, 167]. Raman spectroscopic technique has been developed for the monitoring of Raman hemoglobin bands to evaluate oxygenation capability, oxidative stress and deformities of thalassemic erythrocytes and to assess the responses to drug therapies [168]. Consistent with the study, in reference [169], serum PON activity and total antioxidant capacity were significantly lower in patients with the β-thalassemia trait patients, MDA and carotid artery intima-media thickness were significantly higher in β-thalassemia trait. The total antioxidant capacity, MDA, and CIMT levels were correlated with serum PON1 (r = 0.945, -0.900, 0.940 and -0.922 respectively). Additionally, serum total antioxidant capacity and MDA levels were well correlated (r = -0.979) [170].

An earlier study in 1986 showed that patients with Hb H diseases, including α-thalassemia 1 or α-thalassemia 2 and 21 with α-thalassemia 1/Hb Constant Spring, had increased activities of erythrocyte SOD, GPx, and CAT when compared with those of the controls. The α-thalassemia 1/Hb CS patients had higher SOD and GPx activities, but lower CAT activity than the patients with α-thalassemia 1/2 [171, 172]. One year later, a study of oxidative stress and the antioxidants in β-thalassemia/hemoglobin E patients in Thailand was conducted [173]. Significantly higher levels of urine N-acetyl-β-D-glycosaminidase, MDA and β_2-microglobulin along with aminoaciduria and proximal tubular abnormalities were found in pediatric α-thalassemia patients (Hb H disease and HbS/CS), and this was possibly due to increased oxidative stress [174]. A one-year treatment with DFP significantly decreased serum ferritin, NTBI, and MDA (p <0.05) of transfusion-independent β-thalassemia/HbE patients. Mean pulmonary arterial pressure and pulmonary vascular resistance were diminished significantly (p <0.05). All those parameters were still improved after subgroup analysis was done for the high ferritin group (>2500 ng/ml). The results imply that DFP therapy alone improved iron overload and oxidative stress and the compliance was positive [175]. Oxidative stress was increased in Thai HbE/β-thalassemia patients, as the blood GSH decreased, GSH/GSSG ratio reduced markedly, superoxide anion released from blood cells elevated highly, and γ-glutamylcysteine ligase activity was increased. Additionally, basal forearm blood flow was significantly increased whereas forearm vasodilatory response to reactive hyperemia was depressed [176].

When using ESR spectroscopic quantification of hemin, the serum hemin readily catalyzed free radical reactions and it would be a major pro-oxidant in the blood circulation of β-thalassemia Hb E patients [177]. A previous study showed a precipitous decrease in α-tocopherol and increased TBARS concentrations in both plasma and lipoproteins obtained by Thai β-thalassemia Hb E patients. Cholesteryl linoleate showed a reduction of 70% in LDL, while other cholesterol ester levels showed a lower reduction. A good correlation of NTBI and TBARS (p <0.01) in LDL strongly supported the contention that iron overload is responsible for initiating the lipid peroxidation in thalassemia patients [178]. The ESR results demonstrated a magnitude of increased lipid fluidity in thalassemic lipoproteins. Lipid fluidity at the LDL and HDL cores showed a good correlation with the oxidative stress markers and the α-tocopherol level, suggesting that the hydrophobic region of the thalassemic lipoprotein would be a target site for oxidative damage [179]. Gas chromatography/mass spectrometric (GS/MS) technique has been validated in quantifying ortho- and meta-tyrosine as biomarkers of protein oxidative damage in plasma samples of β-thalassemia patients [180]. Pumala et al. have found that PON1 activity was significantly reduced in association with oxidative stress in the patients with β-thalassemia hemoglobin E, and significant correlations were observed between HDL-PON1 activity and oxidative stress markers (including plasma α-tocopherol and the ratio of cholesteryl linoleate to cholesteryl oleate in HDL, and a marked increased platelet-activating factor/acetylhydrolase (PAF-AH) activity [181]. The GC/MS-based assay showed that the level of urinary and plasma lipid peroxidation poroduct, F(2)-isoprostane in the thalassemic group was significantly increased [182]. An average antioxidant level in Thai thalassemia patients with the HbE trait (3.276±0.209 mM TEAC) was significantly decreased ($p = 0.008$) when compared to the healthy subjects (3.439±0.220 mM TEAC) [183]. It has been reported that Thai thalassemia major patients are associated with an alteration of CYP2E1 and CYP3A4 activities [184], but not CYP1A2 [185]. Anemia was not pronounced in the rescued mice (C57BL/6) with the Hb E transgene mimicing the human β-thalassemia/HbE phenotype; nonetheless, other hematologic parameters in their RBC include highly oxidative stress, no marked changes in PS and vesicles, and a shortened life span, which were abnormally similar to the BKO thalassemic RBC group [136].

7. Conclusions

Under iron overload, oxidative stress plays a major role in the pathophysiologic complications of thalassemia patients. Free extracellular toxic iron (e.g. NTBI and LPI) and intracellular redox iron (e.g. LIP and plasma membrane nonheme iron) that have been identified in thalassemic blood and tissues are responsible for the generation of oxidative stress by catalyzing a formation of oxygen radicals over the antioxidant capacity of the cells. Consequently, there is a rationale to support iron chelation therapy for the elimination of the free-iron species and to promote the free-radical scavenging activity of the antioxidants. Not only synthetic (vitamin C, vitamin E and NAC) but natural (e.g. polyphenolics, flavonoids and fish oils) antioxidants are also capable of ameliorating such increased levels of oxidative stress. Taken together with an effective iron chelator, antioxidants may provide a substantial improvement in hemolytic anemia cases, and particularly in thalassemia patients. Most importantly, natural antioxidants are ubiquitous and very cheap whereas antioxidant supplements are free from the side effects commonly encountered in iron chelation and chemotherapeutic treatments.

Abbreviations

ACE-II = angiotensin-converting enzyme II
AD4 = *N*-acetylcysteine amide
δ-ALA = delta-aminolevulinic acid
ALP = alkaline phosphatase
ALT = alanine aminotransferase

ApoB = apoprotein B
ApoE = apoprotein E AST = aspartate aminotransferase
BKO = beta-knockout
CAT = catalase
CVD = cardiovascular disease
COX = cyclooxygenase
DFO = desferrioxamine
DFP = deferiprone
DFX = deferasirox
eNOS = endothelial nitric oxide synthase
Epo = erythropoietin
EPR = electron paramagnetic resonance
FI = fluorescent intensity
FPP = fermented papaya preparation
GA = gallic acid
GC/MS = gas chromatography/mass spectrometry
GGT = γ-glutamyl transferase
GPx = glutathione peroxidase
GTE = green tea extract
GSH = reduced glutathione
iNOS = inducible nitric oxide synthase
iv = intravenously
im = intramuscularly
IRP = iron-regulatory proteins
LDL = low-density lipoprotein
LIP = labile iron pool
LPI = labile plasma iron
MRI = magnetic resonance imaging
NAC = *N*-acetylcysteine
NAD(P)H = nicotinamide adenine dinucletide (reduced)
nNOS = neuronal nitric oxide synthase
NOX = NAD(P)H oxidase
NTBI = non-transferrin bound iron
PAF-AH = platelet-activating factor/acetylhydrolase
PBMC = peripheral blood mononuclear cells

PMA = phorbol myristyl acetate
PON1 = paraoxonase 1
PMN = polymorphonuclear cells
RBC = red blood cells
RES = reticuloendothelial system
ROS = reactive oxygen species
sc = subcutaneously
SI = serum iron
SOD = superoxide dismutase
TBARS = thiobarbituric acid reactive substances
TBI = transferrin-bound iron
TBRG = Thai black rice grass
TFRG = Thai fragrant rice grass
TRRG = Thai red rice grass
TIBC = total iron-binding capacity
WG = wheat grass
XO = xanthine oxidase

Acknowledgements

This work was partially supported by the Office of Higher Education Commission and Mahidol University under the National Research University Initiative, Thailand Research Fund through Professor Suthat Fucharoen, MD. and by a Research Chair Grant from the National Science and Technology Development Agency (NSTDA) and Mahidol University through Professor Suthat Fucharoen, MD.

Author details

Somdet Srichairatanakool[1] and Suthat Fucharoen[2*]

*Address all correspondence to: suthat.fuc@mahidol.ac.th

1 Department of Biochemistry, Faculty of Medicine, Chiang Mai University, Chiang Mai, Thailand

2 Thalassemia Research Center, Institute of Molecular Bioscience, Mahidol University, Nakornpathom, Thailand

References

[1] Aisen P, Enns C, Wessling-Resnick M. Chemistry and Biology of Eukaryotic Iron Metabolism. International Journal of Biochemistry and Cell Biology 2001;33(10) 940-959

[2] Beutler E. History of Iron in Medicine. Blood Cells, Molecules & Diseases 2002;29(3) 297-308

[3] Hershko C. Iron Loading and Its Clinical Implications. American Journal of Hematology 2007;82(12 Suppl) 1147-1148

[4] Emerit J, Beaumont C, Trivin F. Iron Metabolism, Free Radicals, and Oxidative Injury. Biomedical Pharmacotherapy 2001;55(6) 333-339

[5] Cabantchik ZI, Breuer W, Zanninelli G, Cianciulli P. LPI-Labile Plasma Iron in Iron Overload. Best Practice & Research. Clinical Haematology 2005;18(2) 277-287

[6] Andrews NC. Disorders of Iron Metabolism. New England Journal of Medicine 1999;341(26) 1986-1995

[7] Kohgo Y, Ikuta K, Ohtake T, Torimoto Y, Kato J. Body Iron Metabolism and Pathophysiology of Iron Overload. International Journal of Hematology 2008;88(1) 7-15

[8] Porter JB. A Risk-Benefit Assessment of Iron-Chelation Therapy. Drug Safety 1997;17(6) 407-421

[9] Cranfield LM, Gollan JL, White AG, Dormandy TL. Serum Antioxidant Activity in Normal and Abnormal Subjects. Annual Review of Clinical Biochemistry 1979;16(6) 299-306

[10] Gerli GC, Beretta L, Bianchi M, Pellegatta A, Agostoni A. Erythrocyte Superoxide Dismutase, Catalase and Glutathione Peroxidase Activities in beta-Thalassaemia (Major and Minor). Scandinavian Journal of Haematology 1980;25(1) 87-92

[11] Katerelos C, Constantopoulos A, Agathopoulos A, Constantzas N, Zannos-Mariolea L, Matsaniotis N. Serum Levels of Retinol, Retinol-Binding Protein, Carotenoids and Triglycerides in Children with beta-Thalassemia Major. Acta Haematologica 1979;62(2) 100-105

[12] Rachmilewitz EA, Shohet SB, Lubin BH. Lipid Membrane Peroxidation in beta-Thalassemia Major. Blood 1976;47(3) 495-505

[13] Weatherall DJ, Pressley L, Wood WG, Higgs DR, Clegg JB. Molecular Basis for Mild Forms of Homozygous beta-Thalassaemia. Lancet 1981;1(8219) 527-529

[14] Muncie HL, Jr., Campbell J. Alpha and beta Thalassemia. American Family Physician 2009;80(4) 339-344

[15] Kong WN, Zhao SE, Duan XL, Yang Z, Qian ZM, Chang YZ. Decreased DMT1 and Increased Ferroportin 1 Expression Is the Mechanisms of Reduced Iron Retention in

Macrophages by Erythropoietin in Rats. Journal of Cell Biochemistry 2008;104(2) 629-641

[16] Beutler E. Iron Storage Disease: Facts, Fiction and Progress. Blood Cells, Molecules & Diseases 2007;39(2) 140-147

[17] Hershko C, Konijn AM, Link G. Iron Chelators for Thalassaemia. British Journal of Haematology 1998;101(3) 399-406

[18] Hershko C, Graham G, Bates GW, Rachmilewitz EA. Non-Specific Serum Iron in Thalassaemia: an Abnormal Serum Iron Fraction of Potential Toxicity. British Journal of Haematology 1978;40(2) 255-263

[19] Breuer W, Hershko C, Cabantchik ZI. The Importance of Non-Transferrin Bound Iron in Disorders of Iron Metabolism. Transfusion Science 2000;23(3) 185-192

[20] Esposito BP, Breuer W, Sirankapracha P, Pootrakul P, Hershko C, Cabantchik ZI. Labile Plasma Iron in Iron Overload: Redox Activity and Susceptibility to Chelation. Blood 2003;102(7) 2670-2677

[21] Kushner JP, Porter JP, Olivieri NF. Secondary Iron Overload. Hematology American Society of Hematology Education Program 2001 47-61

[22] Weatherall DJ. Pathophysiology of Thalassaemia. Bailliere's Clinical Haematology 1998;11(1) 127-146

[23] Kalinowski DS, Richardson DR. The Evolution of Iron Chelators for The Treatment of Iron Overload Disease and Cancer. Pharmacology Review 2005;57(4) 547-583

[24] Papanikolaou G, Pantopoulos K. Iron Metabolism and Toxicity. Toxicology and Applied Pharmacology 2005;202(2) 199-211

[25] Schellhammer PF, Engle MA, Hagstrom JW. Histochemical Studies of the Myocardium and Conduction System in Acquired Iron-Storage Disease. Circulation 1967;35(4) 631-637

[26] Kremastinos DT, Toutouzas PK, Vyssoulis GP, Venetis CA, Avgoustakis DG. Iron Overload and Left Ventricular Performance in beta Thalassemia. Acta Cardiology 1984;39(1) 29-40

[27] Sonakul D, Pacharee P, Thakerngpol K. Pathologic Findings in 76 Autopsy Cases of Thalassemia. Birth Defects: Original Article Series 1988;23(5B) 157-176

[28] Bannerman RM, Keusch G, Kreimer-Birnbaum M, Vance VK, Vaughan S. Thalassemia Intermedia, with Iron Overload, Cardiac Failure, Diabetes Mellitus, Hypopituitarism and Porphyrinuria. American Journal of Medicine 1967;42(3) 476-486

[29] Aldouri MA, Wonke B, Hoffbrand AV, Flynn DM, Ward SE, Agnew JE, et al. High Incidence of Cardiomyopathy in beta-Thalassaemia Patients Receiving Regular

Transfusion and Iron Chelation: Reversal by Intensified Chelation. Acta Haematologica 1990;84(3) 113-117

[30] Kremastinos DT, Tiniakos G, Theodorakis GN, Katritsis DG, Toutouzas PK. Myocarditis in beta-Thalassemia Major. A Cause of Heart Failure. Circulation 1995;91(1) 66-71

[31] Rines AK, Ardehali H. Transition Metals and Mitochondrial Metabolism in the Heart. Journal of Molecular and Cellular Cardiology 2012;(55) 50-57

[32] Bartfay WJ, Bartfay E. Iron-Overload Cardiomyopathy: Evidence for a Free Radical-Mediated Mechanism of Injury and Dysfunction in a Murine Model. Biological Research for Nursing 2000;2(1) 49-59

[33] Nienhuis AW, Griffith P, Strawczynski H, Henry W, Borer J, Leon M, et al. Evaluation of Cardiac Function in Patients with Thalassemia Major. Annals of the New York Academy of Sciences 1980;344 384-396

[34] Senior R, Batabyal SK, Dutta RN, Guha S, Dutta S, Bhattacharji TD, et al. An Echo-Cardiographic (M-mode & 2D) Analysis of Thalassaemia Major. Indian Heart Journal 1990;42(1) 73-76

[35] Wielopolski L, Zaino EC. Noninvasive in-Vivo Measurement of Hepatic and Cardiac Iron. Journal of Nuclear Medicine 1992;33(7) 1278-1282

[36] Lattanzi F, Bellotti P, Picano E, Chiarella F, Mazzarisi A, Melevendi C, et al. Quantitative Ultrasonic Analysis of Myocardium in Patients with Thalassemia Major and Iron Overload. Circulation 1993;87(3) 748-754

[37] Lombardo T, Tamburino C, Bartoloni G, Morrone ML, Frontini V, Italia F, et al. Cardiac Iron Overload in Thalassemic Patients: an Endomyocardial Biopsy Study. Annals of Hematology 1995;71(3) 135-141

[38] Anderson LJ, Holden S, Davis B, Prescott E, Charrier CC, Bunce NH, et al. Cardiovascular T2-Star (T2*) Magnetic Resonance for the Early Diagnosis of Myocardial Iron Overload. European Heart Journal 2001; 22(23) 2171-2179

[39] Wolfe L, Olivieri N, Sallan D, Colan S, Rose V, Propper R, et al. Prevention of Cardiac Disease by Subcutaneous Deferoxamine in Patients with Thalassemia Major. New England Journal of Medicine 1985;312(25) 1600-1603

[40] Freeman AP, Giles RW, Berdoukas VA, Talley PA, Murray IP. Sustained Normalization of Cardiac Function by Chelation Therapy in Thalassaemia Major. Clinical and Laboratory Haematology 1989;11(4) 299-307

[41] Halliwell B, Gutteridge JM. Biologically Relevant Metal Ion-Dependent Hydroxyl Radical Generation. An update. FEBS Letters 1992;307(1) 108-112

[42] Rund D, Rachmilewitz E. Pathophysiology of alpha- and beta-Thalassemia: Therapeutic Implications. Seminar in Hematology 2001;38(4) 343-349

[43] Hebbel RP. Auto-Oxidation and a Membrane-Associated 'Fenton Reagent': a Possible Explanation for Development of Membrane Lesions in Sickle Erythrocytes. Clinical Haematology 1985;14(1) 129-140

[44] Hershko CM, Link GM, Konijn AM, Cabantchik ZI. Iron Chelation Therapy. Current Hematologic Malignancy Reports 2005;4(2) 110-116

[45] Henrotin Y, Deberg M, Mathy-Hartert M, Deby-Dupont G. Biochemical Biomarkers of Oxidative Collagen Damage. Advances in Clinical Chemistry 2009;49 31-55

[46] Zhang AS, Sheftel AD, Ponka P. Intracellular Kinetics of Iron in Reticulocytes: Evidence for Endosome Involvement in Iron Targeting to Mitochondria. Blood 2005;105(1) 368-375

[47] Napier I, Ponka P, Richardson DR. Iron Trafficking in the Mitochondrion: Novel Pathways Revealed by Disease. Blood 2005;105(5) 1867-1874

[48] Cappellini MD, Tavazzi D, Duca L, Graziadei G, Mannu F, Turrini F, et al. Metabolic Indicators of Oxidative Stress Correlate with Haemichrome Attachment to Membrane, Band 3 Aggregation and Erythrophagocytosis in beta-Thalassaemia Intermedia. British Journal of Haematology 1999;104(3) 504-512

[49] Carpino A, Tarantino P, Rago V, De Sanctis V, Siciliano L. Antioxidant Capacity in Seminal Plasma of Transfusion-Dependent beta-Thalassemic Patients. Experimental and Clinical Endocrinology and Diabetes 2004;112(3) 131-134

[50] Chakraborty I, Mitra S, Gachhui R, Kar M. Non-Haem Iron-Mediated Oxidative Stress in Haemoglobin E beta-Thalassaemia. Annals of the Academy of Medicine, Singapore 2010;39(1) 13-16

[51] Cheng ML, Ho HY, Tseng HC, Lee CH, Shih LY, Chiu DT. Antioxidant Deficit and Enhanced Susceptibility to Oxidative Damage in Individuals with Different Forms of alpha-Thalassaemia. British Journal of Haematology 2005;128(1) 119-127

[52] Chiou SS, Chang TT, Tsai SP, Jang RC, Lin SK, Lee SC, et al. Lipid Peroxidation and Antioxidative Status in beta-Thalassemia Major Patients with or without Hepatitis C Virus Infection. Clinical Chemistry and Laboratory Medicine 2006;44(10) 1226-1233

[53] Altamentova SM, Shaklai N. Oxidative Stress in beta-Thalassemia: Hemoglobin alpha-Chains Activate Peroxidation of Low Density Lipoproteins. Biofactors 1998;8(1-2) 169-172

[54] Abdalla MY, Fawzi M, Al-Maloul SR, El-Banna N, Tayyem RF, Ahmad IM. Increased Oxidative Stress and Iron Overload in Jordanian beta-Thalassemic Children. Hemoglobin 2011;35(1) 67-79

[55] Bazrgar M, Karimi M, Peiravian F, Fathzadeh M. Apolipoprotein E Gene Polymorphism and Left Ventricular Function in Iranian Patients with Thalassemia Major. Haematologica 2007;92(2) 256-257

[56] Haghpanah S, Davani M, Samadi B, Ashrafi A, Karimi M. Serum Lipid Profiles in Patients with beta-Thalassemia Major and Intermedia in Southern Iran. Journal of Research in Medical Sciences 2011;15(3) 150-154

[57] Afanas'ev IB. Superoxide and Nitric Oxide in Pathological Conditions Associated with Iron Overload: the Effects of Antioxidants and Chelators. Current Medicinal Chemistry 2005;12(23) 2731-2739

[58] Afanas'ev IB. Interplay Between Superoxide and Nitric Oxide in Thalassemia and Fanconi's Anemia. Hemoglobin 2006;30(1) 113-118

[59] Afanas'ev IB, Afanas'ev, II, Deeva IB, Korkina LG. Free Radical Formation and Oxyhemoglobin Oxidation in beta-Thalassemic Red Blood Cells in the Presence of Prooxidants: Effects of the Free Radical Scavenger Rutin and Oral Chelator L1. Transfusion Science 2000;23(3) 237-238

[60] Laksmitawati DR, Handayani S, Udyaningsih-Freisleben SK, Kurniati V, Adhiyanto C, Hidayat J, et al. Iron Status and Oxidative Stress in beta-Thalassemia Patients in Jakarta. Biofactors 2003;19(1-2) 53-62

[61] Amer J, Goldfarb A, Fibach E. Flow Cytometric Analysis of the Oxidative Status of Normal and Thalassemic Red Blood Cells. Cytometry A 2004;60(1) 73-80

[62] Amer J, Fibach E. Oxidative Status of Platelets in Normal and Thalassemic Blood. Thrombosis and Haemostasis 2004;92(5) 1052-1059

[63] Amer J, Fibach E. Chronic Oxidative Stress Reduces the Respiratory Burst Response of Neutrophils from beta-Thalassaemia Patients. British Journal of Haematology 2005;129(3) 435-441

[64] Anderson D, Yardley-Jones A, Vives-Bauza C, Chua-Anusorn W, Cole C, Webb J. Effect of Iron Salts, Haemosiderins, and Chelating Agents on the Lymphocytes of a Thalassaemia Patient without Chelation Therapy as Measured in the Comet Assay. Teratogenesis, Carcinogenesis, and Mutagenesis 2000;20(5) 251-264

[65] Bartfay WJ, Lehotay DC, Sher GD, Bartfay E, Tyler B, Luo X, et al. Erythropoiesis: Comparison of Cytotoxic Aldehyde Generation in Beta-Thalassemia Patients Chelated with Deferoxamine or Deferiprone (L1) Versus NO Chelation. Hematology 1999;4(1) 67-76

[66] Claster S, Wood JC, Noetzli L, Carson SM, Hofstra TC, Khanna R, et al. Nutritional Deficiencies in Iron Overloaded Patients with Hemoglobinopathies. American Journal of Hematology 2009;84(6) 344-348

[67] Awadallah SM, Nimer NA, Atoum MF, Saleh SA. Association of Haptoglobin Phenotypes with Ceruloplasmin Ferroxidase Activity in beta-Thalassemia Major. Clinica Chimica Acta 2011;412(11-12) 975-979

[68] De Franceschi L, Bertoldi M, De Falco L, Santos Franco S, Ronzoni L, Turrini F, et al. Oxidative Stress Modulates Heme Synthesis and Induces Peroxiredoxin-2 as a Novel

Cytoprotective Response in beta-Thalassemic Erythropoiesis. Haematologica 2011;96(11) 1595-1604

[69] Galanello R, Campus S. Deferiprone Chelation Therapy for Thalassemia Major. Acta Haematologica 2009;122(2-3) 155-164

[70] Cappellini MD, Taher A. Deferasirox (Exjade) for the Treatment of Iron Overload. Acta Haematologica 2009;122(2-3) 165-173

[71] Viprakasit V, Lee-Lee C, Chong QT, Lin KH, Khuhapinant A. Iron Chelation Therapy in the Management of Thalassemia: the Asian Perspectives. International Journal of Hematology 2009;90(4) 435-445

[72] Hershko C, Abrahamov A, Konijn AM, Breuer W, Cabantchik IZ, Pootrakul P, et al. Objectives and Methods of Iron Chelation Therapy. Bioinorganic Chemistry and Applications 2003:151-168

[73] Hershko C, Rachmilewitz EA. Iron Chelation in Thalassemia: Mechanism of Desferrioxamine Action. Israel Journal of Medical Science 1978;14(11) 1111-1115

[74] Summers MR, Jacobs A, Tudway D, Perera P, Ricketts C. Studies in Desferrioxamine and Ferrioxamine Metabolism in Normal and Iron-Loaded Subjects. British Journal of Haematology 1979;42(4) 547-555

[75] Porter JB, Jaswon MS, Huehns ER, East CA, Hazell JW. Desferrioxamine Ototoxicity: Evaluation of Risk Factors in Thalassaemic Patients and Guidelines for Safe Dosage. British Journal of Haematology 1989;73(3) 403-409

[76] Freedman MH, Grisaru D, Olivieri N, MacLusky I, Thorner PS. Pulmonary Syndrome in Patients with Thalassemia Major Receiving Intravenous Deferoxamine Infusions. American Journal of Diseases of Children 1990;144(5) 565-569

[77] Olivieri NF, Buncic JR, Chew E, Gallant T, Harrison RV, Keenan N, et al. Visual and Auditory Neurotoxicity in Patients Receiving Subcutaneous Deferoxamine Infusions. New England Journal of Medicine 1986;314(14) 869-873

[78] Olivieri NF, Berriman AM, Tyler BJ, Davis SA, Francombe WH, Liu PP. Reduction in Tissue Iron Stores with a New Regimen of Continuous Ambulatory Intravenous Deferoxamine. American Journal of Hematology 1992;41(1) 61-63

[79] Hoffbrand AV, Cohen A, Hershko C. Role of Deferiprone in Chelation Therapy for Transfusional Iron Overload. Blood 2003;102(1) 17-24

[80] Kolnagou A, Fessas C, Papatryphonas A, Economides C, Kontoghiorghes GJ. Prophylactic Use of Deferiprone (L1) and Magnetic Resonance Imaging T2* or T2 for Preventing Heart Disease in Thalassaemia. British Journal of Haematology 2004;127(3) 360-361

[81] Cohen AR, Galanello R, Piga A, Dipalma A, Vullo C, Tricta F. Safety Profile of the Oral Iron Chelator Deferiprone: a Multicentre Study. British Journal of Haematology 2000;108(2) 305-312

[82] Hoffbrand AV. Iron Chelation Therapy. Current Opinion in Hematology 1995;2(2) 153-158

[83] Nisbet-Brown E, Olivieri NF, Giardina PJ, Grady RW, Neufeld EJ, Sechaud R, et al. Effectiveness and Safety of ICL670 in Iron-Loaded Patients with Thalassaemia: a Randomised, Double-Blind, Placebo-Controlled, Dose-Escalation Trial. Lancet 2003;361(9369) 1597-1602

[84] Galanello R, Piga A, Alberti D, Rouan MC, Bigler H, Sechaud R. Safety, Tolerability, and Pharmacokinetics of ICL670, a New Orally Active Iron-Chelating Agent in Patients with Transfusion-Dependent Iron Overload Due to beta-Thalassemia. Journal of Clinical Pharmacology 2003;43(6) 565-572

[85] Barton JC. Deferasirox Novartis. Current Opinion in Investigational Drugs 2005;6(3) 327-335

[86] Galanello R. Evaluation of ICL670, a Once-Daily Oral Iron Chelator in a Phase III Clinical Trial of beta-Thalassemia Patients with Transfusional Iron Overload. Annals of the New York Academy of Sciences 2005;1054 183-185

[87] Cappellini MD, Cohen A, Piga A, Bejaoui M, Perrotta S, Agaoglu L, et al. A Phase 3 Study of Deferasirox (ICL670), a Once-Daily Oral Iron Chelator, in Patients with beta-Thalassemia. Blood 2006;107(9) 3455-3462

[88] Porter JB. Deferasirox: An Effective Once-Daily Orally Active Iron Chelator. Drugs Today (Barcelona, Spain: 1998) 2006;42(10) 623-637

[89] Wong C, Richardson DR. Beta-Thalassaemia: Emergence of New and Improved Iron Chelators for Treatment. International Journal of Biochemistry and Cell Biology 2003;35(7) 1144-1149

[90] Olivieri NF, Brittenham GM. Iron-Chelating Therapy and the Treatment of Thalassemia. Blood 1997;89(3) 739-761

[91] Balocco M, Carrara P, Pinto V, Forni GL. Daily Alternating Deferasirox and Deferiprone Therapy for "Hard-to-Chelate" beta-Thalassemia Major Patients. American Journal of Hematology 2010;85(6) 460-461

[92] Cappellini MD, Bejaoui M, Agaoglu L, Porter J, Coates T, Jeng M, et al. Prospective Evaluation of Patient-Reported Outcomes during Treatment with Deferasirox or Deferoxamine for Iron Overload in Patients with beta-Thalassemia. Clinical Therapeutics 2007;29(5) 909-917

[93] Merson L, Olivier N. Orally Active Iron Chelators. Blood Review 2002;16(2) 127-134

[94] Brittenham GM, Sheth S, Allen CJ, Farrell DE. Noninvasive Methods for Quantitative Assessment of Transfusional Iron Overload in Sickle Cell Disease. Seminar in Hematology 2001;38(1 Supplement 1) 37-56

[95] Wood JC, Tyszka JM, Carson S, Nelson MD, Coates TD. Myocardial Iron Loading in Transfusion-dependent Thalassemia and Sickle Cell Disease. Blood 2004;103(5) 1934-1936

[96] Westwood M, Anderson LJ, Pennell DJ. Treatment of Cardiac Iron Overload in Thalassemia Major. Haematologica 2003;88(5) 481-482

[97] Fischer R, Piga A, Harmatz P, Nielsen P. Monitoring Long-Term Efficacy of Iron Chelation Treatment with Biomagnetic Liver Susceptometry. Annals of the New York of Academy of Sciences 2005;1054 350-357

[98] Leonardi B, Margossian R, Colan SD, Powell AJ. Relationship of Magnetic Resonance Imaging Estimation of Myocardial Iron to Left Ventricular Systolic and Diastolic Function in Thalassemia. JACC Cardiovascular Imaging 2008;1(5) 572-578

[99] Schramm A, Matusik P, Osmenda G, Guzik TJ. Targeting NADPH Oxidases in Vascular Pharmacology. Vascular Pharmacology 2013;56(5-6) 216-231

[100] Dhaunsi GS, Kaur J, Alsaeid K, Turner RB, Bitar MS. Very Long Chain Fatty Acids Activate NADPH Oxidase in Human Dermal Fibroblasts. Cell Biochemistry and Function 2005;23(1) 65-68

[101] Jung O, Schreiber JG, Geiger H, Pedrazzini T, Busse R, Brandes RP. gp91phox-Containing NADPH Oxidase Mediates Endothelial Dysfunction in Renovascular Hypertension. Circulation 2004;109(14) 1795-1801

[102] Muzykantov VR. Targeting of Superoxide Dismutase and Catalase to Vascular Endothelium. Journal of Controlled Release 2001;71(1) 1-21

[103] Cayatte AJ, Rupin A, Oliver-Krasinski J, Maitland K, Sansilvestri-Morel P, Boussard MF, et al. S17834, a New Inhibitor of Cell Adhesion and Atherosclerosis that Targets NADH Oxidase. Arteriosclerosis Thrombosis and Vascular Biology 2001;21(10) 1577-1584

[104] Zacharski LR, DePalma RG, Shamayeva G, Chow BK. The Statin-Iron Nexus: Anti-Inflammatory Intervention for Arterial Disease Prevention. American Journal of Public Health 2013;103(4) e105-112

[105] Wolf G. Free Radical Production and Angiotensin. Current Hypertension Report 2000;2(2) 167-173

[106] Brosnan MJ, Hamilton CA, Graham D, Lygate CA, Jardine E, Dominiczak AF. Irbesartan Lowers Superoxide Levels and Increases Nitric Oxide Bioavailability in Blood Vessels from Spontaneously Hypertensive Stroke-Prone Rats. Journal of Hypertension 2002;20(2) 281-286

[107] Oelze M, Daiber A, Brandes RP, Hortmann M, Wenzel P, Hink U, et al. Nebivolol Inhibits Superoxide Formation by NADPH Oxidase and Endothelial Dysfunction in Angiotensin II-Treated Rats. Hypertension 2006;48(4) 677-684

[108] Salvemini D, Muscoli C, Riley DP, Cuzzocrea S. Superoxide Dismutase Mimetics. Pulmonary Pharmacology & Therapeutics 2002;15(5) 439-447

[109] Afifi AM, Ellis L, Huntsman RG, Said MI. High Dose Ascorbic Acid in the Management of Thalassaemia Leg Ulcers-a Pilot Study. British Journal of Dermatology 1975;92(3) 339-341

[110] Angelides NS, Angastiniotis C, Pavlides N. Effect of Pentoxifylline on Treatment of Lower Limb Ulcers in Patients with Thalassemia Major. Angiology 1992;43(7) 549-554

[111] Gerli GC, Mongiat R, Sandri MT, Agostoni A, Gualandri V, Orsini GB, et al. Antioxidant System and Serum Trace Elements in alpha-Thalassaemia and Hb Lepore Trait. European Journal of Haematology 1987;39(1) 23-27

[112] Teng CM, Hsiao G, Ko FN, Lin DT, Lee SS. N-Allylsecoboldine as a Novel Antioxidant against Peroxidative Damage. European Journal of Pharmacology 1996;303(1-2) 129-139

[113] Tesoriere L, D'Arpa D, Maggio A, Giaccone V, Pedone E, Livrea MA. Oxidation Resistance of LDL is Correlated with Vitamin E Status in beta-Thalassemia Intermedia. Atherosclerosis 1998;137(2) 429-435

[114] Tesoriere L, D'Arpa D, Butera D, Allegra M, Renda D, Maggio A, et al. Oral Supplements of Vitamin E Improve Measures of Oxidative Stress in Plasma and Reduce Oxidative Damage to LDL and Erythrocytes in beta-Thalassemia Intermedia Patients. Free Radical Research 2001;34(5) 529-540

[115] Alidoost F, Gharagozloo M, Bagherpour B, Jafarian A, Sajjadi SE, Hourfar H, et al. Effects of Silymarin on the Proliferation and Glutathione Levels of Peripheral Blood Mononuclear Cells from beta-Thalassemia Major Patients. International Immunopharmacology 2006;6(8) 1305-1310

[116] Amer J, Atlas D, Fibach E. N-Acetylcysteine Amide (AD4) Attenuates Oxidative Stress in beta-Thalassemia Blood Cells. Biochimica Et Biophysica Acta 2008;1780(2) 249-255

[117] Amer J, Goldfarb A, Rachmilewitz EA, Fibach E. Fermented Papaya Preparation as Redox Regulator in Blood Cells of beta-Thalassemic Mice and Patients. Phytotherapy Research 2008;22(6) 820-828

[118] Amer J, Dana M, Fibach E. The Antioxidant Effect of Erythropoietin on Thalassemic Blood Cells. Anemia 2010;2010 978710

[119] Anderson D, Dhawan A, Yardley-Jones A, Ioannides C, Webb J. Effect of Antioxidant Flavonoids and a Food Mutagen on Lymphocytes of a Thalassemia Patient without

Chelation Therapy in the Comet Assay. Teratogenesis Carcinogenesis and Mutagenesis 2001;21(2) 165-174

[120] Bianco L, Boccaccini R, Capalbo P, Morici G, Maestro M, Mandrino M. [The Role of Vitamin E in the Therapy of Thalassemia]. Pediatria Medica e Chirurgica 1986;8(1) 23-26

[121] Cakmak A, Soker M, Koc A, Erel O. Paraoxonase and Arylesterase Activity with Oxidative Status in Children with Thalassemia Major. Journal of Pediatric Hematology/ Oncology 2009 31(8) 583-587

[122] Cakmak A, Soker M, Koc A, Aksoy N. Prolidase Activity and Oxidative Status in Patients with Thalassemia Major. Journal of Clinical Laboratory Analysis 2010;24(1) 6-11

[123] Das N, Das Chowdhury T, Chattopadhyay A, Datta AG. Attenuation of Oxidative Stress-Induced Changes in Thalassemic Erythrocytes by Vitamin E. Polish Journal of Pharmacology 2004;56(1) 85-96

[124] Kattamis C, Lazaropoulou C, Delaporta P, Apostolakou F, Kattamis A, Papassotiriou I. Disturbances of Biomarkers of Iron and Oxidant-Antioxidant Homeostasis in Patients with beta-Thalassemia Intermedia. Pediatric Endocrinology Reviews 2011;8 Supplemnt 2 256-262

[125] Kontoghiorghes GJ. Prospects for Introducing Deferiprone as Potent Pharmaceutical Antioxidant. Frontiers in Bioscience (Elite Edition) 2009;1 161-178

[126] Suthutvoravut U, Hathirat P, Sirichakwal P, Sasanakul W, Tassaneeyakul A, Feungpean B. Vitamin E Status, Glutathione Peroxidase Activity and the Effect of Vitamin E Supplementation in Children with Thalassemia. Journal of the Medical Association of Thailand 1993;76 Supplement 2 146-152

[127] Vatanavicharn S, Yenchitsomanus P, Siddhikol C. Vitamin E in beta-Thalassaemia and alpha-Thalassaemia (HbH) Diseases. Acta Haematologica 1985;73(3) 183

[128] Phuapradit W, Panburana P, Jaovisidha A, Chanrachakul B, Bunyaratvej A, Puchaiwatananon O. Serum Vitamin A and E in Pregnant Women with Hemoglobinopathies. Journal of Obstetrics and Gynaecology Research 1999;25(3) 173-176

[129] Yenchitsomanus P, Wasi P. Increased Erythrocyte Superoxide Dismutase Activities in beta 0-Thalassaemia/Haemoglobin E and in Haemoglobin H Diseases. Journal of Clinical Pathology 1983;36(3) 329-333

[130] Dissayabutra T, Tosukhowong P, Seksan P. The Benefits of Vitamin C and Vitamin E in Children with beta-Thalassemia with High Oxidative Stress. Journal of the Medical Association of Thailand 2005;88 Supplement 4 S317-321

[131] Kalpravidh RW, Wichit A, Siritanaratkul N, Fucharoen S. Effect of Coenzyme Q10 as an Antioxidant in beta-Thalassemia/Hb E Patients. Biofactors 2005;25(1-4) 225-234

[132] Ciavatta DJ, Ryan TM, Farmer SC, Townes TM. Mouse Model of Human beta Zero Thalassemia: Targeted Deletion of the Mouse beta Maj- and beta Min-Globin Genes in Embryonic Stem Cells. Proceedings of the National Academy of Sciences of the United States of America 1995;92(20) 9259-9263

[133] Jamsai D, Zaibak F, Vadolas J, Voullaire L, Fowler KJ, Gazeas S, et al. A Humanized BAC Transgenic/Knockout Mouse Model for HbE/beta-Thalassemia. Genomics 2006;88(3) 309-315

[134] Jamsai D, Zaibak F, Khongnium W, Vadolas J, Voullaire L, Fowler KJ, et al. A Humanized Mouse Model for a Common beta0-Thalassemia Mutation. Genomics 2005;85(4) 453-461

[135] Vadolas J, Wardan H, Bosmans M, Zaibak F, Jamsai D, Voullaire L, et al. Transgene Copy Number-Dependent Rescue of Murine beta-Globin Knockout Mice Carrying a 183 kb Human beta-Globin BAC Genomic Fragment. Biochimica Et Biophysica Acta 2005;1728(3) 150-162

[136] Wannasuphaphol B, Kalpravidh R, Pattanapanyasat K, Ioannau P, Kuypers FA, Fucharoen S, et al. Rescued Mice with Hb E Transgene-Developed Red Cell Changes Similar to Human beta-Thalassemia/HbE Disease. Annals of the New York Academy of Sciences 2005;1054 407-416

[137] Vogiatzi MG, Tsay J, Verdelis K, Rivella S, Grady RW, Doty S, et al. Changes in Bone Microarchitecture and Biomechanical Properties in the th3 Thalassemia Mouse are Associated with Decreased Bone Turnover and Occur during the Period of Bone Accrual. Calcified Tissue International 2010;86(6) 484-494

[138] Thephinlap C, Phisalaphong C, Fucharoen S, Porter JB, Srichairatanakool S. Efficacy of Curcuminoids in Alleviation of Iron Overload and Lipid Peroxidation in Thalassemic Mice. Medicinal Chemistry 2009;5(5) 474-482

[139] Srichairatanakool S, Thephinlap C, Phisalaphong C, Porter JB, Fucharoen S. Curcumin Contributes to In Vitro Removal of Non-Transferrin Bound Iron by Deferiprone and Desferrioxamine in Thalassemic Plasma. Medicinal Chemistry 2007;3(5) 469-474

[140] Thephinlap C, Phisalaphong C, Lailerd N, Chattipakorn N, Winichagoon P, Vadolus J, et al. Reversal of Cardiac Iron Loading and Dysfunction in Thalassemic Mice by Curcuminoids. Medicinal Chemistry 2011;7(1) 62-69

[141] Kalpravidh RW, Siritanaratkul N, Insain P, Charoensakdi R, Panichkul N, Hatairaktham S, et al. Improvement in Oxidative Stress and Antioxidant Parameters in beta-Thalassemia/Hb E Patients Treated with Curcuminoids. Clinical Biochemistry 2009;43(4-5) 424-429

[142] Weeraphan C, Srisomsap C, Chokchaichamnankit D, Subhasitanont P, Hatairaktham S, Charoensakdi R, et al. Role of Curcuminoids in Ameliorating Oxidative Modifica-

tion in beta-Thalassemia/Hb E Plasma Proteome. Journal of Nutritional Biochemistry 2012;24(3) 578-585

[143] Unchern S, Laohareungpanya N, Sanvarinda Y, Pattanapanyasat K, Tanratana P, Chantharaksri U, et al. Oxidative Modification and Poor Protective Activity of HDL on LDL Oxidation in Thalassemia. Lipids 2010;45(7) 627-633

[144] Srichairatanakool S, Ounjaijean S, Thephinlap C, Khansuwan U, Phisalpong C, Fucharoen S. Iron-Chelating and Free-Radical Scavenging Activities of Microwave-Processed Green Tea in Iron Overload. Hemoglobin 2006;30(2) 311-327

[145] Zuo Y, Chen H, Deng Y. Simultaneous Determination of Catechins, Caffeine and Gallic Acids in Green, Oolong, Black and Pu-erh Teas using HPLC with a Photodiode Array Detector. Talanta 2002;57(4) 307-316

[146] de Alarcon PA, Donovan ME, Forbes GB, Landaw SA, Stockman JA, 3rd. Iron Absorption in the Thalassemia Syndromes and Its Inhibition by Tea. New England Journal of Medicine 1979;300(1) 5-8

[147] Pippard MJ, Callender ST, Warner GT, Weatherall DJ. Iron Absorption and Loading in beta-Thalassaemia Intermedia. Lancet 1979;2(8147) 819-821

[148] Thephinlap C, Ounjaijean S, Khansuwan U, Fucharoen S, Porter JB, Srichairatanakool S. Epigallocatechin-3-gallate and Epicatechin-3-gallate from Green Tea Decrease Plasma NNon-Transferrin Bound Iron and Erythrocyte Oxidative Stress. Medicinal Chemistry 2007;3(3) 289-296

[149] Ounjaijean S, Thephinlap C, Khansuwan U, Phisalapong C, Fucharoen S, Porter JB, et al. Effect of Green Tea on Iron Status and Oxidative Stress in Iron-Loaded Rats. Medicinal Chemistry 2008;4(4) 365-370

[150] Saewong T, Ounjaijean S, Mundee Y, Pattanapanyasat K, Fucharoen S, Porter JB, et al. Effects of Green Tea on Iron Accumulation and Oxidative Stress in Livers of Iron-Challenged Thalassemic Mice. Medicinal Chemistry 2010;6(2) 57-64

[151] Srichairatanakool S, Kulprachakarn K, Pangjit K, Pattanapanyasat K, Fuchaeron S. Green Tea Extract and Epigallocatechin 3-gallate Reduced Labile Iron Pool and Protected Oxidative Stress in Iron-Loaded Cultured Hepatocytes. Advance in Bioscience and Biotechnology 2012;3 1140-1150

[152] Leiro JM, Alvarez E, Arranz JA, Siso IG, Orallo F. In Vitro Effects of Mangiferin on Superoxide Concentrations and Expression of the Inducible Nitric Oxide Synthase, Tumour Necrosis Factor-alpha and Transforming Growth Factor-beta Genes. Biochemical Pharmacology 2003;65(8) 1361-1371

[153] Leiro J, Arranz JA, Yanez M, Ubeira FM, Sanmartin ML, Orallo F. Expression Profiles of Genes Involved in the Mouse Nuclear Factor-kappa B Signal Transduction Pathway are Modulated by Mangiferin. International Immunopharmacology 2004;4(6) 763-778

[154] Pardo-Andreu GL, Sanchez-Baldoquin C, Avila-Gonzalez R, Yamamoto ET, Revilla A, Uyemura SA, et al. Interaction of Vimang (Mangifera indica L. Extract) with Fe(III) Improves Its Antioxidant and Cytoprotecting Activity. Pharmacology Research 2006;54(5) 389-395

[155] Pardo-Andreu GL, Delgado R, Nunez-Selles AJ, Vercesi AE. Mangifera indica L. Extract (Vimang) Inhibits 2-Deoxyribose Damage Induced by Fe (III) Plus Ascorbate. Phytotherapy Research 2006;20(2) 120-124

[156] Engels C, Knodler M, Zhao YY, Carle R, Ganzle MG, Schieber A. Antimicrobial Activity of Gallotannins Isolated from Mango (Mangifera indica L.) Kernels. Journal of Agricultural and Food Chemistry 2009;57(17) 7712-7718

[157] Schieber A, Berardini N, Carle R. Identification of Flavonol and Xanthone Glycosides from Mango (Mangifera indica L. Cv. "Tommy Atkins") Peels by High-Performance Liquid Chromatography-Electrospray Ionization Mass Spectrometry. Journal of Agricultural and Food Chemistry 2003;51(17) 5006-5011

[158] Jariwalla RJ. Rice-Bran Products: Phytonutrients with Potential Applications in Preventive and Clinical Medicine. Drugs under Experimental and Clinical Research 2001;27(1) 17-26

[159] Wang HM, Lo WL, Huang LY, Wang YD, Chen CY. Chemical Constituents from the Leaves of Michelia alba. Natural Product Research 2010;24(5) 398-406

[160] Borrelli R, Di Donato M, Peluso A. Role of Intramolecular Vibrations in Long-Range Electron Transfer between Pheophytin and Ubiquinone in Bacterial Photosynthetic Reaction Centers. Biophysical Journal 2005;89(2) 830-841

[161] Nelson RE, Ferruzzi MG. Synthesis and Bioaccessibility of Fe-Pheophytin Derivatives from Crude Spinach Extract. Journal of Food Science 2008;73(5) H86-H91

[162] Nozoye T, Inoue H, Takahashi M, Ishimaru Y, Nakanishi H, Mori S, et al. The Expression of Iron Homeostasis-Related Genes during Rice Germination. Plant Molecular Biology 2007;64(1-2) 35-47

[163] Marawaha RK, Bansal D, Kaur S, Trehan A. Wheat Grass Juice Reduces Transfusion Requirement in Patients with Thalassemia Major: a Pilot Study. Indian Journal of Pediatrics 2004;41(7) 716-720

[164] Singh K, Pannu MS, Singh P, Singh J. Effect of Wheat Grass Tablets on the Frequency of Blood Transfusions in Thalassemia Major. Indian Journal of Pediatrics 2010;77(1) 90-91

[165] Choudhary DR, Naithani R, Panigrahi I, Kumar R, Mahapatra M, Pati HP, et al. Effect of Wheat Grass Therapy on Transfusion Requirement in beta-Thalassemia Major. Indian Journal of Pediatrics 2009;76(4) 375-376

[166] Filosa A, Valgimigli L, Pedulli GF, Sapone A, Maggio A, Renda D, et al. Quantitative Evaluation of Oxidative Stress Status on Peripheral Blood in beta-Thalassaemic Pa-

tients by Means of Electron Paramagnetic Resonance Spectroscopy. British Journal of Haematology 2005;131(1) 135-140

[167] Jirasomprasert T, Morales NP, Limenta LM, Sirijaroonwong S, Yamanont P, Wilairat P, et al. Pharmaco/Ferrokinetic-Related Pro-oxidant Activity of Deferiprone in beta-Thalassemia. Free Radical Research 2009;43(5) 485-491

[168] De Luca AC, Rusciano G, Ciancia R, Martinelli V, Pesce G, Rotoli B, et al. Spectroscopical and Mechanical Characterization of Normal and Thalassemic Red Blood Cells by Raman Tweezers. Optics Express 2008;16(11) 7943-7957

[169] Selek S, Aslan M, Horoz M, Gur M, Erel O. Oxidative Status and Serum PON1 Activity in beta-Thalassemia Minor. Clinical Biochemistry 2007;40(5-6) 287-291

[170] Labib HA, Etewa RL, Gaber OA, Atfy M, Mostafa TM, Barsoum I. Paraoxonase-1 and Oxidative Status in Common Mediterranean beta-Thalassaemia Mutations Trait, and Their Relations to Atherosclerosis. Journal of Clinical Pathology 2011;64(5) 437-442

[171] Prasartkaew S, Bunyaratvej A, Fucharoen S, Wasi P. Comparison of Erythrocyte Antioxidative Enzyme Activities between Two Types of Haemoglobin H Disease. Journal of Clinical Pathology 1986;39(12) 1299-1303

[172] Prasartkaew S, Bunyaratvej A, Fucharoen S, Wasi P. Oxidative Stress and Antioxidative Enzymes in Hemoglobin H Disease. Birth Defects: Original Article Series 1987;23(5A) 193-198

[173] Ong-Ajyooth S, Suthipark K, Shumnumsirivath D, Likidlilid A, Fucharoen S, Pootrakul P. Oxidative Stress and Antioxidants in beta-Thalassaemia/Haemoglobin E. Journal of the Medical Association of Thailand 1987;70(5) 270-274

[174] Sumboonnanonda A, Malasit P, Tanphaichitr VS, Ong-ajyooth S, Petrarat S, Vongjirad A. Renal Tubular Dysfunction in alpha-Thalassemia. Pediatric Nephrology 2003;18(3) 257-260

[175] Akrawinthawong K, Chaowalit N, Chatuparisuth T, Siritanaratkul N. Effectiveness of Deferiprone in Transfusion-Independent beta-Thalassemia/HbE Patients. Hematology 2011;16(2) 113-122

[176] Kukongviriyapan V, Somparn N, Senggunprai L, Prawan A, Kukongviriyapan U, Jetsrisuparb A. Endothelial Dysfunction and Oxidant Status in Pediatric Patients with Hemoglobin E-beta Thalassemia. Pediatric Cardiology 2008;29(1) 130-135

[177] Phumala N, Porasuphatana S, Unchern S, Pootrakul P, Fucharoen S, Chantharaksri U. Hemin: a Possible Cause of Oxidative Stress in Blood Circulation of beta-Thalassemia/Hemoglobin E Disease. Free Radical Research 2003;37(2) 129-135

[178] Luechapudiporn R, Morales NP, Fucharoen S, Chantharaksri U. The Reduction of Cholesteryl Linoleate in Lipoproteins: an Index of Clinical Severity in beta-Thalassemia/Hb E. Clinical Chemistry and Laboratory Medicine 2006;44(5) 574-581

[179] Morales NP, Charlermchoung C, Luechapudiporn R, Yamanont P, Fucharoen S, Chantharaksri U. Lipid Fluidity at Different Regions in LDL and HDL of beta-Thalassemia/Hb E Patients. Biochemical and Biophysical Research Communication 2006;350(3) 698-703

[180] Matayatsuk C, Poljak A, Bustamante S, Smythe GA, Kalpravidh RW, Sirankapracha P, et al. Quantitative Determination of ortho- and meta-Tyrosine as Biomarkers of Protein Oxidative Damage in beta-Thalassemia. Redox Report 2007;12(5) 219-228

[181] Phumala Morales N, Cherlermchoung C, Fucharoen S, Chantharaksri U. Paraoxonase and Platelet-Activating Factor Acetylhydrolase Activities in Lipoproteins of beta-Thalassemia/Hemoglobin E Patients. Clinical Chemistry and Laboratory Medicine 2007;45(7) 884-889

[182] Matayatsuk C, Lee CY, Kalpravidh RW, Sirankapracha P, Wilairat P, Fucharoen S, et al. Elevated F2-Isoprostanes in Thalassemic Patients. Free Radical Biology and Medicine 2007;43(12) 1649-1655

[183] Palasuwan A, Kittisakulrat T, Amornrit W, Soogarun S, Wiwanitkit V, Pradniwat P. Antioxidant in Plasma of Hemoglobin-E Trait. Southeast Asian Journal of Tropical Medicine and Public Health 2005;36 Supplement 4 271-273

[184] Somparn N, Kukongviriyapan U, Tassaneeyakul W, Jetsrisuparb A, Kukongviriyapan V. Modification of CYP2E1 and CYP3A4 Activities in Haemoglobin E-beta Thalassemia Patients. European Journal of Clinical Pharmacology 2007;63(1) 43-50

[185] Senggunprai L, Kukongviriyapan U, Jetsrisuparb A, Kukongviriyapan V. Drug Metabolizing Enzyme CYP1A2 Status in Pediatric Patients with Hemoglobin E-beta Thalassemia. Journal of the Medical Association of Thailand 2009;92(12) 1675-1680

Chapter 5

General Aspects of Ozone Therapy

Ruhi Cakir

Additional information is available at the end of the chapter

http://dx.doi.org/10.5772/57470

1. Introduction

Ozone is a natural gas consisting of three oxygen atoms that has a distinctive odor. It is intrinsically hazardous over tolerable doses for living organisms. Ozone therapy is a medical therapy that a mixture of oxygen and ozone which is called medical ozone is used as a medical drug, more correctly pro-drug. Medical ozone contains less than 5% of ozone at maximum concentration where rest of it is pure medical oxygen.

The unbelievable versatility of ozone therapy is due to the cascade of ozone-derived compounds able to act on several targets leading to a multifactorial correction of various pathological states. Ozone therapy can improve well-being and delay the negative effects of aging. Aging process basicly related with oxidants and anti-oxidants balance, Advanced Glycoslation End Substances (AGEs), role of genes and immune system, relevance of telomeres and telomerase, hormones, nutrition, environmental factors and some other factors.

2. What is ozone therapy?

Ozone therapy is a general termination of a medical therapy that medical ozone gas is used as drug by several methods. Some of these methods are systemic where many others are local applications. Ozonated autohaemotherapy (O3-AHT) widely known by people firstly described by Wehrli and Steinbart and since 1954 it has been used in millions of patients in different pathologies with apparent clinical benefit. AHT might be applied in two forms, Major AHT simply driving 100-150 ml of venous blood into a sterile bottle made of neutral glass or other ozone resistant material where blood and medical ozone is mixed in therapeutic doses and then reinfused back to the donor without side effects. 3.13 % Natrium Citrate solution is used as an anticoagulant during the procedure with short lasting effect. In some patients Heparin might be used instead of Natrium Citrate depending on the patient's case.

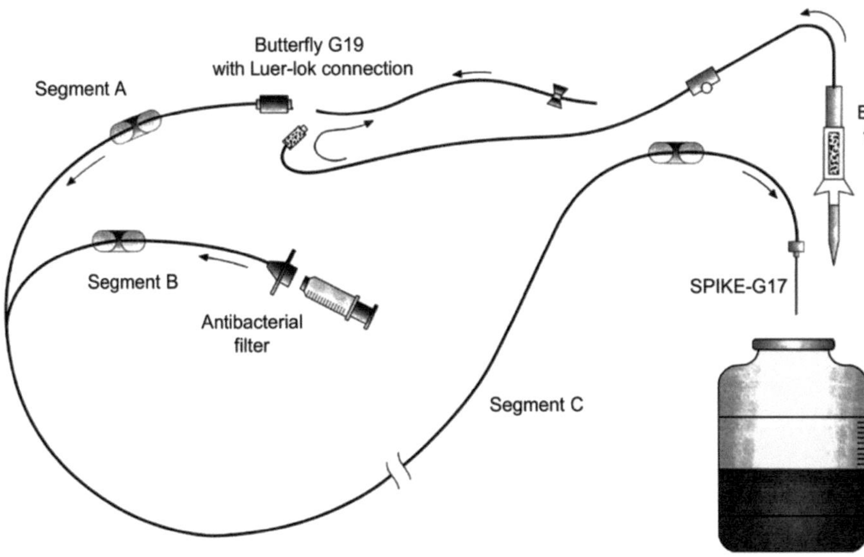

Figure 1. Schematic drawing of the components necessary to perform major autohematherapy

Minor AHT is very similar to major AHT method with a few differences, where 5-10 ml of blood is mixed with precise dose of medical ozone in a syringe and reinjected by intramuscular route to the donor that no anticoagulant is used. Rectal insufflation (RI) of medical ozone gas is another method of systemic ozone therapy that is applied on some cases if others methods cannot be done or this method is preferred over others due to diseases.

Ozone is normally present as gas made of three atoms of oxygen with a cyclic structure. The medical generator of ozone produces it from pure oxygen passing through a high voltage gradient (5-13 mV) according to the reaction.

$$3O_2 + 68{,}400\,\text{cal} \rightarrow 2O_3 \qquad (1)$$

Ozone is 1.6 fold denser and 10-fold more soluble in water (49.0 mL in 100 mL water at 0_C) than oxygen. Although ozone is not a radical molecule, it is the third most potent oxidant (E_5 12.076 V) after fluorine and persulfate. Ozone is an unstable gas that cannot be stored and should be used at once because it has a half life of 40 min at 20_C

2.1. What is the behavior and fate of ozone after coming in contact with body fluids?

The essential concepts to bear in mind are the following;

a. As any other gas, ozone dissolves physically in pure water according to Henry's Law in relation to temperature, pressure and ozone concentration. Only in this situation ozone does not react and in a tightly closed glass bottle, the ozonated water is useful as a disinfectant that remains active for a couple of days

b. On the other hand, at variance with oxygen, ozone reacts immediately as soon as it is dissolved in biological water (physiological saline, plasma, lymph, urine)

$$O_3 + \text{biomolecules} \rightarrow O_2 + O, \tag{2}$$

Where atomic oxygen behaves as a very reactive atom. Contrary to the incorrect belief that ozone penetrates through the skin and mucosae or enters into the cells, it is emphasized that, after the mentioned reaction, ozone does not exist any longer. In order of preference, ozone reacts with polyunsaturated fatty acids (PUFA), antioxidants such as ascorbic and uric acids, thiol compounds with-SH groups such as cysteine, reduced glutathione (GSH) and albumin. Depending upon the ozone dose, carbohydrates, enzymes, DNA and RNA can also be affected. All of these compounds act as electron donor and undergo oxidation.

c. The main reaction:

$$R-CH=CH-R + O_3 + H_2O \rightarrow R-CH=O + R-CH=O + H_2O_2 \tag{3}$$

shows the simultaneous formation of one mole of hydrogen peroxide (included among reactive oxygen species, ROS) and of two moles of lipid oxidation products (LOPs) [12].

The fundamental ROS molecule is hydrogen peroxide, which is a non-radical oxidant able to act as an ozone Messenger responsible for eliciting several biological and therapeutic effects [13,14]. The concept that ROS are always harmful has been widely revised because, in physiological amounts, they act as regulators of signal transduction and represent important mediators of host defense and immune responses. Presence of traces of Fe++should be avoided because, in the presence of hydrogen peroxide, via the Fenton's reaction, they will catalyze the formation of the most reactive OH, (hydroxyl radical).

It is determined [15] that the formation of nitrogen monoxide (NO,) in human endothelial cells exposed to ozonated serum. Attention should be paid to the fact that an excess of ROS can lead to the formation of other toxic compounds such as peroxynitrite (O=NOO-) and hypochlorite anion (ClO-).

Although ROS have a lifetime of less than a second, they can damage crucial cell components and, therefore, their generation must be precisely calibrated to achieve a biological effect without any damage. This can be achieved by regulating the ozone dose (ozone concentration as mg/mL of gas per mL of blood in 1:1 ratio) against the antioxidant capacity of blood that can be measured and, if necessary, strengthened by oral administration of antioxidants before and throughout ozone therapy.

d. LOPs production follows peroxidation of PUFA present in the plasma: they are heterogeneous and can be classified as lipoperoxides (LOO,), alkoxyl radicals (LO,), lipohydroperoxides (LOOH), isoprostanes and alkenals, among which are 4-hydroxy-2,3 transnonenal (HNE) and malonyldialdehyde (MDA). Radicals and aldehydes are intrinsically toxic and must be generated in very low concentrations. They are in vitro far more stable (6) than ROS but fortunately, upon blood reinfusion, they undergo a marked dilution in body fluids, excretion (via urine and bile), and metabolism by GSH-transferase (GSH-Tr) and aldehyde dehydrogenases. Thus, only submicromolar concentrations can reach all organs, particularly bone marrow, liver, central nervous system (CNS), endocrine glands, etc., where they act as signaling molecules of an ongoing acute oxidative stress [16].

If the stage of the disease is not too far advanced, these molecules can elicit the upregulation of antioxidant enzymes such as superoxide dismutase (SOD), GSH-peroxidases (GSH-Px), GSH-reductase (GSH-Rd) and catalase (CAT). Interestingly, Iles and Liu [17] have just demonstrated that HNE, by inducing the expression of glutamate cysteine ligase, causes an intracellular increase of GSH, which plays a key role in antioxidant defense. Furthermore, LOPs induce oxidative stress proteins, one of which is heme-oxygenase I (HO-1 or HSP-32) which, after breaking down the heme molecule, delivers very useful compounds such as CO and bilirubin [18]. Bilirubin is a significant lipophilic antioxidant and a trace of CO cooperates with NO in regulating vasodilation by activating cyclic GMP. Fe++is promptly chelated by upregulated ferritin. The induction of HO-1 after an oxidative stress has been described in hundreds of papers as one of the most important antioxidant defense and protective enzyme. Moreover, LOPs exert a neuroimmunomodulatory effect highlighted by a feeling of well being reported by patients during ozone therapy.

Although it remains hypothetical, it is possible that LOP, throughout the treatments, acting as acute oxidative stressors in the bone marrow microenvironments activate the release of metalloproteinases, of which MP-9 particularly may favor the detachment of staminal cells [11]. These cells, once in the blood circulation, may be attracted and home at sites where a previous injury (a trauma or an ischemic-degenerative event) has taken place. The potential relevance of such an event would have a huge practical importance and will avoid the unnatural, costly and scarcely effective practice of the bone marrow collection with the need of the successive and uncertain reinfusion [19].

It is emphasized that submicromolar LOPs levels can be stimulatory and beneficial, whereas high levels can be toxic. This conclusion, based on many experimental data [16], reinforces the concept that optimal ozone concentrations are critical for achieving a therapeutic result: too low concentrations are practically useless (at best elicit a placebo effect), too high may elicit a negative effect (malaise, fatigue) so that they must be just above the threshold level to yield an acute, absolutely transitory oxidative stress capable of triggering biological effects without toxicity. In conclusion, it must be clear that the ozonation process either happening in blood, or intradiscal or in an intramuscular site represents an acute oxidative stress. However, provided that it is precisely calculated according to a judicious ozone dosage, it is not deleterious but is actually capable of eliciting a multitude of useful biological responses and, possibly, can reverse a chronic oxidative stress due to aging, chronic infections, diabetes, atherosclerosis, degenerative processes and cancer. Indeed, the ozonotherapeutic act is interpreted as an atoxic but real "therapeutic shock" able to restore homeostasis.

2.2. Which are the biological effects elicited by ROS and LOPs?

The ozonation process is therefore characterized by the formation of ROS and LOPs acting in two phases. This process happens either ex vivo (as a typical example in the blood collected in a glass bottle) or in vivo (after an intramuscular injection of ozone) but while ROS are acting immediately and disappear (early and short-acting messengers), LOPs, via the circulation, distribute throughout the tissues and eventually only a few molecules bind to cell receptors. Their pharmacodynamics allow minimizing their potential toxicity and allows them to become late and long-lasting messengers.

Formation of ROS in the plasma is extremely rapid and is accompanied by a transitory and small ozone dosedependent decrease (ranging from 5 to 25%) of the antioxidant capacity. Importantly, this return to normal within 15–20 min owes to the efficient recycling of oxidized compounds such as dehydroascorbate to ascorbic acid [20]. H2O2 diffuses easily from the plasma into the cells and its sudden appearance in the cytoplasm represents the triggering stimulus: depending upon the cell type, different biochemical pathways can be concurrently activated in erythrocytes, leukocytes and platelets resulting in numerous biological effects. It must be noted that between the plasma and the cytoplasm compartments there is a gradient and the intracellular H2O2 concentration is only about 1/10 of the plasmatic one [21]. The rapid reduction to water is operated by the high concentration of GSH, CAT and GSH-Px; nonetheless, H2O2 must be above the threshold concentration for activating several biochemical pathways.

Let us now examine how hydrogen peroxide, now universally recognized as one of the main intracellular signalling molecules [13], acts on the different blood cells. The mass of erythrocytes mops up the bulk of hydrogen peroxide: GSH is promptly oxidized to GSSG and the cell, extremely sensitive to the reduction of the GSH/GSSG ratio, immediately corrects the unbalance by either extruding GSSG or reducing it with GSH-Rd at the expense of ascorbate or of the reduced nicotinamide adenine dinucleotide phosphate (NADPH), which serves as a crucial electron donor. Next, the oxidized NADP is reduced after the activation of the pentose phosphate pathway, of which glucose-6-phosphate dehydrogenase (G-6PD) is the key enzyme. It is determined that a small but significant increase of ATP formation [10,11], but whether this is due to the activation of the pentose cycle or to phosphofructokinase or to both remains to be clarified. Moreover, for a brief period the reinfused erythrocytes enhance the delivery of oxygen into ischemic tissues because of a shift to the right of the oxygen–hemoglobin dissociation curve, due either to a slight decrease of intracellular pH (Bohr effect) or/and an increase of 2,3-diphosphoglycerate (2,3-DPG) levels. Obviously, one AHT treatment has a minimal effect and we need to ozonate at least 2.5–4 L of blood within a period of 30–60 days. During this period, LOPs act as repeated stressors on the bone marrow and these frequent stimuli cause the adaptation to the ozone stress during erythrogenesis with upregulation of antioxidant enzymes. As a consequence, a patient with chronic limb ischemia undergoing ozone therapy can have a clinical improvement due to the formation of successive cohorts of erythrocytes progressively more capable of delivering oxygen to his/her ischemic tissues. However, the final improvement is also due to the localized release of NO, CO and growth factors released from platelets and endothelial cells.

Although ozone is one of the most potent disinfectants, it cannot inactivate bacteria, viruses and fungi in vivo because, paradoxically, the pathogens are well protected, particularly inside the cells, by the powerful antioxidant system. Thus, as it was proposed a long time ago [22,23], ozone acts as a mild enhancer of the immune system by activating neutrophils and stimulating the synthesis of some cytokines (2,5–7). Once again, the crucial messenger is hydrogen peroxide, which after entering into the cytoplasm of blood mononuclear cells (BMC) by oxidizing selected cysteines, activates a tyrosine kinase, which then phosphorylates the transcription factor nuclear factor kB [24], allowing the release of a heterodimer (p50+p65).

This complex moves on to the nucleus and switches on some hundred genes eventually responsible for causing the synthesis of several proteins, among which are the acute-phase reactants and numerous interleukins. In the past, it was measured the release of several cytokines from ozonated blood upon in vitro incubation (2–7). Once the ozonated leukocytes return to the circulation, they home in lymphoid microenvironments and successively release cytokines acting in a paracrine fashion on neighboring cells with a possible reactivation of a depressed immune system [25]. This process, described as the physiological cytokine response, is part of the innate immune system and helps us to survive in a hostile environment.

During ozonation of blood, particularly if it is anticoagulated with heparin, we have noted an ozone dose-dependent increase of activation of platelets [8, 26] with a consequent release of typical growth factors, which will enhance the healing of chronic ulcers in ischemic patients. Whenever possible, the use of heparin as an anticoagulant is preferable to sodium citrate because, by not chelating plasmatic Ca++, it reinforces biochemical and electric events.

During reinfusion of the ozonated blood into the donor, the vast expanse of the endothelial cells will be activated by LOPs, resulting in an increased production of NO, plasma S-nitrosothiols and S-nitrosohemoglobin [15, 27]. Whereas NO has a half-life of less than 1 sec, protein-bound-NO can exert vasodilation also at distant ischemic vascular sites with relevant therapeutic effect.

Moreover, on the basis of the phenomenon of ozone tolerance that says the exposure of an organism to a low level of an agent, harmful at high levels, induces an adaptive and beneficial response [28,29], it is postulated that LOPs, by acting as long-distance messengers, can transmit to all organs the information of an acute oxidative stres [10, 11]. The bone marrow is particularly relevant because it can upregulate antioxidant enzymes during erythrogenesis and allows the release of staminal cells for possibly regenerating infarcted organs. Moreover, the stimulation of the endocrine and central nervous systems may help to understand why most patients during prolonged ozone therapy report a feeling of euphoria and wellness, probably due to an improved metabolism as well as to an enhanced hormonal or neurotransmitter release.

The paradoxical concept that ozone eventually induces an antioxidant response capable of reversing a chronic oxidative stress is common in the animal and vegetal kingdom and there is good experimental evidence [30–34] that this phenomenon is present in the animal and vegetal kingdom. Moreover, it is already supported by findings of an increased level of antioxidant enzymes and HO-1 during ozone therapy [10,11]. It also suggests that a judicious use of ozone, in spite of acting as an oxidant, enhances the antioxidant capacity, which represents the critical factor for overcoming chronic viral infections, ischemia and celldegeneration.

3. A concise summary of biological effects observed after ozone therapy

3.1. Erythrocytes

These cells respond with an activation of glycolysis due to activation of the pentose hosphate pathway. It is found that increased adenosine triphosphate levels (from 13899/260 to 19689/232 mM) in patients with age-related macular degeneration (ARMD) (atrophic form) after a therapeutic cycle (14 sessions) of O3-AHT.26 Moreover, Viebahn [27] reported the same effect in athletes and elderly patients after rectal insufflation of O2_/O3. Ozonation implies a small but consistent oxidation of GSH to glutathione disulfide, and GSH reductase utilizes the reduced form of the coenzyme nicotinamide adenine dinucleotide phosphate supplied by G6PDH to reduce glutathione disulfide to GSH, which indeed returns rapidly to the original level. [28] The increase of 2,3-diphosphoglycerate varies depending on the basic level in ARMD patients and only those who had a low level showed a marked increase with therapy. Viebahn, [27] after a longer cycle of therapy in elderly people, observed a significant increase. An increase of 2,3-diphosphoglycerate level in oxyhemoglobin shifts to the right (p50 value increases); its dissociation curve implies an increased delivery of O2 into the hypoxic tissues. The life-span of ozonated 99Tc-labeled erythrocytes and their uptake by liver and spleen are comparable with oxygenated erythrocytes.(3)

A problem still under study regards the generation of biochemically improved erythrocytes during prolonged ozone therapy. While ROS have an extremely short life, LOPs, during the reinfusion of ozonated blood, return into the donor's circulation. While they are fairly stable in vitro, they rapidly disappear from blood in vivo owing to considerable dilution into body fluids, degradation by aldehyde dehydrogenases, excretion into bile and urine, and uptake in various organs including bone marrow cells. This process is crucial for explaining the mechanism of ozone tolerance: during erythrogenesis, submicromolar LOP concentrations can upregulate the synthesis of antioxidant enzymes and indeed, after appropriate density gradient separation, it is found that young (lighter) erythrocytes contain more G6PDH than older (heavier) cells generated before the therapy. [25] This result suggests that ozone therapy enhances the generation of erythrocytes with improved metabolic characteristics, a sort of 'supergifted erythrocytes' able to correct hypoxia in vascular diseases.

3.2. Leukocytes

These were the cells that were examined first as it is hypothesized that ozone could act as an IFN-g inducer.[29] Since then it is shown [30,31] that ozone behaves as a weak (compared with mitogens) cytokine (such as tumor necrosis factor-a, interleukin-2, interleukin-6, interleukin-8, transforming growth factor-b [TGF-b]) inducer. Several studies [32 - 35] have confirmed that ozone can stimulate bronchoalveolar cells to release proinflammatory cytokines and eicosanoids. Thanks to parallel progress in understanding the role of antioxidants and redox regulation of gene transcription, it has been clarified that, among several signals, H2O2 is one of the most significant cytokine inducers.[36] As already mentioned, after ozonation H2O2 freely diffuses into the leukocyte cytoplasm and activates specific protein kinases that, by phosphorylating IkB bound to the nuclear factor-kB allows the migration of the transcription heterodimer p50_/p65 into the nucleus where it activates gene expression.[37] Obviously H2O2 must reach a concentration able to activate the kinase without being instantaneously reduced by intracellular antioxidants. [38] Therefore the relevance of the response depends on the levels of H2O2, which can act as either 'life or death' signals. The fact that ozone can either be a toxic or a useful signal depends on the minimal antioxidant capacity of the respiratory tract lining fluid, whereas blood has a very potent capacity. The data in fact indicate that too little ozone (hence H2O2) is ineffective and too much (or too little antioxidants) can be toxic. During recent years it is addressed the following questions: first, as ozone acts as a mild cytokine inducer, does reinfusion of ozonated blood modify the plasma cytokine level in vivo? Second, does the induction of oxidative stress proteins, particularly of heme-oxygenase I (HO-I), and of adaptation to the therapeutic oxidative stress have an immunomodulatory effect? And third, can we devise an optimal schedule for improving the immune reactivity in immunodepressed patients?

The classical O3-AHT, usually consisting of 225 ml of blood (plus 25 ml of 3.8% sodium citrate solution) treated with 225 ml of gas (O2_/O3) with ozone concentrations ranging from an initial 20 mg/ml slowly scaled up to 40_/50 mg/ml per ml of blood, continued for several months, twice weekly, is ideal for this purpose. A probable explanation is that, after each blood reinfusion, a small percentage of immune cells are activated and home in several organs: these cells release into the microenvironment cytokines that, in turn, prime or activate neighboring cells thus slowly reinforcing immune responses. Modifications of cytokine plasma levels are hardly detectable so that side effects like the flu-like syndrome, typically observed after administration of immunoadjuvants, are absent [39] and actually most of patients report a sense of well-being during the therapy. There is a wealth of experimental data [40 - 44] showing that both animals and plants can develop ozone tolerance by upregulating the expression of antioxidants, which can correct a chronic imbalance between excessive endogenous oxidation due to viral infections, cancer, chronic inflammations and depressed antioxidants. Both chronic hepatitis C virus and cancer patients have shown a marked improvement of their clinical conditions after several months of O3-AHT treatments, suggesting that this 'calculated and brief oxidative stress' truly merits the term 'therapeutic shock'.

3.3. Platelets

It is known that ROS can induce platelet activation and it was obvious to assume that blood ozonation, by generating H2O2, could cause it. [45 – 46] Moreover H2O2 or other ROS can activate phospholipase C, phospholipase A2, cyclo-oxygenases and lipo-oxygenases and thromboxane synthetase, allowing a step increase of intracellular Ca2_, release of prostaglandin E2, prostaglandin F2a and thromboxane A2 with irreversible platelet aggregation. For these reasons it is studied the behavior of either human platelet rich-plasma anticoagulated with heparin or citrate, either untreated or simply oxygenated, or ozonated at three concentrations (20, 40 and 80 mg/ml). Because the plasmatic Ca2_ level potentiates the ozone effect, we were not surprised to observe a rapid platelet aggregation in heparinized plasma particularly at the highest concentration. [47] Consequently the release of several growth factors like platelet-derived growth factor AB, TGF-b1, interleukin-8 and thromboxane_/2 were significantly higher from heparinized platelets than Ca2_-free platelets. [48] These results taught us that it is better to chelate Ca2_ for performing a safe autohemotherapy. Nonetheless the release of growth factors from Ca2_-free platelets is still important because the reinfusion of ozonated blood implies an elevation of plasma levels of TGF-b that may explain why the healing of necrotic ulcers in hind limb ischemia due to atherosclerosis and diabetes markedly quickens during treatment with both parenteral (O3-AHT) and topical treatments with ozonated water and oil. [49 – 50]

3.4. Endothelial cells and the vascular system

During the reinfusion of ozonated blood, the endothelium comes in contact with traces of LOPs that soon disappear in vivo. It is [51] investigated the effect of addition of ozonated (40 and 80 mg/ml) human plasma to human endothelial cells in culture and it is measured a significant increase of the critical relaxing factor NO+that was ozone dose dependent.

The induction of nitric oxide synthase and the release of NO+was reinforced in the presence of 20 mm of arginine and was abolished by the addition of 20 mM of L-N-omega-nitro-L-arginine methyl ester. In physiological conditions the endothelium regulates the vascular tone [52] by producing some 1_/10 mM of NO+and 1 nM of anion superoxide (one of the contracting factors). The intravascular half-life of NO+is about 2 msec with a strictly localized consumption so that the likelihood of improving vasodilation in remote ischemic areas (the macula or the limbs) seems negligible. However, NO+readily reacts with GSH, cysteine, albumin and hemoglobin (cysteine residue b 93) and the formed S-nitrosothiols and S-nitrosohemoglobin have half-lives of 5_/50 min, allowing a pharmacological effect at distant sites. [53 – 54] It remains to be ascertained whether ozonated blood enhances the release of prostacyclin (PGI2) and angiopoietins, both important factors for improving ischemic vasculopathies.

3.5. Parenchymal cells in other organs

Upon reinfusion of ozonated blood, LOPs can reach other organs such as the hypothalamus, endocrine glands, liver, kidneys and bone marrow. The phenomenon of adaptation to the repeated and acute oxidative stress imposed by O3-AHT is most interesting and able to elicit crucial therapeutic responses. During prolonged treatment, cells throughout the body receive small and gradual pulses of LOPs that are responsible for:

1. Neuro-endocrine responses explaining the reported feeling of wellness, [55]

2. The upregulation of antioxidant enzymes in several cell types that is an excellent way to re-equilibrate the oxidant_/antioxidant unbalance

3. Inducing a number of stress or heat shock proteins (HSPs) such as HSP27, HO-1 (HSP 32), HSP72 and HSP [90 – 56 – 59]

It is observed that HO-1 is a protective enzyme allowing the formation of Fe2_, bilirubin (an antioxidant) and carbon monoxide (CO), a vasodilator that, like NO+, increases the level of cyclic guanosine monophosphate, the reaction catalyzed by guanylate cyclase. Besides gases produced by the gut flora, it is truly remarkable that cells can release other gaseous molecules (NO+, CO and CO2), and it is even more surprising that even ozone can be produced by activated antibody-coated neutrophils. [60] These gases can now be considered as molecules able to deliver crucial physiological and pharmacological effects.

Excessive amounts of these molecules are toxic, causing serious pathological events and possibly death. Nature teaches us that these gases, depending on their concentrations, can be either friends or foes and similarly ozone therapy can be either useful or toxic. If this reasoning is correct, ozone therapy, when judiciously performed, is a simple, inexpensive and atoxic approach with the advantage of activating several biomechanisms in different cells unusually leading to an integrated and often incredible response.

4. The extreme versatility of ozone therapy

The sarcastic comment of the opponents is that ozone therapy looks like a panacea for all diseases. Indeed it seems so, but in reality this is due to the multitude of compounds originated at first from the reaction of ozone with body fluids, and eventually able to display pleiotropic effects delivered by different organs. For the sake of brevity we can only summarize the therapeutic effects so far reported

Specialization	Pathology
Dermatology	Herpes Zoster and simplex, acne, eczema, lipodystrophy (cellulite), mycosis, psoriasis, atopic dermatitis
Internal Medicine	Hepatitis, diabetes, atherosclerosis, arterial hypertension, osteoarthritis, asthma, chronic bronchitis, gastritis, gastric ulcer, Crohn's disease, chronic constipation, hypothyroidism.
Nephrology / Dialysis	Adjuvant in the treatment of ischemic-metabolic pathologies.
Neurology	Migraines, depression, vasomotor cephalea, neuro-vascular disorders.
Dentistry	Treatment of cavities, disinfection of cavities during surgery and post-operatory period. Periodontitis, aphthas.
Orthopedic Rheumatology	Disc-radicular conflicts, disc herniation, articular rheumatism, lumbago, osteoarthritis, arthropathy, periarthritis, rheumatoid arthritis.
Angiology	Venous insufficiency, diabetic ulcer, arthropathy, coronaropathy, gangrene, postphlebitic ulcer, peripheral vasculopathy.
Gynecology	Bacterial infections by protozoa or mycosis, Bartholin's cyst, vaginitis, menopause, chronic pelvic inflammation, infertility.
Immunology	Immuno-modulator, autoimmune disorders, adjuvant in treatments with radiation and in immunodeficiency.

Table 1. Indiciations of Ozone Therapy in General

http://dx.doi.org/10.5772/57470

4.1. Acute and chronic bacterial, viral and fungine infections

Intuitively, ozone therapy is very useful in both acute and chronic bacterial, viral and fungine infections because the generated ROS are the natural and most effective agents to which even antibiotic resistant pathogens do not resist. [3-61] Moreover, improvement of metabolism and immunological functions contribute to a favorable outcome. Abscesses, anal fissures, fistulae, bed sores, furunculosis, inveterate osteomyelitis, vulvovaginitis, necrotizing fasciitis and torpid ulcers of various origin have been shown to improve rapidly, particularly using the combination of O3-AHT with topical treatment using either direct O2_/O3 exposure or the cleansing and stimulating effect of ozonated water and oil. The activity of ozonated solutions in eliminating the infectivity and enhancing healing is almost unbelievable. However, in Western countries accustomed to the use of antibiotic creams (often with corticosteroids) there is no mental attitude to profitably use the inexpensive and most active ozonated oil. [62]

4.2. Ischemic diseases

Chronic limb ischemia (atherosclerosis, diabetes, Burger's disease) is most effectively treated at stage II-b with complete disappearance of pain and claudication. Moreover, since 1981, Rokitansky et al.[49] demonstrated that a cycle of O3-AHT (usually 14 treatments) led to a very good improvement in 70.6% and 53.8% of either stage III or stage IV (Fontaine) patients, respectively. Amputation of toes and limbs could be avoided in pre-terminal phases.

These results have been amply confirmed by Giunta et al.,[63] Mattassi et al. [64] and Tylicki et al.[65] Preterminal patients with chronic heart ischemia and no further susceptibility to conventional treatments have shown marked improvement after a cycle of 14 treatments of extracorporeal circulation of blood against O2_/O3.[66] A randomized controlled study is in progress for establishing the validity of this more invasive method than classical O3-AHT.

4.3. Age-related macular degeneration

A 6-year study in 90 patients with the 'dry' form of ARMD has been carried out performing a cycle of 13_/14 O3-AHT treatments. Mean distance best-corrected visual acuity was significantly improved in the treatment group of patients while in the control group, first treated with oxygenated autohaemotherapy, only a modest and not significant improvement in mean distance visual acuity was observed. No adverse effects have been noted and the patient's compliance has been excellent. [26] Owing to the constant increase of ARMD patients and the lack of an effective conventional treatment, this approach appears mandatory.

4.4. Orthopedic diseases

Until recently it was unthinkable that a mixture of O2_/O3 could be useful in orthopedics. Indeed lumbar disk herniation and osteoarthritis, although having different etiologies, have a common inflammatory background expressed by a localized chronic oxidative stress due to excessive production of ROS, release of proinflammatory cytokines and activation of cyclo-xygenases. Common sense would proscribe the use of ozone, a master generator of free radicals and, as it is well shown, [34 – 67] after pulmonary exposure, a superb inflammatory agent.

Contrary to all expectations, it is now well demonstrated [68] that combined intradiscal and periganglionic injection of medical ozone allows an excellent outcome in 70.3% of patients treated for disk herniation performed after conservative management failed to respond. In the same vein, it appears very surprising that the application of medical ozone in acute and chronic painful diseases of the joints allows rapid pain relief, disappearance of inflammation and improvement of mobility. Thousands of patients have been successfully treated and the lack of side effects is noteworthy. [69] These positive empiric observations need to be explained. Ozone is indeed a surprising gas that paradoxically, after prolonged administration at low concentrations, induces tolerance, a phenomenon termed 'hormesis' by Goldman [70] to indicate 'a beneficial effect of a low level exposure to an agent that is harmful at high levels'. Thus, at this stage, we use the definition of 'ozone paradox' for explaining these excellent therapeutic results. Immediately after O2_/O3 administration in the nucleus pulposus or into inflamed endoarticular cavities; a sort of oxidative shock seems to subvert all the traditional rules by inducing an antioxidative response due to several factors, among which is the cholinergic antiinflammatory pathway. [71] A detailed discussion is reported elsewhere. (3)

4.5. Dentistry

This is another medical specialty where ozone has been recently evaluated with exceedingly interesting results.[72] Primary root carious lesions are being treated with a novel ozone delivery system able to avoid any toxic risk for the mouth cavity and lungs. The tooth's lesion is exposed for 10_/20 sec to a sort of ozone 'hurricane' based on a gas flow of 615 ml/min of O2_/O3 at a low concentration (4 mg/ml), perfectly enclosed in a tightly fitting silicone cup enclosing the tooth. It is not surprising that all bacteria, particularly lactobacilli, are destroyed so that the ozone-sterilized dental surface becomes quickly remineralized, becoming hard and resistant to further bacterial attack. This new approach is simple, inexpensive and well tolerated, as opposed to the conventional and painful 'drilling and filling' management of primary root carious lesions. Dermatological, pulmonary, renal, hematological and neurodegenerative diseases Owing to the ability of ozone to activate a number of biological targets, ozone therapy could be proficiently used in some dermatological, pulmonary, renal, hematological and neurodegenerative diseases. However these pathologies so far have not been evaluated in a controlled fashion. Most of the patients with metastatic cancer resistant to radiotherapy and chemotherapy report a striking improvement of the quality of life with prolonged (twice weekly for months) O3-AHT treatments. [25 – 73] This is a constantly observed result, most probably due to a multifactorial neuroendocrine response.

5. Summary

Finally it must be emphasized that if ozone is judiciously used according to precisely defined guidelines, it causes neither acute, nor chronic side effects. After two decades of practical applications and the results observed in patients after conventional remedies have proved unsatisfactory. One has the feeling that, if ozone therapy could be accepted and used in all hospitals, it would represent a small but important medical revolution able to cure or stabilize several diseases in many patients in both rich and poor countries.

6. Discussion and conclusions

There is no doubt that ozone can be toxic, and even today its hazardous employment by charlatans and unprepared physicians has contributed to a poor consideration of ozone therapy. That is one reason why the use of ozone is prohibited in some states of the USA and why this therapy is still regarded with skepticism by orthodox medicine even in Germany, where this approach was first conceived. Moreover, the following data tend to generalize that ozone is always toxic and should not be used in medicine:

1. Overwhelming evidence shows that the bronchial-pulmonary system is very sensitive to ozone and this gas should never be inhaled. [67]

2. This is very true because the respiratory tract lining fluid is constituted by a very thin, watery film containing a minimal amount of antioxidants that makes mucosal cells extremely vulnerable to oxidation. The opposite situation occurs for blood cells suspended in plasma, which has a potent antioxidant capacity (1.23_/1.83 mmol/l) able to tame any ozone dose within the therapeutic range (10_/80 mg/ml).

3. Saline-washed erythrocytes suspended in saline undergo extensive hemolysis after ozone exposure. [12]

4. Cells in culture, even if exposed to very low ozone concentrations for a long time, undergo apoptosis. [74]

5. One-hour exposure of saline-diluted blood to 5 mM of ozone induces genotoxic effects on leukocyte. [75]

But is ozone always toxic?

As a matter of fact millions of O3-AHT, even if performed in an empirical fashion during the past three decades, has neither yielded acute nor chronic toxic effects. According to Jacobs [76] this procedure has yielded the lowest number of medical complications.

However, four deaths have been recorded due to pulmonary embolism, which occurred during direct intravenous administration of O2_/O3, an application prohibited by the European Society of Ozonetherapy since 1983. Thus ozone seems like Janus and his two faces require an explanation. This is now reasonably clear. Since 1988 we have investigated the problem in a scientific way using precise ozone generators, which allow checking ozone concentration in real time by a photometer calibrated with the classical iodometric method. A review [61] and a critical book (3) have extensively clarified the issue but this does not seem sufficient to dispel the dogma that 'ozone is always toxic'. However, we now consider ozone as a real drug that must be used with caution after having carefully defined its therapeutic window. First, the ozone must be calibrated against the antioxidant capacity of the patient's blood in order to control the potential ozone toxicity

Second, expert scientists in free radicals ought to distinguish the chronic intracellular oxidative stress typical of several pathologies by the transitory (5 min) calculated oxidative stress occurring when a precise volume of blood is exposed ex vivo to an equal volume of gas (O2_/ O3) with well-defined ozone concentrations ranging from 20 up to 40 mg/ml per ml of blood. It needs to be emphasized that the exogenous oxidative stress caused by ozone in blood is due to the fact that ozone, once dissolved in the plasmatic water, instantaneously reacts with biomolecules and disappears but generates ROS, among which are H2O2 and LOPs. These are the effective ozone messengers that interact with a variety of cells and elicit the now-termed 'therapeutic shock' due to the multiform biological responses. That ozone acts as a real chemical drug is proved by the fact that the ozone messengers, to be effective, must reach a threshold because otherwise there are no biological effects and the therapeutic results, if any, are due to a placebo effect. Although we have proven that ozone therapy is not a nebulous approach and has been shown amenable to a precise scientific scrutiny, it is probable that much still remains to be uncovered.

Everyone knows that plasma and blood cells contain an almost redundant antioxidant system made up of hydro-liposoluble compounds and antioxidant enzymes. During aging or pathologic conditions, this is not sufficient to correct the intracellular oxidative stress, but normally it is adequate to tame ozone toxicity while allowing the generation of ROS and LOPs. Thus all data emphasizing ozone toxicity can be easily dismissed because the following is now well proven:

1. Blood is a much more ozone-resistant 'tissue' than the respiratory tract that, for anatomic, biochemical and metabolic reasons, is always at a loss when exposed to ozone, and therefore it is wrong to extrapolate ozone toxicity for the pulmonary system to blood.
2. Washed and saline-resuspended erythrocytes, fully depleted of the plasmatic antioxidants, are obviously very sensitive to ozonation, and all of these unnatural data have neither physiological nor practical significance.
3. The same occurs for cells cultured in antioxidant-poor media and exposed continuously for days to ozone. Surprisingly, cell biologists reported only the ozone concentration but have neither calculated nor taken into account the cumulative dose of ozone that after a long exposure kills the cells.
4. The conclusion is that, although ozone is potentially mutagenic, so far all experimental data performed in physiological conditions and clinical evidence have neithershown any cell damage nor adverse effects in patients. As a matter of fact, blood is exposed to ozone concentrations (0.21_/1.68 mM) lower than the mutagenic ones (1.5_/5.6 mM). The question of whether ozone is genotoxic and mutagenic is a critical one and has been extensively discussed elsewhere. (3) What has never been entirely appreciated is the fact that we can only use an ozone dose that does not overwhelm the antioxidant capacity of blood.

Hopefully this discussion should put an end to the confusion between the endogenously constant oxidative stress due to the oxygen and the transitory and occasional therapeutic 'shock' due to precise blood ozonation. A point that should not be overlooked is that ozone messengers, by acting on different cells, elicit a variety of biological effects that cannot ever be dreamed of with the usual reductionist approach of using a drug for a single target. This consideration can explain the far superior therapeutic effect of parenteral and topical ozone therapy in advanced cases of chronic limb ischemia to the conventional infusion of prostanoids. Another relevant characteristic is that the judicious strategy 'start low, go slow' in using ozone is able to induce in patients the adaptation to the chronic oxidative stress (i.e. ozone) paradoxically upregulates the antioxidant defenses. The scientific evaluation of ozone therapy efficacy remains the crucial point: results accrued during the past 20 years show that is very useful in chronic limb ischemia, ARMD, chronic infectious diseases and, most surprising, in orthopedics and even in dentistry after conventional medicine has failed to provide a real advantage. There are no adverse effects and most of the patients report a feeling of wellness. The efficacy remains uncertain in other pathologies such as neurodegenerative, autoimmune diseases and cancer because clinical experience is fragmentary and anecdotal.

However, orthodox medicine remains skeptical because controlled clinical trials are few and are not considered satisfactory. Unfortunately our good will is not sufficient to overcome prejudice and lack of sponsors. It is distressing to realize that a wrong dogma, commercial interests and the disinterest of Health Authorities delay the application of a medical approach that could help billions of patients, particularly in poor countries. Finally, this paper may serve the purpose of opening a fruitful discussion on the beneficial versus the toxicological actions of ozone, and a referee has proposed that the debate may be hosted as a forum by Mediators of Inflammations.

Author details

Ruhi Cakir

Mediozon Clinics, Istanbul, Turkey

References

[1] Wolff HH. Die behandlung peripherer durchblutungsstorungen mit ozon. Erfahr Hk 1974;23:181–184.

[2] Bocci V, Paulesu L. Studies on the biological effects of ozone: 1. Induction of interferon gamma on human leucocytes. Haematologica 1990;75:510–515.

[3] Bocci V, Luzzi E, Corradeschi F, Paulesu L, Di Stefano A. Studies on the biological effects of ozone: 3. An attempt to define conditions for optimal induction of cytokines. Lymphokine Cytokine Res 1993;12:121–126.

[4] Bocci V, Luzzi E, Corradeschi F, Paulesu L, Rossi R, Cardaioli E, et al. Studies on the biological effects of ozone: 4. Cytokine production and glutathione levels in human erythrocytes. J Biol Regulat Homeost Agent 1993;7:133–138.

[5] Bocci V, Luzzi E, Corradeschi F. Studies on the biological effects of ozone: Evaluation of immunological parameters and tolerability in normal volunteers receiving ambulatory autohaemotherapy. Biotherapy 1994;7:83–90.

[6] Bocci V, Valacchi G, Corradeschi F, Aldinucci C, Silvestri S,Paccagnini E, et al. Studies on the biological effects of ozone: 7. Generation of reactive oxygen species (ROS) after exposure of human blood to ozone. J Biol Regulat Homeost Agent 1998;12:67–75.

[7] Bocci V, Valacchi G, Corradeschi F, Fanetti G. Studies on the biological effects of ozone: 8. Effects on the total antioxidant status and on interleukin-8 production. Mediat Inflamm 1998;7:313–317.

[8] Bocci V, Valacchi G, Rossi R, Giustarini D, Paccagnini E, Pucci AM,et al. Studies on the biological effects of ozone: 9. Effects of ozone on human platelets. Platelets 1999;10:110–116.

[9] Bocci V. Ossigeno-ozono terapia, Comprensione dei meccanismi diazione. Milano: Casa Editrice Ambrosiana;2000.

[10] Bocci V. Oxygen-Ozone Therapy. A critical evaluation. Dordrecht, The Netherlands: Kluwer Academic Publishers;2002.

[11] Bocci V. OZONE. A New Medical Drug. Dordrecht, The Netherlands:Springer;2005.

[12] Pryor WA, Squadrito GL, Friedman M. The cascade mechanism to explain ozone toxicity: the role of lipid ozonation products. Free Radic Biol Med 1995;19:935–941.

[13] Halliwell B, Clement MV, Long LH. Hydrogen peroxide in the human body. FEBS Lett 2000;486:10–13.

[14] Bocci V, Aldinucci C, Bianchi L. The use of hydrogen peroxide as a medical drug. Riv Ital Ossigeno Ozonoterapia 2005;4:30–39.

[15] Valacchi G, Bocci V. Studies on the biological effects of ozone: 11.Release of factors from human endothelial cells. Mediat Inflamm 2000;9:271–276.

[16] Dianzani MU. 4-Hydroxynonenal and cell signalling. Free Radic Res 1998;28:553–560.

[17] Iles KE, Liu R-M. Mechanisms of glutamate cysteine ligase (GCL) induction by 4-hydroxynonenal. Free Radic Biol Med 2005;38: 547–556.

[18] Snyder SH, Baranano DE. Heme oxygenase: a font of multiple messengers.Neuropsychopharmacology 2001;5:294–298.

[19] Wollert KC, Drexler H. Clinical application of stem cells for the heart. Circ Res 2005;96:151–163.

[20] Mendiratta S, Qu Z-C, May JM. Erythrocyte ascorbate recycling:antioxidant effects in blood. Free Radic Biol Med 1998;24:789–797.

[21] Stone JR, Collins T. The role of hydrogen peroxide in endothelial proliferative responses. Endothelium 2002;9:231–238.

[22] BocciV.Areasonable approach for the treatment of HIVinfection in the early phase with ozone therapy (autohemotherapy). How inflammatory cytokines may have a therapeutic role. Mediat Inflamm 1994;3:315–321.

[23] Bocci V. Autohaemotherapy after treatment of blood with ozone. A reappraisal. J Intern Med Res 1994;22:131–144.

[24] Baeuerle PA, Henkel T. Function and activation of NF-kB in the immune system. Annu Rev Immunol 1994;12:141–179.

[25] Bocci V. Roles of interferon produced in physiological conditions. A speculative review. Immunology 1988;64:1–9.

[26] Valacchi G, Bocci V. Studies on the biological effects of ozone: 10:Release of factors from ozonated human platelets. Mediat Inflamm 1999;8:205–209.

[27] Frehm EJ, Bonaventura J, Gow AJ. S-nitrosohemoglobin: an allosteric mediator of NO group function in mammalian vasculature. Free Radic Biol Med 2004;37:442–453.

[28] Goldman M. Cancer risk of low-level exposure. Science 1996;271:1821–1822.

[29] Calabrese EJ, Baldwin LA. Hormesis: U-shaped dose responses and their centrality in toxicology. Trends Pharmacol Sci 2001;22:285–291.

[30] Bocci V. Does ozone therapy normalize the cellular redox balance? Med Hypotheses 1996;46:150–154.

[31] Sharma YK, Davis KR. The effects of ozone on antioxidant responses in plants. Free Radic Biol Med 1997;23:480–488.

[32] Leon OS, Menendez S, Merino N, Castillo R, Sam S, Perez, et al. Ozone oxidative preconditioning: a protection against cellular damage by free radicals. Med Inflamm 1998;7:289–294.

[33] Barber E, Menendez S, Leon OS, Barber MO, Merino N, Calunga JL, et al. Prevention of renal injury after induction of ozone tolerance in rats submitted to warm ischaemia. Mediat Inflamm 1999;8:37–41.

[34] Larini A, Bianchi L, Bocci V. The ozone tolerance: I. Enhancement of antioxidant enzymes is ozone dose-dependent in Jurkat cells. Free Radic Res 2003;37:1163–1168.

[35] Bocci V, Borrelli E, Valacchi G, Luzzi E. Quasi-total body exposure to an oxygen-ozone mixture in a sauna cabin. Eur J Appl Physiol 1999;80:549–554.

[36] Bocci V, Di Paolo N. Oxygenation-ozonation of blood during extracorporeal circulation (EBOO). III. A new medical approach, ozone. Science 2004;26:195–205.

[37] Garber GE, Cameron DW, Hawley-Foss N, Greenway D, Shannon ME. The use of ozone-treated blood in the therapy of HIV infection and immune disease: a pilot study of safety and efficacy. AIDS 1991;5:981–984.

[38] Cooke ED, Pockley AG, Tucker AT, Kirby JDT, Bolton AE. Treatment of severe Raynaud's syndrome by injection of autologous blood pretreated by heating, ozonation and exposure to ultraviolet light (H-O-U) therapy. Int Angiol 1997;16:250–254.

[39] Torre-Amione G, Sestier F, Radovancevic B, Young J. Effects of a novel immune modulation therapy in patients with advanced chronic heart failure. J Am Coll Cardiol 2004;44:1181–1186. 40.

[40] Fadok VA, Bratton DL, Konowal A, Freed PW, Westcott JY, Henson PM. Macrophages that have ingested apoptic cells in vitro inhibit proinflammatory cytokine production through autocrine/paracrine mechanisms involving TGF-b, PGE 2 and PAF. J Clin Invest 1998;101:890–898.

[41] Tremblay J, Chen H, Peng J, Kunes J, Vu MD, Sarkissian SD, et al. Renal ischemia-reperfusion injury in the rat is prevented by a novel immune modulation therapy. Transplantation 2002;74:1425–1433.

[42] Tylicki L, Niew GT, Biedunkiewicz B, Burakowski S, Rutkowski B. Beneficial clinical effects of ozonated autohemotherapy in chronically dialysed patients with atherosclerotic ischemia of the lower limbs. Int J Artif Organs 2001;24:79–82.

[43] Clavo B, Perez JL, Lopez L, Suarez G, Lloret M, Rodriguez V, et al. Effect of ozone therapy on muscle oxygenation. J Altern Compl Med 2003;9:251–256.

[44] Biedunkiewicz B, Tylicki L, Niewegloski T, Burakoski S, Rutkowski B. Clinical efficacy of ozonated autohemotherapy in hemodialyzed patients with intermittent claudication: an oxygen-controlled study. Int J Artif Organs 2004;27:29–34.

[45] De Monte A, van der Zee H, Bocci V. Major ozonated autohemotherapy in chronic limb ischemia with ulcerations. J Alt Compl Med 2005; 11:363–367.

[46] Chan WM, Lam DS, Wong TH, Lai TY, Kwok AK, Tam BS, et al. Photodynamic therapy with verteporfin for subfoveal idiopathic choroidal neovascularization: one-year results from a prospective case series. Ophthalmology 2003;110:2395–2402.

[47] The AMDRT Research Group. The age-related macular degeneration radiotherapy trial (AMDRT): one year results from a pilot study. Am J Ophthalmol 2004;138:818–828.

[48] Gragoudas ES, Adamis AP, Cunningham ET, Feinsod M, Guyer DR. Pegaptanib for neovascular age-related macular degeneration. N Engl J Med 2004;351:2805–2816.

[49] Oxman MN, Levin MJ, Johnson GR, Schmader KE, Straus SE, Gelb LD, et al. A vaccine to prevent herpes zoster and postherpetic neuralgia in older adults. N Engl J Med 2005;352:2271–2284. 50.

[50] BarnesPJ. Scientificrationale for inhaledcombination therapywithlongacting b2-agonists and corticosteroids. Eur Respir J 2002;19:182–191.

[51] Barnes PJ, Liew FY. Nitric oxide and asthmatic inflammation. Immunol Today 1995;16:128–130.

[52] Stamler JS. S-nitrosothiols in the blood: roles, amounts and method of analysis. Circ Res 2004;94:414–417.

[53] Lipsky BA. Medical treatment of diabetic foot infections. Clin Infect Dis 2004;39:S104–S114.

[54] Bocci V, Larini A, Micheli V. Restoration of normoxia by ozone therapy control neoplastic growth: a review and a working hypothesis. J Alt Compl Med 2005;11:257–265.

[55] Gonzalez R, Borrego A, Zamora Z, Romay C, Hernandez F, Menendez S, et al. Reversion by ozone treatment of acute nephrotoxicity induced by cisplatin in rats. Med Inflamm 2004;13:307–312.

[56] Andreula CF, Simonetti L, De Santis F, Agati R, Ricci R, Leonardi M. Minimally invasive oxygen-ozone therapy for lumbar disk herniation. Am J Neuroradiol 2003;24:996–1000.

[57] Baysan A, Whiley RA, Lynch E. Antimicrobial effect of a novel zone-generating device on micro-organisms associated with primary root carious lesions in vitro. Caries Res 2000;34:498–501.

[58] Cianci P. Advances in the treatment of the diabetic foot: is there a role for adjunctive hyperbaric oxygen therapy?Wound Repair Regen 2004; 12:2–10.

[59] Gill AL, Bell CN. Hyperbaric oxygen: its uses, mechanisms of action and outcomes. Q J Med 2004;97:385–395.

[60] Goldstein BD, Balchum OJ. Effect of ozone on lipid peroxidation in the red blood cell. Proc Soc Exp Biol Med 1967;126:356–359.

[61] Couzin J, Kaiser J. As Gelsinger case ends, gene therapy suffers another blow. Science 2005;307:1028.

[62] Maxwell SRJ, Webb DJ. COX-2 selective inhibitors-important lessons learned. Lancet 2005;365:449–451.

[63] Beardsley S. Avoiding another VIOXX. Sci Am 2005;292:9–10.64. Babior BM, Takeuchi C, Ruedi J, Gutierrez A, Wentworth P Jr. Investigating antibody-catalyzed ozone generation by human neutrophils. Proc Natl Acad Sci USA 2003;100:3031–3034.

Chapter 6

Dietary Aspects in Cancer Prevention — A Mini-Review

Mohamed Abdulla and Sangeeta Shukla

Additional information is available at the end of the chapter

http://dx.doi.org/10.5772/57371

1. Introduction

Currently, there are more than 12 million new cancer cases each year worldwide, and it constitutes approximately 12% in mortality statistics. The cancer incidence remains high in south East Asia. In recent years, an alarming increase in cancer incidence has been observed in parts of central and Eastern Europe. A number of studies have implicated chronic inflammations as of the factors involved in cancer development, but the specific ways chronic inflammation lead to cancer is not very clear at the moment. It has been estimated that almost 20% of all cancers are associated with chronic inflammation. Many cancers arise from sites of infection, chronic irritation and inflammation. Tumor necrosis factor (TNF alpha) is a pleiotropic cytokine, is known to regulate multiple inflammatory cells (neutrophils and macrophages). The assumption that nutrition is an important factor in the risk of cancer development dates back to ancient times. Wiseman in 1676 suggested that cancer might arise from "an error in diet" and he recommended restriction of salt and meat in the diet as a means of cancer prevention [1]. During the early decades of twentieth century, the idea of diet modification in cancer prevention gained momentum and several recommendations for the increase or decrease of various dietary components have been tried. Shah in 1907 advocated a prudent dietary regime designed to reduce the risk of cancer development, with more food of vegetable origin, less meat, alcohol and tobacco [2].Along with the scientific advances during the early part of the 20th century, two hypotheses on the environmental cause of cancer were developed. The first one related to occupational exposure of workers to chemical carcinogens and the other one focused on various dietary components. Hoffman in 1931 indicated that increased amounts of fats in diets, sugar and bread as possible contributing factors to some types of cancer development [3]. At the same time, a few epidemiological surveys indicated that a number of dietary components may contribute to the pathogenesis of cancer [4,5]. During the last 50 years, increased attention was focused on the preventive and modifying actions of diet on cancer prevention in general. An early analysis of cancer incidence worldwide indicated that over 50% of cancers is due to external factors and hence theoretically preventable [6-10, 18]. This was further reinforced by a large number of descriptive, ecological and epidemiological studies. Studies by Doll and Peto indicated the importance of antioxidants, leafy vegetables, fish and several other bioactive micronutrients in cancer prevention [7].In 1982, The National Academy of Sciences in USA proposed six interim guidelines to reduce the risk of cancer [8]. This included reduction of dietary fat, increased consumption of food rich in fruits and vegetables, salt restriction, decreased intake of smoked food-stuffs and reduced intake of alcohol. This review will discuss some important concepts in cancer prevention by diet modification.

2. Cancer pattern

As mentioned in the introduction, cancer is a major cause of mortality throughout the world. In developed and fast-growing countries, the mortality due to cancer is generally exceeded only by mortality from cardiovascular diseases. According to a report in the Lancet in 1977, the World Health Organization (WHO) identified the 4 of the 10 leading causes of mortality worldwide. They are from Ischemic heart disease, cerebrovascular disease, chronic obstructive pulmonary disease and lung cancer. In an earlier report, the fourth leading cause of death worldwide was due to nutritional disorders. The authors in that report predicted that even in 2020, the fourth leading cause of death would be due to nutritional disorders [11]. The incidence of lung cancer is likely to increase in the coming decades, especially in fast-growing countries like China, India, Brazil, South Africa and Russia (BRICS) due to smoking, environmental pollution and other unknown factors. The incidence of cancer in our ancestors (gather-hunters and pastoral people) living in remote areas of the globe was very low. The average lifespan on the other hand was very low in those days. According to some experts, the dramatic shift away from the eating habits of our ancestors is probably responsible for fostering many of the "diseases of civilization" including cancer [12]. For males and females taken together, the incidence of most of the common cancers are shown in Table 1.

Cancer site	Males(%)	Females (%)
Lung	18.6	6.7
Stomach	11.9	7.6
Colorectal	8.4	8.6
Prostate	7.5	—
Breast	—	18.6
Oro-Pharyngeal	7.3	3.8
Esophagus	6.1	—
Bladder	4.4	—
Liver	7.1	—
Ovary	—	3.9
Others	28.8	17.4

Table 1. Estimated number of new cases in men and women in 1996

http://dx.doi.org/10.5772/57371

Rank	cancer site	New cases	%of all cancers
1	Lung	1608	12.7
2	Breast	1384	10.9
3	Colorectal	1235	09.8
4	Stomach	989	7.8
5	Prostate	899	7.1
6	Liver	750	5.9
7	cervix uteri	530	4.2
8	Esophagus	482	3.8
9	Bladder	383	3.0
10	Non-Hodgkin lymphoma	356	2.8
11	Leukemia	350	2.0
12	Corpus uteri	288	2.3
13	Pancreas	279	2.2
14	Kidney	274	2.4
15	Others	1879	13.8

Table 2. Cancer statistics. Cases diagnosed in 2008 (100s). Both sexes

As can be observed, lung cancer is the most common cancer worldwide contributing to nearly 13% of the total number of cases diagnosed in 2008. Breast cancer in women is the second common cause of cancer followed by colorectal cancer. The number of lung cancer in man has decreased a little from 18.6% in 1996 to 16.5% in 2008 [20].The global cancer burden doubled in the last three decades of the twentieth century and it is estimated that it will triple by 2030. The major increase would be in low and medium resource countries in Asia, Africa and Latin America. At the same time, there is a clear message of hope that some of the cancers can be prevented with advances in sophisticated technology combined with genetic and other screening techniques.

3. Diet and carcinogenesis

Like many other chronic diseases, the major underlying causes of cancers are environmental in nature. Apart from genetic factors, food and nutrition are important modifiers of cancer risk..Studies of immigrants in various parts of the world support the concept that many human cancers arise from interaction between the environment and constituents of the cells and their membranes. In the past, the concept of etiology of cancer has generally focused on four agents: viruses, radiation, chemical carcinogens and environmental pollutants. Currently, it is estimated that environmental factors are primarily responsible for a significant percent of all human cancers [13].Some of these factors include exogenous chemicals, tobacco smoke and a number of dietary constituents. During the 1930's and 1940's, a number of studies showed repeatedly that diet modification in experimental animals exposed to chemical carcinogens resulted in a beneficial effect [14].During this interval, it was shown that dietary constituents such as vitamins and anti-oxidants had a modifying effect in experimental cancers. Humans are continuously exposed to a variety of carcinogens in their immediate environment. These include carcinogens in the smoke, alcoholic beverages, industrial carcinogens such as asbestos and several non-essentials dietary constituents. The compounds found in diet that are known to be carcinogens include aflatoxins, heterocyclic amines, N-nitroso compounds and similar chemicals and polycyclic aromatic hydrocarbons. With the current advances in transportation and export, it is common to find food articles cultivated throughout the world in most parts of the world. In the fast growing countries, many chemicals and fertilizers are extensively used to increase the food production. When such products are exported to industrialized countries, there is additional risk for the intake of dietary components containing carcinogens and toxic residues even in affluent countries. Carcinogens, heavy metals and toxic residues are known to damage DNA in several ways and that detoxification can be a possibility at the early stage in the metabolic pathway. The efficacy of detoxification can be vital in determining the carcinogen potency. Dietary intervention is probably one way of influencing the carcinogen metabolism.

Food-stuffs containing large amounts of plant materials are good sources of a number of bioactive components. Such compounds and their derivatives are shown to inhibit carcinogenesis in a number of experimental systems involving initiation, promotion and progression. The role of diet in the final carcinogenesis is, however, not very clear at present. Recent studies show that many carcinogens and tumor promoters can produce reactive oxygen species (ROS) that can induce DNA damage and consequent chromosomal breakage. Dietary carcinogens mentioned earlier along with the cooking process and spoiled foods can add further to the body′s carcinogen load. If diets are rich in fruits and vegetables, some of these carcinogens may be detoxified before they become bioactive. During the second stage of cancer development, restriction of energy intake and increased physical activity may have some additional beneficial effect. In the final stage of tumor development when DNA damage plays a crucial role, the amount of single nutrients such as folate, zinc and selenium are known to play some role in the prevention of chromosomal damage and DNA methylation.

4. Reactive oxygen species, antioxidants and cancer prevention

Carcinogenesis encompasses a prolonged accumulation of injuries at several different biological levels and includes both genetic and biochemical changes in the cells. DNA strand breaks are one such injury. Agents that induce DNA damage, and thereby cause cancer include ionizing radiation, ultraviolet light, tobacco smoke, ozone and oxides of nitrogen in the polluted air. As mentioned earlier, reactive oxygen species (ROS) is known to cause damage to the DNA and it is very likely that the carcinogens mentioned above produce cell damage through the action of reactive oxygen species. It is also known that the damaging effect of free radicals (ROS) are encountered by enzymes and small molecules such as glutathione, acetycysteine and uric acid. Certain vitamins like carotene derivatives, minerals and certain trace elements may also counteract the action of free radicals [23]. Under normal circumstances, the defense systems in the body work efficiently and balance the oxidants produced in the cells during various metabolic activities. When oxidant stress is increased, additional antioxidants may be required. The most important antioxidant enzymes are superoxide dismutase, catalase and peroxidases. Among the micronutrient antioxidants, the important ones are vitamin C, Vitamin E, beta–carotene and the essential trace element selenium. The richest source of these nutrients is fresh fruits, vegetable oils, nuts and grain. Most plants contain phytochemicals such as flavanoids and polyphenols. A number of experimental studies have shown that they have antioxidant activities. Flavanoids are water soluble pigments found in exotic fruits, seeds, leaves and bark. These pigments can scavenge reactive oxygen species and thus can prevent breaking lipid peroxide chain reactions.According to Carmia, experimental studies show that the phytochemicals can protect cells from ionizing radiation, inhibit mutations and block prostaglandin synthesis and thus prevent multistage carcinogenesis [16]. Polyphenols found in green tea and grapes have greater antioxidant potential than that exerted by vitamin C and E [17]. Ellagic acid is a phenol found in grapes, various berries and it has been found to protect liver toxicity leading to cancer. Garlic, onions, shallots and leeks also contain several natural antioxidants including flavanoids, vitamin C, selenium and sulfur compounds that increase the metabolic disposal of chemical carcinogens. In recent years, it has been reported that dark chocolate and red wine also contains phytochemicals and may scavenge reactive oxygen species [18]. With the increased pollution of the environment, it is likely that many of these useful components in plant materials may decrease, especially in fast-growing countries.

Until recently, scientists engaged in the study of aging thought that the ROS played a crucial role in aging process. Now, the theory of aging due to oxidative damage is being replaced by other factors. Over the course of past few years, many experiments designed to further support the idea that the ROS and other reactants drive aging have shown very challenging and controversial results. What these results show is that under certain situations, the high energy ROS may not be dangerous but useful and healthy. A final proof, however, for the beneficial effect of free radicals is currently lacking. It is hard to imagine that antioxidants will ever fall out of favor completely. As mentioned earlier, the amounts of natural antioxidants found in plant material, fruits and nuts ought to have a beneficial effect from en evolutionary point of view. There are millions of people in countries like India who survive mainly on food-stuffs of vegetable origin. So are many other species thriving in the forests. Nature must have designed its own mechanisms to deal with environmental factors that influence health and disease.

Table 3 shows a list of various dietary components that have shown to have some beneficial against detoxification of chemical carcinogens.

Nutrient	Active component	Known function
Tea	phytochamicals	Antioxidant
Chocolate	Polyphenols	Antioxidant
Plants	Phytochemicals	Hydroxyl scavenger
Grapes	Catechin	Antioxidant
Olives	Polyphenols	Antioxidant
Soybean	Isoflavones	estrogen-like action
Garlic and Onions	Flavanoids, sulfur	disposal of carcinogens
Vegetables	flavanoids, Indoles	DNA damage protection
Selenium	Antioxidant enzymes	Antioxidant
Vitamin C	Vitamin C	Scavenger of ROS
Vitamin E	Vitamin E	Lipid peroxidation protection
Beta-Carotene	provitamin A	Antioxidant
Tomatoes, salmon	Lycopene	Antioxidant
Red wine	Phenols	Antioxidant

Table 3. List of selected nutrients that have antioxidant potential

As can be seen from table 3, a large number of constituents in fruits, vegetables, green tea, grapes, pepper, red wine and salmon possess substances that have anticancer potential. Apart from the carcinogen exposure from the immediate environment, a number of substances in cooked, grilled and smoked meat can contribute to the carcinogenic load of the cells in the body. The extents to which such carcinogens induce cancer development depend on the quality and quantity of the food consumed regularly and the concentration of scavengers available during the metabolism of cells. During the intermediate stage of cancer development, the restricted energy intake and increased physical activity can have significant additive effect on cancer development through the action of hormones and growth factors.

Reactive oxygen species are also known to be associated with aging process in a number of species, including humans. It is a common observation that the prevalence of many human cancers is high in aging populations. Average life-span in most developed countries as well as in many fast-growing developing countries in Asia, Africa and Latin America has increased tremendously during the last few decades. According to several research groups, cellular damage caused by oxidation is one of the main mechanisms of aging. According to this theory, rampant oxidation in the cells mangles more and more lipids, proteins, and snippets of DNA and other key components of cells over time, eventually compromising tissues and organs and thus resulting in organ failure. Recent studies, however, showed that increase in certain free radicals in mice and worms correlate larger life span. Indeed, in some circumstances, reactive oxygen species seem to signal cellular repair methods. Experimental studies by several groups in the United States of America show that rather than causing aging, some ROS may prove beneficial. One possibility is that certain number of ROS stimulates an organism's internal repair mechanism to get to work. In genetically modified roundworms which produced high levels of certain ROS, it was observed that these worms lived much longer than the normal worms. And further, when these worms were fed with antioxidants, their longevity advantage disappeared. In the February issue of The Scientific American this year, Melinda Moyer has summarized the results of recent studies and her title of her article is "The Myth of Antioxidants" [25].

It appears that the final verdict about the role of ROS in aging and cancer and the beneficial effect, if any, of antioxidants is yet to come. In most developed countries, the consumption of antioxidants as OTC products is very high. These antioxidants include Vitamin E, beta-carotene and Vitamin C. As mentioned earlier, epidemiological studies show that people who eat lots of fruits and vegetables, which are rich in these antioxidants, tend to live longer and are less likely to develop cancer compared to those who eat normal diets. So, it seemed obvious that supplementing daily diets with antioxidants should lead to a better life. But the results of the most rigorously designed studies do not support that hypothesis, Indeed, the evidence shows that some people who take certain vitamin supplements are actually more likely to develop life-threatening illnesses such as lung cancer and heart disease [18]. The influence of mass media is one reason for the high consumptions vitamins and antioxidants. We need more studies and further proof to establish the relation between ROS and antioxidants. Until that time, we have to cope with controversy about ROS, aging. and cancer.

5. Minerals and trace elements

Many of the minerals and trace elements are nutrients that cannot be synthesized by the body. They are involved in all phases of cellular metabolism in one way or another. Trace elements are integral parts of very many enzymes including the ones that scavenge ROS.The minerals and trace elements that are of interest include calcium (together with vitamin D), magnesium, iodine, iron, selenium and zinc. Evidence suggesting the relationship of other minerals and toxic heavy metals with cancer is not substantial and as such, they are not described in this review. The dietary intake of minerals and trace elements in various parts of the world vary significantly due to varied eating habits, culture and tradition, climatic conditions and the amount present in the soil. Studies by the current authors indicate that the intake of a number of important trace elements and minerals is below the current recommended levels [18].The intake levels are especially low in the elderly [18].The richest source of calcium is dairy products and fish. Selenium levels in the soil vary greatly in different regions of the world. Australia, New Zealand and Scandinavian countries have low selenium levels in the soil. Selenium is mainly found in meat, fish and certain cereals [18].Hem iron is mainly found in foods of animal origin. Non-hem iron is found in plant foods and legumes. Zinc is rich in seafood, meat and unprocessed vegetable material. Oysters are one of the richest sources of zinc. Modern food processing destroys significant amounts of trace elements than found in the natural material. For iodine, the best sources are sea food and seaweed.

Evidence on the relationship between calcium and cancer was considered by the 1982 and 1989 reports of the national Academy of Science [19, 20]. According to the report, there are some epidemiological evidence linking high calcium intake and the cancers of colon and rectum. High calcium intake together with vitamin D has also been documented to have some effect in the risk of developing colorectal cancer. Data for other cancer sites linking calcium intake is inconclusive.

With regards to iron and cancer, there is some evidence that diets high in iron may possibly increase the risk of liver and colorectal cancers in humans. In humans, the dietary iron overload is rare except in some ethnic groups in Africa where iron utensils are widely used for cooking. Data from case-control studies are, however, inconsistent. Iodine in the body is related to thyroid function and it has been proposed that a high intake of iodine may induce thyroid cancer. Ecological and experimental studies support the association between high dietary intake and the risk of developing thyroid cancer.

Selenium has attracted consider interest in cancer research during the middle part of twentieth century. During the early 1960′s, it was shown that selenium is an integral part of the antioxidant enzyme, glutathione peroxidase [19]. Currently, selenium is also recognized as an essential component of iodothyronine 5′-deiodinases as well as a few other proteins without any known functions. During the last few decades, a number of experimental studies have indicated the importance of this trace element for cancer prevention. A few epidemiological studies have confirmed such an association even in humans. Several selenium compounds have been found to inhibit or retard carcinogenesis in a variety of experimental animal models using chemical, viral and transplanted tumor models. A prospective case control study in Finland showed a link between selenium status and cancer development. Studies of humans have tended to show selenium status and cancer mortality to be inversely correlated. The soil in Finland was enriched by selenium due to low levels in the environment and studies afterwards did not show any specific pattern on the relationship between selenium and cancer. Other epidemiological studies in low soil areas have failed to show the protective effect of selenium on cancer development. Any potential anticarcinogenic influence of this trace element may relate to its antioxidant properties. This, however, is controversial at present. In some studies, selenium has been shown to suppress cell proliferation, to enhance immune response, and to alter the metabolism of carcinogens to less toxic compounds [21]. The overall interest in selenium as a protective trace element against cancer, however, has faded during the last two decades.

Zinc is another trace element that has attracted considerable interest in human health and disease. Zinc was recognized as an essential nutrient for human growth and development several decades ago. Marginal deficiency of zinc is widespread throughout the world. The prevalence of nutritional zinc deficiency is high in populations consuming large amounts of cereal proteins which contain organic phosphate compounds, such as phytate.Even in affluent countries; it has been observed that mild deficiency of zinc occur in vulnerable groups such as the elderly [18]. Hormonal effects of zinc deficiency include decreased testosterone level in serum of males, increased serum prolactin levels, and decreased activity of serum thymulin, a zinc-dependent thymic hormone. This trace element has attracted much interest in cancer research since Cristo in 1922 showed high amounts in cancer tissues [22].Many research groups in the past have shown that patients with cancer in general have low plasma zinc levels. It is assumed that this decrease is due to the high demand of the tumor tissue, especially when they have a high rate of DNA synthesis. As mentioned earlier, zinc is essential for growth and development of normal tissues and as such it may be needed even more in cancer tissues. Opinion, however, differs regarding the role of zinc in the induction and proliferation of malignant cells. A high zinc intake has been associated with lower incidence of gastric and esophageal cancers in certain parts of the world. Our own studies have shown that low dietary zinc inhibit the growth of oral cancer in experimental animals [22]. Once the tumor starts growing, the requirement becomes high and plasma levels go down. Many essential trace elements like zinc have dual functions: in low concentrations, they show signs of specific disease and at high concentrations, signs of toxicity. Iron is a trace element that shows such a pattern: when the intake is low, it produces anemia and at higher concentrations, it shows toxicity symptoms such as hemochromatosis and liver injury. In general, only little is known about the role of trace elements in carcinogenesis.

6. Summary

Cancer is a major killer throughout human history. In 2008, there were an estimated 12.7 million cancer cases throughout the world. This number is expected to increase to 21 million by 2030. Cancer changed its grasp as humans advanced industrially and technologically. Although the risk of a few cancers has declined significantly in affluent countries during the last few decades, the incidence of other cancers at sites of lung, breast and prostate has increased. Lung cancer is the most common cancer worldwide contributing nearly 13% of the cases diagnosed in 2008.Breast cancer (in women) is the second followed by colorectal cancer. Carcinogenesis encompasses a prolonged accumulation of injuries at several different biological levels and includes both genetic, biochemical and environmental changes in the cells. At each of these levels, there are several possibilities of intervention in order to prevent, slow down or even halt the gradual march of healthy cells to malignancy. Diet modification is one such possibility. A number of natural foodstuffs, especially fruits and vegetables contain significant quantities of molecules that have chemoprotective potential against cancer development. Such molecules include vitamins, certain mineral and trace elements and a variety of other substances with antioxidant properties. Carotenoids, flavanoid polyphenols, osoflavones, catechins, and several other compounds found in cruciferous vegetables are molecules that are thought to protect against the deleterious effect of reactive oxygen species (ROS).A number of epidemiological and experimental studies have shown that some of the abovementioned antioxidants can reduce the risk of cancer. Consistent observations during the last few decades that cancer risk can be reduced by diets rich in fruits and vegetables, legumes, grains, nuts, green tea and red wine have encouraged research to identify several plant components, especially phytochemicals that protect against DNA damage. Many of these substances are known to block specific carcinogen pathways. Very recent studies have, however, questioned the role of ROS, aging and cancer development. Certain reactive oxygen species have been found to be useful as part of the defense mechanism. Other studies have shown that high doses of anti-oxidant supplements may not provide protection against ROS as it was originally thought. We need a lot more proof about the role of ROS in health and disease. The debate on the role of antioxidants as protective agents against cancer is likely to continue. Only little is known about the role of trace elements in cancer.

Author details

Mohamed Abdulla[1] and Sangeeta Shukla[2]

1 Department of Primary care, Swedish Medical Board, Olofström, Sweden

2 Department of Zoology, Jiwaji University, Gwalior, India

References

[1] R.Wiseman. Several Chirgical Treatise, Flesher and Macock 1976.

[2] J.Shah The cure of cancer and surgery blocks the way: Turney, London 1907.

[3] F.Hoffman. Cancer and smoking habits, In: Cancer, F.Adaitr-Lippincott, London 1931

[4] I.M. Orr . Lancet ii 1939, 575-580

[5] P.Stocks . British Empire Cancer Campaign.35th Ann report 1973; 2:1-127

[6] J.Higginson and C.S.Muir. In: JF.Holland and E.Frei 8eds.); Lee and Febiger, Pa. USA 1976.

[7] R.Doll and R.Peto. JNCI 1981; 66 1191-1308.

[8] NAS. Diet, Nutrition and Cancer, National Academy Press, Washington 1982.

[9] E. Wynder and G.Gori. JNCI 1967; 58 825-832.

[10] R.Wynder and T.Shugematsu. Cancer 1967; 20 1520-1561.

[11] Editorial. The Lancet 1997; 1263.

[12] S.B.Eaton, M.Konner and M.Shostak. Am J Med 1988; 739-749.

[13] WHO. The world health report, WHO, Geneva, 1997.

[14] L.A.Poirier. J Clin Nutr 1986; 45:185.

[15] L.A.poirier, P.M. Newberne and M.W.Pariza. Plenum Press, New York, 1986.

[16] B.Carmia. Env Hlth Pers 1993;101(3) 237-245.

[17] B.Carmia. Science and Medicine 1997; 52

[18] M.Abdulla. Thesis, Inorganic chemical elements in prepared meals, University of Lund, 1985.

[19] NAS. National Academy Press, Washington DC, 1989.

[20] Am inst cancer res. World cancer research fund, Washington DC, 1997.

[21] G.F.Combs. In "Antioxidants and disease Prevention, CRC Press, 1997.

[22] A.Mathur and M.Abdulla. Role of zinc in oral cancer, University of Lund, Sweden, 1978.

[23] M.Abdulla and P.Gruber. BioFactors 2000;12 45-51.

[24] P.Boyle and B.Levin IARC. Nonserial publication, World cancer report, 2008.

[25] M.W.Moyer. The myth of Antioxidants. Scientific American 2013, 308(2) 56-61.

Chapter 7

Nutrition, Sleep and Sleep Disorders – Relations of Some Food Constituents and Sleep

Markku Partinen, Tuomas Westermarck and
Faik Atroshi

Additional information is available at the end of the chapter

http://dx.doi.org/10.5772/58345

1. Introduction

Many people suffer from excessive sleepiness during the afternoon hours. In all human individuals the alertness level decreases after the noon peak. This afternoon dip or "postprandial dip" is physiological. The alertness level rises again later in the afternoon and early evening, reaching another peak at about 7 to 8 p.m. Obesity is a recognized public health problem. It is a strong risk factor for type 2 diabetes and cardiovascular disease. Obesity is also the strongest risk factor of obstructive sleep apnea. Nutritional factors are important also in many other sleep disorders. Many patients with restless legs syndrome have low blood ferritin levels. [1] Sleepy patients with hypersomnias should avoid rapidly absorbing carbohydrates at daytime to minimize afternoon sleepiness. Adenosine is accumulating in the brain, notably in the basal forebrain, during wake, increasing the sleep pressure. [2] Caffeine, the most commonly used stimulant, is an adenosine receptor antagonist. During deep slow wave sleep glucose is stored in the glial cells. [3, 4] The brain-gut relationship is important also in the sleep-wake regulation, although well-done studies on that topic are still scarce.

Sleep disorders are a large and under-recognised problem in many parts of the world. The international classification of sleep disorders (ICSD), the most frequent and often the most severe are obstructive sleep apnoea (OSA), narcolepsy, restless legs syndrome (RLS), periodic limb movement disorder, insomnia, parasomnias, circadian rhythm disorders including jet lag and shift work, and sudden infant death syndrome. However, the major research focuses on OSA, insomnia and RLS since they are among the most highly prevalent sleep disorders and there are established links between them and other health conditions, which is the area where the majority of costs are incurred. The health system costs of sleep disorders comprise the cost of the sleep disorders themselves and the share of health costs from other conditions attributed to sleep disorders. The total European cost of brain disorders in 2010 was €798 billion [5], headaches and sleep disorders, meanwhile, only cost 285 and 348 euros respectively [6]. "The human brain is not only the site of our personality, thoughts, feelings and other human characteristics; it is also the seat of many chronic disabling diseases. These diseases have not received the attention that has been devoted to heart disease, cancer or AIDS, but in recent years there has been a growing awareness of their importance" [5]. A growing body of evidence indicates that free radical formation is a mediator of the excessive lipid peroxidation and cell damage seen in neurological disorders [7]. Antioxidant vitamins and trace elements have been shown to have biological activity in acting as scavengers for free radical's delays the onset of defined milestones in the development of a disease. Therefore, micronutrients such as vitamins, minerals or trace elements are supported by evidence that it can delay deterioration of the disease.

Different nutritional factors, and eating, can have an effect on the CNS by different mechanisms: direct nervous connections through the vagus nerve and nucleus tractus solitarius, humoral effects, affecting absorption of different molecules, emotional and cognitive processes.

2. Substances involved in the sleep-wake regulation and food intake

Many different neurotransmitters, neuromodulators and hormones have an important role in regulation of sleep and wakefulness, and in eating behaviour. These substances include (in alphabetical order): acetylcholine, adenosine, alpha-MSH (alpha melanocyte-stimulating hormone), cholecystokinin, dopamine, GABA, ghrelin, glutamate, glycine, insulin, histamine, hypocretin (orexin), leptin, MCH (melanin-concentrating hormone), melatonin, norepinephrine, NPY (neuropeptide Y), prostaglandins, serotonin, somatotrophin and thyrotropin. Little is known about the effect of vitamins and minerals on sleep. They will be discussed shortly later in this review.

3. Neurotransmitters in the Enteric Nervous System (ENS)

The enteric nervous system (ENS) can be considered the body's second brain with more than 100 million neurons of different types. Neural signals may be transmitted from gut to the CNS by neural connection and by humoral mechanisms. The afferent fibers of the gut-brain neural are vagal (parasympathetic) and (ortho)sympathetic. Different sensors respond also to distension of stomach and contractions of the intestine. Chemical stimuli (e.g. spices), gut hormones, neurotransmitters, neuromodulators, cytokines and inflammatory mediators produced by the bacterial flora in the gut-are all important. In the brainstem most afferent vagal fibers terminate on the nucleus tractus solitarius (NTS). There is a viscerotopic representation of different parts of the enteric system in the NTS. The NTS is in connection with hypothalamus and amygdala, which also plays a role in regulation of hunger and satiety. We should not forget the emotional aspects of eating (smell, taste, and situational factors during eating).

Cholecystokinin is secreted by duodenal and jejunal cells after eating food. CCK acts on vagal neurons projecting to the brainstem, giving a signal of satiety inhibiting further need for eating.

Ghrelin is secreted when a person is hungry and it increases appetite. It acts on the hypothalamus stimulating feeding, counteracting the inhibitory effects of leptin.

Leptin is manufactured mainly in fat cells in adipose tissue. Leptin counteracts the effects of neuropeptide Y and inhibits secretion of alpha-MSH (alpha melanocyte-stimulating hormone). Leptin decreases appetite and inhibits food intake contrary to ghrelin.

Alpha-MSH is in the arcuate nucleus in the brain where it acts to suppress appetite. Alpha-MSH may have also some function in the sleep-wake regulation.

Serotonin is an important neurotransmitter in the central nervous system (CNS) with important effects on sleep-wake regulation. Serotonin also has an important role in regulation of the gastrointestinal (GI) function through an interaction with the ENS. Up to 60-90 % of the total body amount of serotonin is in the GI tract, and 2-20% of all enteric neurons express serotonin. Stimulatory receptors include β-adrenoceptors, muscarinic and nicotinic Ach receptors and 5-HT3 receptors. Inhibitory receptors include alpha2-adrenceptors, histamine H3, GABA-B, adenosine A2, and 5-HT4 receptors. In the GI tract 5-HT is eliminated mainly by monoamine oxidase metabolism. [8]

Hypocretin (orexin) was originally considered to be important especially in central control of food intake [9, 10] but it is essential also in control of sleep and wakefulness. There are about 70 000 hypocretin neurons in the lateral hypothalamus. Narcolepsy, a central hypersomnia with excessive daytime sleepiness and cataplexy, is characterized by destruction of the hypocretin neurons. [11, 12] Hypocretin is involved also in energy homeostasis, nociception, reward seeking behavior, and drug addiction. [13-19] In addition to brain, hypocretins are also widely present in the gastrointestinal tract12 where they have a role in regulation of peristaltic GI motility, and in gastric, intestinal and pancreatic secretions. The hypothalamic hypocretin cells are intermingled with MCH neurons. Both hypocretin-and MCH-cells are glucose-sensing neurons. Decrease of glucose increases activity of hypocretin neurons and decreases activity of the MCH cells, producing wakefulness. Respectively, increase of glucose decreases activity of hypocretin and increases activity of MCH, producing sleepiness. These interactions explain at least partly the alerting effects of fasting and the observations that eating rapidly absorbing carbohydrates, provoking fast increase of blood glucose, increase sleepiness.

4. Caffeine and sleep

Coffee is the world's most common psychoactive drug. Coffee includes caffeine, which is also present in coffee, tea, cola and chocolate. The stimulant and wake-producing properties of caffeine depend on its ability to reduce adenosine transmission in the brain. Caffeine acts as an antagonist to adenosine A1 and especially to adenosine A2 receptors. [20, 13]

In experimental studies the concentration of adenosine is higher during wakefulness than during sleep, it accumulates in the brain during prolonged wakefulness, and local perfusions as well as systemic administration of adenosine and its agonists induce sleep and decrease wakefulness.2, 18 Supportive findings have been observed in humans. The longer the previous wakefulness period is, the longer and deeper is the following sleep. [22] The increase in extracellular adenosine concentration decreases the activity of the wakefulness-promoting cell groups, especially the cholinergic cells in the basal forebrain. [2, 22]

In addition to coffee caffeine is found in tea (20-100 mg per 3.5 dl cup of tea), Cola-drinks (30-50 mg per 3.3 dl bottle), energy drinks and chocolate. In chocolate also theobromine is present in large quantities. Dark chocolate is stimulating and 100 grams of 70% chocolate corresponds to 1-2 cups of coffee depending on strength of the coffee and size of the cup.

One small cup (30 ml) of espresso contains 30-50 mg of caffeine, and one large cup (2-4 dl) of ordinary coffee contains 75-150 mg of caffeine. Caffeine is absorbed rapidly and the peak of action occurs in 30 to 60 minutes. The duration of action is usually 4 to 6 hours, but in elderly subjects with slower metabolism the duration may last up to more than 16 hours. A large amount of caffeine, usually over 300-500 mg, i.e. more than 4 to 8 cups of coffee, depending on individual sensitivity, causes restlessness, anxiety, trembling, tinnitus and feelings of euphoria / delirium. Everyday use of more than 500 mg caffeine leads to caffeinism with insomnia, fatigue, and different psychosomatic symptoms. Some chronic coffee drinkers have developed tolerance to caffeine, and may drink more than 10 cups of coffee daily. They have withdrawal symptoms if they do not have their coffee.

Coffee is a well-known factor disturbing sleep. [23-31]Two or three cups (or in sensitive persons just one cup of coffee) in the evening is followed by difficulty falling asleep and restless sleep. Insomniacs are usually advised to avoid coffee after 6 p.m. but in some sensitive persons with insomnia coffee at noon or early afternoon may disturb falling asleep in the evening. It is important to recognize that energy drinks such as Battery and Red Bull contain large amounts of caffeine, which is a known cause for insomnia in adolescents. [31] Paradoxically, in some persons one or two cups of coffee may ameliorate quality of sleep. The reason can be behavioral conditioning, but it is also known that caffeine is inotropic and it stimulates respiratory functions.

5. Neurohormetic phytochemicals

Mediterranean diets rich in fibres, vegetables, fruits and olive oils are associated with reduced risk of cardiovascular disease and many neurological diseases. [32-34]Some effects are explained by antioxidative effects of different phytochemicals, but there is also evidence that some effects may be due to subtoxic effects of some neurotoxic molecules in the gut.

Hormesis is the paradoxical, stimulatory or beneficial action of toxins. Hormetic effects explain why, sometimes, low doses of a given toxic substance, or radiation, may induce beneficial effects while larger doses of the same substance or radiation are toxic to cells and organisms.

[35, 36] Examples of endogenous molecules with neurohormetic actions are nitric oxide, carbon monoxide, glutamate and calcium. Examples of neuroprotective substances include alpha-tocopherol, lycopene, resveratrol (red grapes, red wine, peanuts and soy), sul-foraphanes (broccoli), catechins (green tea), allicin and allium (garlic), curcumin (turmeric) and hypericin (St John's Wort).

Hot spices may disturb sleep. Tabasco and mustard in the evening may reduce slow wave and reduce total time awake and increase time to fall asleep. The spicy food in the evening elevated body temperature during the first sleep cycle, which explains probably some of the effects of capsaicin on sleep. [37]

6. Free radicals, oxidative stress and sleep

Increasing evidence associates sleep deprivation and sleep-related disorders with oxidative stress. Oxidative metabolism and energy production in the body generate free radicals and nonradical derivatives of oxygen and of nitrogen [38]. Normally, the mitochondrial respiratory chain generates a low level of free radicals during the process of making ATP. These free radicals, in turn, may cause further damage to the mtDNA creating a vicious cycle of damage and free radical production. It's unclear exactly how large a role the generation of free radicals plays in causing or worsening the symptoms of mitochondrial disease. Antioxidants, usually in the form of vitamins or trace elements, help neutralize free radicals. Although these products are involved in normal cell regulation and signal transduction, an imbalance between their generation and the antioxidant defense system results in oxidative stress. At the cellular level, the stress response can be initiated by external environmental factors that cause damage to biological macromolecules including lipids, proteins, and nucleic acids [39]. Oxidative stress in sleep apnea is thought to be produced by hypoxic events and by hypoxia-reperfusion injury, and in this way it contributes to cardiovascular complications and inflammatory processes [40, 41]. A role for disrupted sleep itself in the metabolic complications of sleep apnea has been implied by some of the evidence but not fully explored [42]. Ramanathan et al. [43] reported a significant decrease in superoxide dismutase (SOD) activity in the hippocampus and brain stem, but not in the cerebral cortex, hypothalamus, or cerebellum in rats sleep deprived for 5–11 days.

7. Prostaglandins and sleep

Prostaglandins (PGs) are synthesized from arachidonic acid by activated cyclo-oxygenase (COX) in response to various stimuli in various types of cells. When synthesized, PGs are immediately released and exert their actions on cells in the vicinity of their synthesis [44]. PGs act in many parts of the body, including the reproductive system, the nervous system, the cardiovascular system, the immune system and gastrointestinal system [45]. Due to their diverse biological activity, there is potential for prostaglandin analogs (prostanoids) to function as effective therapeutic agents.

Sleep, a complex phenomenon, is not merely the result of physical fatigue or decrease in activity; instead it is a complicated behavioural state requiring the integration of several neuronal processes. Prostaglandins (PGs) are ubiquitously distributed in mammalian tissues, exerting a variety of physiological and pathological effects such as disaggregation of blood platelets [46], relaxation of smooth muscle [47] and pain and inflammation [48]. It is generally accepted that PGD2 is one of the major PGs unique to the CNS, when compared to the relatively low concentrations present in peripheral tissue [49]. Studies have revealed a variety of endogenous substances that convincingly induce sleep. Among the multitude of sleep-promoting substances, PGD2 has been described as a somnolence promoting substance in the adult rat by acting on the traditional sleep centres of the VLPO area. PGD2 is produced from PGH2 precursor by enzyme PGDS that is predominately synthesised in the leptomeningeal layers and CP of the brain.

Prostaglandin D2 (PGD2) is a biologically active primary prostaglandin and a common product of arachidonic metabolism in mammals. As a major eicosanoid product of mast cells PGD2 is released in large quantities during allergic and asthmatic anaphylaxis. Several studies have reported a crucial role for the prostaglandin D system in sleep regulation. This PGD2 accumulates in the cerebrospinal fluid (CSF), where it induces physiologic sleep in rats and humans. PGD2 and PGE2 are found in high concentrations in the hypothalamus compared to other regional areas of the brain [50, 51]. In addition, marked elevations of endogenous PGD2 concentrations in CSF occur in patients who suffer African sleeping sickness [52]. Continuous infusion of PGD, into the lateral cerebral ventricle of monkeys during the diurnal period induced a sleep pattern similar to physiological night sleep [53]. It is involved in the regulation of reducing body temperature in sleep [54]. It is also produced in the brain via an alternative pathway involving a soluble, secreted PGD-synthase also known as β-trace [55]. PGD2 acts in the central nervous system in sleep induction and lowering of body temperature [51].Further pharmacological actions include inhibition of platelet aggregation and relaxation of vascular smooth muscle [56].

8. Glutathione and sleep

Glutathione is a tripeptide (gamma-glutamylcysteinylglycine) that performs many vital functions in every cell of the body [57]. It is present in two forms in the body; in a "reduced (GSH)" or an "oxidized (GSSG)" form. The majority of glutathione in the body is present in its reduced form because this is the only way it can perform its critical role. Certain tissues are more susceptible to GSH depletion than others. The reduced form of glutathione is the most active form and is found in healthy cells. GSH plays an important role in the protection of cells against damage from free radicals and other electrophiles. Several steps in the metabolism of arachidonic acid may be normally regulated by GSH-enzymes [58]. It was an early observation that GSH may function as a chemical cofactor or coenzyme in the formation of some PGs, particularly PGEs [59]. Measuring glutathione levels in specific areas of the brain of sleep-deprived animals reveals that the thalamus and hypothalamus are particularly susceptible [60]. It is essential for detoxifying cells and this process is more active during sleep [61]. The vulnerability of these tissues may contribute to some of the functional effects of sleep deprivation. The relationship between Glutathione (GSH) and sleep has been shown that it defends the cells from destructive agents such as free radicals, chemical toxins, and heavy metals that constantly assault the cells and inhibit their optimum function, causing disease and accelerating the aging process. Studies have shown that sleep deprived animals have lower glutathione levels in certain parts of the brain. The two brain areas involved in sleep are the thalamus and hypothalamus. These areas are particularly vulnerable to glutathione depletion and can lead to sleeping problems [60]. It has been reported that GSH is the only antioxidant that does not become a free radical itself after donating a free electron [62]. Further research suggested that high blood GSH concentrations correlates with long lifespan both in animals and humans [63]. Mancuso et al [64] observed that GSH levels were lower in patients with OSAS than in controls and suggests that antioxidant defences are impaired in patients with Obstructive sleep apnea syndrome (OSAS). Recently, Ntalapascha et al (2012) reported that overnight changes (%) in plasma biomarkers were significantly different between OSAS and controls for GSH/GSSG, controls had increased GSH levels overnight whereas OSAS did not.

9. Dietary nutrients and sleep

In a recent large survey on more than 4500 people the association of many different nutrients to sleep were studied. [66] The nutrients associated with difficulty falling asleep in order of importance were lack of alpha carotene, lack of selenium, lack of dodecanoic acid, lack of calcium and increased hexadecanoic acid. [66]Difficulty maintaining sleep was associated with increased use of salt, less butanoic acid, less carbohydrates, less dodecanoic acid, less vitamin D, less lycopene, more hexanoic acid and more moisture. Non-restorative sleep was associated with more butaneoic acid less calcium, less vitamin C, less plain water, more moisture and more cholesterol. In the same survey increased daytime sleepiness was associated more moisture, more theobromine (see above for caffeine), less potassium and less plain water. [66]

10. Vitamins and minerals and sleep

Management of sleep disturbances combines nonpharmacologic and pharmacologic approaches individualized for the patient. According to the International Classification of Sleep Disorders (ICSD-2, 2005) [67] there are around 90 distinct sleep disorders. The cumulative effects of sleep loss and sleep disorders have been associated with a wide range of deleterious health consequences including an increased risk of hypertension, diabetes, obesity, depression, heart attack, stroke and nutritional status of an individual could play a major role on sleep quality. Observational studies have shown a link between sleep [68] and vitamins and minerals, whether taken in combination or individually, are the most frequently consumed dietary supplements among people today. Unlike other dietary supplement ingredients, vitamins and certain minerals are considered essential nutrients for which standards of adequacy are needed.

10.1. Vitamins B

B vitamins are essential micronutrients and have many important functions in the body. The B vitamins generally are coenzymes in the energy metabolism in the body. They are needed for the syntheses and release of certain neurotransmitters and neurohormones that are involved in the regulation of sleep and the circadian cycle. B vitamins have been advanced as a preventive for insomnia based on research that suggests deficiencies in vitamin B6 promote psychological distress and ensuing sleep disturbance [69]. Folic acid and vitamin B12 are both B vitamins. Folic acid is often used in combination with other B vitamins [70]. Although the direct link between vitamins and insomnia is unclear, there are studies that show an association between vitamins and sleep disorders.

10.2. Vitamin B12, B6 and Folic Acid

Vitamin B12 deficiency has been linked to various neuropsychiatric disorders including slow cerebration; confusion; memory changes; delirium, with or without hallucinations and/or delusions; depression; acute psychotic states; sleep, and reversible manic and schizophreniform states affective illness [71, 72]. It has been shown that depressed subjects have low serum vitamin B12 levels [73]. It has been reported that high levels of vitamin B12 are associated with good treatment outcome in patients with MDD [74]. However, others did not found any association [75]. It has been reported that both folate and vitamin B12 are essential in several metabolic pathways in the central nervous system, and their metabolism is intimately connected [76]. A deficiency of either vitamin causes impaired methylation in the central nervous system and may result in neurological and psychiatric disease that becomes irreversible if not treated properly [71]. Furthermore, vitamin B12 has been shown to modulate human melatonin secretion [77]. Vitamin B6 is involved in the same metabolic pathways in the central nervous system as vitamin B12 and folate. Earlier studies found a low level of plasma vitamin B6 associated with symptoms of depression [78]. Other reported that vitamin B6 supplementation has positive effects on memory performance, but not on mood [79].

10.3. Vitamin D

Vitamin D is a group of fat-soluble prohormones synthesised in response to sunlight. The major source of vitamin D in humans is exposure to UV radiation. The active form of vitamin D in the body is 1,25-dihydroxyvitamin D, or calcitriol. Vitamin D has received a great deal of attention recently. It has long been recognized as primarily a regulator of calcium and phosphorus, helping to protect bone density. In recent years, however, our understanding of the functions of Vitamin D in the body has expanded with numerous health outcomes. Vitamin D is now understood to play an important role in metabolic and immune system functions. Vitamin D deficiency has been linked to a number of illnesses and chronic conditions, including high blood pressure, diabetes; metabolic syndrome, pulmonary disease, and chronic pain. Vitamin D supplementation during winter improve mood in healthy volunteers [80]. One possible mechanism of action is that serum 1,25-dihydroxyvitamin D levels affect the levels of serotonin in the hypothalamus [81] and thereby enhance the synthesis and transmission of serotonin, leading to improvement in mood. Novel associations between sleep symptoms and vitamin D have been reported [82, 83, 84]. Further evidence suggest that low vitamin D levels increase the risk for autoimmune disease, chronic rhinitis, tonsillar hypertrophy, cardiovascular disease, and diabetes [85]. McCarty et al. [86] reported that persistent inadequacy of vitamin D may also increase the risk for obstructive sleep apnea via promotion of adenotonsillar hypertrophy, airway muscle myopathy, and/or chronic rhinitis.

10.4. Vitamin A

Vitamin A is the parent compound of retinoid, which regulate gene transcription by binding to nuclear retinoid receptors. It is involved in immune function, vision, reproduction, and cellular communication. Vitamin A is very important for the mucous membranes as it is needed for the proper production of mucopolysaccharides, which help to protect against infections. Barceló et al. [87], reported that patients with obstructive sleep apnoea syndrome have a decreased antioxidant capacity of vitamin A and E levels. Study of sleep in mouse models of ageing, Ransom et al [88] showed further clues as to the involvement of vitamin A in the regulation of delta oscillations. It has been suggested that retinoid signalling pathways are important for adult neural function in health and disease [89]. A definitive role for vitamin A signalling however is evident in the regulation of delta oscillations. This was first proposed by Maret et al. [90], who observed that the relative contribution of the delta wave to slow move sleep (SWS) is determined by the RA receptor RARb1. Moreover, vitamin A deficiency is known to significantly reduce the power of the delta oscillation in mice [91].

10.5. Vitamin C

Vitamin C prevents some oxidative damage brought on by endurance exercise to the fat and muscle tissue. It is required for the transformation of dopamine into noradrenalin [92], and the function of this vitamin has been suggested to extend to neuromodulation of dopamine, regulation of acetylcholine and catecholamine release, and glutamate and GABA mediated neurotransmission [93]. Sleep symptoms are associated with weight gain and cardio metabolic disease. The potential role of diet including vitamin C that was associated independently with non-restorative sleep has been reported [82, 94], they suggest a novel associations between sleep symptoms and diet/metabolism, potentially explaining associations between sleep and cardiometabolic disease. Singh et al. [95], supplementing OSA patients with vitamins E and C concluded that that antioxidant treatment (oral vitamin E and C) reduced oxidative stress in OSA patients. Furthermore, decreased levels of antioxidants (superoxide dismutase, catalase, glutathione and homocysteine, as well as vitamins E, C, B11 and B12) and lower performance on the neuropsychological tasks were observed in patients with obstructive sleep apnea [96]. The authors suggest that an imbalance between antioxidants and pro-oxidants may contribute to neuropsychological alterations in this patient population. In restless leg syndrome (RLS), vitamins C and E and their combination are used as safe and effective treatments for reducing the severity of RLS in hemodialysis patients [97]. Ascorbic acid and sodium-dependent vitamin C transporters (SVCT) have been shown to have important functions in the peripheral nervous system (PNS) [98].

10.6. Vitamin E

Vitamin E has active ingredients of tocopherols and tocotrienols. It exists in eight different natural forms, all of which have antioxidant properties When supplemented it may reduce damage to cell DNA and cell and it has neuroprotective effect on the brain. Vitamin E may stabilize peripheral blood circulation, suppressing abrupt deformation of vessels [99], acceleration of blood flow in vessels would increase the pressure of blood on the vessel walls, and subtle changes in vessel tension or shape might stimulate nerve fibres that are in anatomical proximity to the vessels [99]. Vitamin E normalized chronic sleep deprivation-induced reduction in the hippocampus GSH/GSSG ratio, and activity of catalase, super oxide dismutase (SOD), and glutathione peroxidase (GPx) [100]. Decreased levels of antioxidants and lower performance on the neuropsychological tasks were observed in patients with obstructive sleep apnea [10][1]. This study suggests that an imbalance between antioxidants and pro-oxidants may contribute to neuropsychological alterations in this patient population.During eight-year follow-up study to investigate the link between vitamin E, namely α-tocopherol, and memory disorders, it was found that higher total serum levels of vitamin E, and higher levels of γ-tocopherol, β-tocotrienol and total tocotrienols in particular, seemed to protect against memory disorders [102]. Their results show that the entire vitamin E family plays a role in memory processes. Accordingly, measuring the levels of vitamin E from serum is the most reliable way to determine whether they are sufficiently high. Limited research indicates that supplemental vitamin E may reduce symptom occurrence in restless leg syndrome [103].

10.7. L-carnitine and Sleep

Acetyl-L-carnitine (ALC) is a naturally occurring compound that facilitates the transport of fatty acids into mitochondria for β-oxidation [104]. Acetyl-L-carnitine can enter the brain, and the acetyl group helps form acetylcholine, an important neurotransmitter. L-carnitine enhances resistance to oxidative stress by reducing DNA damage in Ataxia telangiectasia cells [105]. Positive results were seen in carnitine supplementation in depression, dysthymia, mental and physical energy, with less fatigue, muscle pain, and sleep problems [106,107,108]. Muscle weakness and hepatic dysfunction can also been noted [109]. Supplementation of carnitine has also been shown to be a mood elevator in the elderly [110]. Acetyl L-Carnitine helps the brain form acetylcholine, a neurotransmitter needed for memory and thinking [111].

Evidence for the effectiveness of L-carnitine in attention deficit and hyperactivity disorder (ADHD) has been studied [112]. Other studies in animals and human have shown that a combination of acetyl-L-carnitine and alpha-lipoic acid reversed many of the signs of aging and restored both physical and mental vigor. Low levels of carnitine are associated with a higher frequency of fragmented wakefulness [113].

L-Carnitine has been demonstrated to be therapeutic for individuals with narcolepsy. A recent study investigated the contribution of a gene polymorphism found in narcolepsy called CPT1B, which is important in fatty acid oxidation [114]. They found that individuals with narcolepsy had very low levels of serum acylcarnitine [115]. L-carnitine was given (510 mg/day) to patients with narcolepsy it was revealed that total time for dozing off during daytime in narcolepsy patients, the primary endpoint, was significantly decreased by L-carnitine

http://dx.doi.org/10.5772/58345

supplementation compared with placebo [114]. Although narcolepsy is a rather rare disorder, daytime sleepiness is not. It is possible that low levels of carnitine could be a cause of fatigue and daytime sleepiness. For example, low serum carnitine levels have been observed in patients with chronic fatigue syndrome (CFS) – a clinically defined condition characterized by severe disabling fatigue and a combination of symptoms, such as musculoskeletal pain, difficulty in concentration and sleep disturbances.

L-carnitine supplementation also increased serum carnitine levels and reduced serum triglycerides concentration indicating improvement in the burning of fat as energy. Other researchers found that ALC treatment reduced symptoms of depression in older people [116]. It also improved dysthymia, a milder form of depression, about as well as a common medication. Several studies show that ALC may help improve certain behaviours in boys with fragile X syndrome (FXS), such as their social skills and hyperactivity. The study has linked ALC with less pain or less-intense pain in people with nerve problems from these causes. ALC is a compound of great interest in various neurological disorders such as in treating Alzheimer's dementia, HIV-infection, diabetic neuropathies and aging [117,118,119,120]. A decrease of sleep disorders, a muscle discomfort, and of the prolonged fatigue after exercise has also been shown [121]. Carnitine supplementation could be helpful in mitochondrial disorders as the sleep problems are commonly reported in patients with mitochondrial myopathies [122,123].

11. Fatty acids

There is a growing consensus that omega-3 fatty acids are essential nutrients for humans. Much of the evidence is based on physiological measurements such as neurological development and visual acuity. To better understand why this class of polyunsaturated fatty acids is required, we must determine the biochemical basis for the essentiality. Of the eight fatty acids that comprise the omega-3 metabolic pathway, the two that are most likely to have essential biochemical functions are eicosapentaenoic acid (EPA) and docosahexaenoic acid (DHA).

EPA can be converted to prostaglandins, thromboxanes and lipoxygenase products [124]. However, no essential role for these EPA-metabolites has been reported, and it seems unlikely that the formation of these products is the reason that omega-3 fatty acids are essential. When elevated amounts of EPA are available, the incorporation of arachidonic acid (AA) into cell phospholipids and its conversion to eicosanoid mediators is reduced. Thus, EPA acts as a competitive inhibitor of AA, and this probably accounts for some of the beneficial effects of omega-3 fatty acids in the treatment of cardiovascular and inflammatory diseases. While the possibility that EPA is essential in order to modulate the effects of AA cannot be ruled out, the amounts ordinarily present in the plasma and tissues probably are too low to competitively inhibit the actions of AA. Therefore, modulation of AA metabolism is more likely to be a pharmacological effect of omega-3 fatty acid supplements rather than an essential physiological function.

The basis for considering DHA as the biochemically essential omega-3 component is much more compelling. DHA is the most abundant omega-3 fatty acid in most tissues, and it is present in large amounts in the brain and retina. DHA is the omega-3 fatty acid required for normal development of the nervous system and optimum visual acuity. Furthermore, when an omega-3 fatty acid deficiency exists, the body compensates by replacing it with the corresponding fatty acid of the omega-6 series, omega-6 docosapentaenoic acid (DPAn-6). These findings strongly suggest that DHA has an essential biochemical function. The most likely possibility is a membrane structural effect involving the packing of phospholipid head groups or the interaction of the lipid domains with membrane proteins. The lipids that contain the highest percentages of DHA are ethanolamine plasmalogen, phosphatidylethanolamine and phosphatidylserine. Therefore, it is likely that the function of DHA involves the metabolism, trafficking or physical properties of these phospholipids. Other possibilities that must be considered include the conversion of DHA to a lipid mediator, binding of DHA to a nuclear receptor that regulates gene expression, or formation of a DHA-centered free radical. It is thought that omega-3 fatty acids in fish oils may reduce inflammation of the brain and play a part in brain development and nerve cell regeneration [125]. However, there has been mixed evidence as to the benefits of omega-3 fish oils on the brain and whether they may protect against memory decline and dementia [126,127]. A combination of omega-3 fatty acid and vitamin B12 enriched diet may exert beneficial effects on synaptic plasticity and cognition, which may prove beneficial for mental health, particularly in preventing neurocognitive disorders [128].

A central question concerning the essentiality of omega-3 fatty acids is why DHA rather than the corresponding member of the omega-6 series, DPAn-6, fulfils this purpose. The usual Western diet contains 10-to 20-times more omega-6 fatty acid, and the same metabolic pathway is utilized by both fatty acid classes. One possibility is that DHA is utilized more efficiently than DPAn-6.

However, studies with neural cells in culture indicate that there is no appreciable difference in the uptake, retention or incorporation into phospholipids of DHA as compared with DPAn-6. While more detailed measurements may reveal a functional difference between DHA and DPAn-6, no such evidence is currently available. This suggests that DHA is utilized rather than DPAn-6 because it is more available to the tissues. Although the absolute amounts of these fatty acids in the plasma lipids are very small, there ordinarily is about five-times more DHA than DPAn-6. Furthermore, the main product formed by cultured astrocytes from omega-3 fatty acid precursors is DHA, whereas the main omega-6 product is AA. Astrocytes are the site where most of the polyunsaturated fatty acid precursors are elongated and desaturated in the brain. Thus, much more DHA than DPAn-6 appears to be available in the central nervous system [129].

11.1. Fish oils and omega-3 fatty acids

Polyunsaturated fatty acids (PUFA) are essential fatty acids in many mammals including humans. Both docosahexaenoic acid (DHA) and eicosapentaenoic acid (EPA) are omega-3 acids and they may also be obtained by eating fish oils. There is some evidence showing that a reduced amount of ingested omega-3 fatty acids is associated with fatigue, depression and problems of attention. [130-136] A sufficient amount of PUFA from food is necessary for health and well-being. Fatty fish is the best source of omga-3 acids. One hundred grams of salmon contains about 1000 mg of omega-3 acids and 100 grams of herring contains about 2000 mg. White fish meat contains much less of these essential fatty acids than fish with fatty meat. Omega-3 acids have been tested in the treatment of subjects with attention deficit disorder and in subjects with depression, female subjects with borderline personality, fatigue in multiple sclerosis, memory disturbances, dementia and some other neuropsychiatric diseases. Some randomized controlled studies have shown that omega-3 fatty acids may ameliorate mental functions, but they are also conflicting results. [130 - 137]

There is only little evidence showing that essential fatty acids may modulate sleep. In a small studied eight children. They were fed by total parenteral nutrition without essential lipids and seven other children who received a daily supplement of essential lipids in their parenteral nutrition. Slow wave sleep was significantly decreased in the group of children who did not receive fatty acids as compared to those who did. [138]No randomized clinical trials have been done in primary insomnia or in central hypersomnias.

12. Trace elements and sleep

Certain nutritional imbalances appear to influence sleep quality and play an important role in the maintenance of redox homeostasis:

12.1. Zinc

Zinc is an important cofactor for metabolism relevant to neurotransmitters, prostaglandins, and melatonin, and indirectly affects dopamine metabolism [139]. The role of zinc is thought to transduce oxidative stress and other signals converging at the production of nitric oxide into an specific intracellular response, suggesting an intriguing task of "signal transducer" [140]. It contributes to structure and function of brain [141], and low levels of zinc can cause a range of symptoms including hyperactivity and jitters [142]. Epidemiological studies on the influence of zinc/diet and lifestyle implications on degenerative disease and in particular on autism has been documented. Interestingly, antioxidant and micronutrients in the diet, such as zinc, influence the development and function of immune cells, the activity of stress-related proteins and antioxidant enzymes and help to maintain genomic integrity and stability [143, 144]. Zinc is included in many enzymatic processes. [145, 146] In CNS zinc is abundant in the so-called "zinc containing" synapses of glutamatergic neurons. Such neurons are located mainly in the prefrontal lobe. Frontal dysfunction may follow lack of zinc. On the other hand, bivalent zinc may cause excitotoxic damage. Also other minerals (e.g., magnesium, manganese) are important for proper functioning of the CNS. [145, 147, 148]

Zinc was shown to play a role in inducing the synthesis of metallothionein that acts as a scavenger of metals and free radicals [149]. It is necessary for 100 different metalloenzymes and metal–enzyme complexes [150], many of them in the central nervous system. Zinc supplementation of young children in low income countries improves their neurophysiological performance [151], also in combination with iron supplements [152]. Some behavioural abnormalities in adults also seem to respond favourably to zinc supplementation, such as mood changes, emotional lability, anorexia, irritability and depression [153]. All these physiological functions occur through the action of proteins involved in the regulation of zinc homeostasis, such as metallothioneins, which bind zinc with high affinity but, at the same time, release free zinc ions in response to oxidative/nitrosative stress to modulate the expression of zinc-dependent genes and to activate antioxidant enzymes and impact immune response [154].

12.1.1. Antioxidant properties of zinc

Zinc deficiency is difficult to evaluate due to the lack of sensitive and specific biomarkers [155]. Studies observed improved neurophysiologic performance, positive growth response, and significantly reduced mortality and morbidity with zinc supplementation in Chinese children [156]. Zinc effect on immune/inflammation responses has been reported [157]. It has been suggested that the bioavailability of zinc ion regulates the expression of pro-inflammatory cytokines and heat shock proteins such as IL-6, TNF-α and Hsp70 [158], and affects TH1/TH2 balance [159]. Several mechanisms could be involved in antioxidant function of zinc. One, zinc may protect protein sulfhydryl groups from oxidative modification by influencing the conformation and reducing potential of thiol groups. Since the sulfhydryl groups are required for the catalytic activities of several enzymes, zinc protects the enzyme's activity from oxidative inactivation.

Second, zinc may antagonize the activity of transition metals such as iron and copper. A number of studies have linked RLS to deficiencies of dopamine and iron. The disorder may result from inefficient processing of iron in certain brain cells [160]. A decrease in iron levels in the substantia nigra and, to a lesser degree, in idiopathic RLS patients was reported [161]. Ferritin levels were lower in cerebrospinal fluid, whereas transferrin levels were higher in patients with RLS compared to controls [162]. Connor et al. [163] found that receptors which help cells absorb iron are abnormally regulated in cells that produce the nerve-signaling chemical dopamine. Zago and Oteiza [164] showed that zinc may compete with copper and iron ions and prevent transition metal mediated oxidative modifications, and third mechanism for the antioxidant property of zinc is that zinc may reduce oxidative damage indirectly by modulating antioxidant defence including (a) enzymes which catalytically remove free radicals and reactive species, like superoxide dismutase, catalase, and glutathione peroxidase; (b) proteins which minimize the availability of pro-oxidants, like transferrins, ceruloplasmin and metallothioneins; (c) low-molecular-mass ROS and RNS scavengers, like glutathione, ascorbic acid, uric acid and alpha-tocopherol.

Antioxidant enzymes such as CuZn superoxide dismutase (CuZnSOD), glutathione peroxidase (GPX) and catalase are located in different cellular compartments and have different functions. Mice defective in CuZnSOD develop neurological damage and cancer at an accelerated rate as they age [165]. GPX-1 knockout mice are much more sensitive to paraquat toxicity than the wide type mice [166]. One human study done in a European population observed that the erythrocyte SOD activities were negatively associated with the plasma zinc concentrations, and positively associated with age. They also observed that the plasma catalase and GPX activities were similar among groups having different plasma zinc concentrations [158].

Zinc is one of the micronutrients involved in behavior, learning and mental functions. Zinc is necessary for proper immune function, and to create protein and DNA. The administration of nightly melatonin, magnesium, and zinc appears to improve the quality of sleep and the quality of life in long-term care facility residents with primary insomnia [167]. micronutrients such as zinc and magnesium may play a role in facilitating sleep. Zinc exhibits an antidepressant-like activity, as stated in a preclinical model of depression [168]. Significant clinical correlates were shown by Sowa-Kućma et al. [169] related to its action as an antagonist of the glutamate/N-methyl-D-aspartate receptor. Magnesium has beneficial effects on mood and is crucial, together with zinc, in the endogenous synthesis of melatonin [170].

Zinc is an essential bio-element, which plays a fundamental role in a wide range of biochemical processes. This metal is a major component of various proteins and is an important modulator of the mammalian immune and nervous systems [171]. Zinc is one of the mineral that has such a wide application in human health. A deficiency may result in sleep disturbances. Most sleeping pills, especially when taken over long periods of time, can have multiple side effects. Alterations of blood zinc homeostasis may accompany mood disturbances as well as affect functions of the immune system [172]. Recent data indicate that alterations in zinc (a natural modulator of amino-acidergic neurotransmission) homeostasis may contribute to mood disorders and may be involved in antidepressant-like actions in laboratory models [171].

12.2. Iron

Iron has an important role in many enzymatic processes. Sufficient iron in the CNS is necessary for normal functioning of the dopamine system. Iron has an effect on functioning of the dopamine receptors. Tyrosine hydroxlase regulates dopamine synthesis. Iron and tetrahydrobiopterin are cofactors of tyrosinehydroxylase. Iron is also linked to functions of GABA, serotonin and opidiod-peptides. In experimental cell cultures dopaminergic cells of the substantia nigra can be destroyed by chelation of iron by desferoxamine. Adding opioids in these cell cultures is protective. Iron also has a catalytic effect in oxidative mechanisms of the CNS and epilepsy [173]. Measuring serum ferritin and soluble transferring receptor from a venous blood sample allows estimation of tissue iron levels. In restless legs syndrome S-ferritin is often low, in which case, giving iron per os, or intravenously in more severe cases, should be part of the treatment.

In patients with RLS 45 μg/L is usually used as a limit when one should consider giving iron supplement even if hemoglobin is normal. Usually the soluble transferrin receptor values are also low. Iron should be gioven as Fe2+(bivalent iron) together with vitamin C to increase absorption of iron from the gut. If ferritin levels do not rise and the symptoms are bothersome one might consider IV iron. Iron dextrane should be avoided because of potential risks but safe formulations exist, such as Venofer®. Several studies have already shown the benefits of IV iron starting from the early experiences from Sweden in the 1950's. [174, 175]

Yehuda has noted that in young children sleep disturbances, fatigue and possible learning disturbances may be related to iron deficiency early in life. These findings require further studies. [176] To determine if there is a relationship between low serum ferritin and sleep disturbance in children with autism spectrum disorder, an eight-week open-label treatment trial on 33 children with oral iron supplementation has been done. Seventy-seven percent had restless sleep at baseline, which improved significantly with iron therapy, suggesting a relationship between sleep disturbance and iron deficiency in children with autism spectrum disorder. Sixty-nine percent of preschoolers and 35% of school-aged children had insufficient dietary iron intake. Mean ferritin increased significantly (16 μg/L to 29 μg/L). It may be that children with autism spectrum disorder should be screened for iron deficiency. [177]

Kuhn et al. studied the effects of five days of sleep deprivation on the circadian rhythm of serum iron in a group of six healthy male volunteers. The results were compared with a control group of five individuals, whose normal sleep cycle was preserved, but whose daily regimen was otherwise identical with the sleep deprivation group. Their biorhythm was analyzed using cosinor analysis. Sleep deprivation markedly reduced the mean level of iron, diminished the absolute and relative amplitude of oscillations, disturbed the shape of the daily course of serum iron and gradually decreased the computative acrophase, i.e., shortened the period of rhythm. Forty-eight hours of recovery resulted in only a partial normalization of all the observed changes. The potential mechanisms of the observed changes are discussed. [178]

12.3. Copper

Copper acts as a cofactor in many enzymatic processes including ceruloplasmin, monoaminexidases, cytochromoxidase, and superoxide dismutase. The largest part of copper (96%) is binded into cerluloplasmin and ferro-oxidase, which is needed in many phases of iron metabolism. [179] Lack of copper can manifest as neutropenia, microcytic anemia, growth disturbances or slowing of erythropoiesis. Large amount of vitamine C, zinc, iron and cysteine worsen the absorption of copper from the gut. Menkes syndrome is an example of a genetic disturbance of copper metabolism causing deficiency of copper. Wilson's disease is an autosomal recessive disease that causes accumulation of copper in the liver and brain [180]. It is practically impossible to have too much copper from a normal diet. Lack of copper may follow poor diet or excessive consumption of zinc tablets.

12.4. Selenium

Selenium (Se) is a natural antioxidant which delays the oxidation of polyunsaturated fatty acids and preserves the elasticity of tissue [181, 182]. Se is an essential component of thioredoxinreductase and glutathione peroxidases, with strong antioxidative and antiinflammatory properties, and there is particular interest in the potential of Se to modulate oxidative stress and induce anticancer activity [183, 184]. Selenium is required for the production of certain prostaglandins which decrease platelet aggregation [185]. Selenium deficiency has been linked to adverse mood states [183]. Several lines of evidence have shown that selenium is crucially important in the maintenance and modulation of different brain functions. [186-189] Selenium may have some role in regulation of sleep and in development of insomnia as lack of selenium was statistically significantly associated with difficulty falling asleep in a recent large survey. [130]

Selenium supplementation together with other vitamins has been found beneficial in the treatment of mood lability [190, 191].In synergy with vitamin E, selenium promotes normal growth and fertility, and improves the function of certain energy producing cells [192, 193]. Also, selenium also plays a role in your immune system and thyroid function and may contribute to sleeping abnormalities. Infusion of selective inhibitors of PGDS, e.g., tetravalent selenium compounds, reversibly, time-and dose-dependently inhibited both non-rapid eye movement (NREM) and rapid eye movement (REM) sleep during the daytime [194], which shows that PGDS plays a crucial role in the regulation of physiological sleep. Selenium deficit may result in severe disorders [195, 196], including mood disorders. Gosney et al [197] reported the effects of micronutrient supplementation on mood in nursing home residents; selenium supplementation was directly correlated with decreases in depression scores and increases in serum levels. Supplementation with selenium resulted in reduced serum thyroid hormone T4 and increased serum thyroid hormone T3, suggesting that the additional selenium helped the rather boring T4 become the metabolically active T3. Effects of sleep deprivation (SD) and selenium (Se) on wound healing were studied [198], the number of fibroblasts and capillary vessels were higher in control and Se groups than in sleep deprivation groups, and the number of PNLs and the radiolabeled polyvalent IgG levels were higher in SD groups than in control and Se groups. OSA patients had lower concentrations of plasma Zn and erythrocyte Se [199]. Furthermore, the effect of selenium on restless leg syndrome treatment was studied [200, 201], selenium supplementation would be an alternative treatment in improvement of RLS symptoms.

13. In summary

Little is still known about the effects of different constituents of meals on sleep. There is evidence that a heavy lunch and rapidly absorbing carbohydrates enhance sleepiness in the afternoon. This may add to daytime sleepiness and for that reason they should be avoided when one wants to avoid fatigue. On the contrary, a light evening meal which is rich in carbohydrates may help one to fall asleep in the evening. The relationships between the enteric nervous system and CNS, and different roles of dietary nutrients and CNS need to be studied much more in the future.

Author details

Markku Partinen[1,2*], Tuomas Westermarck[3] and Faik Atroshi[4]

*Address all correspondence to: markpart@mac.com

1 Helsinki Sleep Clinic, Vitalmed Research Centre, Sitratori, Helsinki, Finland

2 Haartman Institute, University of Helsinki, Helsinki, Finland

3 Rinnekoti Research Centre, Espoo, Finland

4 Pharmacology & Toxicology, University of Helsinki, Finland

References

[1] Allen RP, Earley CJ. The role of iron in restless legs syndrome. Mov Disord 2007.

[2] Porkka-Heiskanen T, Kalinchuk AV. Adenosine, energy metabolism and sleep homeostasis. Sleep Med Rev 2011; 15(2): 123-35.

[3] Magistretti PJ, Pellerin L. Cellular mechanisms of brain energy metabolism and their relevance to functional brain imaging. Phil Trans Royal Soc London 1999; 354: 1155-63.

[4] Pellerin L, Magistretti PJ. Neuroenergetics: calling upon astrocytes to satisfy hungry neurons. Neuroscientist 2004; 10(1): 53-62.

[5] Olesen J, Gustavsson A, Svensson M, Wittchen HU, Jönsson B; CDBE2010 study group; European Brain Council. The economic cost of brain disorders in Europe. Eur J Neurol. 2012 Jan;19(1):155-62

[6] Wittchen HU, Jacobi F, Rehm J, Gustavsson A, Svensson M, Jönsson B, Olesen J, Allgulander C, Alonso J, Faravelli C, Fratiglioni L, Jennum P, Lieb R, Maercker A, van Os J, Preisig M, Salvador-Carulla L, Simon R, Steinhausen HC. The size and burden of mental disorders and other disorders of the brain in Europe 2010. Eur Neuropsychopharmacol. 2011 Sep;21(9):655-79.

[7] Jerzy Majkowski, Tuomas Westermarck, Faik Atroshi. Oxygen stress: epilepsy and antiepileptic drugs. EPILEPTOLOGIA, 2011, 19:143-157.

[8] McLean PG, Borman RA, Lee K. 5-HT in the enteric nervous system: gut function and neuropharmacology. Trends Neurosci 2007; 30(1): 9-13.

[9] de Lecea L, Kilduff TS, Peyron C, Gao X, Foye PE, Danielson PE, Fukuhara C, Battenberg EL, Gautvik VT, Bartlett FS, 2nd, Frankel WN, van den Pol AN, Bloom FE,

Gautvik KM, Sutcliffe JG. The hypocretins: hypothalamus-specific peptides with neuroexcitatory activity. Proc Natl Acad Sci U S A 1998; 95(1): 322-7.

[10] Sakurai T, Amemiya A, Ishii M, Matsuzaki I, Chemelli RM, Tanaka H, Williams SC, Richardson JA, Kozlowski GP, Wilson S, Arch JR, Buckingham RE, Haynes AC, Carr SA, Annan RS, McNulty DE, Liu WS, Terrett JA, Elshourbagy NA, Bergsma DJ, Yanagisawa M. Orexins and orexin receptors: a family of hypothalamic neuropeptides and G protein-coupled receptors that regulate feeding behavior. Cell 1998; 92(4): 573-85.

[11] Peyron C, Faraco J, Rogers W, Ripley B, Overeem S, Charnay Y, Nevsimalova S, Aldrich M, Reynolds D, Albin R, Li R, Hungs M, Pedrazzoli M, Padigaru M, Kucherlapati M, Fan J, Maki R, Lammers GJ, Bouras C, Kucherlapati R, Nishino S, Mignot E. A mutation in a case of early onset narcolepsy and a generalized absence of hypocretin peptides in human narcoleptic brains. Nat Med 2000; 6(9): 991-7.

[12] Nishino S. The hypothalamic peptidergic system, hypocretin/orexin and vigilance control. Neuropeptides 2007; 41(3): 117-33.

[13] Burdakov D, Gerasimenko O, Verkhratsky A. Physiological changes in glucose differentially modulate the excitability of hypothalamic melanin-concentrating hormone and orexin neurons in situ. J Neurosci 2005; 25(9): 2429-33.

[14] Harris GC, Aston-Jones G. Arousal and reward: a dichotomy in orexin function. Trends Neurosci 2006; 29(10): 571-7.

[15] Grimaldi D, Silvani A, Benarroch EE, Cortelli P. Orexin/hypocretin system and autonomic control: New insights and clinical correlations.Neurology. 2014 Jan 21;82(3): 271-8.

[16] Korczynski W, Ceregrzyn M, Matyjek R, Kato I, Kuwahara A, Wolinski J, Zabielski R. Central and local (enteric) action of orexins. J Physiol Pharmacol 2006; 57 Suppl 6: 17-42.

[17] Watson CJ, Baghdoyan HA, Lydic R. Neuropharmacology of sleep and wakefulness. Sleep Medicine Clinics 2010; 5(4): 513-28.

[18] Parker JA, Bloom SR. Hypothalamic neuropeptides and the regulation of appetite. Neuropharmacology 2012; 63(1): 18-30.

[19] Burdakov D, Karnani MM, Gonzalez A. Lateral hypothalamus as a sensor-regulator in respiratory and metabolic control. Physiol Behav 2013.

[20] Fisone G, Borgkvist A, Usiello A. Caffeine as a psychomotor stimulant: mechanism of action. Cell Mol Life Sci 2004; 61(7-8): 857-72.

[21] Huang ZL, Qu WM, Eguchi N, Chen JF, Schwarzschild MA, Fredholm BB, Urade Y, Hayaishi O. Adenosine A2A, but not A1, receptors mediate the arousal effect of caffeine. Nat Neurosci 2005; 8(7): 858-9.

[22] Porkka-Heiskanen T. Sleep homeostasis. Curr Opin Neurobiol 2013.

[23] Hauri P, S. L. No More Sleepless Nights. New York: John wiley & Sons, Inc; 1990.

[24] Curless R, French JM, James OF, Wynne HA. Is caffeine a factor in subjective insomnia of elderly people? Age Ageing 1993; 22(1): 41-5.

[25] Brown SL, Salive ME, Pahor M, Foley DJ, Corti MC, Langlois JA, Wallace RB, Harris TB. Occult caffeine as a source of sleep problems in an older population. J Am Geriatr Soc 1995; 43(8): 860-4.

[26] Riedel BW, Lichstein KL. Insomnia and daytime functioning. Sleep medicine reviews 2000; 4(3): 277-98.

[27] Gyllenhaal C, Merritt SL, Peterson SD, Block KI, Gochenour T. Efficacy and safety of herbal stimulants and sedatives in sleep disorders. Sleep Med Rev 2000; 4(3): 229-51.

[28] Stepanski EJ, Wyatt JK. Use of sleep hygiene in the treatment of insomnia. Sleep Med Rev 2003; 7(3): 215-25.

[29] Boutrel B, Koob GF. What keeps us awake: the neuropharmacology of stimulants and wakefulness-promoting medications. Sleep 2004; 27(6): 1181-94.

[30] Roehrs T, Roth T. Caffeine: Sleep and daytime sleepiness. Sleep Medicine Reviews 2008; 12(2): 153-62.

[31] Wolk BJ, Ganetsky M, Babu KM. Toxicity of energy drinks. Curr Opin Pediatr 2012; 24(2): 243-51.

[32] Estruch R, Ros E, Salas-Salvado J, Covas MI, Corella D, Aros F, Gomez-Gracia E, Ruiz-Gutierrez V, Fiol M, Lapetra J, Lamuela-Raventos RM, Serra-Majem L, Pinto X, Basora J, Munoz MA, Sorli JV, Martinez JA, Martinez-Gonzalez MA. Primary prevention of cardiovascular disease with a Mediterranean diet. N Engl J Med 2013; 368(14): 1279-90.

[33] Lourida I, Soni M, Thompson-Coon J, Purandare N, Lang IA, Ukoumunne OC, Llewellyn DJ. Mediterranean diet, cognitive function, and dementia: a systematic review. Epidemiology 2013; 24(4): 479-89.

[34] Psaltopoulou T, Sergentanis TN, Panagiotakos DB, Sergentanis IN, Kosti R, Scarmeas N. Mediterranean diet, stroke, cognitive impairment, and depression: A meta-analysis. Ann Neurol 2013; 74(4): 580-91.

[35] Calabrese EJ. Hormesis and medicine. Br J Clin Pharmacol 2008; 66(5): 594-617.

[36] Doss M. Evidence supporting radiation hormesis in atomic bomb survivor cancer mortality data. Dose-response : a publication of International Hormesis Society 2012; 10(4): 584-92.

[37] Edwards SJ, Montgomery IM, Colquhoun EQ, Jordan JE, Clark MG. Spicy meal disturbs sleep: an effect of thermoregulation? Int J Psychophysiol 1992; 13(2): 97-100.

[38] Halliwell B and Gutteridge JMC (1999) Free Radicals in Biology and Medicine, 3rd edn. Oxford: Clarendon Press.

[39] Kültz D. Molecular and evolutionary basis of the cellular stress response. Annu Rev Physiol. 2005;67:225-57

[40] Carpagnano GE, Kharitonov SA, Resta O, Foschino-Barbaro MP, Gramiccioni E, Barnes PJ. 8-Isoprostane, a marker of oxidative stress, is increased in exhaled breath condensate of patients with obstructive sleep apnea after night and is reduced by continuous positive airway pressure therapy. Chest. 2003 Oct;124(4):1386-92

[41] Lavie L. Obstructive sleep apnoea syndrome--an oxidative stress disorder. Sleep Med Rev. 2003 Feb;7(1):35-51

[42] Tasali E, Van Cauter E. Sleep-disordered breathing and the current epidemic of obesity: consequence or contributing factor? Am J Respir Crit Care Med. 2002 Mar 1;165(5):562-3.

[43] Ramanathan L, Gulyani S, Nienhuis R, Siegel JM. Sleep deprivation decreases superoxide dismutase activity in rat hippocampus and brainstem. Neuroreport. 2002 Aug 7;13(11):1387-90.

[44] Busija DW. Prostaglandins and other Eicosanoids. In: Edvinsson L, Krause D, ed. Cerebral blood flow and metabolism. Lippincott Williams and Wilkins, 325-338, 2002.

[45] Roberts SM, Newton RF. Prostaglandins and Thromboxanes by Stanley M. Roberts and Roger F. Newton,1982, 143 pages, Elsevier Science & Technology Books. I ISBN-10: 0408107731 I ISBN-13: 978040810773.

[46] Schrör K. Aspirin and platelets: the antiplatelet action of aspirin and its role in thrombosis treatment and prophylaxis. Semin Thromb Hemost. 1997;23(4):349-56.

[47] Walch L, Labat C, Gascard JP, de Montpreville V, Brink C, Norel X. Prostanoid receptors involved in the relaxation of human pulmonary vessels. Br J Pharmacol. 1999 Feb;126(4):859-66.

[48] Adelizzi RA. COX-1 and COX-2 in health and disease. J Am Osteopath Assoc. 1999 Nov;99(11 Suppl):S7-12.

[49] Narumiya S, Ogorochi T, Nakao K, Hayaishi O. Prostaglandin D2 in rat brain, spinal cord and pituitary: basal level and regional distribution.Life Sci. 1982 Nov 8;31(19): 2093-103.

[50] Ogorochi T, Narumiya S, Mizuno N, Yamashita K, Miyazaki H, Hayaishi O. Regional distribution of prostaglandins D2, E2, and F2 alpha and related enzymes in postmortem human brain. J Neurochem. 1984 Jul;43(1):71-82.

[51] Hayaishi O. Sleep-wake regulation by prostaglandin D2 and E2. J Biol Chem. 1988, 263:14593–6.

[52] Pentreath VW, Rees K, Owolabi OA, Philip KA, Doua F. The somnogenic T lymphocyte suppressor prostaglandin D2 is selectively elevated in cerebrospinal fluid of advanced sleeping sickness patients.Trans R Soc Trop Med Hyg. 1990 Nov-Dec;84(6): 795-9.

[53] Onoe H, Ueno R, Fujita I, Nishino H, Oomura Y, Hayaishi O. Prostaglandin D2, a cerebral sleep-inducing substance in monkeys.Proc Natl Acad Sci U S A. 1988 Jun; 85(11):4082-6.

[54] Satoh, S., Matsumura, H., Suzuki, F. and Hayaishi, O. Promotion of sleep mediated by the A2a-adenosine receptor and possible involvement of this receptor in the sleep induced by prostaglandin D2 in rats. Proc. Natl. Acad. Sci. U S A, 1996, 93: 5980–5984.

[55] Onoe H, Ueno R, Fujita I, Nishino H, Oomura Y, and Hayaishi O. Prostaglandin D2, a cerebral sleep-inducing substance in monkeys. Proc Natl Acad Sci U S A. 1988 June; 85(11): 4082–4086.

[56] Giles, H. & Leff, P. The biology and pharmacology of prostaglandin D2. Prostaglandins,1988, 35, 277 ± 300.

[57] Atroshi F., Sankari S., Työppönen J. and Parantainen J. Inflammation related changes in trace elements, GSH-metabolism, prostaglandins and sialic acid. In: Trace Elements in Man and Animals 6 (Hurly LS ; Keen CL; Lonnerdal Bo, & Rucker RB, Editors), Plenum Press, New York & London, 1988, pp.97-99.

[58] Rouzer, C. A., Scott, W. A., Hamill, A. L., Liu, F. T., Katz, D. H. & Cohn, Z. A. Secretion of leukotriene C and other arachidonic acid metabolites by macrophages challenged with immunoglobulin E immune complexes. J. Exp. Med.1982, 156:1077-1086

[59] Mimata H, Tanigawa T, Ogata J, Takeshita M. Regulation of prostaglandin synthesis by reduced glutathione in urinary bladder epithelium.J Urol. 1988 Mar;139(3):616-20.

[60] D'Almeida V, Lobo LL, Hipólide DC, de Oliveira AC, Nobrega JN, Tufik S. Sleep deprivation induces brain region-specific decreases in glutathione levels. Neuroreport. 1998 Aug 24;9(12):2853-6.

[61] Lang CC. When is a nightmare really a nightmare? Pacing Clin Electrophysiol. 2001 Sep;24(9 Pt 1):1415-6.

[62] Dickinson, D.A., Moellering, D.R., Iles, K.E., Patel, R.P., Levonen, A.-L., Wigley, A., Darley-Usmar, V.M., and Forman, H.J., Cytoprotection against oxidative stress and the regulation of glutathione synthesis, Biol. Chem. (2003) 384:527-537.

[63] Lang CA, Mills BJ, Mastropaolo W, Liu MC. Blood glutathione decreases in chronic diseases.J Lab Clin Med. 2000 May;135(5):402-5.

[64] Mancuso M, Bonanni e, LoGerfo a, orsucci D, Maestri M, Chico L et al. oxidative stress biomarkers in patients with untreated obstructive sleep apnea syndrome. Sleep Med 2012;13:632-636.

[65] Ntalapascha M, Makris D, Kyparos A, Tsilioni I, Kostikas K, Gourgoulianis K, Kouretas D, Zakynthinos E (2012) Oxidative stress in patients with obstructive sleep apnea syndrome. Sleep Breath. doi:10. 1007/s11325-012-0718-y.

[66] Grandner MA, Jackson N, Gerstner JR, Knutson KL. Sleep symptoms associated with intake of specific dietary nutrients. J Sleep Res 2013.

[67] International Classification of Sleep Disorders – Second Edition (ICSD-2), 298 pages. ©2005 American Academy of Sleep Medicine, ISBN 0965722023 ISBN 978-0965722025.

[68] Partinen M. Nutrition and sleep. Sleep Disorders Medicine, ed SC (Butterworth/Elsevier), 3rd Ed, pp:307-318, 2009.

[69] Baldewicz T, Goodkin K, Feaster DJ, Blaney NT, Kumar M, Kumar A, Shor-Posner G, Baum M. Plasma pyridoxine deficiency is related to increased psychological distress in recently bereaved homosexual men. Psychosom Med. 1998 May-Jun;60(3):297-308.

[70] Durga J, van Boxtel MP, Schouten EG, Kok FJ, Jolles J, Katan MB, Verhoef P. Effect of 3-year folic acid supplementation on cognitive function in older adults in the FACIT trial: a randomised, double blind, controlled trial. Lancet. 2007 Jan 20;369(9557): 208-16.

[71] Hector M, BurtonJR: What arc th e psychi atric mani fest ations of vitamin B-12 deficien cy?JAGS, 1988, 36: 1105-1112.

[72] Okawa M, Takahashi K, Egashira K, Furuta H, Higashitani Y, Higuchi T, Ichikawa H, Ichimaru Y, Inoue Y, Ishizuka Y, Ito N, Kamei K, Kaneko M, Kim Y, Kohsaka M, Komori T, Kotorii T, Matsumoto M, Mishima K, Mizuki Y, Morimoto K, Nagayama H, Ohta T, Okamoto N, Takahashi S, et al. Vitamin B12 treatment for delayed sleep phase syndrome: a multi-center double-blind study. Psychiatry Clin Neurosci. 1997 Oct;51(5):275-9.

[73] Syed EU, Wasay M, Awan S. Vitamin B12 supplementation in treating major depressive disorder: a randomized controlled trial. Open Neurol J. 2013 Nov 15;7:44-8. doi: 10. 2174/1874205X01307010044.

[74] Hintikka J, Tolmunen T, Tanskanen A, Viinamäki H. High vitamin B12 level and good treatment outcome may be associated in major depressive disorder.BMC Psychiatry. 2003 Dec 2;3:17.

[75] Morris MS, Fava M, Jacques PF, Selhub J, Rosenberg IH. Depression and folate status in the US Population. Psychother Psychosom. 2003 Mar-Apr;72(2):80-7.

[76] Chanarin I, Deacon R, Lumb M, Perry J. Cobalamin-folate interrelations. Blood Rev. 1989 Dec;3(4):211-5

[77] Yamazaki J, Sugishita M, Moriya Y, Isojima G, Ohshima H, Yamazaki O, Takeda Y, Yamauchi T, Takashima M, Takahashi K. The effects of vitamin B12 on the suppression of melatonin secretion under illumination. Jpn J Psychiatry Neurol. 1991 Mar; 45(1):169-70.

[78] Hvas AM, Juul S, Bech P, Nexø E. Vitamin B6 level is associated with symptoms of depression. Psychother Psychosom. 2004 Nov-Dec;73(6):340-3.

[79] Bryan J, Calvaresi E, Hughes D. Short-term folate, vitamin B-12 or vitamin B-6 supplementation slightly affects memory performance but not mood in women of various ages. J Nutr. 2002 Jun;132(6):1345-56.

[80] Lansdowne AT, Provost SC. Vitamin D3 enhances mood in healthy subjects during winter. Psychopharmacology (Berl). 1998 Feb;135(4):319-23.

[81] Privette TH, Stumpf WE, Mueller RA, Hollis BW. Serum 1,25 dihydroxyvitamin D3 (soltriol) levels influenceserotonin levels in the hypothalamus of the rat Abstr. Soc Neurosci 1991;17:498 (197. 9).

[82] Grandner MA, Jackson N, Gerstner JR, Knutson KL. Dietary nutrients associated with short and long sleep duration. Data from a nationally representative sample. Appetite. 2013 May;64:71-80.

[83] Gominak SC, Stumpf WE. The world epidemic of sleep disorders is linked to vitamin D deficiency. Med Hypotheses. 2012 Aug;79(2):132-5. doi: 10. 1016/j.mehy.2012. 03. 031. Epub 2012 May 13.

[84] Shiue I. Low vitamin D levels in adults with longer time to fall asleep: US NHANES, 2005-2006. Int J Cardiol. 2013 Oct 12;168(5):5074-5.

[85] Rosen CJ, Adams JS, Bikle DD, Black DM, Demay MD, Manson JE, Murad M,Kovacs CS. The nonskeletal effects of vitamin D: an Endocrine Society Scientific statement. Endocr Rev. 2011;33:456–492.

[86] McCarty DE, Chesson AL Jr, Jain SK, Marino AA. The link between vitamin D metabolism and sleep medicine. Sleep Med Rev. 2013 Sep 25. pii: S1087-0792(13)00073-7.

[87] Barceló A, Barbé F, de la Peña M, Vila M, Pérez G, Piérola J, Durán J, Agustí AG. Antioxidant status in patients with sleep apnoea and impact of continuous positive airway pressure treatment. Eur Respir J. 2006 Apr;27(4):756-60.

[88] Ransom J, Morgan PJ, McCaffery PJ, Stoney PN. The rhythm of retinoids in the brain. J Neurochem. 2013 Nov 24. doi: 10. 1111/jnc.12620.

[89] Sei H. Vitamin A and sleep regulation. J Med Invest. 2008 Feb;55(1-2):1-8.

[90] Maret S, Franken P, Dauvilliers Y, Ghyselinck NB, Chambon P, Tafti M. Retinoic acid signaling affects cortical synchrony during sleep.Science. 2005 Oct 7;310(5745):111-3.

[91] Kitaoka K, Hattori A, Chikahisa S, Miyamoto K, Nakaya Y, Sei H. Vitamin A deficiency induces a decrease in EEG delta power during sleep in mice.Brain Res. 2007 May 30;1150:121-30.

[92] Bourre JM. Effects of nutrients (in food) on the structure and function of the nervous system: update on dietary requirements for brain. Part 1: micronutrients.J Nutr Health Aging. 2006 Sep-Oct;10(5):377-85.

[93] Harrison FE, May JM. Vitamin C function in the brain: vital role of the ascorbate transporter SVCT2. Free Radic Biol Med. 2009 Mar 15;46(6):719-30.

[94] Grandner MA, Jackson N, Gerstner JR, Knutson KL. Sleep symptoms associated with intake of specific dietary nutrients. J Sleep Res. 2014 Feb;23(1):22-34. doi: 10. 1111/jsr. 12084. Epub 2013 Sep 2.

[95] Singh TD, Patial K, Vijayan VK, Ravi K. Oxidative stress and obstructive sleep apnoea syndrome. Indian J Chest Dis Allied Sci. 2009 Oct-Dec;51(4):217-24.

[96] Sales LV, Bruin VM, D'Almeida V, Pompéia S, Bueno OF, Tufik S, Bittencourt L. Cognition and biomarkers of oxidative stress in obstructive sleep apnea. Clinics (Sao Paulo). 2013 Apr;68(4):449-55.

[97] Sagheb MM, Dormanesh B, Fallahzadeh MK, Akbari H, Sohrabi Nazari S, Heydari ST, Behzadi S. Efficacy of vitamins C, E, and their combination for treatment of restless legs syndrome in hemodialysis patients: a randomized, double-blind, placebo-controlled trial. Sleep Med. 2012 May;13(5):542-5. doi: 10. 1016/j.sleep.2011. 11. 010. Epub 2012 Feb 7.

[98] Gess B, Röhr D, Young P. Ascorbic Acid and sodium-dependent vitamin C transporters in the peripheral nervous system: from basic science to clinical trials. Antioxid Redox Signal. 2013 Dec 10;19(17):2105-14. doi: 10. 1089/ars.2013. 5380. Epub 2013 Jul 31.

[99] Sugita Y. Is restless legs syndrome an entirely neurological disorder? Eur J Gen Pract. 2008;14(1):45-6. doi: 10. 1080/13814780802095550.

[100] Alzoubi KH, Khabour OF, Rashid BA, Damaj IM, Salah HA. The neuroprotective effect of vitamin E on chronic sleep deprivation-induced memory impairment: the role of oxidative stress. Behav Brain Res. 2012 Jan 1;226(1):205-10.

[101] Sales LV, Bruin VM, D'Almeida V, Pompéia S, Bueno OF, Tufik S, Bittencourt L. Cognition and biomarkers of oxidative stress in obstructive sleep apnea. Clinics (Sao Paulo). 2013 Apr;68(4):449-55.

[102] Mangialasche F, Solomon A, Kåreholt I, Hooshmand B, Cecchetti R, Fratiglioni L, Soininen H, Laatikainen T, Mecocci P, Kivipelto M. Serum levels of vitamin E forms

and risk of cognitive impairment in a Finnish cohort of older adults.Exp Gerontol. 2013 Dec;48(12):1428-35.

[103] Sagheb MM, Dormanesh B, Fallahzadeh MK, Akbari H, Sohrabi Nazari S, Heydari ST, Behzadi S. Efficacy of vitamins C, E, and their combination for treatment of restless legs syndrome in hemodialysis patients: a randomized, double-blind, placebo-controlled trial. Sleep Med. 2012 May;13(5):542-5.

[104] Goa KL, Brogden RN. l-Carnitine. A preliminary review of its pharmacokinetics, and its therapeutic use in ischaemic cardiac disease and primary and secondary carnitine deficiencies in relationship to its role in fatty acid metabolism. Drugs. 1987 Jul;34(1): 1-24.

[105] Berni A, Meschini R, Filippi S, Palitti F, De Amicis A, Chessa L. L-carnitine enhances resistance to oxidative stress by reducing DNA damage in Ataxia telangiectasia cells. Mutat Res. 2008 Feb 29;650(2):165-74.

[106] Garzya G, Corallo D, Fiore A, Lecciso G, Petrelli G, Zotti C. Evaluation of the effects of L-acetylcarnitine on senile patients suffering from depression. Drugs Exp Clin Res. 1990;16(2):101-6.

[107] Kuratsune H, Yamaguti K, Takahashi M, Misaki H, Tagawa S, Kitani T. Acylcarnitine deficiency in chronic fatigue syndrome. Clin Infect Dis. 1994 Jan;18 Suppl 1:S62-7.

[108] Schneider JE, Tyler DJ, ten Hove M, Sang AE, Cassidy PJ, Fischer A, Wallis J, Sebag-Montefiore LM, Watkins H, Isbrandt D, Clarke K, Neubauer S. In vivo cardiac 1H-MRS in the mouse. Magn Reson Med. 2004 Nov;52(5):1029-35.

[109] Răşanu T, Mehedinţi-Hâncu M, Alexianu M, Mehedinţi T, Gheorghe E, Damian I. Carnitine deficiency. Rom J Morphol Embryol. 2012;53(1):203-6.

[110] Soczynska JK, Kennedy SH, Chow CS, Woldeyohannes HO, Konarski JZ, McIntyre RS. Acetyl-L-carnitine and alpha-lipoic acid: possible neurotherapeutic agents for mood disorders? Expert Opin Investig Drugs. 2008 Jun;17(6):827-43. doi: 10. 1517/13543784. 17. 6. 827.

[111] Villardita C, Smirni P, Vecchio I. L-Acetylcarnitine in depressed elderly patients. Eur Rev Med Pharmacol Sci 1984;62:341-4.

[112] Van Oudheusden LJ, Scholte HR. Efficacy of carnitine in the treatment of children with attention-deficit hyperactivity disorder. Prostaglandins Leukot Essent Fatty Acids. 2002 Jul;67(1):33-8.

[113] Van Hove JL, Kishnani P, Muenzer J, Wenstrup RJ, Summar ML, Brummond MR, Lachiewicz AM, Millington DS, Kahler SG. Benzoate therapy and carnitine deficiency in non-ketotic hyperglycinemia. Am J Med Genet. 1995 Dec 4;59(4):444-53.

[114] Miyagawa T, Kawamura H, Obuchi M, Ikesaki A, Ozaki A, Tokunaga K, Inoue Y, Honda M. Effects of oral L-carnitine administration in narcolepsy patients: a

randomized, double-blind, cross-over and placebo-controlled trial. PLoS One. 2013;8(1):e53707. doi: 10. 1371/journal.pone.0053707. Epub 2013 Jan 17.

[115] Miyagawa T, Miyadera H, Tanaka S, Kawashima M, Shimada M, Honda Y, Tokunaga K, Honda M. Abnormally low serum acylcarnitine levels in narcolepsy patients. Sleep. 2011 Mar 1;34(3):349-53A.

[116] Pettegrew JW, Levine J, McClure RJ. Acetyl-L-carnitine physical-chemical, metabolic, and therapeutic properties: relevance for its mode of action in Alzheimer's disease and geriatric depression. Mol Psychiatry. 2000 Nov;5(6):616-32.

[117] Rai G, Wright G, Scott L, Beston B, Rest J, Exton-Smith AN. Double-blind, placebo controlled study of acetyl-l-carnitine in patients with Alzheimer's dementia. Curr Med Res Opin. 1990;11(10):638-47.

[118] Patrick L. Nutrients and HIV: part three-N-acetylcysteine, alpha-lipoic acid, L-glutamine, and L-carnitine. Altern Med Rev. 2000 Aug;5(4):290-305

[119] De Grandis D, Minardi C. Acetyl-L-carnitine (levacecarnine) in the treatment of diabetic neuropathy. A long-term, randomised, double-blind, placebo-controlled study. Drugs R D. 2002;3(4):223-31.

[120] Calabrese P, Gambassi A. Aging at criticality in model-C dynamics. Phys Rev E Stat Nonlin Soft Matter Phys. 2003 Mar;67(3 Pt 2):036111. Epub 2003 Mar 20.

[121] Malaguarnera M, Vacante M, Bertino G, Neri S, Malaguarnera M, Gargante MP, Motta M, Lupo L, Chisari G, Bruno CM, Pennisi G, Bella R. The supplementation of acetyl-L-carnitine decreases fatigue and increases quality of life in patients with hepatitis C treated with pegylated interferon-α 2b plus ribavirin. J Interferon Cytokine Res. 2011 Sep;31(9):653-9

[122] Campos Y, Huertas R, Lorenzo G, Bautista J, Gutiérrez E, Aparicio M, Alesso L, Arenas J. Plasma carnitine insufficiency and effectiveness of L-carnitine therapy in patients with mitochondrial myopathy. Muscle Nerve. 1993a Feb;16(2):150-3.

[123] Campos Y, Huertas R, Bautista J, Gutiérrez E, Aparicio M, Lorenzo G, Segura D, Villanueva M, Cabello A, Alesso L, et al. Muscle carnitine deficiency and lipid storage myopathy in patients with mitochondrial myopathy.Muscle Nerve. 1993b Jul;16(7): 778-81.

[124] Atroshi F., Rizzo A, Österman T, Parantainen J. Free fatty acids and lipid peroxidation in normal and mastitic milk. J. Vet Med A 36, 321-330.

[125] Morley JE. Nutrition and the brain. Clin Geriatr Med. 2010 Feb;26(1):89-98.

[126] Innis SM. Dietary omega 3 fatty acids and the developing brain. Brain Res. 2008 Oct 27;1237:35-43.

[127] Chang CY, Ke DS, Chen JY. Essential fatty acids and human brain. Acta Neurol Taiwan. 2009 Dec;18(4):231-41.

[128] Rathod R, Khaire A, Kemse N, Kale A, Joshi S. Maternal omega-3 fatty acid supplementation on vitamin B₁₂ rich diet improves brain omega-3 fatty acids, neurotrophins and cognition in the Wistar rat offspring. Brain Dev. 2014 Jan 10. pii: S0387-7604(13)00350-1. doi: 10. 1016/j.braindev.2013. 12. 007.

[129] Moriguchi T, Lim SY, Greiner R, Lefkowitz W, Loewke J, Hoshiba J, Salem N Jr. Effects of an n-3-deficient diet on brain, retina, and liver fatty acyl composition in artificially reared rats.J Lipid Res. 2004 Aug;45(8):1437-45.

[130] Chiu C-C, Huang S-Y, Shen Winston W, Su K-P. Omega-3 fatty acids for depression in pregnancy. American journal of psychiatry 2003; 160((2)): 385.

[131] Haag M. Essential fatty acids and the brain. Canadian journal of psychiatry Revue canadienne de psychiatrie 2003; 48^((3)^): 195-203.

[132] Portwood MM. The role of dietary fatty acids in children's behaviour and learning. Nutr Health 2006; 18(3): 233-47.

[133] Williams AL, Katz D, Ali A, Girard C, Goodman J, Bell I. Do essential fatty acids have a role in the treatment of depression? J Affect Disord 2006; 93(1-3): 117-23.

[134] Tsaluchidu S, Cocchi M, Tonello L, Puri BK. Fatty acids and oxidative stress in psychiatric disorders. BMC Psychiatry 2008; 8 Suppl 1: S5.

[135] Riediger ND, Othman RA, Suh M, Moghadasian MH. A systemic review of the roles of n-3 fatty acids in health and disease. J Am Diet Assoc 2009; 109(4): 668-79.

[136] Lavialle M, Denis I, Guesnet P, Vancassel S. Involvement of omega-3 fatty acids in emotional responses and hyperactive symptoms. J Nutr Biochem 2010; 21(10): 899-905.

[137] Hakkarainen R, Partonen T, Haukka J, Virtamo J, Albanes D, Lonnqvist J. Food and nutrient intake in relation to mental wellbeing. Nutr J 2004; 3: 14.

[138] Fagioli I, Baroncini P, Ricour C, Salzarulo P. Decrease of slow-wave sleep in children with prolonged absence of essential lipids intake. Sleep 1989; 12(6): 495-9.

[139] Prasad AS. Clinical and biochemical manifestation zinc deficiency in human subjects. J Pharmacol. 1985 Oct-Dec;16(4):344-52.

[140] Maret W. Zinc coordination environments in proteins as redox sensors and signal transducers. Antioxid Redox Signal. 2006 Sep-Oct;8(9-10):1419-41.

[141] Black MM. Zinc deficiency and child development.Am J Clin Nutr. 1998 Aug;68(2 Suppl):464S-469S.

[142] Aggett PJ, Harries JT. Current status of zinc in health and disease states.Arch Dis Child. 1979 Dec;54(12):909-17.

[143] Mecocci P, Polidori MC, Troiano L, Cherubini A,Cecchetti R, Pini G, Straatman M, Monti D, Stahl W, Sies H, Franceschi C, Senin U (2000) Plasma antioxidants and longevity: a study on healthy centenarians.Free Radic Biol Med 28(8):1243–1248.

[144] Sensi SL, Jeng JM. Rethinking the excitotoxic ionic milieu: the emerging role of Zn(2+) in ischemic neuronal injury. Curr Mol Med. 2004 Mar;4(2):87-111.

[145] Mulder TP, van der Sluys Veer A, Verspaget HW, Griffioen G, Peña AS, Janssens AR, Lamers CB. Effect of oral zinc supplementation on metallothionein and superoxide dismutase concentrations in patients with inflammatory bowel disease.J Gastroenterol Hepatol. 1994 Sep-Oct;9(5):472-7.

[146] Toren P, Eldar S, Sela BA, Wolmer L, Weitz R, Inbar D, Koren S, Reiss A, Weizman R, Laor N. Zinc deficiency in attention-deficit hyperactivity disorder. Biol Psychiatry. 1996 Dec 15;40(12):1308-10.

[147] Bentley ME, Caulfield LE, Ram M, Santizo MC, Hurtado E, Rivera JA, Ruel MT, Brown KH. Zinc supplementation affects the activity patterns of rural Guatemalan infants. J Nutr. 1997 Jul;127(7):1333-8.

[148] Black MM, Baqui AH, Zaman K, Ake Persson L, El Arifeen S, Le K, McNary SW, Parveen M, Hamadani JD, Black RE. Iron and zinc supplementation promote motor development and exploratory behavior among Bangladeshi infants.Am J Clin Nutr. 2004 Oct;80(4):903-10.

[149] Lehto SM, Ruusunen A, Tolmunen T, Voutilainen S, Tuomainen TP, Kauhanen J. Dietary zinc intake and the risk of depression in middle-aged men: a 20-year prospective follow-up study. J Affect Disord. 2013 Sep 5;150(2):682-5.

[150] Hijova E. Metallothioneins and zinc: their functions and interactions. Bratisl Lek Listy. 2004;105(5-6):230-4.

[151] Lowe NM. In search of a reliable marker of zinc status-are we nearly there yet? Nutrition. 2005 Jul-Aug;21(7-8):883-4.

[152] Sandstead HH, Penland JG, Alcock NW, Dayal HH, Chen XC, Li JS, Zhao F, Yang JJ. Effects of repletion with zinc and other micronutrients on neuropsychologic performance and growth of Chinese children. Am J Clin Nutr. 1998 Aug;68(2 Suppl): 470S-475S.

[153] Mocchegiani E, Malavolta M, Marcellini F, Pawelec G. Zinc, oxidative stress, genetic background and immunosenescence: implications for healthy ageing. Immun Ageing. 2006 Jun 26;3:6

[154] Mariani E, Cattini L, Neri S, Malavolta M, Mocchegiani E, Ravaglia G, Facchini A. Simultaneous evaluation of circulating chemokine and cytokine profiles in elderly subjects by multiplex technology: relationship with zinc status. Biogerontology. 2006 Oct-Dec;7(5-6):449-59.

[155] Uciechowski P, Kahmann L, Plümäkers B, Malavolta M, Mocchegiani E, Dedoussis G, Herbein G, Jajte J, Fulop T, Rink L. TH1 and TH2 cell polarization increases with aging and is modulated by zinc supplementation. Exp Gerontol. 2008 May;43(5): 493-8.

[156] Connor JR, Boyer PJ, Menzies SL, Dellinger B, Allen RP, Ondo WG, Earley CJ. Neuropathological examination suggests impaired brain iron acquisition in restless legs syndrome. Neurology. 2003 Aug 12;61(3):304-9.

[157] Allen RP, Barker PB, Wehrl F, et al. MRI measurement of brain iron in patients with restless legs syndrome. Neurology 2001;56:263–5.

[158] Earley CJ, Connor JR, Beard JL, et al. Abnormalities in CSF concentrations of ferritin and transferrin in restless legs syndrome. Neurology 2000;54:1698–700.

[159] Connor JR, Ponnuru P, Wang XS, Patton SM, Allen RP, Earley CJ. Profile of altered brain iron acquisition in restless legs syndrome. Brain. 2011 Apr;134(Pt 4):959-68.

[160] Zago MP, Oteiza PI. The antioxidant properties of zinc: interactions with iron and antioxidants. Free Radic Biol Med. 2001 Jul 15;31(2):266-74.

[161] Reaume AG, Elliott JL, Hoffman EK, Kowall NW, Ferrante RJ, Siwek DF, Wilcox HM, Flood DG, Beal MF, Brown RH Jr, Scott RW, Snider WD. Motor neurons in Cu/Zn superoxide dismutase-deficient mice develop normally but exhibit enhanced cell death after axonal injury. Nat Genet. 1996 May;13(1):43-7.

[162] Cheng WH, Ho YS, Valentine BA, Ross DA, Combs GF Jr, Lei XG. Cellular glutathione peroxidase is the mediator of body selenium to protect against paraquat lethality in transgenic mice. J Nutr. 1998 Jul;128(7):1070-6.

[163] Rondanelli M, Opizzi A, Monteferrario F, Antoniello N, Manni R, Klersy C. The effect of melatonin, magnesium, and zinc on primary insomnia in long-term care facility residents in Italy: a double-blind, placebo-controlled clinical trial. J Am Geriatr Soc. 2011 Jan;59(1):82-90. doi: 10. 1111/j.1532-5415. 2010. 03232. x.

[164] Siwek M, Dudek D, Paul IA, Sowa-Kućma M, Zieba A, Popik P, Pilc A, Nowak G. Zinc supplementation augments efficacy of imipramine in treatment resistant patients: a double blind, placebo-controlled study. J Affect Disord. 2009 Nov;118(1-3): 187-95.

[165] Sowa-Kućma M, Legutko B, Szewczyk B, Novak K, Znojek P, Poleszak E, Papp M, Pilc A, Nowak G. Antidepressant-like activity of zinc: further behavioral and molecular evidence. J Neural Transm. 2008 Dec;115(12):1621-8.

[166] Laires, M.J., Monteiro, C.P. & Bicho, M. (2004) Role of Cellular Magnesium in Human Health and Disease. Frontiers in Bioscience, 9, p.262-276.

[167] Nowak G, Szewczyk B. Mechanisms contributing to antidepressant zinc actions. Pol J Pharmacol. 2002 Nov-Dec;54(6):587-92.

[168] Nowak G. Does interaction between zinc and glutamate system play a significant role in the mechanism of antidepressant action? Acta Pol Pharm. 2001 Jan-Feb;58(1): 73-5.

[169] Ounjaijean S, Westermarck T, Partinen M, Plonka-Poltorak E, Kaipainen P, Kaski M, Fucharoen S, Srichairatanakool S, Atroshi F. Increase in non-transferrin bound iron and the oxidative stress status in epilepsy patients treated using valproic acid monotherapy. Int J Clin Pharmacol Ther. 2011,49(4):268-76.

[170] Nordlander SB. Intravenous iron in treatment of restless legs. Acta Med Scand 1953; 145: 453-7.

[171] Ekbom K. Restless legs syndrome after partial gastrectomy. Acta Neurol Scand 1966; 42: 79-89.

[172] Yehuda S, Yehuda M. Long lasting effects of infancy iron deficiency--preliminary results. J Neural Transm Suppl 2006; (71): 197-200.

[173] Dosman CF, Brian JA, Drmic IE, Senthilselvan A, Harford MM, Smith RW, Sharieff W, Zlotkin SH, Moldofsky H, Roberts SW. Children with autism: effect of iron supplementation on sleep and ferritin. Pediatr Neurol 2007; 36(3): 152-8.

[174] Kuhn E, Brodan V. Changes in the circadian rhythm of serum iron induced by a 5-day sleep deprivation. Eur J Appl Physiol Occup Physiol 1982; 49(2): 215-22.

[175] Woimant F, Trocello JM. Disorders of heavy metals. Handb Clin Neurol. 2014;120:851-64.

[176] Kaler SG. Inborn errors of copper metabolism. Handb Clin Neurol. 2013;113:1745-54.

[177] Atroshi F, Westermarck T. Antioxidants and diseases: Can we find the ideal approach through nutritional pharmacology? Trace Elements in Medicine 6 (2): 37-40, 2005

[178] Harrison, J. P., D. D. Hancock and H. R. Conrad, 1984. Vitamin E and selenium for reproduction of the dairy cow. J. Dairy Sci., 67: 123–132.

[179] Rayman MP. The importance of selenium to human health. Lancet. 2000 Jul 15;356(9225):233-41

[180] Lovell MA, Xiong S, Lyubartseva G, Markesbery WR. Organoselenium (Sel-Plex diet) decreases amyloid burden and RNA and DNA oxidative damage in APP/PS1 mice. Free Radic Biol Med. 2009 Jun 1;46(11):1527-33.

[181] Perona G, Schiavon R, Guidi GC, Veneri D, Minuz P. Selenium dependent glutathione peroxidase: a physiological regulatory system for platelet function. Thromb Haemost. 1990 Oct 22;64(2):312-8.

[182] Gosney MA, Hammond MF, Shenkin A, Allsup S. Effect of Micronutrient Supplementation on Mood in Nursing Home Residents. Gerontology 2008.

[183] Tang YL, Wang SW, Lin SM. Both inorganic and organic selenium supplements can decrease brain monoamine oxidase B enzyme activity in adult rats. Br J Nutr 2008; 100(3): 660-5.

[184] Grandner MA, Kripke DF, Naidoo N, Langer RD. Relationships among dietary nutrients and subjective sleep, objective sleep, and napping in women. Sleep Med 2010; 11(2): 180-4.

[185] Bourre JM. The role of nutritional factors on the structure and function of the brain: an update on dietary requirements. Rev Neurol (Paris) 2004; 160(8-9): 767-92.

[186] Reilly C. Selenium in food and health. 2nd Edition. New York: Springer 2006. here: pp. 46ff

[187] Tinggi U. Selenium: its role as antioxidant in human health. Environ Health Prev Med. 2008 March; 13(2): 102–108.

[188] Sundström H, Korpela H, Sajanti E, Kauppila A. Supplementation with selenium, vitamin E and their combination in gynaecological cancer during cytotoxic chemotherapy. Carcinogenesis. 1989 Feb;10(2):273-8.

[189] Moslemi MK, Tavanbakhsh S. Selenium-vitamin E supplementation in infertile men: effects on semen parameters and pregnancy rate. Int J Gen Med. 2011 Jan 23;4:99-104. doi: 10. 2147/IJGM.S16275.

[190] Matsumura H, Takahata R, Hayaishi O. Inhibition of sleep in rats by inorganic selenium compounds, inhibitors of prostaglandin D synthase. Proc Natl Acad Sci U S A. 1991 Oct 15;88(20):9046-50.

[191] Ingen-Housz-Oro S, Blanchet-Bardon C, Vrillat M, Dubertret L. Vitamin and trace metal levels in recessive dystrophic epidermolysis bullosa. J Eur Acad Dermatol Venereol. 2004 Nov;18(6):649-53.

[192] Sopjani M, Föller M, Gulbins E, Lang F. Suicidal death of erythrocytes due to selenium-compounds. Cell Physiol Biochem. 2008;22(5-6):387-94.

[193] Gosney MA, Hammond MF, Shenkin A, Allsup S. Effect of micronutrient supplementation on mood in nursing home residents.Gerontology. 2008;54(5):292-9.

[194] Gümüştekín K, Seven B, Karabulut N, Aktaş O, Gürsan N, Aslan S, Keleş M, Varoglu E, Dane S. Effects of sleep deprivation, nicotine, and selenium on wound healing in rats. Int J Neurosci. 2004 Nov;114(11):1433-42.

[195] Chen PC, Guo CH, Tseng CJ, Wang KC, Liu PJ. Blood trace minerals concentrations and oxidative stress in patients with obstructive sleep apnea. J Nutr Health Aging. 2013;17(8):639-44

[196] Rahimdel AG, Ayatollahi P, Zeinali A, Mehrabanian N, Mellat-Ardekani A. The effect of selenium administration on restless leg syndrome treatment. Iran Red Crescent Med J. 2012 Jan;14(1):14-9.

[197] Brahme-Isgren M, Stenhammar L. Muscular symptoms common in selenium deficiency. Association with growth pain, restless legs and calf cramps. Lakartidningen. 2007 Jan 24-30;104(4):214.

Chapter 8

Bioelements and Bioelementology in Pharmacology and Nutrition: Fundamental and Practical Aspects

A.V. Skalny

Additional information is available at the end of the chapter

http://dx.doi.org/10.5772/57368

1. Introduction

The development of bioelementological approach can open the new perspectives in creation of integrative diagnostics of the health status and provision by "blocks of life" of the humans and provide the real personalized nutrition and therapy of diseases at etiological niveau – imbalance of bioelements.

Despite the biological role of chemical elements has come under intensive studying in the last decades, the "lack of multidisciplinary approach has been the Achilles heel of biological trace element research" [1]. The desire to integrate the "organic" and "inorganic" approach in studying the biological role of chemical elements is observed in a number of fundamental works. Since 2003 we put forward and develop the concept of bioelements and bioelementology as an integrative scientific direction [2, 3]. Bioelement is the elemental functioning unit of living matter, which is a biologically active complex of chemical elements as atoms, ions and nanoparticles with organic compounds of exogenous (primary) or biogenous (secondary) origin. Bioelements include any chemical structures found in living nature, but which do not have a set of fundamental properties of living things: metabolism, variability, reproduction and heredity. The assembly of bioelements can be called "bioelementome". We propose to subdivide bioelements into simple (atoms, ions, among them structural elements C, H, N, O, P, S, Si, Ca, electrolytic K, Na, Ca, Cl, Mg, enzymatic Mg, Fe, Zn, Cu, Mn, Co, Cr, Mo, Se, Sn, F, I, Ni, V, B, and water as the universal solvent), and complicated ones, consisting of the above-mentioned 68 molecules (8 of them are nucleosides, which compose DNA and RNA, 20 are natural amino acids necessary for protein synthesis, at least 32 glycans, 8 types of lipids). Also, bioelements can be subdivided into primary, i.e. those which could exist before the origin of life, and secondary, i.e. those which have formed as production of living organisms.

In principle, bioelements include any chemical structures found in living nature, but which do not have a set of fundamental properties of living things: metabolism, variability, reproduction and heredity. Primarily, these are organogens (C, H, N, O), P, S and representatives of four classes of small organic molecules which compose the cells: amino acids, nucleotides, sugars, fatty acids, – and coordination structures, aquated ions of vital macro and trace elements and water as well. Bioelements can continuously form from ionic compounds when they enter the cell. Inside the cell, biopolymers and their complexes create a complicated, coordinated and regulated system for transformation of substances. Cell is the main place of natural birth of secondary bioelements and their destruction. Biosphere is an assembly of bioelements and living organisms existing under permanent regulatory influence of physico-chemical factors of terrestrial and cosmic origin. The evolution of living organisms on Earth was accompanied by a broadening and deepening of the utilization of chemical elements and their compounds, i.e., in fact, by diversification, improvement and complication of bioelements. This process continues today in both natural and artificial environment, if allowing for the development of biotechnology, genetic engineering and pharmacy. The scientific discipline, which study bioelements, is proposed to be called bioelementology. This discipline could lay the foundation for the integration of bioorganic chemistry, bioinorganic chemistry, biophysics, molecular biology and other parts of life sciences.

2. Terminology and classification of bioelements and bioelementology

It is known that the chemical element exists in the organism not by itself, but in close interaction with other components. There are no any particular elements in cell, which are typical of only living nature. On the level of atom, there are no differences between chemical composition of organic and inorganic matter. The differences are found on higher, molecular level of organization.

Thus, the position and classification of the chemical elements in the Periodic System of Elements (PSE) does not permit any statement to be made about their functional essentiality or their acute or chronic toxicity for living organisms. This is due to the fact that the Periodic System is based on purely physicochemical aspects [4]. Therefore B.Markert developed an idea about a Biological System of Elements (BSE), which primarily considers aspects of basic biochemical and physiological research. As the author said, "Biological processes on the molecular level are frequently based on physical and chemical conditions… However, these physical and chemical regularities are frequently modified in biological systems". The BSE of B.Markert is obtained from data on correlation analysis, physiological function of individual elements in the living organism, evolutional development out of the inorganic environment and with respect to their uptake by the living organism as a neutral molecule or charged ion.

Atoms, atomic nuclei, elementary particles and fields that bind them, which have independent significance at the physicochemical stage of evolution, after being included in biological molecules lose this self-importance and play their role in the ensemble, called by me bioelement, where everything is interdependent, more complicated and at the same time more

http://dx.doi.org/10.5772/57368

vulnerable to external influence. Since the general conditions of biological evolution (the composition of biosphere), are continuously changing, a set of bioelements in a living organism can also change. This distinguishes them from chemical elements as objects of physicochemical stage, which remain identical to themselves along the course of evolution. So, bioelement is the elemental functioning unit of living matter, which is a biologically active complex of chemical elements as atoms, ions and nanoparticles with organic compounds of exogenous (primary) or biogenous (secondary) origin [3].

In principle, bioelements include any chemical structures found in living nature, but which do not have a set of fundamental properties of living things: metabolism, variability, reproduction and heredity. Primarily, these are organogens (C, H, N, O), P, S and representatives of four classes of small organic molecules which compose the cells: amino acids, nucleotides, sugars, fatty acids, – and coordination structures, aquated ions of vital macro and trace elements and water as well.

Bioelement is not a chemical element inside a molecular compound, but it is temporarily formed biocomplex, where the chemical element is bound by covalent (chelate) bond to the organic molecule. They should not be considered separately, because, interacting, together they produce biological effect of new quality [5].

If chemical element is a physicochemical unit of the matter's evolution, then bioelement – is a precursor of a biological unit, which has physicochemical nature. Fundamental differences between chemical elements and their compounds in abiogenic media and bioelements are described in Table 1.

Bioelements can continuously form from ionic compounds when they enter the cell. Inside the cell, biopolymers and their complexes create a complicated, coordinated and regulated system for transformation of substances. Cell is the main place of natural birth of secondary bioelements and their destruction.

According to modern views, the life processes cannot occur outside the cell. Therefore, the cell is considered as the smallest quantum of life, which, for managing its internal parameters and performing cell-cell interactions, use information, energy and substances, including bioelements, obtaining them from the environment. Bioelement is yet a substance. Cell (organism) is already a being. In our opinion (Figure 1), bioelements are precursors of living matter, a successful combination of which, particularly of polymer-ion reactions running autocatalytically, led to the formation of cells.

We proposed to call the assembly of bioelements "bioelementome" unlike elementome as an assembly of chemical elements and their compounds. Bioelementome is a particular continuum of molecules for the maintenance of biological units of evolution, possessing the ability to control the process, and biological objects [3].

However, when considering the biological role of bioelements, we should clearly distinguish two questions. The first is a question of initial formation and participation of bioelements in the origin of life. The second is a question concerning the role of bioelements in the modern

Chemical element	Bioelement
There in the biosphere and beyond. Weight is virtually unlimited.	There is mainly in biosphere. Outside biosphere, existence is temporary or impossible. Weight limited.
No quantitative limits.	The quantitative limit exists (depends on the space of the biosphere), as space available for organisms is limited.
	Limit of bioelements in the "mass of life" is constant in the course of geological time.
Exists in 2000-3000 species of minerals and corresponding chemical compounds.	Exists in millions of biological compounds.
Involved in formation of biologically inert natural objects by physico-chemical and geological processes, regardless of the previously existed natural objects.	Like a living organism is born only from another living organism, the new bioelement appears in biochemical transformations of the previous compounds (living objects, containing bioelements). In the course of geological time, some qualitative changes in forms of bioelements happen, which lead to the evolution of species or loss of some of them.
Its formation may occur in living bodies, varying in its manifestations and giving inert natural bodies elements incorporated in living natural body (e.g., concretions in kidneys).	Bioelements are formed not only during natural biochemical transformations of other living bodies, containing bioelements, but also can be created as a result of human activities (industrial synthesis of bioelements, biotech processes) from abiotic substances or other bioelements (from simple to complicated).
The process of turning abioelements in inorganic matter, as the processes that created the inert natural object, is reversible in time.	Formation of bioelement (i.e., form of existence of a chemical element in the biosphere), as well as the creation of a natural living body, is process irreversible in time.
Number of elements as components of inert natural objects, does not depend on size of the planet, but is determined by the properties of planetary matter – by energy.	Number of bioelements and number of living natural bodies are limited by the size of the biosphere (Earth).

Table 1. The fundamental main characteristics of chemical elements and bioelements (modified from ideas of V.I.Vernadsky [5] about abiotic and botic matter) [3]

biosphere, at the anthropogenic stage of its development. I.e., one should separate the role of bioelements during early formation of the biosphere, and the modern role of bioelements.

On our opinion, as a result of chemical evolution on the Earth there appeared the "pre-biological organic world" [7], a variety of living systems, which consists of the same set of molecules (bioelements), work by the same laws, have the metabolism based on the same principles, and the system of homeostasis that can control the flows of food, energy and information.

http://dx.doi.org/10.5772/57368

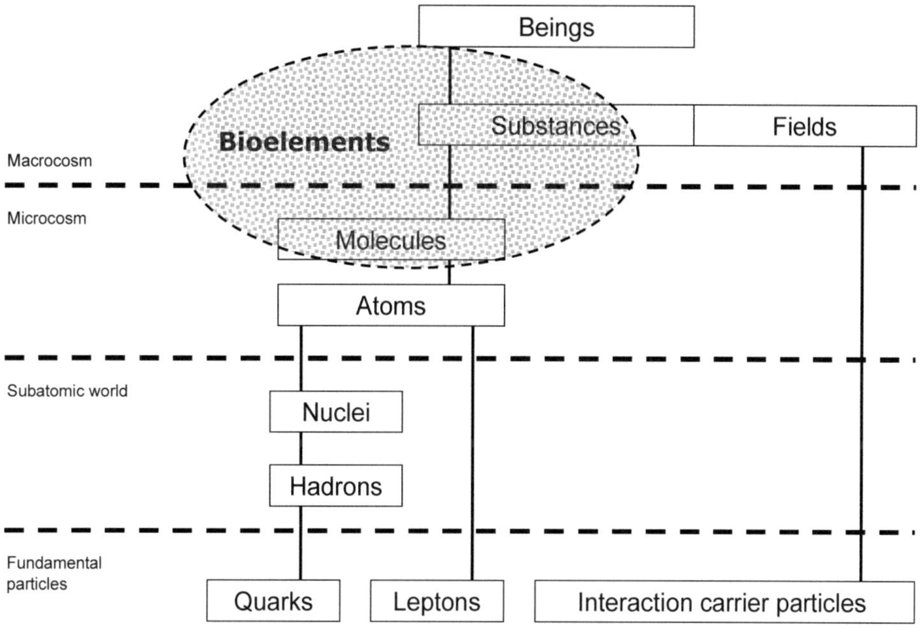

Figure 1. Structural levels of the matter (by Yu.N.Orlov [6], expanded by A.V.Skalny)

The biological evolution has led to a sharp increase in mass and diversity of the living substance on the planet, including formation of new chemical compounds and molecules, the novel (secondary) bioelements (in cells) [3].

So called "simple bioelements" produced four fundamental components of cellular life, which, according to J.D.Marth [8], divided into 68 molecular building blocks ("building blocks of life"). I.e., the simplest bioelements formed more complicated, macromolecular bioelements.

We proposed to subdivide bioelements into simple (atoms, ions and water as the universal solvent), and complicated ones, consisting of the above-mentioned 68 molecules (8 of them are nucleosides, which compose DNA and RNA, 20 are natural amino acids necessary for protein synthesis, at least 32 glycans, 8 types of lipids, see Table 2) [8].

Thus, bioelements can be subdivided into primary, i.e. those which could exist before the origin of life, and secondary, i.e. those which have formed as production of living organisms. This division is necessary for us to better understand the nature and role of bioelements. For example, the fact that life is a self-sustaining process that can produce "raw material" for new living structures. This agrees with the theory of natural self-organization of pre-biological processes by M.Eigen [9] and ideas of I.Prigogine [10] about self-organization in open systems.

In recent years, along with the evolution of our knowledge and understanding of bioelements, the definitions of bioelementology evolved [2, 11-12]. Currently, we guess the most appropriate definition of bioelementology is the following:

Primary	Simple	C, H, N, O, P, S, Si, Ca (structural)
		K, Na, Ca, Cl, Mg (electrolytic)
		Mg, Fe, Zn, Cu, Mn, Co, Cr, Mo, Se*, Sn*, F*, I*, Ni*, V*, B** (enzymatic)
		H_2O, O_2, N_2 etc.
	Complicated	Nucleic acids (deoxyadenosine, deoxycytidine, deoxyguanosine, deoxythymidine, adenosine, cytidine, guanosine, uridine)
		Glycans (Fucose, galactose, glucose, glucuronic acid, mannose, N-acetylgalactosamine, N-acetylglucosamine, neuraminic acid, xylose, nononic acid, octulosonic acid, arabinose, arabinofuranose, colitose, fructose, galactofuranose, galacturonic acid, glucolactilic acid, heptose, legionaminic acid, mannuronic acid, N-acetylfucosamine, N-acetylgalacturonic acid, N-acetylmannosamine, N-acetylmannosaminuronic acid, N-acetylmuramic acid, N-acetylperosamine, N-acetylquinovosamine, perosamine, pseudaminic acid, rhamnose, talose)
		Proteins (Alanine, arginine, aspartic acid, asparagine, cysteine, glutamic acid, glutamine, glycine, histidine, isoleucine, leucine, lysine, methionine, phenylalanine, proline, serine, threonine, tryptophan, tyrosine, valine)
		Lipids (Fatty acyls, glycerolipids, glycerophospholipids, polyketides, prenol lipids, saccharolipids, sphingolipids, sterol lipids)
Secondary	Complicated (components of bioelemental systems, "omes")	Metabolome (components)
		Metallome
		Lipidome
		Proteome
		Genome
		Transcriptome
		(...?)

Table 2. Classification of bioelements

Bioelementology is a science, which can unite all the "omics", probably including genomics. Authors of the term "genomics", V.A.McKusick and F.H.Riddle, in the editorial article to the first issue of the journal "Genomics" have explained introduction of the new term as follows: "...logies" are very academic, while "...omics" are more aggressive and democratic [13] in style of live matter studying.

Thus, bioelementology is a part of biology (and of the "life science" in terms of V.I.Vernadsky), a science about biological role of substances, important for building and existence of the living matter [3].

http://dx.doi.org/10.5772/57368

Bioelementology is a direction of fundamental science studying the transition state of the matter (evolution from biologically inert to living), formation and change of bioelements, which are vital or conditionally essential for the living matter, under influence of various physical interactions and matrix effect of water.

Bioelementology as an integrative science, based on the ideas of V.I.Vernadsky, will bring us closer to understanding the origin of life. Unlike the currently prevailing molecular approach, which unfortunately does not solve the problem of the life origin despite the involvement in consideration of new biochemical factors – nucleic acids, matrix mechanisms of continuity and biochemical memory [14], – bioelementology, in our view, will help to consider the conditions of life more holistically as the presence of bioelements is already the most important condition for its maintenance. The planetary environment, which surrounds the living substance, and the extraplanetary space environment which influence it, together provide the necessary material and energy flows for the proper functioning and continual renewal of the structure of living matter.

The ideas of autotrophy of the mankind and noosphere, suggested by V.I.Vernadsky in 1923 [5], have fostered the epoch of nanobiology, the living matter of Universe. We believe that bioelementology can help to solve the main problem of the mankind – achievement of the autotrophy – through solving the problem of essence of the living matter of Earth and identification of this essence with wider principle of life existence in Universe [15].

The bioelementology combines the systemic and integrative approaches in life science and is a possible precursor to systemic biology.

3. Practical aspects

The materials above illustrates that the evolution of living organisms on Earth was accompanied by a broadening and deepening of the utilization of chemical elements and their compounds, i.e., in fact, by diversification, improvement and complication of bioelements. This process continues today in both natural and artificial environment, if allowing for the development of biotechnology, genetic engineering and pharmacy.

Diversification of bioelements is a natural tool of the evolution aimed at adaptation of living organisms to the changing conditions of their existence. The emergence of new bioelements accompanies the process of evolution from simple prokaryotic cells (universal) to specialized cells within multicellular organisms with longer duration of individual life at a deceleration of reproduction rate. Changing the composition of the extracellular environment, such as the concentration of key ions or gases, it is possible to cause a cascade of formation of new bioelements. More diverse set of bioelements is observed in organisms with relatively low reproduction rates, but with a longer individual life.

It must be remembered that a set of bioelements is a necessary but not sufficient condition for the formation of life. In many cases in medicine, in our opinion, it is possible to use bioelements for maintaining organs and tissues instead of using cell cultures and tissues, because it is not always necessary or possible (including for financial reasons) to recover the function by a substance, organ or tissue, completely identical to the living one (e.g., in transplantology, orthopedics, in treatment of osteoporosis, diseases of skin, hair, etc.).

The development of bioelementology may lead to appearance of modified cells or technologies for creation of new cells which can be used for medical purposes. Without going into details, we only note that this tale may sooner become a reality with the correct formulation of tasks, based on the correct understanding of the hierarchy of "pre-living" processes and of the life itself, on the formation of new methodological approaches on its basis, on the proper division of essential substances in necessary and sufficient, primary and secondary, with a better understanding of the boundary between "pre-living" and "living", between the set of bioelements and life.

It is reasonable that the deficiency of only one primary bioelement can due to the extinction of living organism in Earth. According to US Department of Energy (2010), in not far future chemical (elemental) diversity may be sacrified (Table 3). The lack of rare earths can stop the "Clean green future", but deficiency f only one trace element (cobalt) can have the dramatic effect on a lot of species, for which this element and the vitabin B12 are essential.

Level	Elements
Critical	Y, Nd, Eu, Tb, Dy, In
Near-critical	La, Ce, Te
Non-critical (but not far future)	Co, Li, Ga

Table 3. Risk of supply disruption by 2015 (US Department of Energy, 2010)

This is why the mankind needs to plan and realize the emergent actions. Below we present our point of view on the strategy of survival.

Strategy of survival:

1. Reducing of resources consumption (?)
2. Free redistribution of resources between countries (nations) (?)
3. Restoring of resources:
   a. Conservation of nature (±)
   b. Biotechnological (microbial etc.) production of resources (+)
4. Artificial life technology developing (protocells etc.) (±)

Of course, today the mankind is not ready to reduce its resource consumptions, which leads to decreasing of number of bioelements. Also, on a pity, the nations are not ready to agree with free redistribution of resources between them. The conservation of nature has also a lot of limitations because of decreasing of forests and desertization intensive use of more and more soils and water for agriculture etc. Only the biotechnological (or pharmaceutical) production of secondary bioelements which are more effective, better available and safe is a fruitful direction toward provision of humans and animals by "blocks of life". The developing of so-called artificial life technologies is a controversial way for accumulation of bioelements, because such experiments can produce undesirable effects from unknown protocells and other modified organisms.

An example of technology for enlargement of food density for future use is enrichment of algae (Spirulina, Nostoc) [16]. We have managed to obtain the greatest possible accumulation of some essential trace elements by cell cultures of S. platensis and S. maxima. This could considerably increase the value and applicability of spirulina biomass in human health care nutrition. The work has begun from registering a patent [17] for a method of obtaining selenium-containing preparation of spirulina biomass enriched with selenium in organic form with pronounced antioxidant properties. The content of selenium in the cells was determined by atomic-adsorption and fluorometric methods, the total elemental composition of the cell – by developed complex of ICP-AES methods [18].

The possibility to obtain spirulina biomass enriched with selenium in organic form, which has increased bioavailability, has promptly caused the appearance of works extending this direction. In some works a spirulina preparation enriched with bioavailable selenium in combination with reduced glutathione was administered to rats, allowing normalization of intestinal permeability, impaired after systemic anaphylaxis. In other studies it was shown that effective regulation of homeostasis was possible by addition of selenium-rich spirulina to rats' feed. Also there were reports about successful use of selenium-enriched spirulina and yeast as a dietary supplement for patients with non-specific ulcerative colitis and for patients with coronary heart disease [19-20].

The material demonstrates that electromagnetic radiation of millimeter range (EHF) at low non-thermal intensity, which can be characterized as extremely weak and possibly even superweak physical influence, can affect various aspects of metabolism of phototrophic cyanobacteria and microalgae, stimulate growth and yield of biomass of the cultures etc. It can also influence the accumulation of some essential trace elements in cells of cyanobacteria. It is shown that EHF radiation can reduce the toxicity of trace elements introduced into the medium. And, for the first time, it is established that the entering of elevated concentrations of certain trace elements into cultural medium causes shifts in general mineral profile of the cyanobacterial cells.

4. Novel paradigm of the nutrition and pharmacology

As it is ahown in Figure 2, for the effective prevention and treatment of human disease it is essential to control and correct the initial imbalances of bioelements, caused by suboptimal nutrition, ecological influence, stress etc. We can do this for relatively healthy people that to prevent their disease. If we missed the possibility of the correction of human health by bioelements in stages I-II, we need to start the treatment but also with the restoration of basic defects of metabolism (stable deficiency of bioelements).

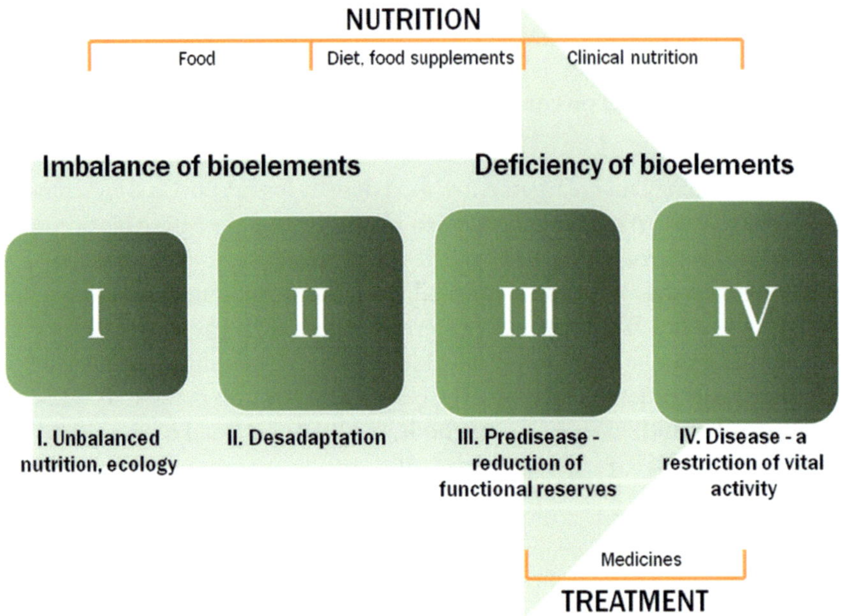

Figure 2. Levels of bioelement imbalances and their correction

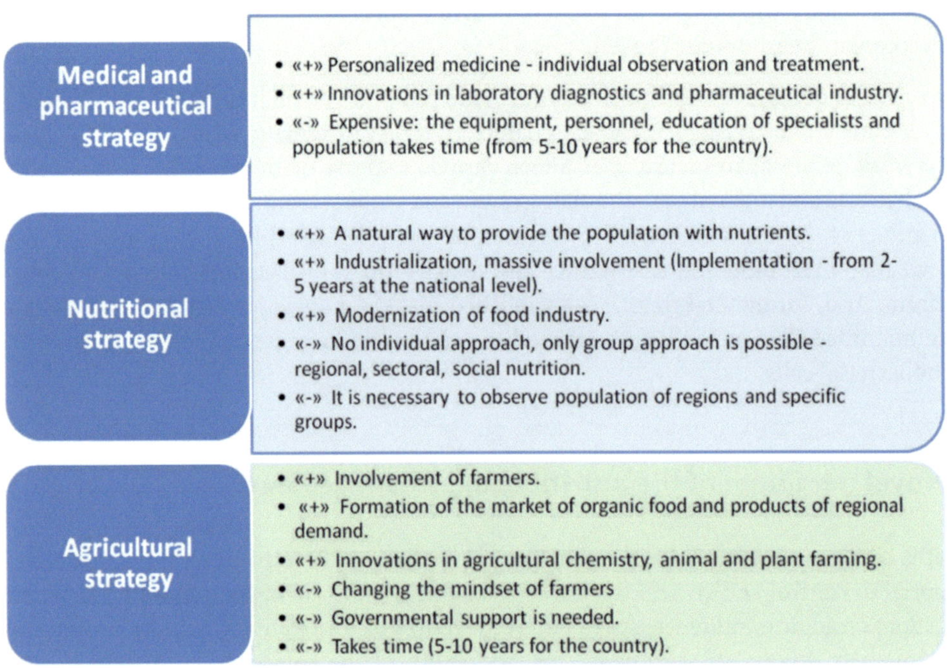

Figure 3. Approaches to solving the problem of bioelements provision for human health

So, there are few directions to serve and develop the "life set" of bioelements. As demonstrated in Figure 3, the mankind can use medical and pharmacological therapy for detection of individual and populational provision by bioelements (primary and secondary). This is the most expensive way, but realistic for rich countries, which needs to develop the technological diagnostics ("omics"), personalized healthy nutrition and treatment.

The second direction is more natural – improvement of nutrition on the basis of fortified foods, "high food density" products. It is appreciable for almost all countries and layers of population, if the governments and international organizations (FAO, IMF, UNIDO etc.) will support the development of food industry and support authorities to manage the social nutrition, for example. The last strategy is most natural, but needs a lot of efforts in agricultural sector of industry and science. More detailed description of the strategies is presented below.

1. Medical and pharmaceutical strategy

   - Development of personalized medicine and medical geography, epidemiology and ecology
   - Improving methods of laboratory and clinical diagnostics of micronutrient deficiencies and intoxications
   - Creation (reconstruction and development) of resource base for food and pharmaceutical industry
   - Creation and production of adapted means for nutraceutical and pharmaceutical correction of deficiency/surplus of micronutrients (based on physiological, regional and professional needs)
   - Creation and production of new drugs for treatment of genetic and other rare diseases related to metabolic disorders of micronutrient exchange

2. Nutritional strategy

   - Fortification (enrichment) of food with micronutrients at the production stage - focused and strictly bound to the elemental status of the population (massive involvement)
   - Choice among existing products the required (enriched) ones to complete rations
   - Exchange of products between the regions
   - Dietary supplements - an individual approach - 10% of the population, in developed countries - up to 80%
   - Functional food
   - Forming assortment of food products - information policy
   - Creation of functional beverages, artificial water mineralization
   - Exchange of products between regions according to regional needs in micronutrient
   - Improving the quality of tap water

- Social nutrition (water consumption) on the basis of physiological and professional groups of the population

Food fortification as a long-term regional program "Development of a regional system for detection and prevention of natural and technogenic deficiencies and surpluses of macro and trace elements in the population"

Project

- Formation of scientific and methodological basis for monitoring of elemental status of the population and correction of deviations

Regional program for monitoring elemental status of the population

- Determination of deficiencies and surpluses of macro and trace elements
- Development of recommendations for correction of deviations

Formation of regional regulations based on governmental policy in the field of healthy nutrition

- Increasing the proportion of production for mass consumption, rich in vitamins and minerals, including mass varieties of bakery products, and dairy products - up to 40% of total production

Consolidated ordering of fortification ingredients for the regional food producers

- Formation of joint supply of fortification ingredients for the regional producers of products for social and mass feeding in accordance with results of the monitoring

Sectoral nutrition

- Scientific and methodological support of diets for different groups of people in the region: pupils, students, workers etc.
- Regional standards for food products
- System of targeted subsidies for fortification (enrichment of food with micronutrients)

3. Agricultural strategy
    - Agrochemical service: targeted introduction of *micro*fertilizers
    - Variety zonation
    - Breeding
    - Specialized mixed feeds, premixes for animals, mineralized water
    - Development of industry: fertilizers, animal feed, etc.

Before the realization of the presented strategies it is needed to estimate the balance of bioelements in population or individuals. Below we present an example of evaluation of bioelement (macro and trace elements) status of population.

http://dx.doi.org/10.5772/57368

1. Screening of the region

   - Screening (assessment of the current state)

     - Organizational period (1-3 months)
     - Collection of biological material (2 months)
     - Investigations (3-6 months)
     - Data processing, development of recommendations (1-2 months): factor analysis, identification of basic dependencies
     - Preliminary report (1-2 months): organizational policy

In the result of the screening we get the identification of factors and control parameters, forming mineral profile of the region. Further step is analysis of obtained data and creation of database for public health, agriculture, social services of a region.

2. Creation of database on directions:

   - Updatable database on physical media
   - Medical information
   - Epidemiological information
   - Database of technologies, measures, activities, management decisions
   - Regional standards of the consumer basket (nutrients)

The efforts of correction of bioelement status can be insufficient if medical doctors, social workers in population do not understand the aims of such studies and do not participate actively in the prophylactic activity. So, we need organize an information campaign in the region with a support of local medical, public health and social organizations and authorities.

3. Information policy in the field of healthy living

   - Educational lectures
   - Declaration of human responsibility
   - Creation of an independent "guild" of doctors
   - Lack of proper information policy - exit to informational diseases
   - Training program for students on nutriciology
   - Organization of club structure (stimulation of involvement)

Feedback

- Control of elemental status of the population - influence on medical and demographic indices
- Quality of life: formation of focus groups for continuous monitoring of the life quality

- Analysis of statistical data (demography, health, employment, etc.)
- Monitoring (repeated screening every 3-5 years) of a representative sample of the population.
- Update of data banks and databases with identification of trends and forecasting
- One-time studies connected to emergencies, disease outbreaks of unknown etiology, etc. Determination of non-obvious causes of emergencies.

5. Conclusion

So, the evolution of living organisms on Earth was accompanied by a broadening and deepening of the utilization of chemical elements and their compounds, i.e., in fact, by diversification, improvement and complication of bioelements. This process continues today in both natural and artificial environment, if allowing for the development of biotechnology, genetic engineering and pharmacy.

In many cases in medicine, it is possible to use bioelements for maintaining organs and tissues instead of using cell cultures and tissues, because it is not always necessary or possible (including for financial reasons) to recover the function by a substance, organ or tissue, completely identical to the living one (e.g., in transplantology, orthopedics, in treatment of osteoporosis, diseases of skin, hair, etc.).

The development of bioelementology may lead to appearance of modified cells or technologies for creation of new cells which can be used for medical purposes.

On our opinion, the progress in trace element research will be due to interdisciplinary approach such as bioelementology. It needs change in educational programs for high school students of biological, chemical and physical specialties, creation of special programs for biotechnologists, medical researchers, ecologists and pharmacists. And this will demand united efforts of scientists and specialists from adjacent fields. Integration of scientific researches without division into separate parts, studied by only one of the "omics", though this will demand deeper and more global planning of scientific investigations on the basis of the multidisciplinary concept. Also, it is necessary to change the paradigm of diseases' prevention and treatment from mainly symptomatic to basics to prevent and normalize the balance of bioelements by nutrition and use of sources of bioelements in pharmacotherapy.

Author details

A.V. Skalny[1]

1 Russian Society of Trace Elements in Medicine, Russia

Trace Element – Institute for UNESCO, France

References

[1] Iyengar V. Elemental analysis of biological systems. Vol.1. Boca Raton: CRC Press; 1989.

[2] Skalny AV, Rudakov IA. Bioelementology – a new term or a new research direction? Vestnik OSU 2005; 2 4-8 [in Russian].

[3] Skalny AV. Bioelementology as an interdisciplinary integrative approach in life science: terminology, classification, perspectives. J Trace Elem Med Biol. 2011; 25S S3-S10.

[4] Markert B. Instrumental element and multi-element analysis of plant samples – methods and applications. 2nd ed. Wiley, New York; 1996.

[5] Vernadsky VI. Russian cosmism: anthology of philosophical thought. Moscow: Rolf; 2002 [in Russian].

[6] Orlov YuN. Study of the rhythmics of life. Moscow: AMNT; 2009 [in Russian].

[7] Galimov EM. Phenomenon of life: between equilibrium and non-linearity. Origin and principles of evolution. Moscow: Librokom; 2009 [in Russian].

[8] Marth JD. A unified vision of the building blocks of life. Nat Cell Biol. 2008; 10(9) 1015-6.

[9] Eigen M. Selforganization of matter and the evolution of biological macromolecules. Naturwissenschaften 1971; 58(10) 465-523.

[10] Prigogine I. From Being To Becoming. New York: W.H.Freeman & Co Ltd; 1980.

[11] Skalny AV, Rudakov IA. Bioelements in medicine. Moscow: Onix 21 vek: Mir; 2004 [in Russian]

[12] Skalny AV. Development of the concept of bioelements and the prospects of bioelementology. Trace Elements in Medicine (Moscow) 2009; 10(3-4) 1-6 [in Russian].

[13] McKusick VA, Riddle FH. A new discipline, a new name, a new journal. Genomics 1987; 1(1) 1-2.

[14] Kaznacheev VP, Spirin EA. Cosmoplanetary phenomenon of the human: problems of a comprehensive study. Novosibirsk: Nauka; 1991 [in Russian]

[15] Kaznacheev VP, Akulov AI, Kiselnikov AA. Survival of the population of Russia: problems of "Sphinx of the XXI century". 2nd Ed. Novosibirsk: Novosibirsk University Press; 2002 [in Russian].

[16] Tambiev A, Skalny A. Electromagnetic radiation and life: bioelementological point of view. Biophysics / ed.by A.N.Misra. Rijeka: InTech; 2012.

[17] Tambiev AKh, Kirikova NN, Mazo VK, Skalny AV. A method of obtaining selenium-containing preparation of spirulina biomass: Patent RF 2096037 from 17.04.1996. 1997.

[18] Sedykh EM, Lyabusheva OA, Tambiev AKh, Bannykh LN. Determination of the elemental composition of cyanobacteria cells and individual cell fractions by atomic emission and atomic absorption spectrometry. Journal of Analytical Chemistry 2005; 60(1) 35-40 [in Russian].

[19] Mazo VK, Gmoshinski IV, Parfenov AI, Ekisenina NI, Safonova SA, Shahovskaya AK, Popova YuP, Nizov AA(jr). Selenium status in some groups of patients suffering from gastrointestinal diseases. Trace Elements in Medicine (Moscow) 2001; 2(1) 28-31 [in Russian].

[20] Notova SV, Baranova OV, Barysheva ES, Nigmatullina JF, Frolova OO, Gubajdullina SG. Modern conditions and ways of correcting the nutritional status in various age and industrial groups in the population of Orenburg region. Proc Int Kongress Hannover 2006.

Chapter 9

Impact of CoQ_{10}, L-Carnitine and Cocktail Antioxidants on Oxidative Stress Markers in HIV Patients — Mini Review and Clinical Trial

M Sauka, G Selga, A Skesters, A Silova,
T Westermarck, A Latvus and F Atroshi

Additional information is available at the end of the chapter

http://dx.doi.org/10.5772/58415

1. Introduction

Nutritional deficiencies have long been recognized as an important problem among HIV-1-seropositive individuals. They have a great demand for nutrients because of the stress placed on their immune systems. Moreover, poor nutrition may also affect drug effectiveness or increased toxicity [34-37]. It has been shown that micronutrient deficiencies are associated with more rapid HIV-disease progression and higher HIV-1 related mortality [38-40]. Supplementation of micronutrient has delayed time to AIDS and improved survival, suggesting that supplementation could offer a simple and relatively inexpensive strategy to slow HIV-1 progression [41, 42].

HIV infected patients present changes in components of the antioxidant defense system, which may be the result of excessive production of oxygen-derived species during the development of the disease (Pace and Leaf, 1995) and that cells infected with HIV can enhance production of $O_2^{\bullet-}$ [43]. This phenomenon combined with a deficiency in key antioxidant enzymes superoxide dismutase and catalase, and a decreased concentrations of the antioxidant vitamins [44] may lead to severe oxidative stress in HIV-infected patients. Humans infected with human immunodeficiency virus (HIV) have been shown to be under chronic oxidative stress [44-46], which is the result of imbalance between free radical (or pro-oxidant) production and antioxidant action. In HIV infection, oxidative stress may be caused by both overproduction of reactive oxygen species (ROS) and a simultaneous deficiency of antioxidant defenses [47, 48]. Oxidative stress induced by ROS play a critical role in the stimulation of HIV replication and the development of immunodeficiency [49, 50].

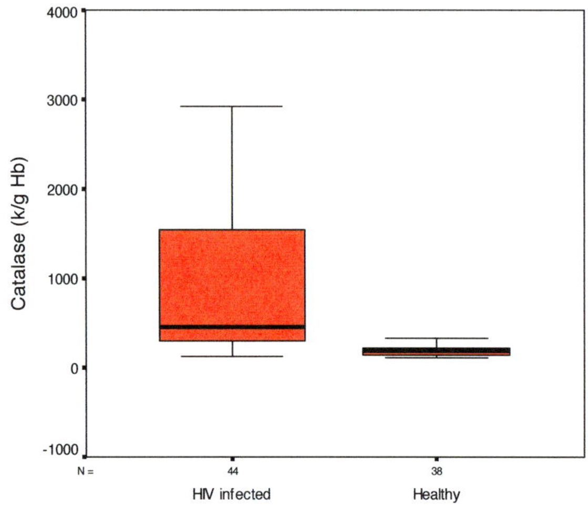

Figure 1. Catalase level of HIV infected individuals and healthy subjects (k/g Hb)Catalase level of

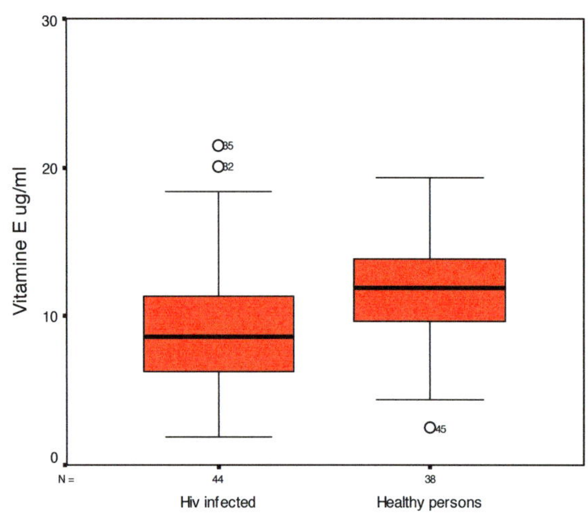

Figure 2. Vitamin E level of HIV infected individuals and healthy subjects (μg /ml)

Many studies have focused on the role of nutritional supplements to attenuate signs and symptoms of HIV. Of these, some have reported favorable results, while many others have reported no benefit of the selected nutrient. Despite these mixed findings, recommendations for the use of nutritional supplements for the purposes of attenuating HIV are rampant. Based on this background, we have assessed the antioxidant status among HIV-infected patients on oxidative stress after antioxidant supplementation.

http://dx.doi.org/10.5772/58415

2. Subjects and methods

2.1. Subjects

Open clinical trial study was implemented to access antioxidant status among HIV-infected male volunteers in Latvia. Twenty six HIV-positive males (age 35.3 ± 2.5) whose serostatus are known were studied. They were recruited among two non-governmental HIV infected patients' support organizations by "snow-ball" methodology using gatekeepers as contact persons. All participants in the research study were volunteers and their agreement to participate was get through their gatekeepers. The HIV-infected subjects represented a broad range of disease progression. None of the screened subjects had (CD4) T cell counts less than $200x10^9/L$.

Exclusion criteria for the study groups were as follows: they were over 18 years old, have not used antioxidants as food supplement two months before the study, had no active opportunistic infections or malignancies, had readily mobile, and were no drug users. Any information of partner identifications was not used in the written information

For the control group 10 uninfected males were selected among uninfected friends and relatives of HIV-infected individuals. Control subjects had no acute or chronic illness and were not taking any medications or nutritional supplements.

HIV-infected individuals used food supplements– antioxidant cocktail for 6 month, including 250 mg L-carnitine (Bio-Carnitine$^{TM)}$, 800 μg vitamin A, 15 mg vitamin E, 90 mg vitamin C, 2 mg vitamin B_6, 15 mg Zn, 100 mg CoQ_{10} and 75 μg selenium (organic) (Bio-Selenium^{TM+}Zn) a day. All subjects underwent an initial screening and after 6 months that included an anthropometric (weight and height) and biochemical (complete blood count, bilirubin, albumin, from liver panel-alanine aminotranferase (ALT) and alkaline aminotranferase (), from lipid profile total holesterol and triglicerides. All patients were evaluated with regard to the blood antioxidant system, specifically superoxide dismutase (SOD), catalase (CAT) selenium-dependent glutathione peroxidase (GSH-Px, trace element selenium, and α-tocopherol).

Participants will be involved in the study only after obtaining informed consent. The study protocol was approved by the ethics committee of the Latvian Institute of Cardiology for Clinical and Physiological Research, Drug and Pharmaceutics Product Clinical Investigation.

2.2. Laboratory analysis

After overnight fasting, venous blood samples were collected from all study subjects. Biochemical determinations were done at the hospital laboratory. CD4+and CD8+cell count was estimated by FACSscan flowcytometry (BD Becton Dickimon). Alanine aminotranferase (ALT) and alkaline aminotranferase were estimated by kinetic reaction (Hitachi 917, Roche Diagnostics), bilirubin, albumin and total protein by two point colour reaction (Hitachi 917, Roche Diagnostics). From lipid profile total holesterol and triglycerides were estimated by using fermentative colour reaction (Hitachi 917, Roche Diagnostics). Blood antioxidant system was evaluated at Riga Stradinš University laboratory. Selenium and α-Tocophrol concentrations in plasma were measured using fluorometric method. Other measurements were also included such as catalase and GSHPX.

2.3. Statistical analyses

Using the SPSS 14.0 for Windows software standard version, statistical analyses were performed. All group data are expressed as means ± SEMs. The HIV-positive group was compared with the seronegative control subjects by using one way ANOVA. The minimal level of significance was identified at $P < 0.05$. All patients were evaluated with regard to the blood antioxidant system, specifically superoxide dismutase (SOD) and glutathione peroxidase.

3. Results

Subject characteristics, including CD4+cell count, CD8+cell count, and CD4/CD8 ratio, weight, body mass index (BMI, in kg/m^2), are shown in Table 1. At initial screening HIV-infected subjects were significantly lower weight and BMI compared to healthy subjects. There were insignificant changes between initial screening and after 6 months. The range of CD4+cell counts was broad, from 282 to 1830 x 10^6 cells/L at the initial screening and from 323 to 1687 after 6 months CD4/CD6 ratio was from 0.1 to 1.7 at the initial screening and from 0.1 to 3.4 after 6 months of using food supplements, CD8+cell counts was from 272 to 4525 at the initial screening and from 222 to 4851 after 6 months.

			Baseline		After 6 months
		n	Mean±SE	n	Mean±SE
Weight	HIV-infected	26	73.1±2.1	13	74.7±2.8
	healthy uninfected	10	82.4±2.6	9	83.3±2.7
			p<0.05		p<0.05
BMI	HIV-infected	26	22.5±0.6	13	23.0±0.8
	Healthy	10	24.7±0.7	9	25.1±0.7
			p<0.05		NS
CD4+	HIV-infected	25	698.4±74.3	21	743.6±87.4
CD8+	HIV-infected	25	1641.9±188.1	21	1341.0±216.1
CD4+/CD8	HIV-infected	25	0.6±0.1	21	0.9±0.2

Table 1. Effect of antioxidant supplementation on body weight, body mass index and immune function in HIV patients.

Antioxidant status is shown in Table 2. At the baseline HIV-positive patients had significantly lower GSHPX and CAT concentrations compare to healthy subjects (p<0.05), but did not differ after 6 months using food supplements. There were insignificant differences in SOD and MDA

http://dx.doi.org/10.5772/58415

measurements and α-Tocopherol concentration at the initial screening, but differed significantly after 6 months compare to HIV-infected and healthy individuals. Changes of biochemical measurements (alanine aminotranferase, alkaline aminotranferase, bilirubin, albumin and total protein, total holesterol and triglicerides) were not significant between groups of HIV-infected and healthy individuals as well as at the initial screening and after 6 months after use of food supplements. Additionally, two HIV-infected individuals from 26 involved in the study reported that after the use of antioxidant cocktail, gingival bleeding was stopped. One reported this symptom for two years before the study and one reports half a year this problem before study.

Measuremetns	**groups**	**Baseline**		**After 6 months**		
		n	Mean±SE	n	Mean±SE	p
GSHPX	infected	25	46.5±1.1	19	45.6±1.3	NS
	healthy	10	50.9±1.6	9	49.5±0.7	NS
	p		0.036		NS	
CAT	infected	26	1023.5±164.1	19	350.3±22.3	0.01
	healthy	10	317.4±34.6	9	377.7±13.1	NS
			0.013		NS	
SOD	infected	25	1074±68.3	19	1419.3±56.6	0.001
	healthy	10	1293.7±36.6	9	1172.8±30.4	0.023
			NS		0.008	
TAS	infected	24	1.0±0.0	17	1.5±0.0	0.001
	healthy	10	1.4±0.0	9	1.4±0.0	NS
			NS		NS	
VITE	infected	26	10.8±0.8	19	13.2±1.2	NS
	healthy	10	9.2±1.0	9	7.4±0.1	NS
			NS		0.003	
SE	infected	25	47.4	21	64.0±3.7	0.000
	healthy	10	51±3.0	9	53.9±3.1	NS
			NS		NS	
MDA	infected	24	3.5±0.1	17	5.1±0.3	0.000
	healthy	10	3.4±0.2	9	3.4±0.2	NS
			NS		0.000	

Table 2. Effect of antioxidants supplementation on antioxidant enzymes, selenium, vitamin E and lipid peroxidation in HIV patients.

4. Discussion

There has been increasing interest in the application of antioxidants to many diseases as information is constantly gathered linking the development of HIV to oxidative stress [51]. Antioxidants are believed to function interactively and synergistically to neutralize reactive oxygen species (ROS). Reactive oxygen species include molecules like hydrogen peroxide; ions like the hypochlorite ion; radicals like the hydroxyl radical; and the superoxide anion, which are an ion and a radical.

All subjects from the current study are at low serum selenium level (which is about 80 – 120 μg /L in Europe), and stayed as that even after use of antioxidants supplements, including selenium. Similar trend was also notice in the selenoenzyme glutathione peroxidase (GSHPx) level among HIV patients. Low serum selenium was defined as a serum level ≤ 85 μg/l [52]. Selenium deficiency, more than any other nutrient, has been documented to correlate with progression and mortality of HIV [53]. Selenium is needed for the proper functioning of the immune system, and appears to be a key nutrient in counteracting the development of virulence and inhibiting HIV progression to AIDS [54]. When taken as a supplement, selenium modulates the cellular response to oxidative stress, inducing a faster restoration of the endogenous antioxidative defence system against the production of reactive oxygen species [55]. Glutathion peroxidase controls the interacellular level of hydrogen peroxide, reducing the formation of reactive oxygen species that can induce lipid peroxidations with consequent damage to the cellular membranes [56].

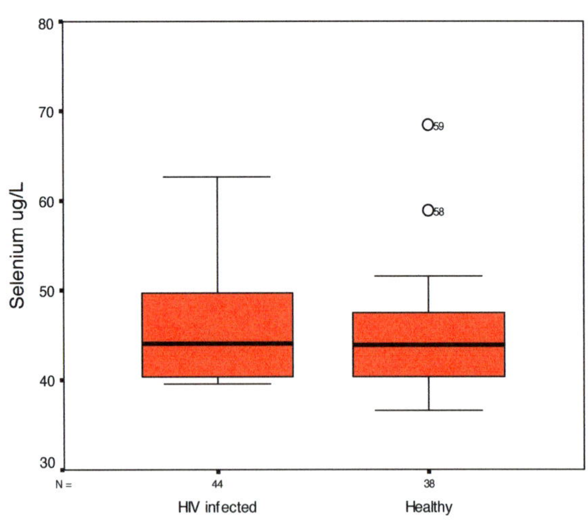

Figure 3. Selenium level of HIV infected individuals and healthy subjects (μ/g Hb)

The loss of CD4 T lymphocytes is a central factor in the progression of HIV infection to AIDS. The key role of these cells in regulating and amplifying the immune response means that any decline in their number results in deficits in both humoral and cell-mediated immunity [57]. Both the CD4 percentage and the CD4:CD8 ratio are also affected by changes in the number of CD8 cells, which tends to rise through the course of HIV infection [58].This study demonstrates that after supplementation, there is an increase in CD4 T cells in HIV patients. Several research studies have indicated that the apoptosis of CD4 cells contributing to HIV progression does not result solely from HIV infection, but largely from antioxidant imbalances in the host [43, 59, 60]. Activation of latent HIV state can be stimulated in the presence of reactive oxygen species (ROS) through the stimulation of oxygen-responsive transcription factors, specifically NF-kB, which induces HIV replication in the infected T-lymphocyte.

The mean serum malondialdehyde (MDA) concentrations in this study were significantly elevated in HIV infected patients. Serum concentration of total serum antioxidant status (TAS) was increased after supplementation. Our data indicate that severe oxidative stress occurs in the serum of HIV patients in comparison with controls ones and the inclusion of antioxidants in the therapeutic approach in managing HIV patients may prevent the additional free radicals damage. It has been shown that cells infected with the HIV undergo a significant amplification of O_2^- generation. This phenomenon combined with a deficiency in key antioxidant enzymes (SOD and CAT) and a decreased concentration of the antioxidant vitamins, may lead to severe oxidative stress in HIV-infected patients. Consequently these conditions may in turn be responsible for the DNA base modifications observed in this study [43]. Serum MDA adducts also tended to correlate inversely with expression of CD127 on T cells was shown [61]. Study in placenta, umbilical cord blood and infant blood in HIV/ART-exposed infants compared with uninfected controls [62] showed that placental mitochondria malondialdehyde (MDA) concentrations and mtDNA content in placenta and cord blood were similar between groups. Supplementation with antioxidant vitamins prevents oxidative modification of DNA in lymphocytes of HIV-infected patients [44]. Furthermore, as an antioxidant, vitamin E [63]and atherosclerotic lesions contain oxidized lipids [64], therefore, supplementation with vitamin E would decrease heart disease risk. It has been reported that α-tocopherol concentrations in serum are regulated by the α-tocopherol transfer protein and are dependent on serum lipid concentrations because α-tocopherol is non-specifically transported by lipoproteins [63]. Serum micronutrient concentrations along with surrogate markers of atherosclerosis in a cohort of HIV infected adults were studied [65](Falcone et al. 2010), the highest tertile of serum vitamin E concentration was associated with higher common and internal carotid intima-media thickness (c-IMT) and coronary artery calcium (CAC) scores [65]. The authors concluded that elevated serum vitamin E values may increase the risk of cardiovascular complications in HIV-infected adults [65].

There appears to be a possible role for antioxidants supplements. However, these supplements cannot effectively eliminate HIV signs and symptoms and the optimal dosage of these nutrients is (whether used alone or in combination) has to defined

Author details

M Sauka[1], G Selga[1], A Skesters[1], A Silova[1], T Westermarck[2], A Latvus[3] and F Atroshi[4]

1 Rīga Stradiņš University, Rīga, LV, Latvia

2 Rinnekoti Research Center, Espoo-Finalnd, Finland

3 Hankintatukku Oy, Museokatu, Helsinki, Finland

4 Pharmacology &Toxicology, University of Helsinki, Finland

References

[1] WHO. HIV/AIDS.Global situation and trends, 2013.

[2] Sicotte M, Langlois EV, Aho J, Ziegler D, Zunzunegui MV. Association between nutritional status and the immune response in HIV + patients under HAART: protocol for a systematic review. Syst Rev. 2014 Feb 10;3(1):9. [Epub ahead of print]

[3] Kaio DJ, Rondó PH, Souza JM, Firmino AV, Luzia LA, Segurado AA. Vitamin A and Beta-Carotene Concentrations in Adults with HIV/AIDS on Highly Active Antiretroviral Therapy. J Nutr Sci Vitaminol (Tokyo). 2013;59(6):496-502.

[4] Fawzi, W. Micronutrients and human immunodeficiency virus type 1 disease progression among adults and children. Clin. Infect. Dis., 2003, 37 Suppl 2, S 112 – 6.

[5] Nkengfack GN, Torimiro JN, Englert H. Effects of antioxidants on CD4 and viral load in HIV-infected women in sub-Saharan Africa - dietary supplements vs. local diet. nt J Vitam Nutr Res. 2012 Feb;82(1):63-72.

[6] van Lettow M, Harries AD, Kumwenda JJ, Zijlstra EE, Clark TD, Taha TE, Semba RD. Micronutrient malnutrition and wasting in adults with pulmonary tuberculosis with pulmonary tuberculosis with and without HIV co-infection in Malawi. BMC Infect Dis 2004;4:61.

[7] Stone CA, Kawai K, Kupka R, Fawzi WW. Role of selenium in HIV infection. Nutr Rev 2010; 68:671–81.

[8] Campa A, Baum MK. Micronutrients and HIV infection. HIV Ther 2010;4:437–69.

[9] Rayman MP. Selenium and human health. Lancet 2012;379:1256–68.

[10] Odeh M. The role of zinc in acquired immunodeficiency syndrome. J Intern Med. 1992 May;231(5):463-9.

[11] Baum MK, Shor-Posner G, Lu Y, Rosner B, Sauberlich HE, Fletcher MA, Szapocznik J, Eisdorfer C, Buring JE, Hennekens CH. Micronutrients and HIV-1 disease progression. AIDS. 1995 Sep;9(9):1051-6.

[12] Graham NM, Sorensen D, Odaka N, Brookmeyer R, Chan D, Willett WC, Morris JS, Saah AJ. Relationship of serum copper and zinc levels to HIV-1 seropositivity and progression to AIDS. J Acquir Immune Defic Syndr. 1991;4(10):976-80.

[13] Tang AM, Graham NM, Saah AJ. Effects of micronutrient intake on survival in human immunodeficiency virus type 1 infection. Am J Epidemiol. 1996 Jun 15;143(12): 1244-56.

[14] Miyamoto H, Araya Y, Ito M, Isobe H, Dosaka H, Shimizu T, Kishi F, Yamamoto I, Honma H, Kawakami Y. Serum selenium and vitamin E concentrations in families of lung cancer patients. Cancer. 1987 Sep 1;60(5):1159-62.

[15] Delmas-Beauvieux MC, Peuchant E, Couchouron A, Constans J, Sergeant C, Simonoff M, Pellegrin JL, Leng B, Conri C, Clerc M. The enzymatic antioxidant system in blood and glutathione status in human immunodeficiency virus (HIV)-infected patients: effects of supplementation with selenium or beta-carotene. Am J Clin Nutr. 1996 Jul;64(1):101-7. Erratum in: Am J Clin Nutr 1996 Dec;64(6):971.

[16] Flax VL, Bentley ME, Combs GF Jr, Chasela CS, Kayira D, Tegha G, Kamwendo D, Daza EJ, Fokar A, Kourtis AP, Jamieson DJ, van der Horst CM, Adair LS. Plasma and breast-milk selenium in HIV-infected Malawian mothers are positively associated with infant selenium status but are not associated with maternal supplementation: results of the Breastfeeding, Antiretrovirals, and Nutrition study. Am J Clin Nutr. 2014 Feb 5. [Epub ahead of print].

[17] Mburu S, Marnewick JL, Abayomi A, Ipp H. Modulation of LPS-induced CD4+ T-cell activation and apoptosis by antioxidants in untreated asymptomatic HIV infected participants: an in vitro study. Clin Dev Immunol. 2013;2013:631063. doi: 10.1155/2013/631063. Epub 2013 Nov 21.

[18] Hillesheim E, Lima LR, Silva RC, Trindade EB. Dietary intake and nutritional status of HIV-1-infected children and adolescents in Florianopolis, Brazil. Int J STD AIDS. 2013 Dec 18. [Epub ahead of print].

[19] Kaiser JD, Campa AM, Ondercin JP, Leoung GS, Pless RF, Baum MK. Micronutrient supplementation increases CD4 count in HIV-infected individuals on highly active antiretroviral therapy: a prospective, double-blinded, placebo-controlled trial. J Acquir Immune Defic Syndr. 2006 Aug 15;42(5):523-8

[20] Baeten JM, McClelland RS, Richardson BA, Bankson DD, Lavreys L, Wener MH, Overbaugh J, Mandaliya K, Ndinya-Achola JO, Bwayo JJ, Kreiss JK. Vitamin A deficiency and the acute phase response among HIV-1-infected and -uninfected women in Kenya. J Acquir Immune Defic Syndr. 2002 Oct 1;31(2):243-9.

[21] Guo Y, Pino-Lagos K, Ahonen CA, Bennett KA, Wang J, Napoli JL, Blomhoff R, Sockanathan S, Chandraratna RA, Dmitrovsky E, Turk MJ, Noelle RJ. A retinoic acid--rich tumor microenvironment provides clonal survival cues for tumor-specific CD8(+) T cells. Cancer Res. 2012 Oct 15;72(20):5230-9.

[22] Irlam JH, Visser MM, Rollins NN, Siegfried N. Micronutrient supplementation in children and adults with HIV infection. Cochrane Database Syst Rev. 2010 Dec 8;(12):CD003650. doi: 10.1002/14651858.CD003650.

[23] Thorne-Lyman AL, Fawzi WW. Vitamin A and carotenoids during pregnancy and maternal, neonatal and infant health outcomes: a systematic review and meta-analysis. Paediatr Perinat Epidemiol. 2012 Jul;26 Suppl 1:36-54. doi: 10.1111/j.1365-3016.2012.01284.

[24] Forrester JE, Wang XD, Knox TA, Borek CG, Tang AM, Johnson EJ. Factors associated with serum retinol, alpha-tocopherol, carotenoids, and selenium in Hispanics with problems of HIV, chronic hepatitis C, and drug use. J Public Health Policy. 2009 Sep;30(3):285-99.

[25] Monteiro JP, Freimanis-Hance L, Faria LB, Mussi-Pinhata MM, Korelitz J, Vannucchi H, Queiroz W, Succi RC, Hazra R. Both human immunodeficiency virus-infected and human immunodeficiency virus-exposed, uninfected children living in Brazil, Argentina, and Mexico have similar rates of low concentrations of retinol, beta-carotene, and vitamin E. Nutr Res. 2009 Oct;29(10):716-22.

[26] Villamor E, Koulinska IN, Aboud S, Murrin C, Bosch RJ, Manji KP, Fawzi WW. Effect of vitamin supplements on HIV shedding in breast milk. Am J Clin Nutr. 2010 Oct;92(4):881-6.

[27] Dror DK, Allen LH. Vitamin E deficiency in developing countries. Food Nutr Bull. 2011 Jun;32(2):124-43.

[28] Isanaka S, Mugusi F, Fawzi WW. Standard-dose vs high-dose multivitamin supplements for HIV--reply. JAMA. 2013 Feb 13;309(6):546. doi: 10.1001/jama.2012.216995.

[29] Sudfeld CR, Isanaka S, Mugusi FM, Aboud S, Wang M, Chalamilla GE, Giovannucci EL, Fawzi WW. Weight change at 1 mo of antiretroviral therapy and its association with subsequent mortality, morbidity, and CD4 T cell reconstitution in a Tanzanian HIV-infected adult cohort. Am J Clin Nutr. 2013 Jun;97(6):1278-87.

[30] Abrams B, Duncan D, Hertz-Picciotto I. A prospective study of dietary intake and acquired immune deficiency syndrome in HIV-seropositive homosexual men. J Acquir Immune Defic Syndr. 1993 Aug;6(8):949-58.

[31] Folkers K, Langsjoen P, Nara Y, Muratsu K, Komorowski J, Richardson PC, Smith TH. Biochemical deficiencies of coenzyme Q10 in HIV-infection and exploratory treatment. Biochem Biophys Res Commun. 1988 Jun 16;153(2):888-96.

[32] Cherry CL, Mobarok M, Wesselingh SL, Fain R, Weinstock S, Tachedjian G, Srivastava S, Tyssen DP, Glass JD, Hooker DJ. Ubisol-Aqua: coenzyme Q10 prevents antiretroviral toxic neuropathy in an in vitro model. Curr HIV Res. 2010 Apr;8(3):232-9.

[33] Xue SY, Hebert VY, Hayes DM, Robinson CN, Glover M, Dugas TR. Nucleoside reverse transcriptase inhibitors induce a mitophagy-associated endothelial cytotoxicity that is reversed by coenzyme Q10 cotreatment. Toxicol Sci. 2013 Aug;134(2):323-34.

[34] Hickey, M. S. Nutritional support of patients with AIDS. Surg.Clin.North Am. 71:645-664, June 1991.

[35] Karter DL, Karter AJ, Yarrish R, Patterson C, Kass PH, Nord J, Kislak JW. Vitamin A deficiency in non-vitamin-supplemented patients with AIDS: a cross-sectional study. J Acquir Immune Defic Syndr Hum Retrovirol. 1995 Feb 1;8(2):199-203.

[36] Timbo BB, Tollefson L. Nutrition: a cofactor in HIV disease. J Am Diet Assoc. 1994 Sep;94(9):1018-22.

[37] Augustus LJ. Nutritional care for patients with HIV. Am J Nurs. 1997 Oct;97(10):62-5.

[38] Beach RS, Mantero-Atienza E, Shor-Posner G, Javier JJ, Szapocznik J, Morgan R, Sauberlich HE, Cornwell PE, Eisdorfer C, Baum MK: Specific nutrient abnormalities in asymptomatic HIV-1 infection. AIDS 1992, 6:701-708.

[39] Semba RD, Graham NM, Caiaffa WT, Margolick JB, Clement L, Vlahov D: Increased mortality associated with vitamin A deficiency during human immunodeficiency virus type 1 infection. Arch Intern Med 1993, 153:2149-2154.

[40] Tang AM, Graham NM, Semba RD, Saah AJ: Association between serum vitamin A and E levels and HIV-1 disease progression. AIDS 1997, 11:613-620.

[41] Jiamton S, Pepin J, Suttent R, Filteau S, Mahakkanukrauh B, Hanshaoworakul W, Chaisilwattana P, Suthipinittharm P, Shetty P, Jaffar S: A randomized trial of the impact of multiple micronutrient supplementation on mortality among HIV-infected individuals living in Bangkok. AIDS 2003, 17:2461-2469.

[42] Fawzi WW, Msamanga GI, Spiegelman D, Wei R, Kapiga S, Villamor E, Mwakagile D, Mugusi F, Hertzmark E, Essex M, Hunter DJ: A randomized trial of multivitamin supplements and HIV disease progression and mortality. N Engl J Med 2004, 351:23-32.

[43] Kameoka M, Kimura T, Ikuta K. Superoxide enhances the spread of HIV-1 infection by cell-to-cell transmission. FEBS Lett. 1993 Sep 27;331(1-2):182-6.

[44] Jaruga P, Jaruga B, Gackowski D, Olczak A, Halota W, Pawlowska M, Olinski R. Supplementation with antioxidant vitamins prevents oxidative modification of DNA in lymphocytes of HIV-infected patients. Free Radic Biol Med. 2002, 32(5):414-20.

[45] Peterhans E. Oxidants and antioxidants in viral diseases: disease mechanisms and metabolic regulation.J Nutr. 1997 May;127(5 Suppl):962S-965S.

[46] Pace GW, Leaf CD. The role of oxidative stress in HIV disease. Free Radic Biol Med. 1995 Oct;19(4):523-8.

[47] Smit E, Tang A. Nutritional assessment in intravenous drug users with HIV/AIDS. J Acquir Immune Defic Syndr. 2000 Oct 1;25 Suppl 1:S62-9.

[48] Tang AM, Smit E, Semba RD, Shah N, Lyles CM, Li D, Vlahov D. Improved antioxidant status among HIV-infected injecting drug users on potent antiretroviral therapy.J Acquir Immune Defic Syndr. 2000 Apr 1;23(4):321-6.

[49] Wong GHW, McHugh T, Weber R, Goeddel DV. Tumor necrosis factor alpha selectively sensitizes human immunodeficiency virus infected cells to heat and radiation. Proc Natl Acad Sci U S A 1991;88:4372–6.

[50] Kotler DP. Nutritional management of patients with AIDS-related anorexia. Semin Gastrointest Dis. 1998 Oct;9(4):189-99.

[51] Kupka R, Msamanga GI, Spiegelman D, Morris S, Mugusi F, Hunter DJ, Fawzi WW: Selenium status is associated with accelerated HIV disease progression among HIV-1-infected pregnant women in Tanzania. J Nutr 2004, 134:2556-2560.

[52] Hardy G, Hardy I. Selenium: the Se-XY nutraceutical. Nutrition. 2004 Jun;20(6):590-3.

[53] Baum MK, Shor-Posner G, Lai S, et al. High risk of HIV-related mortality is associated with selenium deficiency. J Acquir Immune Defic Syndr Hum Retrovirol 1997;15:370–4.

[54] Rayman M.P. (2000).The importance of selenium to human health. Lancet. 15;356(9225):233-41.

[55] Jozanov-Stankov O, Demajo M, Djujić I, Mandić M. Selenium intake as a modulator of responsiveness to oxidative stress. J Environ Pathol Toxicol Oncol. 1998;17(3-4): 251-7.

[56] Levander OA, Beck MA. Selenium and viral virulence. Br Med Bull. 1999;55(3): 528-33.

[57] Grossman Z, Meier-Schellersheim M, Sousa AE, Victorino RM, Paul WE. CD4+ T-cell depletion in HIV infection: are we closer to understanding the cause? Nat Med 2002; 8:319–323.

[58] Highleyman, L. (2003). Monitoring tests for people with HIV. Bulletin of Experimental Treatments for AIDS: Retrieved July 2003 from Hogg, R. et. al. (2001). Rates of disease progression based on CD4 cell count and viral load after initiating drug therapy. Journal of the American Medical Association, 286(20). 2568-2577.

[59] Sandstrom PA, Murray J, Folks TM, Diamond AM. Antioxidant defenses influence HIV-1 replication and associated cytopathic effects. Free Radic Biol Med 1998;24:1485-1491.

[60] Droge W, Eck HP, Gmunder H, Mihm S. Requirement for prooxidant and antioxidant states in T cell mediated immune responses. Relevance for the pathogenic mechanisms of AIDS? Klin Wochenschr 1991;69:118-122.

[61] Kalinowska M, Bazdar DA, Lederman MM, Funderburg N, Sieg SF. Decreased IL-7 responsiveness is related to oxidative stress in HIV disease. PLoS One. 2013;8(3):e58764. doi: 10.1371/journal.pone.0058764. Epub 2013 Mar 7.

[62] Ross AC, Leong T, Avery A, Castillo-Duran M, Bonilla H, Lebrecht D, Walker UA, Storer N, Labbato D, Khaitan A, Tomanova-Soltys I, McComsey GA. Effects of in utero antiretroviral exposure on mitochondrial DNA levels, mitochondrial function and oxidative stress. HIV Med. 2012 Feb;13(2):98-106.

[63] Traber MG. Vitamin E regulatory mechanisms. Annu Rev Nutr 2007;27:347–62.

[64] Diaz MN, Frei B, Vita JA, Keaney JFJ. Antioxidants and atherosclerotic heart disease. N Engl J Med 1997;337:408–16.

[65] Falcone EL, Mangili A, Tang AM, et al. Micronutrient concentrations and subclinical atherosclerosis in adults with HIV. Am J Clin Nutr , 2010;91:1213–9

Chapter 10

Pharmacological and Clinical Effectiveness of *Zingiber officinale* and *Alpinia galanga* in Patients with Osteoarthritis

Guntars Selga, M. Sauka, L. Aboltina, A. Davidova,
P. Kaipainen, D. Kheder, T. Westermarck and
F. Atroshi

Additional information is available at the end of the chapter

http://dx.doi.org/10.5772/58417

1. Introduction

Osteoarthritis (OA) is a progressive degenerative joint disease that has a major impact on joint function and quality of life. OA is a painful condition caused by a gradual loss of cartilage from the joints and, in some people, joint inflammation [1]. Pain, stiffness, and difficulty moving the joint easily are common symptoms of OA. Non-drug treatments for osteoarthritis have gained popularity according to the American College of Rheumatology (ACR) [2] and can often reduce the symptoms. Therefore, there is a significant need to improve current osteoarthritis therapies and to search for novel therapies. Nutraceuticals and dietary supplements derived from herbs have long been used in traditional medicine. Though they aren't recognized as drugs, herbal and natural remedies are used for a drug-like effect, and they can potentially cause the same reactions and complications prescription drugs can cause. There is considerable evidence that nutraceuticals may play an important role in inflammation and joint destruction in OA. The World Health Organization (WHO) [3] has taken an interest in the indigenous system of medicine; particularly, plant remedies. Ginger is widely used as a spice, an antiemetic and carminative agent, and for its essential oils. Gingerols, in particular 6-gingerol, are the active components of ginger. Proposed mechanisms include direct stimulation of the gastro-intestinal tract, or serotonin antagonism in the gut or central nervous system [4, 5]. A study on 6-gingerol was shown to significantly inhibit the production of nitric oxide, a highly reactive nitrogen molecule that quickly forms a very damaging free radical called peroxynitrite and greatly lessened depletion of glutathione [6]. Other reports suggest that ginger produces its anti-inflammatory effect by inhibiting arachidonic acid metabolism [4, 7], induce apoptosis in HL-60 leukemia [8], non-small cell lung cancer cells [9] and against acute monocytic leukemia [10]. It is also reported to be chemopreventive and anti-inflammatory [11, 12]. The antioxidant, antimicrobial and cytotoxic activities of Zingiber officinale displayed specific inhibition on Escherichia coli was also studied [13]. Gingerols also promoted significant reduction in mRNA transcription of TNF-α, IL-2 and INF-γ [14]. Ginsenoside Rg5 (Rg5), an abundant natural compound in Panax ginseng, has been found to be beneficial in treating AD [15]. Pharmacologic studies in the last decades have shown that ginsenosides (ginseng saponins) are primarily responsible for the actions of ginseng [16]. In diabetes ginger supplementation in oral administration reduced inflammation in type 2 diabetic patients [17]. Other studies have shown that ginger may benefits musculoskeletal disorder treatment [18] nausea and vomiting [19], inflammation or inflammatory states [20, 21] such as osteoarthritis [20-22], migraine [23], cancer [24], hyperlipidemia and hyperglycemia [25, 26]. In vitro studies suggest that ginger produces its anti-inflammatory effect by inhibiting arachidonic acid metabolism[4], [7]. This chapter intends to give a brief outline of ginger health benefit and to investigate the ability of ginger tablets to reduce postoperative pain in patients with osteoarthritis.

1.1. History

The earliest evidence of humans' use of plants for healing dates back to the Neanderthal period [27]. In the 16th century, botanical gardens were created to grow medicinal plants for medical schools [28]. Herbal medicine practice flourished until the 17th century when more "scientific" pharmacological remedies were favoured [29]. The use of plants for healing purposes predates human history and forms the origin of much modern medicine. Many conventional drugs originate from plant sources: a century ago, most of the few effective drugs were plant based. Examples include aspirin (from willow bark), digoxin (from foxglove), quinine (from cinchona bark), and morphine (from the opium poppy). The development of drugs from plants continues, with drug companies engaged in large scale pharmacological screening of herbs.

1.2. Therapeutic scope

Although herbal preparations are widely used as self-medication for acute conditions, practitioners of herbal medicine tend to concentrate on treating chronic conditions. A typical caseload might include asthma, eczema, premenstrual syndrome, rheumatoid arthritis, migraine, menopausal symptoms, chronic fatigue, irritable bowel syndrome and lately to treat mental or musculoskeletal disorders.

1.3. Safety

Many plants are highly toxic. Herbal medicine probably presents a greater risk of adverse effects and interactions than any other complementary therapy. There are case reports of serious adverse events after administration of herbal products. In most cases the herbs involved were self-prescribed and bought over the counter or obtained from a source other than a registered practitioner. In the most notorious instance, several women developed rapidly progressive interstitial renal fibrosis after taking Chinese herbs prescribed by a slimming clinic

2. Method and subjects

2.1. Method

Fourthly patients with OA of the knee and moderate-to-severe pain were enrolled in a randomised, double –blind, placebo-controlled, two-center, parallel group, 12-week study. The primary efficacy variable was the proportion of responders experiencing a reduction in "knee pain on standing" using a visual analog scale.

The study was approved by the ethics committee of the Latvian Institute of Cardiology for clinical and physiological research, drug and pharmaceutics product clinical investigation.

Only those willing to participate and after getting their informed consent will be involved in the investigation

2.2. Subjects

Elderly patients with clinical diagnosis of osteoarthritis (OA) of the knee, defined as knee (articular and not periarticular or referred) pain for most days of the prior month and radiographic osteophytes at the tibiofemoral joint margins were involved in the study. All involved patients had a baseline pain score > 40 mm and < 90 mm on a 100-mm Visual Analogue Scale (VAS) at the time of randomization, when evaluating pain on standing during the last 24 hours. Both men and women were included.

Exclusion Characteristics

- No NSAID's or other medication before intervention start-or consider including one week wash-out period.
- History of allergy to ginger;
- History of rheumatoid disease;
- History of asthma, if the patient needs treatment with steroids;
- Treatment with oral corticosteroids within four weeks prior to screening;
- Treatment with intra-articular corticosteroids;
- Treatment with intra-articular hyaluronic acid within 6 months prior screening;
- Prior treatment with immuno-suppressive drugs, cytostatic drugs, gold or peniciilamine;
- Other investigational drugs within one month prior to screening;
- History or clinical signs of impaired kidney function;

- Clinical signs of liver disorders;
- Severe neurological diseases;
- Increased oral temperature, (37,5 C) at the time of screening;
- Affection of the hip to an extent that would influence the ratings done at the visits";
- History of fibromyalgia;
- Gout;
- Recurrent or active pseudo-gout;

2.2.1. Study design

The study was 12 weeks, double blind, and placebo-controlled, parallel group trial performed in two social care centres for elderly people. The study was approved by the ethics committee of the Latvian Institute of Cardiology for clinical and physiological research, drug and pharmaceutics product clinical investigation. Only those willing to participate and after getting their informed consent will be involved in the investigation. Patients were randomised to receive treatment and both investigators and the patients were blind to treatment assignment.

2.2.2. Treatment

During the 12-week period, patients ingested 1 capsule twice daily, morning and evening. Each capsule contained 150 mg Ginger rhizome *(lat. Zingiberis officinale rhizome)* powdered extract and 125 mg Galangae rhizome (*Alpinia officinarum rhizome)* dry extract. 22 patients were got tablets with "A" and 18 patients got tablets with "B". Examination was done at the baseline, after 6 weeks and after 12 weeks.

2.2.3. Results

Characteristics of the subjects

Forty patients were included in the study (for group "A"-mean age ± SD 69±13,7 and for group "B"-mean age ± SD 75 ± 8,6). There were ten males (35 %) and thirty females (75%). The patients in both groups were generally overweight, since the average was >28 kg/m^2 (range 43 – 120 kg).

2.2.4. Assessments

The primary efficacy parameter was proportion of respondents experiencing at least a 15-mm reduction in pain between baseline and the final examination for knee pain on standing and walking during preceding 24 hours, as measured by a 100-mm, VAS.

The secondary measurement was mean ±SE of measurements for knee pain on standing and walking.

	" A" group (n=22)	"B "group (n=18)
Age, mean ± SD years	69 ± 13,7	75 ± 8,6
Sex %		
Men	23	28
Women	77	72
Body mass index ± SD kg/m²	29.31 ± 7,7	28 ± 7,0
Waste/hip ratio ± SD	0,88 ± 0,04	0,91 ± 0,04

Table 1. Demographic characteristics

	Baseline data		After 6 weeks		after 12 weeks	
	A	B	A	B	A	B
	n=22	n=18	n=20	n=18	n=20	n=18
Pain on standing and walking (%)						
> 15 mm	-	-	-	-	50	44
0 – 15 mm	-	-	-	-	41	50
≤ 0	-	-	-	-	9	6
Pain on standing, mean ± SE (mm)	62.95±2.2	57.11±+2.5	56.65±2.3	49.52±2.5	51.2±2.3	43.88±2.5
Pain on walking, mean ± SE (mm)	61.68±2.4	60.64±2.7	54.85±2.5	54±2.7	49.25±2.5	49.23±2.7

Table 2. Measurements for knee pain between group "A" and group "B"

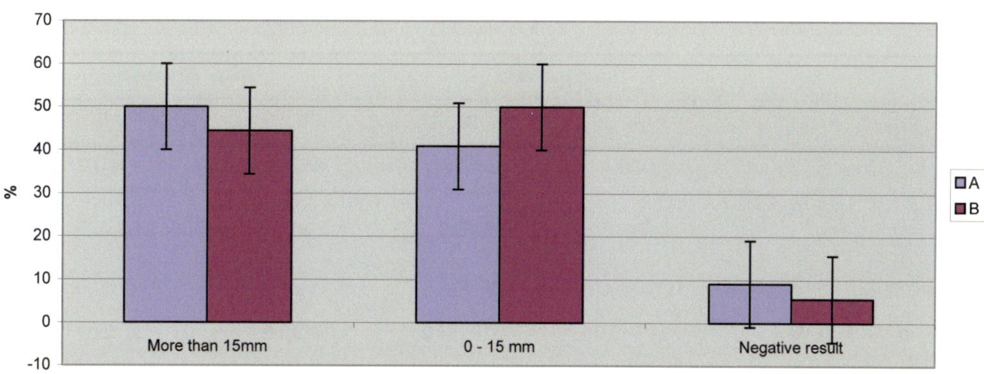

Figure 1. Pain on standing and walking after using of Ginger containg food supplements

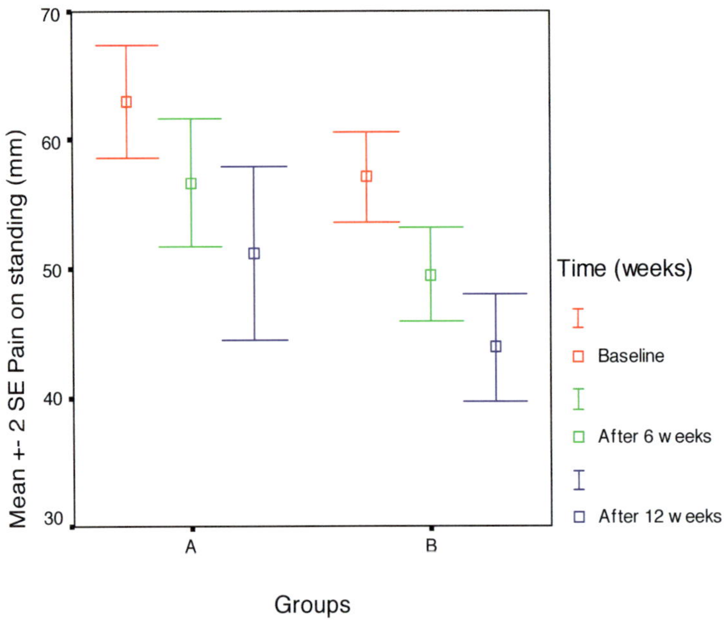

Figure 2. Knee pain on standing as measured by 100-mm visual analog scale at baseline and after 6 weeks and 12 weeks. Bars shows means with 2 SE (mm)

Additionally blood sample was checked in both groups. There were no statistically significant changes between groups.

	Baseline data		**After 12 weeks**	
	A	**B**	**A**	**B**
	n=22	**n=18**	**n=20**	**n=18**
Erytrocytes, Mean±SE, (10 [12]/L)	4.42±0.9	4.46±1	4.31±0,09	4.2±1
Hb Mean±SE, (g/L)	131.66±5.8	135.8±6.5	134.8+5.9	113.15±6.5
Hematocrit Mean±SE (%)	39.28±0.9	40.03±1.0	38.8±0.9	37.85±1.0
WBC Mean±SE (10^9/L)	7.7±0.5	6.4±0.5	6.38±0.5	5.6±0.5
ESR Mean±SE (mm/h)	23.77±3.6	20.06±4.0	19.31±3.8	18.76±4.1

Table 3. Comparison of blood samples between both groups in the study.

http://dx.doi.org/10.5772/58417

3. Discussion and conclusion

Ginger (Zingiber officinale Roscoe), a well-known spice plant, has been used traditionally in a wide variety of ailments including hypertension and osteoarthritis. Gingerol, the active components of ginger, derivatives are currently under investigation as potential drug therapy for disorders of platelet function, but the small amounts consumed in the diet are unlikely to influence platelet function. We report here the osteoarthritis effects of Zingiber officinale and Alpinia galanga tablets under controlled experimental conditions.

Osteoarthritis, the most common form of arthritis, is a debilitating progressive disease principally affecting the elderly. Osteoarthritis therapy has evolved in the past few decades from symptomatic treatment to possible disease-modifying solutions. Osteoarthritis continues to be a difficult disorder to treat, as there is no cure as such and current treatments focus mainly on relieving pain and maintaining joint function. The search nevertheless continues for management regimens that can slow, alter or reverse the degenerative processes of osteoarthritis. Experimental therapies that seek to modify the course of osteoarthritis. These include such medications as colchicine, bisphosphonates and hormones. Dietary therapeutics, such as ginger extract also has been suggested. Current approaches to treating osteoarthritis-i.e. medications; nonpharmacological modalities, such as physical therapy, exercise, weight management and orthotics; and (as a last resort) surgery-focus on reducing pain and improving (or at least maintaining) mobility

Musculoskeletal conditions are prevalent and their impact is pervasive. They are the most common cause of severe long-term pain and physical disability. The prevalence of many of these conditions increases markedly with age, and many are affected by lifestyle factors, such as obesity and lack of physical activity. The increasing number of older people and the changes in lifestyle throughout the world mean that the burden on people and society will increase dramatically. This has been recognized by the United Nations and WHO, with their endorsement of Bone and Joint Decade 2000–2010 [30]. Osteoarthritis was estimated to be the eighth leading non-fatal burden of disease in the world in 1990, accounting for 2.8% of total years of living with disability, around the same percentage as schizophrenia and congenital anomalies [31]. It was the sixth leading cause of years of living with disability at the global level, accounting for 3% of the total global years of living with disability [32], [33], [34]. According to the American Holistic Medical Association it is believed that the spiritual element should also be taken into account when assessing a person's overall well-being [35], [36]. Ginger is an herb which has been used for centuries in Ayurdevic medicine to relieve the pain of arthritis although few studies are available to demonstrate its benefits. There appears to be good evidence from epidemiological studies and clinical trials that Zingiber officinale and Alpinia galanga tablets lower osteoarthritis tendency. The mechanism of action is believed to be due to the inhibition of prostaglandin and leukotriene synthesis. Zingiber officinale and Alpinia galanga was also tested for antibacterial activities by evaluating growth delays using human strains of the genera Staphylococcus and Micrococcus. Staphylococcus aureus was found to be sensitive to the ginger extract. When the extract was tested for the haemolytic effect, no lytic effects on procaryotic cells were found. Patients suffering from such disorders reported relief in pain and associated symptoms on extract administration. No significant side effects of supplementation were noted, which may be considered as adjuvant therapy in patients with osteoarthritis of the knee. In this study ginger extract may have a beneficial effective in treatment for osteoarthritis. However, more observational studies, with a larger sample size, are needed to confirm the encouraging preliminary data on effectiveness and safety. The use of Zingiber officinale and Alpinia galanga in osteoarthritis will reduce the symptoms to an equivalent extent in elderly people with osteoarthritis.

Author details

Guntars Selga[1], M. Sauka[1], L. Aboltina[1], A. Davidova[1], P. Kaipainen[2], D. Kheder[1], T. Westermarck[2] and F. Atroshi[3]

1 Department of Oral and Maxillofacial Surgery, Faculty of Dentistry, Rīga Stradiņš University, Rīga, Latvia

2 Rinnekoti Research Center, Espoo, Finland

3 Pharmacology &Toxicology, University of Helsinki, Finland

References

[1] Kraus JF, D'Ambrosia RD, Smith EG, Van Meter J, Borhani NO, Franti CE, Lipscomb PR. An epidemiological study of severe osteoarthritis. Orthopedics. 1978 Jan-Feb; 1(1):37-42.

[2] ACR, Recommendations for the medical management of osteoarthritis of the hip and knee: 2000 update. American College of Rheumatology Subcommittee on Osteoarthritis Guidelines. Arthritis Rheum. 2000;43(9):1905.

[3] WHO. "Fact sheet no. 134: Traditional medicine". World Health Organization. 2008-12-01. Retrieved 2009-05-02.

[4] Grant KL, Lutz RB. Ginger. American Journal of Health-System Pharmacy 2000; 57: 945–7.

[5] Ernst E, Pittler MH. Efficacy of ginger for nausea and vomiting: a systematic review of randomised controlled clinical trials. British Journal of Anaesthesia 2000; 84: 367–71.

[6] Jagetia GC, Baliga MS, Venkatesh P, Ulloor JN. Influence of ginger rhizome (Zingiber officinale Rosc) on survival, glutathione and lipid peroxidation in mice after whole-body exposure to gamma radiation. Radiat Res. 2003 Nov;160(5):584-92. 2003

[7] Koo KL, Ammit AJ, Tran VH, Duke CC, Roufogalis BD. Gingerols and related analogues inhibit arachidonic acid-induced human platelet serotonin release and aggregation. Thrombosis Research 2001; 103: 387–97.

[8] Lee E, Surh YJ: Induction of apoptosis in HL-60 cells by pungent vanilloids, [6]-gingerol and [6]-paradol. Cancer Lett 1998;134:163–168.

[9] Wang G, Li X, Huang F, Zhao J, Ding H, Cunningham C, Coad JE, Flynn DC, Reed E, Li QQ: Antitumor effect of β-elemene in non-small cell lung cancer cells is mediated via induction of cell cycle arrest and apoptotic cell death. Cell Mol Life Sci 2005;62:881–893.

[10] Omoregie SN, Omoruyi FO, Wright VF, Jones L, Zimba PV. Antiproliferative activities of lesser galangal (Alpinia officinarum Hance Jam1), turmeric (Curcuma longa L.), and ginger (Zingiber officinale Rosc.) against acute monocytic leukemia. J Med Food. 2013 Jul;16(7):647-55.

[11] Nonn L, Duong D, Peehl, DM: Chemopreventive anti-inflammatory activities of curcumin and other phytochemicals mediated by MAP kinase phosphatase-5 in prostate cells. Carcinogenesis 2007;28:1188–1196.

[12] Zick SM, Djuric Z, Ruffin MT, Litzinger AJ, Normolle DP, Alrawi S, Feng MR, Brenner DE: Pharmacokinetics of 6-gingerol, 8-gingerol, 10-gingerol, and 6-shogaol and conjugate metabolites in healthy human subjects. Cancer Epidemiol Biomarkers Prev 2008;17:1930–1936.

[13] Lu CL, Zhao HY, Jiang JG. Evaluation of multi-activities of 14 edible species from Zingiberaceae. Int J Food Sci Nutr. 2013 Feb;64(1):28-35.

[14] Rodrigues FA, Prata MM, Oliveira IC, Alves NT, Freitas RE, Monteiro HS, Silva JA, Vieira PC, Viana DA, Libório AB, Havt A. Gingerol Fraction from Zingiber officinale Protects Against Gentamicin-Induced Nephrotoxicity. Antimicrob Agents Chemother. 2014 Jan 6. (Epub ahead of print).

[15] Chu S, Gu J, Feng L, Liu J, Zhang M, Jia X, Yao D, Liu M. Ginsenoside Rg5 improves cognitive dysfunction and beta-amyloid deposition in STZ-induced memory impaired rats via attenuating neuroinflammatory responses.Int Immunopharmacol. 2014 Feb 3. pii: S1567-5769(14)00032-0. doi: 10. 1016/j.intimp.2014. 01. 018.

[16] Im DS, Nah SY. Yin and Yang of ginseng pharmacology: ginsenosides vs gintonin. Acta Pharmacol Sin. 2013 Nov;34(11):1367-73.

[17] Mahluji S, Ostadrahimi A, Mobasseri M, Ebrahimzade Attari V, Payahoo L. Anti-inflammatory effects of zingiber officinale in type 2 diabetic patients. Adv Pharm Bull. 2013;3(2):273-6.

[18] Srivastava KC, Mustafa T. Ginger (zingiber officinale) in rheumatism and musculoskeletal disorders. Med Hypotheses. 1992;39(4):342–8.

[19] Bryer E. A literature review of the effectiveness of ginger in alleviating mild-to-moderate nausea and vomiting of pregnancy. J Midwifery Womens Health. 2005;50(1):e1–3.

[20] Leach MJ, Kumar S. The clinical effectiveness of ginger (zingiber officinale) in adults with osteoarthritis. Int J Evid Based Healthc. 2008;6(3):311–20.

[21] Altman RD, Marcussen KC. Effects of a ginger extract on knee pain in patients with osteoarthritis. Arthritis Rheum. 2001;44(11):2531–8.

[22] Therkleson T. Ginger Therapy for Osteoarthritis: A Typical Case. J Holist Nurs. 2014 Jan 29. [Epub ahead of print].

[23] Mustafa T, Srivastava KC. Ginger (Zingiber officinale) in migraine headache. J Ethnopharmacol. 1990;29(3):267–73.

[24] Shukla Y, Singh M. Cancer preventive properties of ginger: A brief review. Food Chem Toxicol. 2007;45(5):683–90.

[25] Ali BH, Blunden G, Tanira MO, Nemmar A. Some phytochemical, pharmacological and toxicological properties of ginger (Zingiber officinale Roscoe): a review of recent research. Food Chem Toxicol. 2008;46(2):409–20.

[26] White B. Ginger: An overview. Am Fam Physician. 2007;75(11):1689–91.

[27] Kleiner SM. The true nature of herbs. Phys Sports Med. 1995;23:13-14.

[28] Akerele O. Nature's medicinal bounty: don't throw it away. World Health Forum. 1993;14:390-395.

[29] Trevelyan J. Herbal medicine. Nurs Times. 1993;89:36-38.

[30] Woolf AD. The bone and joint decade 2000-2010. Ann Rheum Dis. 2000 Feb;59(2):81-2

[31] Murray CJ, Lopez AD. Evidence-based health policy--lessons from the Global Burden of Disease Study. Science. 1996 Nov 1;274(5288):740-3.

[32] Lau EM, Symmons DP, Croft P. The epidemiology of hip osteoarthritis and rheumatoid arthritis in the Orient. Clin Orthop Relat Res. 1996 Feb;(323):81-90.

[33] Symmons DP. Safety profile of low-dose aspirin. Lancet. 1996 Nov 23;348(9039): 1394-5.

[34] Akhtar N and Haqqi TM. Current nutraceuticals in the management of osteoarthritis: a review. Ther Adv Musculoskelet Dis. 2012 June; 4(3): 181–207.

[35] Roberts M, American Holistic Medical Association 02/05/2014.

[36] Strandberg, E; Ovhed, I; Borgquist, L; Wilhelmsson, S. "The perceived meaning of a (w) holistic view among general practitioners and district nurses in Swedish primary care: A qualitative study". BMC Family Practice, 2007, 8: 8. doi:10. 1186/1471-2296-8-8.

Chapter 11

Trace Elements, Antioxidant Enzymes and Free Carnitine Levels Among Epileptic Patients Treated with Valproate Monotherapy

Elżbieta Płonka-Półtorak, Tuomas Westermarck, Pekka Kaipainen, Markus Kaski and Faik Atroshi

Additional information is available at the end of the chapter

http://dx.doi.org/10.5772/57613

1. Introduction

1.1. Epilepsy and oxidative stress

Epilepsy is a common chronic neurological disorder with a prevalence of 0, 4 – 1 % of the general population [1]. The highest incidence rates are in children and elderly. Epilepsy is characterized by recurrent unprovoked seizures, generalized or focal. The epileptic seizure is a clinical manifestation of transient excessive and hyper synchronous activity of neurones in the brain. It may include alterations of consciousness, motor or autonomic components or subjective sensory or psychic phenomena. An epilepsy syndrome is a complexity of signs and symptoms defining a unique condition. One of the most common syndromes is Juvenile myoclonic epilepsy accounting for up to 10% of all epilepsies [2].

Etiology of epilepsy in the majority is not identified [3]. Genetic defect or structural-metabolic disorder of the brain may be the cause of some chronic seizures. The commonest acquired causes of epilepsy include vascular diseases, tumours, trauma, and infections of the central nervous system [2]. However, the mechanisms of epileptogenesis are not well understood.

Experimental and human studies suggested that the homeostasis of trace elements and membrane lipid peroxidation due to increase of free radicals or decreased of antioxidant defence mechanisms have been causally involved in some forms of epilepsies. They were directly or indirectly implicated as taking part in the pathophysiology of neuronal excitability, neuronal excitotoxicity, seizure recurrence and its resistance to treatment with antiepileptic drugs [4].

Oxidative stress is a common pathogenic mechanism in neurodegenerative disorders. The central nervous system is particularly susceptible to reactive oxygen species (ROS) due to high oxygen demands of the brain, low concentration of endogenous antioxidants and concomitant accumulation of reactive iron. Furthermore, the abundance of polyunsaturated fatty acids and excess of predominant neurotransmitter glutamate, favour cell toxicity [5]. ROS can activate a self-accelerating vicious cycle leading to mitochondrial damage and neuronal cell death [6].

In epilepsy, the oxidative/antioxidative balance can have a role in both seizure controls and side effects of often life-long pharmacotherapy.

2. Pharmacotherapy of epilepsy-Valproic acid

There are a large range of antiepileptic drugs with different mechanisms of action, pharmacokinetics, pharmacology, and important side effects. Pharmacotherapy of epilepsy is symptomatic.

Valproic acid (VPA) which is an eight-carbon branched-chain fatty acid, is one of the most widely used effective antiepileptic drugs. The main mechanism of the action includes a blockade of sodium channels, activating calcium dependent potassium conductance and GABAergic effect [7]. VPA is metabolized by microsomal glucuronide conjugation, mitochondrial beta-oxidation and cytochrome P450-dependent omega-, (omega-1)-and (omega-2)-oxidation [8]. Therefore, an involvement of lipid peroxidation seems to be probable during pharmacotherapy with VPA.

Serious side effects are relatively rare but include fatal hepatotoxicity and acute haemorrhagic pancreatitis. They occur mainly in children on polypharmacy and those with organic brain disease. Hyperammonaemic encephalopathy has been reported in patients with urea cycle disorder. Benign elevation of liver enzymes is common during valproate therapy and dose depended. Thrombocytopenia and other haematological abnormalities should be controlled. Other troublesome adverse effects are weight gain, gastrointestinal disturbances, hair loss and tremors. Hormonal disturbances with polycystic ovary syndrome and risk of teratogenicity, including a 1 to 3% risk of neural tube defects, make the use of VPA in some women undesirable [7].

In numerous studies there was found to be an imbalance in oxidative status of the patient with epilepsy treated with VPA [9].

3. Role of trace elements and antioxidant enzymes in epilepsy

3.1. Iron

In several neurodegenerative diseases, iron accumulates in brain tissues. Since post-mortem examinations cannot distinguish whether iron accumulation is a cause or consequence of brain damage, it is necessary to manipulate iron to assess its causal role. In the animal model of epilepsy, iron supplementation increased damage in various brain regions, and a tight relationship between iron and zinc in micro gliosis was found [10]. In general, iron is kept safe by binding itself to protein; transported in form of transferrin-bound iron or stored in form of ferritin. The liberation of free iron can augment generation of active free radicals and it appears to play a crucial role in the posttraumatic epilepsy [11]. Iron deposition results in tissue damage by either directly damaging cells or changing the cellular environment so that it is more susceptible to toxins or other pathologic processes. On the other hand, iron is a cofactor of catalase (CAT), which plays a role in antioxidant defence systems by catalysing the decomposition of hydrogen peroxide. The proper balance of iron without excessive supplementation is very important for oxidant status.

The surrogate markers of iron status may be non-transferrin bound iron (NTBI). There was found an increase in NTBI in patients treated due to epilepsy with VPA [12].

3.2. Selenium, cooper, zinc

The trace elements selenium (Se), cooper (Cu) and zinc (Zn) are important cofactors of antioxidant enzymes such as superoxide dismutase (Cu-SOD, Zn-SOD), glutathione peroxidise (GPX) as well as protein with antioxidant properties, ceruloplasmin (CRL, copper-binding protein). SOD and GPX play a predominant role as free radical scavengers in the brain tissue, whilst CAT is deficient [13]. SOD and GPX are also important for detoxification of xenobiotics, and may be involved in the oxidative injury caused by antiepileptic drugs [14].

Results of various studies on trace elements levels and activities of main antioxidant enzymes during pharmacotherapy of epilepsy are conflicting. A selected bias of patients and different laboratory methods might be responsible, as well as the influence of lifestyle with consumption of natural antioxidants or their supplementation [4, 15, 16].

A decrease in the trace elements selenium and copper was reported in epileptic patients receiving sodium valproate [17]. One of the main selenium status marker is plasma glutathione peroxidise (GPX3). The product of plasma SOD (pSOD) activity, H_2O_2, is the major substrates for GPX3. An involvement of lipid peroxidation seems to be probable and the elevated activity of pSOD in some studies may be explained by this induction. Significant effects of duration of VPA therapy, activity of seizures and gender were found on Zn, pSOD, and erythrocyte SOD (eSOD) levels [4, 9]. Also in prospective studies [18, 19] were reported increased levels of eSOD in epileptic children after implementation of VPA treatment. Some other authors did not find a significant difference in enzyme activity or even a reduced level of pSOD was found in young people with epilepsy treated using valproate [20].

pSOD is a sensitive index of Cu status, while plasma Cu is not a reliable marker of copper status [21]. Zinc supplements can decrease SOD activity, primarily due to the antagonistic relationship between high zinc intakes and copper absorption [22, 23]. A few authors reported lower or normal Zn concentrations in persons with epilepsy [24, 25]

4. Carnitine and cellular energy

L-carnitine is the key factor in mitochondrial beta oxidation of fatty acids for the generation of metabolic energy. Apart from carrying the long-chain fatty acids into the mitochondrial matrix, it takes part in transporting from peroxysomes into mitochondria the products of oxidation of very long-chain fatty acids and in removing from mitochondria medium and short-chain fatty acids, which can be toxic at a high level. As a donor of acetyl group, it participates in the synthesis of neurotransmitter acetylocholine. It also takes part in the reaction of detoxication, including the removal of some drugs, and in chelation of iron [26].

L-carnitine is synthesized in the liver, kidneys and brain from essential amino acids lysine and methionine, with participation of the vitamins C, B_6, PP, and iron. The main source of L-carnitine in the diet is meat and dairy products. When the diet is rich in the aforementioned products and there are no liver and kidney diseases, the risk of carnitine deficiency is low. Bioavailability of carnitine from medical preparations is only ca. 20% [27].

Carnitine deficiency can result from fatty acid oxidation disorders, organic acidemias, renal insufficiency, and treatment with some drugs, as valproic acid. The clinical symptoms of L-carnitine deficiency involve brain with enhanced risk of hypoketonic-hypoglycemic and hepatic encephalopathy, or skeletal and cardiac myopathy. Carnitine deficiency in case of fatty acids oxidative disorders can cause epileptic seizures. The seizures may result from cerebral bioenergetic failure associated with acute episodes of hypoglycemic, hypoketotic encephalopathy, or hypoxic-ischemic encephalopathy due to cardiac arrhythmias and/or cardiomyopathy [28].

In numerous studies, reduced carnitine levels were found during VPA therapy, especially with prolonged use and with high dosage levels [29]. The mechanism of this may include: 1) the formation of valproylcarnitine, 2) the reduction of tubular reabsorption of carnitine in the kidneys, 3) the inhibition of selected enzymes, which take part in biosynthesis of carnitine, 4) the inhibition of the membrane carnitine transporter and 5) the impairment of recycling of carnitine from long-chain acylcarnitines by the VPA-induced decrease of mitochondrial free Co-A level. Deficiency of carnitine is one possible mechanism which explains the VPA induced hepatotoxity. Carnitine depletion can impair the urea cycle (by influence on its enzymes) and cause accumulation of ammonia, what can be found in hepatic failure [30]. The impairment of beta-oxidation can shift the metabolism of VPA toward predominantly peroxisomal gamma-oxidation, resulting in excessive production and accumulation of toxic metabolite 4-en-VPA. It is postulated that carnitine supplementation may increase the beta-oxidation of VPA and limit production of its toxic metabolites. Carnitine inhibits free radicals generation preventing the impairment of fatty acid betaoxidation in mitochondria and protects tissues from damage by repairing oxidized membrane lipids [31].

http://dx.doi.org/10.5772/57613

5. New therapeutic approaches

Some of side effects of therapy with VPA have been suggested by alteration the homeostasis of trace elements and antioxidants. Seriously increase membrane lipid peroxidation at the expense of protective antioxidants; this may lead to an increase in the frequency of seizures and an idiosyncratic drug effect.

Adequate trace elements and antioxidants supply is essential for normal brain functions, and is particularly important for protection against neurological disorders. To elucidate the mechanism of action such substances in the brain should result in new safe therapeutic approaches.

Author details

Elżbieta Płonka-Półtorak[1], Tuomas Westermarck[2], Pekka Kaipainen[2], Markus Kaski[2] and Faik Atroshi[3]

1 Antiepileptic Outpatient Clinic, Provincial Hospital No. 2, Lwowska, Rzeszow, Poland

2 Rinnekoti Research Center, Espoo, Finland

3 Pharmacology & Toxicology, University of Helsinki, Finland

References

[1] http://www.who.int/mediacentre/factsheets/fs999/en/

[2] Shorvon S. Epilepsy. ONL Series. Oxford Neurology Library. Oxford University Press, 2009.

[3] Banerjee PN, Filippi D, Allen Hauser W. The descriptive epidemiology of epilepsy-a review. Epilepsy Res 2009; 85(1):31-45.

[4] Hamed S, Abdullah M. Trace elements and electrolytes homeostasis and their relation to antioxidant enzyme activity in brain hyperexcitability of epileptic patients. J Pharmacol Sci 2004; 96:349-59.

[5] Naziroglu M. (New molecular mechanism on the activation of TRPM2 channels by oxidative stress and ADP-ribose. Neurochem Res 2007; 32:1990-2001.

[6] Patel M. Mitochondrial dysfunction and oxidative stress: cause and consequence of epileptic seizures. Free Radic Biol Med 2004; 37(12):1951–1962.

[7] Panayiotopoulos CP. Pharmacopoeia of prophylactic antiepileptic drugs. In: The epilepsies: seizures, syndromes and management. Bladon Medical Publishing, Oxfordshire (UK) 2005;pp 504-506.

[8] Perucca E. Pharmacological and therapeutic properties of valproate: a summary after 35 years of clinical experience. CNS Drugs 2002; 16:695-714.

[9] Płonka-Półtorak E, Zagrodzki P, Chłopicka J, Bartoń H, Westermarck T, Kaipainen P, Kaski M, Atroshi F. Valproic acid modulates superoxide dismutase, uric acid-independent FRAP and zinc in blood of adult epileptic patients. Biol Trace Elem Res 2011;143(3):1424-34.

[10] Shoham, S, Youdim MBH. Iron involvement in neural damage and microgliosis in models of neurodegenerative diseases. Cell. Mol. Biol 2000; 46: 743–760.

[11] Choi, BH. Oxygen, antioxidants and brain dysfunction. Yonsei Med J 1993; 34(1):1–10.

[12] Ounjaijean S, Westermarck T, Partinen M, Plonka-Poltorak E, Kaipainen P, Kaski M, Fucharoen S, Srichairatanakool S, Atroshi F. Increase in non-transferrin bound iron and the oxidative stress status in epilepsy patients treated using valproic acid monotherapy. Int J Clin Pharmacol Ther 2011; 49(4): 268-7

[13] Halliwell B, Gutteridge JM. Free radicals in biology and medicine. Oxford University Press,1999, Oxford.

[14] Maertens P, Dyken P, Graf W, et al. Free radicals, anticonvulsants, and the neuronal ceroid-lipofuscinoses. Am J Med Genet 1995; 57:225-228.

[15] Sudha K, Rao AV, Rao A. Oxidative stress and antioxidants in epilepsy. Clin Chim Acta 2001; 303:19-24.

[16] Cengiz M, Yüksel A, Seven M. The effects of carbamazepine and valproic acid on the erythrocyte glutathione, glutathione peroxidase, superoxide dismutase and serum lipid peroxidation in epileptic children. Pharmacol Res 2000;41:423-425

[17] Armutcu F, Ozerol E, Gurel A, et al. Effect of long-term therapy with sodium valproate on nail and serum trace element status in epileptic children. Biol Trace Elem Res 2004; 102:1-10.

[18] Yiş U, Seçkin E, Kurul SH, Kuralay F, Dirik E. Effects of epilepsy and valproic acid on oxidant status in children with idiopathic epilepsy. Epilepsy Res 2009; 84:232-237

[19] Yüksel A, Cengiz M, Seen M, Ulutin T Erythrocyte glutathione, glutathione peroxidase, superoxide dismutase and serum lipid peroxidation in epileptic children with valproate and carbamazepine monotherapy.J Basic Clin Physiol Pharmacol 2000; 11:73-81

[20] Solowiej E, Sobaniec W. The effect of antiepilepticdrug therapy on antioxidant enzyme activity and serum lipid peroxidation in young patients with epilepsy. Neurol Neurochir Pol 2003; 37:991-1003

[21] Harvey LJ, McArdle HJ. Biomarkers of copper status: a brief update. Brit J Nutr 2008; 99:S10–S13

[22] Mariani E, Mangialasche F, Feliziani FT, et al. Effects of zinc supplementation on antioxidantenzyme activities in healthy old subjects. Exp Gerontol 2008; 43:445-451

[23] Hughes S, Samman S. The effect of zinc supplementation in humans on plasma lipids, antioxidant status and thrombogenesis. J Am Coll Nutr 2006; 25:285-291

[24] Barbeau A, Donaldson J. Zinc, taurine, and epilepsy. Arch Neurol 1974; 30: 52-58

[25] Higashi A, Ikeda T, Matsukura M, Matsuda I. Serum zinc and vitamin E concentrations in handicapped children treated with anticonvulsants. Dev Pharmacol Ther 1982; 5:109-113

[26] Arrigoni-Martelli E, Caso V. Carnitine protects mitochondria and removes toxic acyls from xenobiotics. Drugs Exp Clin Res 2001; 27: 27–49.

[27] Verrotti A, Greco R, Morgese G, Chiarelli F. Carnitine deficiency and hyperammonemia in children receiving valproic acid with and without other anticonvulsant drugs. Int J Clin Lab Res 1999; 29(1):36-40.

[28] Tein I, Xie ZW. Reversal of valproic acid-associated impairment of carnitine uptake in cultured human skin fibroblasts. Biochem Biophys Res Commun1994; 28, 204(2): 753-8.

[29] Płonka-Półtorak E, Zagrodzki P, Chłopicka J, Bartoń H, Westermarck T, Kaipainen P, Kaski M, Atroshi F. Valproic acid modulates superoxide dismutase, uric acid-independent FRAP and zinc in blood of adult epileptic patients. Biol Trace Elem Res. 2011; 143(3):1424-34

[30] Lheureux PE, Penaloza A, Zahir S, Gris M. Science review: carnitine in the treatment of valproic acid-induced toxicity-what is the evidence? Crit Care 2005; 9(5):431-40

[31] Gulcin I. Antioxidant and antiradical activities of L-carnitine. Life Sci 2006; 78:803-811.

Chapter 12

Clinical and Hematological Profiles During Valproate Treatment of Epileptic Patients with Intellectual Disability — Case Study and Mini Review

P. Kaipainen, T. Westermarck, F. Atroshi,
M. Kaski and M. Iivanainen

Additional information is available at the end of the chapter

http://dx.doi.org/10.5772/57369

1. Introduction

Valproic acid or sodium valproate (VPA) is an antiepileptic drug commonly used for treatment of epilepsies [Aldenkamp et al. 2006; Ben-Menachem et al. 2006; Iivanainen & Alvarez 1998; Perucca et al. 2006). It affects the function of the neurotransmitter GABA in the human brain by enhancing the neurotransmission of GABA (Rosenberg, 2007). VPA is known to cause many harmful side effects such as hepatotoxicity (Koenig et al. 2006) and carnitine deficiency (Coppola et al. 2006). Carnitine as a healing agent has begun to play an important role in VPA-induced hepatotoxicity. When signs of hepatotoxicity occur, it is important to discontinue VPA immediately and substitute carnitine i.v (Koenig et al. 2006). Inhibitions of the β-oxidation, oxidative phoshorylation and urea synthesis and a decrease of intracellular carnitine are supposed to induce hepatopathy (Cotarlu & Zaldman 1988; Hjelm et al. 1987; Murakami et al. 1996). It has been reported that urinary concentration of a VPA metabolite, 4-en VPA, is markedly increased in acute VPA intoxication (Murakami et al. 1996). It is believed that this metabolite of VPA is responsible for developing hepatotoxicity. VPA metabolism returns to normal after L-carnitine supplementation (Murakami et al. 1996). Thurston & Hauhart 1993 reported that a reduction of intracellular CoA may be the central common pathway for VPA-induced hepatotoxicity.

The clinical relevance of coagulopathies, known as side effects of VPA, especially thrombocytopenia, von Willebrand disease and a decrease of factor XIII, is still unclear (Gerstner et al. 2006). The incidence of coagulation disorders related to VPA in children is estimated to be nearly 4% (Gerstner et al. 2006).

It has been reported that VPA may be associated with hyperammonemia and thrombocytopenia, but the aetiology of valproic acid-induced thrombocytopenia has not been elucidated (Mallet et al. 2004). In patients receiving long-term VPA VPA-induced hyperammonaemic encephalopathy may occur (Lheureux et al. 2005). It is suggested that this severe side-effect may be promoted by a pre-existing carnitine deficiency or by deficiency induced by VPA (Lheureux et al. 2005). Because the onset of the clinical symptoms of VPA-associated hepatotoxicity, especially in patients with intellectual disability, is sudden and unpredictable, the aim of our study was to find out suitable biochemical and haematological markers to prevent this state of illness.

2. Case presentation

Blood samples for assays of sodium (Na), potassium (K), aspartate aminotransferase (ASAT), alanine aminotranferase (ALAT), amylase, alkaline phosphatase, c-reactive protein (CRP), creatinine, haemoglobin, mean cell volume, haematocrit, erythrocytes, thrombocytes and leukocytes were obtained from ID patients with epilepsy and on VPA and from healthy persons of hospital staff after overnight fasting. All patients in this study used VPA as a monotherapy. Vacuette serum tubes were used to obtain serum samples and vacuette K_2EDTA tubes were used to obtain haematological samples. All assays were made immediately after sampling in the same day. The whole large patient material was from Rinnekoti hospital, Espoo-Finland. Sex and age varied in the VPA and control groups. Approximately 50% from the whole patient and control material was male. The mean ages for the VPA group and the control group were 37±15 years and 50±10 years, respectively. Laboratory determinations and reagents:Serum sodium (Na), potassium (K), aspartate aminotransferase (ASAT), alanine aminotransferase (ALAT), amylase, alkaline phosphatase, c-reactive protein (CRP) and creatinine were analyzed with Cobas Mira analyzer. Haemoglobin, mean cell volume (MCV), hematocrit, erythrocytes, thrombocytes and leukocytes were assayed with Sysmex KX-21N analyzer. All used reagents were reagent grade. All laboratory determinations were controlled with the control samples from Labquality Ltd, Helsinki, Finland.

3. Discussion and review

The levels of CRP and potassium (K) were higher while haematocrit and contents of thrombocytes and erythrocytes and the levels of sodium (Na), creatinine and haemoglobin were lower in the VPA group compared with the control group. All results of 14 clinical and haematological markers are shown in table 1. The results showed that thrombocyte and erythrocyte counts, haematocrit and the levels of sodium (Na), creatinine and hemoglobin were lower in the VPA group compared with the control group. Differences in haematocrit and thrombocyte and erythrocyte counts were statistically extremely significant so that these determinations besides assay of serum free carnitine can be used as markers to evaluate VPA toxicity. The haematological profile is the most common investigations patients undergo.

http://dx.doi.org/10.5772/57369

Many structural, biochemical and physiological changes take place in the brain following head trauma which in turn account for epileptogenesis (Katayama et al. 1990). For example, seizures occur in rats shortly after traumatic injury lead to increase in glutamate and aspartate levels which explain possible involvement in epileptogenesis (Nilson et al. 1994). Antiepileptic drugs affect hepatic enzyme levels in patients known to have a coexisting hepatic abnormality, those who develop symptoms of hepatic involvement while receiving AEDs, and perhaps those receiving bitherapy with high serum AED levels (Verma & Haidukewych, 1994). Rao et al. (1993) reported 72% of the AED-treated patients and 33% of the unmedicated patients showed an increase in one or several serum liver enzymes [alanine aminotransferase (ALT), aspartate aminotransferase (AST), and/or gamma-glutamyl transferase (gamma-GT)]; particularly gamma-GT.

The World Health Organisation defines anaemia as < 13 g Hb/dL for men and < 12 g Hb/dL for women (2001), accepting that women generally have lower haemoglobin concentrations than men. However, when ferritin levels (Waalen et al. 2002), is considered then the difference may be due to hormonal influences on red cell production (Shahidi, 1973), the do not support this (Waalen et al. 2002). Platelet counts have been found to be significantly higher in women (Butkiewicz et al.2006), with possible explanations of increased thrombopoietin in women being reported. Total leukocyte count showed to be significantly higher in women than men due to a highly significant difference in neutrophil count, with no significant correlation between monocytes, basophils and gender (Bain & England, 1975).

This study is in line with the earlier observations that VPA may induce thrombocytopenia (Koenig et al. 2006; Gerstner et al. 2006; Mallet et al. 2004). According to Gerstner et al. 2006 thrombocytopenia is the most common haematological adverse effect of VPA. An incidence varies from 5% to 60% (Gerstner et al. 2006; Zeller et al. 1999). It is suggested that there are two possible mechanisms inducing thrombocytopenia. First mechanism is that VPA have a direct toxic effect on bone marrow (Gertsner et al. 2006). Second mechanism is that VPA seems to induce the formation of autoantibody against platelets (Sandler et al. 1978). We found that contents of thrombocytes and erythrocytes lowered approximately 30 % and 10 %, respectively, in patients on VPA monotherapy. This observation supports the hypothesis that VPA seems to have a direct toxic effect on bone marrow (Gerstner et al. 2006).

To prevent severe hepatotoxicity in patients on long-term VPA therapy, it is important to control contents of thrombocytes and erythrocytes and to determine the level of serum free carnitine, regularly. If the level of serum free carnitine and the thrombocyte counts are lowered, addition of carnitine to long-term VPA regimen of epileptic patients may be indicated. Further investigations are needed to evaluate appropriate dosages of L-carnitine supplementation to epileptic patients on long-term VPA therapy.

Valproic acid (N-dipropylacetic acid, or 2-propylpentanoic acid) is one of the mainstays of therapy for epilepsy and bipolar mood disorders, due to its anticonvulsant and mood-stabilizing effects (Blaheta & Cinatl, 2002). It is a branched short-chain fatty acid with a half-life of 9 to 16 hours. Clinically, VPA is usually administered as uncoated tablets, but may also be administered in the form of syrup, capsules and enteric-coated tablets. Ninety per cent of VPA in the blood is bound to albumin (Cramer & Mattson, 1979), and despite its hydrophilic nature enters the CNS by crossing the blood brain barrier via passive diffusion and bidirectional carrier-mediated transport, such as an anion exchanger at the brain capillary endothelium (Perucca, 2002). VPA crosses into the brain parenchyma utilizing another set of transporters which results in higher neuronal and glial concentrations than interstitial fluid concentrations (Perucca, 2002). VPA, in addition to being an effective anticonvulsant and mood-stabilizing agent has been shown to be an effective anxiolytic (Lal et al., 1980), antidystonic and antinociceptive (Loscher, 1999), in animal studies. Clinically, VPA is effective in clinical depression (Delucchi & Calabrese, 1989), absence seizures (Coppola et al., 2004), tonic-clonic seizures, complex partial seizures (Dean & Penry, 1988), and juvenile myoclonic epilepsy (Calleja et al., 2001).

4. Haematological toxicity of valproic acid

Valproic acid has been shown to have some haematological toxicity. Acute toxicity is not common and the most adverse effects are nausea, vomiting, anorexia, thrombocytopenia, von Willebrand disease type 1, decreased factor XIII, abnormal platelet function, bleeding, haemolytic anaemia, leukopenia, leucocytosis, eosinophilia, thrombocytosis, prolonged prothrombin and thromboplastin times, fibrinogen and hematoma (Kreuz et al 1992; Gerstner et al. 2006; Gerstner et al, 2008; Pan et al 2007; Mazaira, 2008; Chen et al. 2013). However, some of these effects may lead to adverse effects and life-threatining complications such as bone marrow toxicity (Acharya & Bussel, 2000). Pharmacokinetics drug interaction involves a drug displacement from protein binding sites causing drug redistribution (McQueen & Wardell, 1971). Valproic acid is commonly used in the treatment of seizures and as a mood stabilizer in the treatment of manic depression.

Our study presents interesting clinical findings. Laboratory tests confirmed macrocytic anaemia. Thrombocytes concentrations were decreased, but other biochemical measurements such as haemoglobin were within the normal range (Table1). However, Taher et al. (2009) reported an association between divalproex sodium (DVPX) therapy and total Hb level. It has been reported that in patients treated with VAP 18% experienced at least one episode of thrombocytopenia (Nasreddine &, Beydoun, 2008). However, Rahman et al. (2009) reported 26% of his patients experienced leukopenia. The haematological complications in patients treated with VAP appear to be heterogenic depending on the period of treatment, taking other anticonvulsants, or additional medications (Hemingway et al. 1999; Antoniou et al. 2004). Valporic acid is able to alter hematopoiesis by inhibition of erythroid differentiation in the experimental K562 cell linkage (Chateauvieux et al. 2011). Ladd et al (2009) reported that an elevated level of creatinine phosphokinase is not required for a DSM-IV diagnosis of neuroleptic malignant syndrome (Ladds et al.2009). In our study creatinine phosphokinase was at levels 70 U/l compared to 82 U/l in controls. A creatinine phosphokinase level of 800,000 U/l was reported for a patient who was being treated with a conventional antipsychotic (Sanai et al. 2006).

Determinations	Patients (M±SD) (n)	Controls (M±SD) (n)	p-value	
Thrombocytes (E9/l)	186±67 (141)	259±59 (367)	1.4×10^{-23}	↓↓
Erythrocytes (E12/l)	4.1±0.43 (140)	4.5±0.4 (217)	2.1×10^{-10}	↓↓
Hematocrit	0.38±0.04 (142)	0.4±0.03 (217)	4.0×10^{-7}	↓↓
Sodium (Na) (mmol/l)	136±5.5 (49)	140±1.4 (49)	0.000016	↓
Potassium (K) (mmol/l)	4.4±0.4 (49)	4.1±0.3 (49)	0.000038	↑
Hemoglobin (g/l)	132±15 (142)	138±12 (217)	0.000100	↓
C-reactive protein (CRP) (mg/l)	28±32 (64)	10±18 (136)	0.000130	↑
Creatinine (μmol/l)	70±13 (13)	82±14 (50)	0.007600	↓
Mean cell volume (MCV) (fl)	92±3.9 (142)	91±5.0 (217)	0.028500	↑
Alanine aminotransferase (ALAT) (U/L)	21±18 (65)	41±90 (86)	0.044850	↓
Alkaline phosphatase (AFOS) (U/L)	150±53 (16)	125±41 (25)	0.134720	↑
Leukocytes (E9/l)	6.2±2.5 (140)	6.5±2.5 (217)	0.197680	↓
Aspartate aminotransferase (ASAT) (U/L)	26±14 (38)	31±22 (29)	0.330570	↓
Amylase (U/L)	205±45 (42)	192±75 (29)	0.399700	↑

M=mean value

SD=standard deviation

n=number of observations

Table 1. The levels of eight clinical and six hematological markers in patients on VPA and in control

Author details

P. Kaipainen[1], T. Westermarck[1], F. Atroshi[2], M. Kaski[1] and M. Iivanainen[1,3]

1 Rinnekoti Research Centre, FIN Espoo, Finland

2 Department of Clinical Sciences, Pharmacology & Toxicology, University of Helsinki, Finland

3 Department of Child Neurology, University of Helsinki, Finland

References

[1] Acharya S, Bussel JB. Hematologic toxicity of sodium valproate. J Pediatr Hematol Oncol. 2000 ;22(1):62-5.

[2] Aldenkamp A., Vigevano F., Arzimanoglou A & Covanis A. Role of valproate across the ages.Treatment of epilepsy in children. Acta neurological Scandinavica Supplementum;2006,184,1-13.

[3] Antoniou T, Gough K, Yoong D, Arbess G. Severe anemia secondary to a probable drug interaction between zidovudine and valproic acid.Clin Infect Dis. 2004,1;38(5): 38-40.

[4] Bain B, England J: Normal haematological values: sex difference in neutrophil count. BMJ 1975, 1:306-309.

[5] Ben-Menachem E., Schmidt B., Tomson T & Vajda F. Role of valproate across the ages. Treatment of epilepsy in adults. Acta neurologica Scandinavica Supplementum; 2006,184: 14-27.

[6] Blaheta, R. A., & Cinatl, J.,Jr. Anti-tumor mechanisms of valproate: A novel role for an old drug. Medicinal Research Reviews,2002; 22(5), 492-511.

[7] Butkiewicz AM, Kemona H, Dymicka-Piekarska V, Matowicka-Karna J, Radziwon P, Lipska A: Platelet count, mean platelet volume and thrombopoietic indices in healthy women and men. Thrombosis Res 2006, 118:199-204.

[8] Calleja, S., Salas-Puig, J., Ribacoba, R., & Lahoz, C. H. Evolution of juvenile myoclonic epilepsy treated from the outset with sodium valproate. Seizure: The Journal of the British Epilepsy Association,2001; 10(6), 424-427.

[9] Chateauvieux S, Eifes S, Morceau F, Grigorakaki C, Schnekenburger M, Henry E, Dicato M, Diederich M. Valproic acid perturbs hematopoietic homeostasis by inhibition of erythroid differentiation and activation of the myelo-monocytic pathway.Biochem Pharmacol. 2011,15;81(4):498-509.

[10] Chen HF, Xu LP, Luo ZY, Yu ZQ, Li ZY, Cui QY, Qin LM, Ren YY, Shen HS, Tang JQ, Jin LJ, Zhu JJ, Wang J, Wang KY, Wu TQ, Wang ZY. Valproic acid-associated low fibrinogen and delayed intracranial hemorrhage: case report and mini literature review. Drug Des Devel Ther. 2013,13;7:767-70.

[11] Coppola G, Auricchio G, Federico R, Carotenuto M, Pascotto A. Lamotrigine versus valproic acid as first-line monotherapy in newly diagnosed typical absence seizures: an open-label, randomized, parallel-group study.Epilepsia. 2004 ;45(9):1049-53.

[12] Coppola G., Epifanio G., Auricchio G., Federico RR., Resicato G & Pascotto A. Plasma free carnitine in epilepsy children, adolescents and young adults treated with old and new antiepileptic drugs with or without ketogenic diet. Brain & Development. 2006; 28: 358-65.

[13] Cotarlu D & Zaldman L. Valproic acid and the liver. Clinical chemistry. 1988; 34:890-897.

http://dx.doi.org/10.5772/57369

[14] Cramer, J. A., & Mattson, R. H. Valproic acid: In vitro plasma protein binding and interaction with phenytoin. Therapeutic Drug Monitoring,1979; 1(1), 105-116.

[15] Dean, J. C., & Penry, J. K. Valproate monotherapy in 30 patients with partial seizures. Epilepsia, 1988; 29(2): 140-144.

[16] Delucchi, G. A., & Calabrese, J. R. Anticonvulsants for treatment of manic depression. Cleveland Clinic Journal of Medicine,1989; 56(8): 756-761.

[17] Gerstner T, Bell N, Koenig SA. Valproate-associated reversible encephalopathy in a 3-year-old girl with Pallister-Killian syndrome. Ther Clin Risk Manag. 2008 ;4(3): 645-7.

[18] Gerstner T, Buesing D, Longin E, Bendl C, Wenzel D, Scheid B, Goetze G, Macke A, Lippert G, Klostermann W, Mayer G, Augspach-Hofmann R, Fitzek S, Haensch CA, Reuland M, Koenig SA. Valproic acid induced encephalopathy--19 new cases in Germany from 1994 to 2003--a side effect associated to VPA-therapy not only in young children. Seizure. 2006 ;15(6):443-8.

[19] Gerstner T., Teich M., Bell N., Longin E., Dempfle CE., Brand J & König S. Valproate-associated coagulopathies are frequent and variable in children. Epilepsia, 2006; 47, 1136-43.

[20] Hartwig A. Cadmium and cancer. Met Ions Life Sci. 2013;11:491-507.

[21] Hemingway C, Leary M, Riordan G, Schlegal B, Walker K. The effect of carbamazepine and sodium valproate on the blood and serum values of children from a third-world environment.J Child Neurol. 1999 Nov;14(11):751-3.

[22] Hjelm M., Oberholzer V., Seakins J., Thomas S & Kay JDS. Valproate inhibiton of urea cycle. Lancet. 1987; 923.

[23] Iivanainen M & Alvarez N. (eds). Drug treatment of epilepsy in people with intellectual disability. Journal of Intellectual Disability Research. 1998; 42 (suppl. 1), 1-92.

[24] Katayama Y, Becker DP, Tamura T, Hovda DA. Massive increases in extracellular potassium and the indiscriminate release of glutamate following concussive brain injury. J Neurosurg. 1990 ;73(6):889-900.

[25] Koenig SA, Buesing D, Longin E, Oehring R, Häussermann P, Kluger G, Lindmayer F, Hanusch R, Degen I, Kuhn H, Samii K, Jungck A, Brückner R, Seitz R, Boxtermann W, Weber Y, Knapp R, Richard HH, Weidner B, Kasper JM, Haensch CA, Fitzek S, Hartmann M, Borusiak P, Müller-Deile A, Degenhardt V, Korenke GC, Hoppen T, Specht U, Gerstner T. Valproic acid-induced hepatopathy: nine new fatalities in German from 1994 to 2003. Epilepsia. 2006;47, 2027-31.

[26] Kreuz W, Linde R, Funk M, Meyer-Schrod R, Föll E, Nowak-Göttl U, Jacobi G, Vigh Z, Scharrer I. Valproate therapy induces von Willebrand disease type I. Epilepsia. 1992;33(1):178-84.

[27] Ladds B, Thomas P, Mejia C, Hauser D. Extreme elevation of creatinine phosphokinase levels in neuroleptic malignant syndrome associated with atypical antipsychotics. Am J Psychiatry. 2009;166(1):114-5.

[28] Lal, H., Shearman, G. T., Fielding, S., Dunn, R., Kruse, H., & Theurer, K. Evidence that GABA mechanisms mediate the anxiolytic action of benzodiazepines:A study with valproic acid. Neuropharmacology,1980;19(8), 785-789.

[29] Lheureux PHR., Penaloza A., Zahir S & Gris Mireille. Science review:Carnitine in the treatment of valproic acid-induced toxicity-what is the evidence? Critical Care.2005; 9, 431-440.

[30] Loscher, W. Valproate: A reappraisal of its pharmacodynamic properties and mechanisms of action. Progress in Neurobiology,1999; 58(1), 31-59.

[31] Mallet L., Babin S & Morais JA. Valproic acid-induced hyperammonemia and thrombocytopenia in an elderly woman. The Annals of Pharmacotherapy. 2004; 38, 1643-7.

[32] Mazaira S. Haematological adverse effects caused by psychiatric drugs. Vertex, 2008; 19(82):378-86.

[33] McQueen EG, Wardell WM. Drug displacement from protein binding: isolation of a redistributional drug interaction in vivo.Br J Pharmacol. 1971;43(2):312-24.

[34] Murakami K., Sugimoto T., Woo M., Nishida N & Muro H. Effect of L-carnitine supplementation on acute valproate intoxication. Epilepsia,1996; 37, 687-689.

[35] Nasreddine W, Beydoun A. Valproate-induced thrombocytopenia: a prospective monotherapy study. Epilepsia. 2008;49(3):438-45.

[36] Nilsson P, Ronne-Engstrom E, Flink R, Ungerstedt U, Carlson H, Hillered L. Epileptic seizure activity in the acute phase following cortical impact trauma in rat. Brain Res. 1994; 637: 227–232.

[37] Pan CF, Shen MY, Wu CJ, Hsiao G, Chou DS, Sheu JR. Inhibitory mechanisms of gabapentin, an antiseizure drug, on platelet aggregation. J Pharm Pharmacol. 2007;59(9):1255-61.

[38] Perucca E., Aldenkamp A., Tallis R & Kramer G. Role of valproate across the ages. Treatment of epilepsy in the elderly. Acta neurologica Scandinavica Supplementum. 2006; 184, 28-37.

[39] Perucca, E. Pharmacological and therapeutic properties of valproate: A summary after 35 years of clinical experience. CNS Drugs,2002; 16(10), 695-714.

[40] Rahman A, Mican LM, Fischer C, Campbell AH. Evaluating the incidence of leukopenia and neutropenia with valproate, quetiapine, or the combination in children and adolescents. Ann Pharmacother. 2009 ;43(5):822-30.

[41] Rao ML, Stefan H, Scheid C, Kuttler AD, Fröscher W. Serum amino acids, liver status, and antiepileptic drug therapy in epilepsy. Epilepsia. 1993 ;34(2):347-54

[42] Rosenberg, G. "The mechanisms of action of valproate in neuropsychiatric disorders: Can we see the forest for the trees?". Cellular and Molecular Life Sciences; 2007, 64 (16): 2090–2103.

[43] Sanai T, Matsui R, Hirano T, Torichigai S, Yotsueda H, Higashi H, Hirakata H, Iida M. Successful treatment of six patients with neuroleptic malignant syndrome associated with myoglobulinemic acute renal failure.Ren Fail. 2006;28(1):51-5.

[44] Sandler RM., Emberson C., Roberts GE, Voak D., Darnborough J & Heeley AF. IgM platelet autoantibody due to sodium valproate. British Journal of Medicine.1978; 2, 1683-4.

[45] Shahidi N: Androgens and erythropoesis. NEJM 1973, 289:72.

[46] Taher AT, Musallam KM, Nasreddine W, Perrine SP, El-Hajj TI, Beydoun A. Effects of divalproex sodium on hemoglobin level.Blood Cells Mol Dis. 2009;43(1):49-52.

[47] Thurston JH & Hauhart RE. Reversal of the adverse chronic effects of the unsaturated derivative of valproic acid - 2-n-propyl-4-pentenoic acid - on ketogenesis and liver coenzyme A metabolism by a single injection of pantothenate, carnitine and acetylcysteine in developing mice. Pediatric Research.1993; 33, 72-76.

[48] Verma NP, Haidukewych D. Differential but infrequent alterations of hepatic enzyme levels and thyroid hormone levels by anticonvulsant drugs. Arch Neurol. 1994 ;51(4):381-4.

[49] Waalen J, Felitti V, Beutler E: Haemoglobin and ferritin concentrations in men and women: cross sectional study. BMJ 2002, 325:137.

[50] World Health Organization: Iron deficiency anaemia: assessment, prevention, and control; A guide for programme manager; 2001.

[51] Zeller JA., Schlesinger S., Runge U & Kessler C. Influence of valproate monotherapy on platelet activation and hematologic values. Epilepsia, 1999; 40,186-9.

Chapter 13

Anti Oxidative, Anti Peroxidative and Hepatoprotective Potential of *Phyllanthus amarus* Against Anti Tb Drugs

Sangeeta Shukla, Neelu Sinha and Amita Jaswal

Additional information is available at the end of the chapter

http://dx.doi.org/10.5772/57373

1. Introduction

The liver plays an astonishing array of vital functions in the maintenance and performance of the body. Additionally, it is also handling the metabolism and excretion of drugs and other xenobiotics from the body thereby providing protection against foreign substances by detoxifying and eliminating them (saleem et al., 2010). Large numbers of xenobiotics are reported to be potentially hepatotoxic. Free radicals generated from the xenobiotic metabolism can induce lesions of the liver and react with the basic cellular constituents such as proteins, lipids, RNA and DNA (Ajith *et al.,* 2007). A growing international health concern is Tuberculosis caused by *Mycobacterium tuberculosis* (Abdelaal *et al.,* 2009).India is the highest TB burden country accounting for one fifth (21%) of the global incidence (WHO, 2010). The first line anti-tuberculosis drugs isoniazid (INH), rifampicin (RIF), pyrazinamide (PZA) and Ethambutol(ETH)continues to be the effective drugs in the treatment of tuberculosis, however, the use of these drugs is associated with toxic reactions in tissues, particularly in the liver, leading to hepatitis (Eminzade *et al.,* 2008). This is one of the most serious adverse effects of anti-tuberculosis drugs (ATD). Liver injury or liver dysfunction is a major health problem that challenges not only health care professionals but also the pharmaceutical industry and drug regulatory agencies (saleem *et al.,* 2010). It has great capacity to detoxify and synthesize useful substances, and therefore damage to the liver has grave consequences (Devaraj *et al.,* 2011). Currently, there is no effective treatment against ATD induced hepatic damage. Plants are an important component of the health care system in India and have been found to be effective in the treatment of different diseases and are the beacon of the therapeutic sources for curing diseases from times immemorial (Merina *et al.*, 2012). *Phyllanthus amarus* Linn. is commonly known as *bhumi amla* (Joshi&Parle2007). It is reported to possess antiviral (Lee *et al.*, 1996), anticancer (Rajeshkumar *et al.*, 2002). But there is no scientific evidence for its hepatoprotective activity against ATD induced liver injury. Hence the present study was undertaken to explore the key behind the use of *P.amarus* as a hepatoprotective formulation against xenobiotics induced hepatic adverse effect.

2. Materials and methods

2.1. Chemicals

Anti TB drug *i.e,* Rifampicin, Isoniazid, Pyrazinamide as anti TB kit was generously obtained from Government TB hospital, Gwalior (M.P.). All the other chemicals used in this study were of analytical grade and were procured from Sigma–Aldrich (USA), E Merck (Germany), Ranbaxy Pvt. Ltd. and BDH Company (India).

2.2. Preparation of plant extract

Whole plant of *Phyllanthus amarus* was obtained from the authenticated ayurvedic dealer and was identified by the experts of Botany Department, Jiwaji University Gwalior, India. The shade dried plant was pulverized and extracted with 75% alcohol for 10 days with concomitant shaking and then filtered. The filtrate was evaporated in vacuum to yield a brownish powder (P. amarus) powder it was stored in refrigerator at 4°C and administered orally according to body weight of animals at different concentration.

2.3. Animal maintenance and feeding

Female albino rats of *Sprague Dawley* strain (160±10 g, b.w.) were used for the present investigation. Animals were housed in polypropylene cages under standard conditions (25±2°C temperature, 60%-70% relative humidity and 14 h light and 10 h dark) and were fed on standard pellet diet (Pranav Agro Industries Ltd., New Delhi, India) and drinking water *ad libitum*. Animals used in this study were treated and cared for in accordance with the guidelines recommended by the Committee for the Purpose of Control and Supervision of Experiments on Animals (CPCSEA), Government of India, Ministry of Culture, Chennai.

2.4. Experimental design

Animals were divided into various groups of six animals each. *P.amarus* and anti TB drugs were given alternatively for 8 weeks (3 days/week). The groups were treated as follows:

Group I: Control (normal saline, 0.9%).

Group II: *Per se* - 400mg/kg, b.w., *P.amarus* (p.o.), daily.

Group III: Experimental control-RIF+INH+PZA+ETH at 52, 70,175,140 mg/kg, b.w., (p.o.), 3days/week.

Group VI- VII: INH+RIF+PZA (as in group III) + *P.amarus* at 100, 200, 300 and 400 mg/kg, b.w., (p.o) 3days/week.

Group VIII: Positive control-Silymerin -50mg/kg b.w. (p.o.), daily.

All the animals were euthanized 24hours after the last treatment to perform various biochemical and histological analysis.

2.4.1. Blood biochemical investigations

Blood was drawn from retro-orbital venous sinus and serum was isolated. Serum Urea, Uric acid and Creatinine determined by commercially prepared kit method (E-Merck, Germany). Serum AST and ALT activity were determined with Reitman and Frankel, 1957.

2.4.2. Tissue biochemical investigations

The tissues viz., liver and kidney were quickly excised, washed in ice cold, normal saline and blotted individually freed from extraneous material on ash-free filter paper. The tissues were then homogenized separately in hypotonic buffer (0.008% NaHCO3), pH 7.4, using a Potter-Elvejham homogenizer at 600-1000 rpm in ice cold conditions.

The crude tissue homogenate was centrifuged at 2000 rpm for 15 min (0-4°C). The supernatant was collected and stored at- 20°C until used for estimating tissue biochemical parameters. Lipid Peroxidation (LPO) was determined by measuring thiobarbituric acid reactive substances (TBARS) in tissues according to Sharma and Krishnamurthy, 1968.SOD and Catalase activity were determined according to Misra and Fridovich, 1972 and Aebi, 1974 respectively.

2.4.3. Histopathological investigations

Tissues were fixed with Bouin's solution. They were later sectioned using a microtome, dehydrated in graded alcohol, embedded in paraffin section, and stained with hemotoxylin and Eosin (H & E).

2.5. Statistical analysis

Results are presented as mean ± S.E. of six animals used in each group. Data were subjected to statistical analysis through one-way analysis of variance (ANOVA) at 5% significance level followed by Student's t-test at $p \leq 0.05$(Snedecor and Cochran,1989).

3. Results — Table 1-6 and histopathology

Treatment	AST (IU/L)	ALT (IU/L)
Group I	69 ± 3.81	52 ± 2.87
Group II	74 ± 4.09	53.6±2.96
Group III	345±19.07#	188 ± 10.39#
Group IV	120.22 ± 6.65* (81.44%)	81 ± 4.48* (78.67%)
Group V	112.34 ± 6.21* (84.29%)	71 ± 3.92* (86.02%)
Group VI	100.7 ± 5.57* (88.51%)	63 ± 3.48* (91.91%)
Group VII	94.4± 5.22* (90.79%)	60 ± 3.32* (94.11%)
Group VIII	83 ± 4.59* (94.92%)	59 ± 3.26* (94.85%)
ANOVA F Value	**141.88@**	**90.172@**

Data are mean ± S.E., n=6.ANOVA (F Values at 5% level). # P≤0.05 vs. Control,*P ≤0.05 vs. ATD, @ Significant

Table 1. Therapeutic effect of *P.amarus* against ATD induced blood biochemical alterations

Treatment	SALP (U/L)	Albumin (g/dl)	Bilirubin(mg/dl)
Group I	193.3±10.68	4.1 ± 0.23	0.19 ± 0.010
Group II	220±12.16	4.0 ± 0.22	0.2±0.011
Group III	462±25.54#	3.0±0.17#	0.8± 0.044#
Group IV	381.3±21.08* (30.03%)	3.5 ± 0.19 (45.45%)	0.65± 0.036* (24.59%)
Group V	305.25±16.87* (58.33%)	3.6 ± 0.199 (54.54%)	0.58 ± 0.032* (36.06%)
Group VI	257±14.21* (76.29%)	3.7 ± 0.20* (63.63%)	0.34± 0.018* (75.4%)
Group VII	236±13.05* (84.10%)	3.8± 0.21* (72.72%)	0.32 ± 0.017* (78.68%)
Group VIII	216±11.94* (91.55%)	4.0± 0.22* (90.9%)	0.3 ± 0.016* (81.96%)
ANOVA F Value	**39.135@**	**3.631@**	**89.61@**

Table 2. Curative effect of *P.amarus* against ATD on selected serological parameters serum

Treatment	Urea (mg/dl)	Uric acid (mg/dl)	Creatinine (mg/dl)
Group I	19.5±1.08	5.3± 0.292	0.4± 0.022
Group II	24±1.33	5.6± 0.309	0.5±0.027
Group III	52.6±2.91#	10±0.552#	0.8± 0.044#
Group IV	47±2.59 (16.91%)	7.6± 0.420* (51.06%)	0.7± 0.038* (25%)
Group V	44.1±2.44* (25.67%)	6.22± 0.343* (80.42%)	0.66± 0.036* (35%)
Group VI	35.7±1.97* (51.05%)	6.1± 0.337* (82.97%)	0.6± 0.033* (66%)
Group VII	30.7±1.70* (66.16%)	6± 0.331* (88.90%)	0.575± 0.032* (75%)
Group VIII	27.8±1.544* (74.92%)	5.8± 0.320* (89.36%)	0.55± 0.030* (83%)
ANOVA F Value	**32.005@**	**20.642@**	**16.887@**

Data are mean ± S.E., n=6.ANOVA (F Values at 5% level).# P≤0.05 vs. Control,*P ≤0.05 vs. ATD,@ Significant

Table 3. *P.amarus* efficiency in reducing Anti TB drugs induced renal alterations.

Treatment	Lipid Peroxidation (n mole of TBARS/mg protein)		Reduced glutathione (μ mole / g)	
	Liver	Kidney	Liver	Kidney
Group I	0.31±0.017	0.3± 0.016	7.97± 0.441	7.5± 0.441
Group II	0.341±0.018	0.33± 0.018	8.136±0.449	7.78± 0.449
Group III	1.94±0.107#	1.28±0.071#	6.8± 0.376#	6.17± 0.376#
Group IV	0.69±0.038* (76.68%)	1.096± 0.061* (18.77%)	7.08± 0.391 (23.93%)	6.69± 0.391 (39.09%)
Group V	0.57±0.034* (84.04%)	1.096± 0.061* (18.77%)	7.18± 0.396 (32.47%)	7.0± 0.397 (62.40%)
Group VI	0.44±0.0243* (92.02%)	0.737± 0.041* (55.47%)	7.4± 0.409 (51.28%)	7.25± 0.409 (81.20%)
Group VII	0.431±0.0238* (92.57%)	0.721± 0.039* (57.04%)	7.75± 0.428 (81.19%)	7.33± 0.428 (87.21%)
Group VIII	0.335±0.018* (98.46%)	0.665± 0.037* (62.75%)	7.85± 0.434 (89.74%)	7.34± 0.434 (87.96%)
ANOVA F Value	**174.79@**	**70.42@**	**1.566**	**1.971**

Data are mean ± S.E., n=6.ANOVA (F Values at 5% level).# P≤0.05 vs. Control,*P ≤0.05 vs. ATD,@ Significant

Table 4. Effect of *P.amarus* against AT drugs treated animals in tissue biochemical estimations.

Treatment	SOD (U/min./mg protein)		Catalase (μ mole of H_2O_2 oxidised/min/mg protein)	
	Liver	Kidney	Liver	Kidney
Group I	70.7±3.908	48.78± 2.696	50.7± 2.802	70.1± 3.875
Group II	76±4.201	51.2± 2.830	51.8±2.863	62.14± 3.435
Group III	37.52±2.074#	24.39±1.348#	38.1± 2.106#	50.8± 2.808#
Group IV	44±2.432 (19.52%)	33.3± 1.840* (36.53%)	42.02± 2.322 (31.11%)	59.67± 3.298 (45.95%)
Group V	45.6±2.520 (24.35%)	35.9± 1.984* (47.19%)	42.5± 2.349 (34.92%)	59.97± 3.315 (47.51%)
Group VI	55±3.040* (52.68%)	41.15± 2.274* (68.71%)	44.05± 2.435 (47.22%)	61.96± 3.425* (57.82%)
Group VII	60.9±3.366* (70.46%)	43.13± 2.384* (76.83%)	45.2± 2.498 (56.34%)	62.1± 3.432* (58.54%)
Group VIII	68±3.759* (91.86%)	41.83± 2.312* (71.50%)	50.6± 2.775* (96.03%)	62.57± 3.458* (58.54%)
ANOVA F Value	**22.664@**	**12.569@**	**4.464@**	**2.911@**

Data are mean ± S.E., n=6.ANOVA (F Values at 5% level).# P≤0.05 vs. Control,*P ≤0.05 vs. ATD,@ Significant

Table 5. Effect of *P.amarus* on SOD, Catalase activity in liver and kidney against anti TB drugs.

Treatment	ATPase Liver	ATPase Kidney
	(mgPi/100gm/min)	
Group I	1971±108.95	2449.99±135.44
Group II	2114±116.86	2257.14±124.77
Group III	1335.71±73.84#	1785.7±98.72#
Group IV	1721.4± 95.16* (60.71%)	1814.28±100.29 (4.30%)
Group V	1864.28±103.06* (83.02%)	1907.14±105.43 (18.28%)
Group VI	1889±104.43* (87.09%)	2042.85±112.93 (38.71%)
Group VII	1966.06±108.69* (99.22%)	2149.99±118.85* (54.83%)
Group VIII	1969±108.85* (99.68%)	2107.14 ±116.48 (48.38%)
ANOVA F Value	**6.350@**	**4.696@**

Data are mean ± S.E., n=6.ANOVA (F Values at 5% level). # P≤0.05 vs. Control,*P ≤0.05 vs. ATD, @ Significant.

Table 6. Therapeutic Effect of *P.amarus* on ATPase against ATD

4. Discussion

The liver diseases remain one of the serious health problems as variedly exposed to xenobiotics. Modern medicines have little to offer for alleviation of hepatic diseases. Although *P. amarus is* reported to possess varied medicinal properties such as antiviral, anticancer, antioxidant, anti-inflammatory, hepatoprotective (Joshi and Parle, 2007), there is no previous report about the hepatoprotective activity of this plant against anti TB drugs. The present investigation reports the hepatoprotective effect of *P.amarus*. In the present study, hepatotoxicity model in albino rats was successfully produced by administering RIF, INH and PZA.

Effects of administration of Anti TB Drugs and *Phyllanthus amarus* orally on selected biochemical parameters in rat tissue and blood serum is presented in Table 1-6.

Significant rise above the normal upper limits in the measured serum transaminases in toxicant group on day 60 of the experiment was a biochemical indication of liver injury. Elevated levels of serum enzymes, AST and ALT are indicative of cellular leakage, and loss of functional integrity of cell membrane in liver (Ranawat *et al.,* 2010). Oral administration of *P. amarus* extract at doses (100, 200, 300 and 400 mg/kg) showed significant recoupment in a dose dependent manner ($P \leq 0.05$) (Table1).

The increased level of serum alkaline phosphatase is reliable marker of liver damage, which occurs due to the *de novo* synthesis by the liver cells (Muriel and Escobar, 2003). Serum albumin concentration is affected by hepatic protein and its synthesis is a typical function of normal liver cells (Thirunavukkarasu and Skthisenkaran, 2003). Bilirubin is one of the most frequent clinical test to evaluate the extent of chemically induced hepatotoxicity (Zimmerman, 1973). Toxicants administration caused significant increase in the serum alkaline phosphatase activity. Stabilization of SALP and bilirubin levels by the treatment of *P.amarus* is clear indication of improvement in functional status of liver cells. Results suggested that *P.amarus* at a dose of 400mg/kg, b.w., have protective effect on plasma membrane of hepatocytes. (Table2)

As a measure of renal function status, serum urea, uric acid and creatinine are often regarded as reliable markers (Adebisi *et al.*, 2000). Serum creatinine has been used to estimate glomerular filtration rate. Thus, elevations in the serum concentrations of these markers are indicative of renal injury (Adebisi *et al.*, 2000; Adewole *et al.*, 2007).The same was observed after toxicant administration. It may be due to dysfunctional and dystrophic changes in the liver and kidney. Experiment has shown that *P.amarus* at different doses, showed significant protective but the highest protection was obsereved at 300 and 400 mg/kg with mere difference indicating normal glomerular filtration rate thereby improved functional status of kidney. (Table 3)

Various biochemical parameters were measured in liver and kidney tissues. The levels of TBARS in liver and kidney tissues of ATD intoxicated rats were significantly elevated when compared to the level of TBARS in control animals. The increased lipid peroxidation results in changes in cellular metabolism of the hepatic and extra hepatic tissues, which ultimately leads to the whole cell deformity and cell death (Arun and Balasubramanian, 2011). The administration of herbal drug *P. amarus* at the different therapeutic doses showed reduction in TBARS level. The standard hepatoprotective drug Silymarin maintained the decreased lipid peroxidation level to the normal limits in the liver.

Concomitant cellular oxidative stress was manifested by reduced GSH levels and increased lipid peroxidation. The inverse linear relationship between the ROS level and the GSH level indicated that free radical species were generated by exposure to anti TB drugs which reduced intracellular antioxidant levels. The results indicate that, the herbal drug *Phyllanthus amarus* has very good hepatoprotective effect in liver damage. The results were presented in the Table 4.

Superoxide dismutase and Catalase mutually function as important enzymes in elimination of Reactive oxygen species (ROS). SOD is the major attractive metalloprotein in the antioxidant family. The defensive antioxidant enzyme next to SOD is CAT. CAT is an enzymatic antioxidant widely distributed in all animal tissues, and the highest activity is found in the red cells and liver. Both are the key component of the antioxidant defense system. In the present study, the observed decrease in SOD and CAT activities were presumably associated with the increased oxidative stress caused by these toxicants that might be due to low level of zinc (a metal constituent of the enzyme SOD) in liver tissue (Arun and Balasubramanian, 2011) Therapy at 200-400 mg/kg b.w. reversed the SOD and CAT activity in the liver tissues and protected from free radical induced oxidative stress. These observations are substantiated by author (Gnanadesigan *et al.*, 2011).(Table 5)

ATPase is a membrane bound enzyme. Since, phosphatase is a constituent of all the body tissues; it plays an important role in inorganic pyrophosphates activity. ATPase activity may be considered as a marker for assessing hepatocellular damage induced by hepatotoxic agents. (Table 6)

In our experiment, a concurrent fall was found in ATPase in liver after toxicants exposure. It might be due to dysfunctional and dystrophic changes in the mitochondria and cell membrane permeability. This damage was also very clearly visible in histopathological studies after toxicant administration. These observations are substantiated by other authors (Gao and Zhou, 2005; Krithika and Verma, 2009).The effect of the extracts on ATPase was as pronounced with 100mg/kg as with 200-400mg/kg b.w.

Liver damage induced by toxicant was associated with a variety of biochemical abnormalities following loss of integrity of the cell membrane or interference with normal hepatocytes metabolism and function.

The reason for hepatoprotective effect of the extracts may be due to presence of lignans and flavonoids which might have scavenged the free radical offering hepato protection.

5. Conclusion

The results of this study showed that common medicinal plant, *P. amarus* even at minimal dose 300mg/kg was found to have beneficial hepatoprotective properties in albino rats as all the major parameters showed percent protection level above 50% at dose levels 300 and 400mg/kg. All these properties make *P. amarus*, a novel herb for treating oxidative stress and anti Tb drug associated hepatic toxicity. There is, however, the need of further experiments for chronic study to exercise on excessive and prolonged use of this plant.

6. Histopathological studies

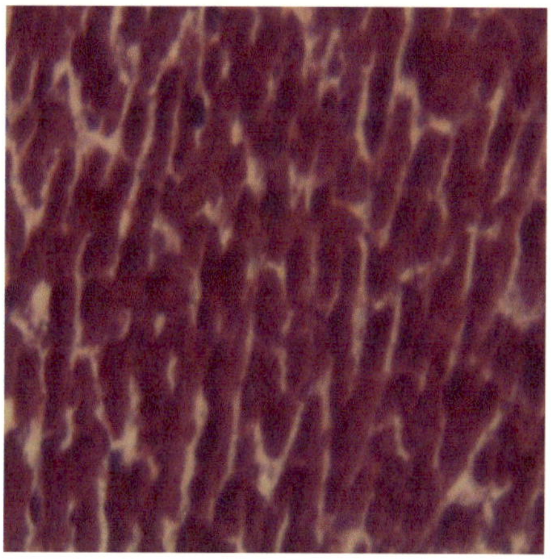

Figure 1. Hepatocytes of the normal control group showed a normal lobular architecture of the liver (400 x).

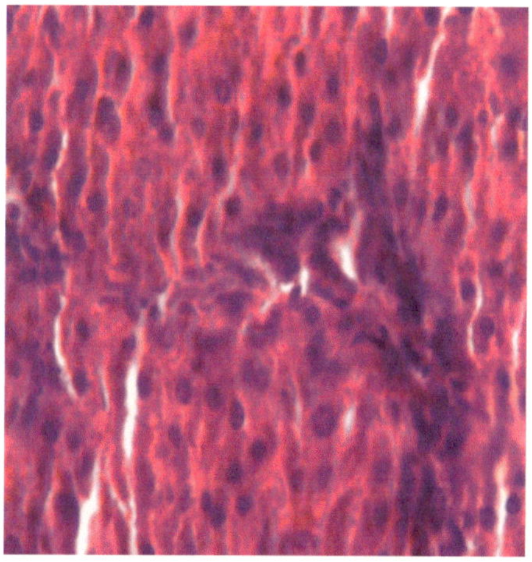

Figure 2. Hepatocytes of the INH + RIF+ PZA treated group showed liver cell necrosis and inflammation also observed in the centrilobular region with portal triaditis (400 x).

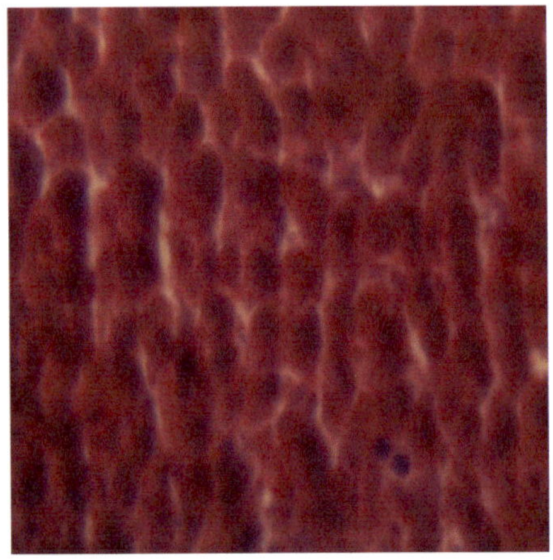

Figure 3. Hepatocytes of the *P.amarus* treated group showed cuboidal hepatocytes with moderate portal triaditis and their lobular architecture was normal (400 x).

Acknowledgements

Authors are grateful to Jiwaji University for providing lab facility and UGC for financial assistance.

Author details

Sangeeta Shukla*, Neelu Sinha and Amita Jaswal

*Address all correspondence to: profsshukla@gmail.com

School of Studies in Zoology, Jiwaji University, Gwalior, India

References

[1] Saleem TSM, Chetty CM, Ramkanth S, Rajan VST, Kumar KM, Gauthaman K (2010).Hepatoprotective Herbs – A Review. Int. J. Res. Pharm. Sci.1:1, 1-5.

[2] Ajith TA, Hema U and Aswathy MS (2007). Zingiber officinale Roscoe prevents acetaminophen-induced acute hepatotoxicity by enhancing hepatic antioxidant status. Food Chem. Toxicol.; 45(11): 2267-72.

[3] Abdelaal A, El-Ghaffar HA, Hosam M, Zaghloul E, El mashad N, Badran E and Fathy A (2009).Genotypic detection of rifampicin and isoniazid resistant Mycobacteri-

um tuberculosis strains by DNA sequencing: a randomized trial. Annals of Clinical Microbiology and Antimicrobials, 8:4.

[4] Eminzade S, Uras F and Izzettin FV. (2008). Silymarin protects liver against toxic effects of anti-tuberculosis drugs in experimental animals. Nutrition & Metabolism, 5:18.

[5] Devaraj VC, Gopala KB, Viswanatha GL, Kamath JV, Kumar S (2011). Hepatoprotective activity of Hepax-A polyherbal formulation. Asian Pacific Journal of Tropical Biomedicine. 142-146.

[6] Joshi H, Parle M (2007). Pharmacological evidences for antiamnesic potentials of *Phyllanthus amarus* in mice. African Journal of Biomedical Research, Vol. 10; 165 – 173.

[7] Lee S B, Bablanian R and Esteban M. (1996). Regulated expression of the interferon-induced protein kinase p68 (PKR) by vaccinia virus recombinants inhibits the replication of vesicular stomatitis virus but not that of poliovirus. Journal of Interferon and Cytokine Research 16, 1073-1078.

[8] Reitman and Frankel. (1957). A colorimetric method for the determination of serum glutamic oxalacetic and glutamic pyruvic transaminases. Amer. J. Clin. Pathol. 28: 56-63.

[9] Sharma SK and Krishnamurthy CR (1968). Production of lipidperoxides of brain. J Neurochem; 15: 147-9.

[10] Misra HP and Fridovich I (1972). The role of superoxide anion in the autoxidation of epinephrine and a simple assay for superoxide dismutase. J Biol Chem. 247: 3170–3175.

[11] Aebi H (1984). Catalase in vitro; Methods Enzymol. 105. 121–126

[12] Ranawat L, Bhatt J and Patel J. (2010). Hepatoprotective activity of ethanolic extracts of bark of Zanthoxylum armatum DC in CCl4 induced hepatic damage in rats. J. Ethnopharmacol. 127(3):777-780.

[13] Muriel P, EscobarY (2003). Kupffer cells are responsible for liver cirrhosis induced by carbon tetrachloride. J. App. Toxicol., 23(2):103-108.

[14] Thirunavukkarasu C, Sakthisekaran D (2003).Influence of sodium selenite on glycoprotein contents in normal and N-nitrosodiethylamine initiated and Phenobarbital promoted rat liver tumors. Pharmacol Res 48(2):167-73.

[15] Zimmerman L (1973).Podiatry and the law.J Am Podiatry Assoc, 63; 691-3.

[16] Adebisi SA, Oluboyo PO, Okesina AB (2000).Effect of drug-induced hyperuricaemia on renal function in Nigerians with pulmonary tuberculosis. Afr J Med Med Sci. 3-4:297-300.

[17] Adewole SO, Salako AA, Doherty OW, Naicker T (2007). Effect of melatonin on carbon tetrachloride-induced kidney injury in Wistar rats. Afr. *J. Biomed. Res.,* 10: 153-164.

[18] Arun K and Balasubramanian U (2011).Comapartive study on hepatoprotective activity of *phyllanthus amarus* and *eclipta prostrata* against alcohol induced in albino rats. International journal of environmental sciences volume 2:1.

[19] Gnanadesigan M, Ananad M, Ravikumar S, Maruthupandy M, Syed Ali M, Vijayakumar V, Kumaraguru AK (2011).Antibacterial potential of biosynthesized silver nanoparticles using *Avicennia marina* mangrove plant, Applied Nanoscience.

[20] Gao H, Zhou YW (2005).World. J. Gastroenterol.11, 3671.

[21] Krithika R and VERMA R J (2009). Ameliorative potential of phyllanthus amarus against carbon tetrachloride-induced hepatotoxicity. Acta Poloniae Pharmaceutica ñ Drug Research, 66(5)-579-583.

[22] Snedecor GW, Cochran, WG (1989).Statistical method.8th edition Ames,IA:Affiliated east-West Press;217-36.

[23] Rajeshkumar NV, Joy KL, Kuttan G, Ramsewak RS, Nair MG, Kuttan R (2002). Antitumour and anticarcinogenic activity of Phyllanthus amarus extract. J Ethnopharmacol.81(1):17-22.

[24] Narah M, Kalita JC, Kotoky J (2012). Medicinal plants with potential anticancer activities: a review. International Research Journal of Pharmacy.3 (6)

Chapter 14

The Pharmacology and Biochemistry of Selenium in Cancer

T. Westermarck, Arno Latvus and Faik Atroshi

Additional information is available at the end of the chapter

http://dx.doi.org/10.5772/58425

1. Introduction

Cancer is the leading cause of death in economically developed countries and the second leading cause of death in developing countries (WHO)[1]. It is extraordinarily complex with novel mutations and phenotypes that are often unique to an individual. It is a disease of the chromosomes and the problem is, in almost all cancers, it isn't just one mutation but may be much more. Cancer may be regarded as a complex metabolic deficiency disease [9, 10, 11, 12, 13, 14]

Cancer diet is also used as a complementary approach to cancer that involves the use of special nutritional supplements. Selenium (Se) and cancer is a term that can be referred to the approach or associations between cancer and nutrition that is to lower an individual's risk of cancer. Selenium was first recognized as having some nutritional importance almost six decades ago [15]. Selenium is found in food as selenoamino acids or selenoproteins, and as selenide, selenite, or selenate [16]. Selenium is a critical cofactor in the activity of gluthathione peroxidase and is also important in the management of peroxynitrite. The selenium content of food depends upon soil content and varies regionally and nationally, with soil levels relatively low in most European countries [17, 18, 19]. Soil conditions have been associated with clinical selenium toxicity in animals (selenosis) in some areas with very high selenium content, and with selenium deficiency syndromes in animals and humans in areas of low soil selenium [17].

Selenium is essential nutrient that act as cofactor in enzyme oxidation–reduction reactions (e.g. iodothyronine deiodinase and glutathione peroxidases) [20]. It maintains the specific configuration of proteins, is incorporated into the structure of hormones, and plays a structural and catalytic role in gene expression and transcriptional regulation. The trace element selenium is contained in soil and drinking water varies from area to area, which determines the variation in intake seen in different communities and the amount and chemistry of dietary constituents eaten with the this element affect the absorption efficiency of the selenium is said be 'the only trace element to be specified in the genetic code' [21].

Selenocysteine is a vital component of 35 or more selenoproteins, some of which are important enzymes [22]. Selenium functions as a redox centre, an example of which is the reduction of hydrogen peroxide and lipid and phospholipid hydroperoxides to nondamaging water and alcohols by the glutathione peroxidases [23]. Functions of this kind help maintain membrane integrity, and protect prostacyclin production. Prevention of the oxidative chain reactions in this way prevents further damage to lipids, lipoproteins, and DNA; hence its antioxidant function helps prevent atheroma and cancer, among other things [24, 25, 26].

2. Clinical applications

Selenium deficiency results in impaired immunity [27], and supplementation is immune stimulant. Deficiency increases the virulence of some viruses such as in Keshan disease [28, 29] by altering their genome to a more virulent one. Deficiency may also be associated with low mood [30], increased cognitive decline in older people, and susceptibility to epilepsy [31], exacerbates hypothyroidism in iodine deficiency [32], protective against cardiovascular disease and cancer [33, 34], beneficial in a variety of inflammatory conditions by reducing oxidative stress, and in male fertility [35] through testosterone synthesis and spermatozoa function.

The conventional cancer therapies currently available are surgery, radiotherapy, and chemotherapy. Chemotherapy is typically the main regimen for most cancers. However, many tumours develop resistance to these harsh drugs, known as chemo resistance, which can lead to other complications [36]. A number of natural products and compounds have been shown to act as effective chemo sensitizers. However, taking antioxidants during cancer treatment could interfere with the way chemotherapy work and diminish their benefits to the patient [37]. It was conclude that the use of supplemental antioxidants during chemotherapy and radiation therapy should be discouraged because of the possibility of tumour protection and reduced survival [37].This is because radiation and some chemotherapy agents work by generating free radicals, which then kill rapidly dividing cancer cells. Since antioxidants scavenge free radicals, they might interfere with the therapeutic effects of these treatments. However, oxidation supports the proliferation of malignant cells and may itself interfere with treatment [38]. People who hold this view maintain that antioxidants may counter the harmful effects of oxidation in the malignant process and thereby increase the effects of drugs or radiation therapy to the benefit of the patient. Moreover, they note that some evidence suggests that antioxidant supplements offer patients protection from the toxic effects of therapy [39].

The balance between oxidants and antioxidants can be a key issue in the development of cancer [40] and reactive oxygen species (ROS) are involved in aging, chronic illness, and cancer. Oxidants also cause free radical damage, thus the body generates large amounts of antioxidants to prevent harm and maintain health. However, Watson [41] reported that antioxidants can promote cancer growth of late stage metastatic cancers. The process is explained in terms of redox signalling, redox being a term used for reduction and oxidation. Healthy cells and also malignant ones benefit from intact Keap1/Nrf2 signalling, making a dysregulated hydroperoxide signaling a plausible explanation for the increased cancer risk in selenium deficiency [42]. Therefore, a research agenda to investigate the synergistic operation of such substances in cancer treatment is required.

3. Cancer and oxidation

Cancer is a generic term for a large group of diseases that can affect any part of the body and it can exist in many different forms and types, some of which are brought on by the destructive choices people make while others are less predictable and are not the result of destructive decisions. It can be broadly grouped into different types (Carcinomas, Sarcomas, Lymphomas and Leukaemia's), depending on which tissues they come from [43, 44]. Cancer develops when cells multiply in the presence of oxidation and other damage. According to micro-evolutionary models, cells become damaged and change their behaviour, growing uncontrollably, and act like the single-celled organisms from which they originally evolved. The cancer cells' individualism overwhelms the cooperative control processes that are essential to a complex multicellular organism [45, 46]. As cancers become malignant, they exhibit incredible genetic diversity. Whereas a benign tumour is like a colony of similar abnormal cells, a malignant tumour is a whole ecosystem. At this late stage, some (but not all) antioxidants can indeed promote cancer cell growth. Thousands of different cell types coexist: cooperating, competing, and struggling to survive. A consequence of the anaerobic conditions that prevail during the early development of a malignancy is that cancer cells differ from healthy cells, in that they have been selected for the way they generate energy (i.e. anaerobically, using glucose) [47, 48].

The sulfhydryl group is the most sensitive to the oxidizing effects of ROS among the amino acid side chains in protein; it is often involved in the intracellular transduction machinery of redox signals in response to physiological and oxidative stimuli. In fact, a variety of biological functions, not directly related to peroxidase activity, have also been reported for the Prx family [49]. Oxidative damage in DNA can cause cancer. Several antioxidant enzymes such as superoxide dismutase, catalase, glutathione peroxidase, glutathione reductase, glutathione S-transferase etc. protect DNA from oxidative stress. It has been proposed that polymorphisms in these enzymes are associated with DNA damage and subsequently the individual's risk of cancer susceptibility [50].

Nutrition and physical activity and major lifestyle changes can reduce the risk of cancer [51, 52]. Antioxidants are becoming an increasingly common choice as a hopeful cancer prevention agent. Importantly, antioxidants limit oxidative damage and thus inhibit early benign cancer growth, preventing cancer from developing. Selenium has received publicity over the past decades based on some confusing and contradictory research about whether low-selenium diets are implicated in cancer risk. To date, this is still a question without a clear answer. However, selenium is required for the proper activity of a group of enzymes collectively called glutathione peroxidase. Each of these enzymes helps to turn toxic hydrogen peroxide into harmless water. Of the eight known glutathione peroxidase enzymes, five of them require selenium. It is a necessary component for appropriate function of the immune system, muscle function, successful reproduction, and peak brain function. Also, selenium produces valuable antioxidant enzymes. Deficiencies in selenium have been linked to decreased thyroid function, cardiovascular disease, and cancers [24]. Research shows selenium, especially when used in conjunction with vitamin C, vitamin E and beta-carotene, works to block chemical reactions that create free radicals in the body (which can damage DNA and cause degenerative change in cells, leading to cancer). Also research has demonstrated that selenium is also linked to reduction in risk to some carcinomas [6, 7].

4. Pathophysiology of cancer and causes

Cancer is a disease of regulation of tissue growth. In this disease, the cells of the body display uncontrolled growth, invasion that intrudes and destroys adjacent tissues and spreads to other body locations. In order for a normal cell to transform into a cancer cell, genes which regulate cell growth and differentiation must be altered and DNA repair genes are altered and turned off [53, 54]. The pathophysiology of cancer is a complicated issue. Genes that are influenced in the pathogenesis of cancer are proteins that are involved in a variety of processes including cell growth and differentiation, cell cycle processes, and angiogenesis, which is the formation of new blood vessels [55]. These proteins also play a role in tumour progression, immune regulation, and apoptosis. Since the cells involved are complex and have such a broad range of functions, the pathophysiology of cancer has been hard to determine precisely.

Understanding what causes cancer is a complex process. Cancer has been linked to many factors, such as environmental exposures, lifestyle practices, medical interventions, genetic traits, viruses, familial susceptibility, and aging. Cancer is most probably the result of interactions between repeated carcinogenic exposures and an individual's susceptibility status [56]. Environmental exposures and lifestyle practices have been determined to be the major risk factors in the development of cancer [57, 58]. The major lifestyle factors that contribute to cancer include smoking, alcohol, diet, medical practices, and ultraviolet exposures.

Genes that are influenced in the pathogenesis of lung cancer are proteins that are involved in a variety of processes including cell growth and differentiation, cell cycle processes, and angiogenesis, which is the formation of new blood vessels. The proteins also play a role in tumour progression, immune regulation, and apoptosis [59, 60]. Since the cells involved are complex and have such a broad range of functions, the pathophysiology of lung cancer has been hard to determine precisely. A healthy cell becomes a cancer cell by undergoing the following processes in which proto-oncogenes are changed to oncogenes. Proto-oncogenes are genes that are coded to maintain normal cell growth. In cases of a developing cancer, oncogene takes its place. Oncogene is a gene that makes cells grow and divide rapidly [61]. Pharmaceutical companies are continuing to develop approaches for targeting oncogene activity in the ongoing war on cancer [61]. Pathology of cancers and other complex disorders have undergone a big change after development of technologies like immunohistochemistry, flow cytometry, and molecular biologic approaches to cancer diagnosis. Cancer is not a singular, specific disease but a group of variable tissue responses that result in uncontrolled cell growth [56].

5. Selenium mechanism

The biochemistry of selenium differs from other dietary minerals and trace elements. Selenium is not a structural component nor a metal coordination complex and the biosynthesis of selenocysteine is regulated by four genes and begins with the aminoacylation of the amino acid serine by the enzyme serine synthetase to produce Ser-tRNASec [62, 63]. However, selenocysteine is the active site in which, at physiological pH, selenium is fully ionized and is a very efficient redox catalyst [64]. Selenium exists in elemental, organic, and inorganic forms, with four important oxidation states: selenide (Se 2−), elemental (Se0) selenite (Se+4), and selenate (Se+6) [62, 65]. Selenium compounds inhibit signaling enzymes such as protein kinase C (PKC) [66] that play crucial roles in tumor promotion. The selenium-containing nutrient, selenomethionine has been shown to regulate the tumor suppresser p53 by the redox factor refl-dependent redox mechanism. Studies continue to support evidence that one important pathway is that many selenium-containing nutrients can be converted in the body to methylselenol. Methylselenol has been shown to block expansion of pre-malignant cells forming into fully developed cancers [67]. Several pathways have been proposed that could explain how selenium-containing compounds could block mutated cells from progressing to cancer. Methylseleninic acid has been shown to inhibit NF-kappa B and regulate I kappa B in prostate cancer cells [68]. Selenium compounds inhibit signaling enzymes such as protein kinase C (PKC) [66] that play crucial roles in tumor promotion. A representative of the hydrogen selenide metabolic pool has been found to protect liver cells against damage to DNA. The cellular redox-milieu involves several metabolic, antioxidative and regulatory aspects that are maintained and regulated largely by two enzyme-based systems: the glutathione and thioredoxin systems [69] The thioredoxin and glutathione systems constitute a balanced redox network. The thioredoxin system may influence virtually all phases of tumorgenesis via its involvement in transcription and translation [69].

There are several possible mechanisms for the protective effect of selenium. Selenium activates an enzyme in the body called glutathione peroxidase that protects against the formation of free radicals—those loose molecular cannons that can damage DNA. There appear to be at least two distinct families of selenium-containing enzymes [70, 71]. The first includes glutathione peroxidases Bermano et al [72] and thioredoxin reductase [73], which are involved in controlling tissue concentrations of highly reactive oxygen-containing metabolites. These metabolites are essential at low concentrations for maintaining cell-mediated immunity against infections but highly toxic if produced in excess.

The role of selenium in the cytosolic enzyme glutathione peroxidase (GPx) was first illustrated [74, 75]. During stress, infection, or tissue injury, selenoenzymes may protect against the damaging effects of hydrogen peroxide or oxygen-rich free radicals. This family of enzymes catalyses the destruction of hydrogen peroxide or lipid hydroperoxides according to the following general reactions:

Selenium-containing glutathione peroxidases (GPx) constitute a family of anti-oxidative enzymes that are capable of reducing organic and inorganic hydroperoxides to the corresponding hydroxy compounds utilizing glutathione or other hydrogen donors as reducing equivalents

$$\begin{aligned} &H_2O_2 + 2GSH \cdots\cdots\cdots\cdots 2H_2O + GSSG \\ &ROOH + 2GSH \cdots\cdots\cdots\cdots ROH + H_2O + GSSG \end{aligned} \tag{1}$$

Where GSH is glutathione and GSSG is its oxidized form. At least four forms of GPx exist; they differ both in their tissue distribution and in their sensitivity to selenium depletion [72]. The GPx enzymes of liver and blood plasma fall in activity rapidly at early stages of selenium deficiency. In contrast, a form of GPx associated specifically with phospholipid-rich tissue membranes is preserved against selenium deficiency and is believed to have broader metabolic roles (e.g., in prostaglandin synthesis) [76]. In concert with vitamin E, selenium is also involved in the protection of cell membranes against oxidative damage. The selenoenzyme thioredoxin reductase is involved in disposal of the products of oxidative metabolism [77]. It contains two selenocysteine groups per molecule and is a major component of a redox system with a multiplicity of functions, among which is the capacity to degrade locally excessive and potentially toxic concentrations of peroxide and hydroperoxides likely to induce cell death and tissue atrophy [76].

There is strong evidence that oxidative free radicals have a role in the development of degenerative diseases including CHD [78]. Oxidative free radicals increase the peroxidation of low density lipoprotein thereby increasing its uptake by macrophages with increased foam cell formation and atherosclerosis [79], though other mechanisms may exist. Anti-oxidants in the diet include vitamin A (carotenoids, which are metabolised to retinol), vitamin C (ascorbate), vitamin E (tocopherol), and selenium, which is an integral part of the antioxidant enzyme glutathione peroxidase:

6. Selenium function

Despite an evident progress in cancer diagnosis and treatment, there is a constant need of a drug which could arrest the premalignant process, thus reducing the risk of cancer. However, the role of selenium (Se) as an antioxidant and anticancer agent is well documented [80]. In addition, it has been proven that an adequate concentration of selenium can restore the sensitivity to chemotherapeutic agents of cytostatic-resistant malignant cells [81]. Selenium can exist with oxidation state-2,+2,+4,+6, and Se (II) is the dominant form in organoselenium chemistry [82]. The highest activity as a free radical scavenger and anticancer agent is assigned to selenium compounds containing selenium at the+4 oxidation level [83]. Other essential role of selenium in human and animal nutrition is well established. In humans, it has been demonstrated that an endemic cardiomyopathy (Keshan disease) prevalent in certain areas of China is correlated with selenium deficiency [84, 85]. Selenium is often thought to be a dietary antioxidant, but the antioxidant effects of selenium are most likely due to the antioxidant activity of proteins that have this element as an essential component (i.e., selenium-containing proteins), and not to selenium itself [86]. The damage to cells caused by free radicals, especially the damage to DNA, may play a role in the development of cancer and other health conditions [40]. Many observational studies, including case–control studies and cohort studies, have been conducted to investigate whether the use of dietary antioxidant supplements is associated with reduced risks of cancer in humans. Overall, these studies have yielded mixed results [87]. Healthy Chinese men and women at increased risk of developing esophageal cancer and gastric cancer were randomly assigned to take a combination of 15 milligrams (mg) beta-carotene, 30 mg α-tocopherol, and 50 micrograms (μg) selenium daily for 5 years or to take no antioxidant supplements. The initial results of the trial showed that people who took antioxidant supplements had a lower risk of death from gastric cancer but not from oesophageal cancer. However, their risks of developing gastric cancer and/or esophageal cancer were not affected by antioxidant supplementation [88].

As an essential trace element in humans [89], it's only established function is its presence in the enzyme glutathione peroxidase [90]. Using GSH2 as the reducing equivalent, this enzyme plays a significant role in detoxification of peroxides induced by oxygen radicals. As such it may be important in the toxicity of anticancer treatments that generate such reactive molecules [91]. In addition, epidemiological and experimental data suggest an anti-carcinogenic activity by selenium [92]. Considerable epidemiological data suggests that cancer mortality is inversely correlated with selenium consumption. Chemoprotective effect of diphenylmethyl selenocyanate against cyclophosphamide (CP) induced cellular toxicity and antitumor efficacy was evaluated in mice bearing Ehrlich ascites carcinoma [93], their results indicate that diphenylmethyl selenocyanate has the potential to reduce the cellular toxicity of CP at the same time improving its antitumor efficacy. Supplementation of a torula yeast-based diet with 2.5 or 5.0 ppm Selenium as Na_2SeO_3 also significantly increased the survival time of EAT-bearing mice [94]. Their data show that the form and mode of administration of selenium influence the antitumorigenic properties of this trace element. In addition, they suggested that some intermediate in the normal pathway for selenium detoxification is probably responsible for this trace element's antitumorigenic properties [94]. The ability of selenium to inhibit or prevent the growth of Ehrlich as cites tumour cells was highly dependent upon the form and quantity of selenium administered [95]. The only significant alteration that has been observed in mice treated with quantities of selenium at dosages of 4μg 3 times weekly was a slight reduction in intestinal weights. The reduction in intestinal weights was not attributable to a reduction in the intestinal macro constituents, suggesting that selenium may have altered rapidly dividing cells [95]. In fact selenocystine was used in the treatment of human leukaemia in 1956 with some short term success [96, 97]. The mechanism of its effect was thought to be competitive deprivation of cystine, but this was not proven. Others have shown that selenium compounds can cause chromosome breaks and inhibit critical DNA synthetic enzymes [98]. Specific incorporation of selenium into RNA molecules has been observed in several bacterial species. Since in a number of instances modified bases in RNAs have been shown to be involved in regulatory functions of the RNAs, the selenium-modified bases may have similar roles.

Furthermore, some RNA viruses, as well as leader mRNAs contain RNA-like segments that may interact with specific enzymes and, thus, play regulatory roles [99]· Hence, it is reasonable to assume that detailed information concerning selenium-modified RNAs may contribute to the understanding of the biological roles of selenium [100]. Near toxic levels of selenium have been reported to produce tumours in rats but other studies indicated that these concentrations of selenium created chronic toxic hepatitis that resembled hyperplasia.

In mammals glutathione peroxidase is the only selenium-dependent enzyme so far identified, but it seems unlikely that the complicated biological effects of selenium in man and animals are attributable solely to variations in the level of this enzyme. In fact, at least two other seleno proteins of unknown catalytic activity have been detected in animals. Investigations in a variety of animal systems have suggested that there is a significant interaction of selenium with glutathione independent of the enzyme glutathione peroxidase [101]. White muscle disease (WMD), a degenerative muscle disease, found in domestic animals [102, 103]. It is caused by a deficiency of selenium and/or vitamin E. Selenium and vitamin E deficiencies can produce symptoms of ill thrift and reproductive losses: lower conception rates, fetal reabsorption, dystocia, retained placenta, reduced milk production, and reduced semen quality, poor rate of growth or ill thrift in young lambs, low wool yields and have increased incidence of periodontal disease [102, 103]. Selenium appears to be a key nutrient in counteracting the development of virulence and inhibition of HIV progression to AIDS. It is required for sperm motility and may reduce the risk of miscarriage. Selenium deficiency has been linked to adverse mood states and some findings suggest that selenium deficiency may be a risk factor in cardiovascular diseases [104]. Studies continue to confirm that people with higher levels of selenium in their blood have lower rates of prostate and lung cancers [105].

Selenium is synergistic with vitamin E; they serve related metabolic functions and share in common the role of endogenous antioxidants [106]. Vitamin E has a free radical Scavenger, and Se as a component of the peroxide reducing enzyme, glutathione peroxidase. Vitamin E restricts the formation of peroxides by neutralizing free radicals, an integral component of glutathione peroxidase, an enzyme responsible for the removal of hydrogen peroxide and organic hydroperoxides [107].

Selenium and vitamin C; CH_3SeH is thought to be a critical metabolite in Se chemoprevention [108, 109]. The family of selenoenzymes called thioredoxin reductases catalyze the NADPH-dependent reduction of oxidized thioredoxin, hyperoxides, dehydroascorbate, ubiquinol and other substrates [110].The action of thioredoxin reductases in recycling dehydroascorbate to ascorbate (vitamin C) now explain the synergistic action of selenium and vitamin C [111]. The thioredoxin system is also capable of regenerating proteins inactivated by ROS. Daily supplementation with vitamin C (120 mg), vitamin E (30 mg), beta-carotene (6 mg), and the minerals selenium (100 μg) and zinc (20 mg) for a median of 7.5 years had no effect on the incidence of cancer or cardiovascular disease or on all-cause mortality [112]. Antioxidant and mineral supplementation was associated with lower total cancer incidence and all-cause mortality among men but not among women, and with an increase in skin cancer incidence, including melanoma, among women but not among men [113].

Selenium and Silver; Selenium serves as a major protective factor in precipitating the silver in a highly insoluble and hence inert form of silver selenide. Although some of this may be taken up in lysosomes in macrophages, the deposits are essentially long lived or permanent [114]. A lack of positive effect of Se supplementation on the prostate cancer incidence was observed in this study.

7. Conclusion

Selenium as non-metals is an essential nutrient that acts as cofactor in enzyme oxidation–reduction reactions. It maintains the specific configurations of proteins, is incorporated into the structure of hormones, and plays a structural and catalytic role in gene expression and transcriptional regulation. In the physiological dosage range, Se appears to function as an antimutagenic agent, preventing the malignant transformation of normal cells and the activation of oncogenes. These protective effects of Se seem to be primarily associated with its presence in the glutathione peroxidases, which are known to protect DNA and other cellular components from damage by oxygen radicals. Selenoenzymes are also known to play roles in carcinogen metabolism, in the control of cell division, oxygen metabolism, detoxification processes, apoptosis induction and the functioning of the immune system. Other modes of action, either direct or indirect, may also be operative, such as the partial retransformation of tumor cells and the inactivation of oncogenes.

Author details

T. Westermarck[1*], Arno Latvus[2] and Faik Atroshi[3]

*Address all correspondence to: tuomas.westermarck@ppa.inet.fi

1 Rinnekoti Research Center, Espoo, Finland

2 Hankintatukku Oy, Museokatu, Helsinki, Finland

3 Pharmacology & Toxicology, University of Helsinki, Finland

References

[1] WHO, World Health Organization. The Global Burden of Disease: 2004 Update. Geneva: World Health Organization; 2008.

[2] Meyskens, F. L., Jr., & Szabo, E. Diet and cancer: the disconnect between epidemiology and randomized clinical trials. Cancer Epidemiol Biomarkers Prev, 2005, 14(6), 1366-1369.

[3] Bjelakovic, G; Nikolova, D; Gluud, LL; Simonetti, RG; Gluud, C (2012). "Antioxidant supplements for prevention of mortality in healthy participants and patients with various diseases". In Bjelakovic, Goran. Cochrane database of systematic reviews (Online) 3: CD007176.

[4] Imlay JA. Pathways of oxidative damage. Annu Rev Microbiol. 2003;57:395-418.

[5] Rayman MP. Food-chain selenium and human health. Br J Nutr. 2008;100:254-268.

[6] Clark LC, Combs GF Jr, Turnbull BW, Slate EH, Chalker DK, Chow J, Davis LS, Glover RA, Graham GF, Gross EG, Krongrad A, Lesher JL Jr, Park HK, Sanders BB Jr, Smith CL, Taylor JR. Effects of selenium supplementation for cancer prevention in patients with carcinoma of the skin. A randomized controlled trial. Nutritional Prevention of Cancer Study Group. JAMA. 1996 Dec 25;276(24):1957-63.

[7] Clark LC, Jacobs ET. Environmental selenium and cancer: risk or protection? Cancer Epidemiol Biomarkers Prev. 1998 Oct;7(10):847-8.

[8] Combs G.F. Selenium in global food systems. Br. J. Nutr. 2001;85:517–547.

[9] Tallberg T, Westermarck T, Atroshi F. Cancer Treatment, Based on Active Nutritional Bio-Modulation, Hormonal Therapy and Specific Autologous Immunotherapy.In: Heavy Metals in the Environment (editors: Zueng-Sang Chen, Dar-Yuan Lee, Tser-Sheng Lin). Publisher, National Taiwan UniversityTaipei, Taiwan.

[10] DeBerardinis RJ. Is cancer a disease of abnormal cellular metabolism? New angles on an old idea. Genet Med. 2008 Nov;10(11):767-77.

[11] Anand P, Kunnumakkara AB, Kunnumakara AB, Sundaram C, Harikumar KB, Tharakan ST, Lai OS, Sung B, Aggarwal BB (September 2008). "Cancer is a preventable disease that requires major lifestyle changes". Pharm. Res. 25 (9): 2097–116.

[12] Seyfried TN, Shelton LM. Cancer as a metabolic disease. Nutr Metab (Lond). 2010 Jan 27;7:7. doi: 10.1186/1743-7075-7-7.

[13] Tallberg, T and Atroshi F. Prostate Cancer, the Long Search for Etiologic and Therapeutic Factors: Dietary Supplementation Avoiding Invasive Treatment. In: Prostate Cancer – From Bench to Bedside, 33-52, 2011.

[14] Crohns M, Westermarck T and Atroshi F. Prostate Cancer, Inflammation and Antioxidants. In :Advances in Prostate Cancer. (Gerhard Hamilton, ed.), 2013, INTECH Publisher, Croatia. 978-953-51-0932-7.

[15] Schwarz, K., and C. M. Foltz. 1957. Se as an integral part of factor against dietary liver degeneration. J. Am. Chem. Society 79:3292-3296.

[16] Sunde RA. Regulation of glutathione peroxidase-1 expression. In: Hatfield DL, Berry MJ, Gladyshev VN, editors. Selenium: its molecular biology and role in human health. 2nd ed. New York: Springer Science Media; 2006. p. 149–60.

[17] Kabata-Pendias A. Geochemistry of selenium. J Environ Pathol Toxicol Oncol. 1998;17(3-4):173-7.

[18] Haug A, Graham RD, Christophersen OA, Lyons GH. How to use the world's scarce selenium resources efficiently to increase the selenium concentration in food. Microb Ecol Health Dis. 2007 Dec;19(4):209-228.

[19] Sioen, I., Boon, P.E., Huybrechts, I. et al. (2010) Long-term dietary exposure to selenium in young children living in different European countries. Scientific Report submitted to EFSA.

[20] Kraus RJ, Prohaska JR, Ganther HE. Oxidized forms of ovine erythrocyte glutathione peroxidase. Cyanide inhibition of a 4-glutathione:4-selenoenzyme. Biochim Biophys Acta. 1980 Sep 9;615(1):19-26.

[21] Hatfield DL, Gladyshev VN. How selenium has altered our understanding of the genetic code. Mol Cell Biol. 2002 Jun;22(11):3565-76.

[22] Johansson L, Gafvelin G, Arnér ES. Selenocysteine in proteins-properties and biotechnological use. Biochim Biophys Acta. 2005 Oct 30;1726(1):1-13.

[23] Stadtman TC. Discoveries of vitamin B12 and selenium enzymes. Annu Rev Biochem. 2002;71:1-16.

[24] Rayman MP. The importance of selenium to human health.Lancet. 2000 Jul 15;356(9225):233-41.

[25] Donovan J, Copeland PR. The efficiency of selenocysteine incorporation is regulated by translation initiation factors. J Mol Biol. 2010 Jul 23;400(4):659-64.

[26] Bjelakovic G, Nikolova D, Gluud LL, Simonetti RG, Gluud C. Antioxidant supplements for prevention of mortality in healthy participants and patients with various diseases. Cochrane Database Syst Rev. 2012 Mar 14;3:CD007176. doi: 10.1002/14651858.CD007176.pub2.

[27] Arthur JR, McKenzie RC, Beckett GJ. Selenium in the immune system. J Nutr. 2003 May;133(5 Suppl 1):1457S-9S.

[28] Diplock AT. Metabolic and functional defects in selenium deficiency. Philos Trans R Soc Lond B Biol Sci. 1981 Aug 14;294(1071):105-17.

[29] Chen X. Selenium and cardiomyopathy (Keshan disease). Acta Pharmacol Toxicol (Copenh). 1986;59 Suppl 7:325-30.

[30] Hawkes WC, Hornbostel L. Effects of dietary selenium on mood in healthy men living in a metabolic research unit. Biol Psychiatry. 1996 Jan 15;39(2):121-8.

[31] Majkowski J, Atroshi F, Westermarck T. Effects of Epileptic Seizures and Antiepileptic Drugs on Oxygen Stress. Factors Attenuating the Effects of Oxygen Stress. EPILEPTOLOGY 2011, 19:143-157.

[32] Zimmermann MB, Köhrle J. The impact of iron and selenium deficiencies on iodine and thyroid metabolism: biochemistry and relevance to public health. Thyroid. 2002 Oct;12(10):867-78.

[33] Whanger PD. Selenium and its relationship to cancer: an update.Br J Nutr. 2004 Jan; 91(1):11-28.

[34] Aboul-Fadl T. Selenium derivatives as cancer preventive agents. Curr Med Chem Anticancer Agents. 2005 Nov;5(6):637-52.

[35] Hansen JC, Deguchi Y. Selenium and fertility in animals and man--a review. Acta Vet Scand. 1996;37(1):19-30.

[36] Gupta D, Raina V, Rath GK, Shukla NK, Mohanti BK, Sharma DN. Clinical and pathological response rates of docetaxel-based neoadjuvant chemotherapy in locally advanced breast cancer and comparison with anthracycline-based chemotherapies: eight-year experience from single centre. Indian J Cancer. 2011 Oct-Dec;48(4):410-4.

[37] Lawenda BD, Kelly KM, Ladas EJ, Sagar SM, Vickers A, Blumberg JB. Should supplemental antioxidant administration be avoided during chemotherapy and radiation therapy? J Natl Cancer Inst. 2008 Jun 4;100(11):773-83. doi: 10.1093/jnci/djn148. Epub 2008 May 27.

[38] Borek C, Ong A, Mason H. In vitro transformation of human cells by radiation. Toxicol Ind Health. 1987 Sep;3(3):397-404.

[39] Casciari JJ, Riordan NH, Schmidt TL, Meng XL, Jackson JA, Riordan HD. Cytotoxicity of ascorbate, lipoic acid, and other antioxidants in hollow fibre in vitro tumours. Br J Cancer. 2001 Jun 1;84(11):1544-50.

[40] Valko M, Rhodes CJ, Moncol J, Izakovic M, Mazur M. Free radicals, metals and antioxidants in oxidative stress-induced cancer. Chem Biol Interact. 2006;160:1–40.

[41] Watson J. Oxidants, antioxidants and the current incurability of metastatic cancers. Open Biol. 2013 Jan 8;3(1):120144.

[42] Brigelius-Flohé R, Kipp AP. Selenium in the redox regulation of the Nrf2 and the Wnt pathway. Methods Enzymol. 2013;527:65-86.

[43] Cancer Research UK "How many different types of cancer are there? CancerHelp UK". Retrieved 11 May 2012.

[44] Lebeau A, Kriegsmann M, Burandt E, Sinn HP. [Invasive breast cancer: the current WHO classification]. Pathologe. 2014 Feb;35(1):7-17. doi: 10.1007/s00292-013-1841-7.

[45] Hanahan, D ; Weinberg, R A. (2011). "Hallmarks of Cancer: The Next Generation". Cell 144 (5): 646–74.

[46] Danaei G, Vander Hoorn S, Lopez AD, Murray CJ, Ezzati M (2005). "Causes of cancer in the world: comparative risk assessment of nine behavioural and environmental risk factors". Lancet 366 (9499): 1784–93

[47] Warburg O. On the origin of cancer cells. Science. 1956 Feb 24;123(3191):309-14.

[48] Villalba M, Rathore MG, Lopez-Royuela N, Krzywinska E, Garaude J, Allende-Vega N. From tumor cell metabolism to tumor immune escape. Int J Biochem Cell Biol. 2013 Jan;45(1):106-13.

[49] Butterfield LH, Merino A, Golub SH, Shau H. From cytoprotection to tumor suppression: the multifactorial role of peroxiredoxins. Antioxid Redox Signal. 1999 Winter; 1(4):385-402.

[50] Asim M, Khan LA, Husain SA, Husain S, Sarma MP, Ahmad I, Sharma JK, Sharma A, Sharma S, Thayumanavan L, Kar P. Genetic polymorphism of glutathione S transferases M1 and T1 in Indian patients with hepatocellular carcinoma.Dis Markers. 2010;28(6):369-76.

[51] Doyle C, Kushi LH, Byers T, Courneya KS, Demark-Wahnefried W, Grant B, McTiernan A, Rock CL, Thompson C, Gansler T, Andrews KS. Nutrition and physical activity during and after cancer treatment: an American Cancer Society guide for informed choices. CA Cancer J Clin. 2006 Nov-Dec;56(6):323-53.

[52] Anand P, Kunnumakkara AB, Sundaram C, Harikumar KB, Tharakan ST, Lai OS, Sung B, Aggarwal BB. Cancer is a preventable disease that requires major lifestyle changes. Pharm Res. 2008 Sep;25(9):2097-116.

[53] Braig M, Schmitt CA. Oncogene-induced senescence: putting the brakes on tumor development. Cancer Res. 2006 Mar 15;66(6):2881-4.

[54] Baylin SB, Ohm JE. Epigenetic gene silencing in cancer-a mechanism for early oncogenic pathway addiction? Nat Rev Cancer. 2006 Feb;6(2):107-16.

[55] Suzuki H, Asakawa A, Amitani H, Fujitsuka N, Nakamura N, Inui A. Cancer cachexia pathophysiology and translational aspect of herbal medicine. Jpn J Clin Oncol. 2013 Jul;43(7):695-705. doi: 10.1093/jjco/hyt075. Epub 2013 Jun 4.

[56] Fraumeni JF Jr. Epidemiologic approaches to cancer etiology. Annu Rev Public Health. 1982;3:85-100.

[57] Chlebowski RT. Reducing the risk of breast cancer. N Engl J Med. 2000 Jul 20;343(3): 191-8.

[58] Lichtenstein GR. Reduction of colorectal cancer risk in patients with Crohn's disease. Rev Gastroenterol Disord. 2002;2 Suppl 2:S16-24.

[59] Wick, M., Dubey, P., Koeppen, H., Siegel, C. T., Fields, P. E., Chen, L., Bluestone, J. A., Schreiber, H. Antigenic cancer cells grow progressively in immune hosts without evidence for T cell exhaustion or systemic anergy J. Exp. Med. 1997,186,229-238.

[60] Rosenberg, S. A. Progress in human tumour immunology and immunotherapy Nature, 2001, 411,380-384.

[61] Chin L, Gray JW. Translating insights from the cancer genome into clinical practice. Nature. 2008 Apr 3;452(7187):553-63. doi: 10.1038/nature06914.

[62] Rotruck JT, Pope AL, Ganther HE, Swanson AB, Hafeman DG and Hoekstra WG. Selenium: biochemical role as a component of glutathione peroxidase. Science 1973 Feb 9;179(73):588-90.

[63] Leinfelder, W., Forchhammer, K., Veprek, B., et al., In vitro synthesis of selenocysteinyl-tRNA (UCA) from seryl-tRNA (UCA): involvement and characterization of the selD gene product. Proc. Natl. Acad. Sci. USA 1990:87;543-547.

[64] Reddy CC, Massaro EJ. Biochemistry of selenium: a brief overview. Fundam Appl Toxicol. 1983 Sep-Oct;3(5):431-6.

[65] Stadtman TC. SELENIUM BIOCHEMISTRY. Annu. Rev. Biochem. 1990. 59:111-127.

[66] Gopalakrishna R, Gundimeda U. Antioxidant regulation of protein kinase C in cancer prevention. J Nutr. 2002 Dec;132(12):3819S-3823S.

[67] Zeng H, Cheng WH, Johnson LK. Methylselenol, a selenium metabolite, modulates p53 pathway and inhibits the growth of colon cancer xenografts in Balb/c mice. J Nutr Biochem. 2013 May;24(5):776-80.

[68] Pillai SS, Sugathan JK, Indira M. Selenium downregulates RAGE and NFκB expression in diabetic rats. Biol Trace Elem Res. 2012 Oct;149(1):71-7.

[69] Gromer S., Arscott L.D., Williams C.H., Jr, Schirmer R.H., Becker K. Human placenta thioredoxin reductase. Isolation of the selenoenzyme, steady state kinetics, and inhibition by therapeutic gold compounds. J. Biol. Chem. 1998, 273:20096–20101.

[70] Chu FF. "The human glutathione peroxidase genes GPX2, GPX3, and GPX4 map to chromosomes 14, 5, and 19, respectively". Cytogenet Cell Genet, 1994, 66 (2): 96–8.

[71] Müller C, Wingler K, Brigelius-Flohé R. "3'UTRs of glutathione peroxidases differentially affect selenium-dependent mRNA stability and selenocysteine incorporation efficiency". Biol. Chem, 2003,384 (1): 11–8.

[72] Bermano G, Arthur JR, Hesketh JE. Role of the 3' untranslated region in the regulation of cytosolic glutathione peroxidase and phospholipid-hydroperoxide glutathione peroxidase gene expression by selenium supply. Biochem J. 1996 Dec 15;320 (Pt 3):891-5.

[73] Lacey BM, Eckenroth BE, Flemer S, Hondal RJ. Selenium in thioredoxin reductase: a mechanistic perspective. Biochemistry. 2008 Dec 2;47(48):12810-21.

[74] Mills GC. Hemoglobin catabolism. I. Glutathione peroxidase, an erythrocyte enzyme which protects hemoglobin from oxidative breakdown. J Biol Chem. 1957 Nov; 229(1):189–197.

[75] Ganther HE, Kraus RJ. Oxidation states of glutathione peroxidase. Methods Enzymol. 1984;107:593-602.

[76] Maiorino M, Chu FF, Ursini F, Davies KJ, Doroshow JH, Esworthy RS. Phospholipid hydroperoxide glutathione peroxidase is the 18-kDa selenoprotein expressed in human tumor cell lines. J Biol Chem. 1991 Apr 25;266(12):7728-32.

[77] Arteel GE, Sies H. The biochemistry of selenium and the glutathione system. Environ Toxicol Pharmacol. 2001 Sep;10(4):153-8.

[78] Ames. B N, Shigenaga MK, and Hagen TM. Oxidants, antioxidants, and the degenerative diseases of aging. Proc. Natl. Acad. Sci. USA,1993, 90:7915-7922.

[79] Aviram, M. (1995) Oxidative modification of low density lipoprotein and its relation to atherosclerosis. Isr. J. Med. Sci. 31:241-249.

[80] Tapiero H, Townsend DM, Tew KD. The antioxidant role of selenium and seleno-compounds. Biomed Pharmacother. 2003 May-Jun;57(3-4):134-44.

[81] Jönsson-Videsäter K, Björkhem-Bergman L, Hossain A, Söderberg A, Eriksson LC, Paul C, Rosén A, Björnstedt M. Selenite-induced apoptosis in doxorubicin-resistant cells and effects on the thioredoxin system. Biochem Pharmacol. 2004 Feb 1;67(3): 513-22.

[82] Wallschläger D, Feldmann J. Formation, occurrence, significance, and analysis of organoselenium and organotellurium compounds in the environment. Met Ions Life Sci. 2010;7:319-64. doi: 10.1039/BK9781847551771-00319. Epub 2010 Jan 30.

[83] Suchocki P, Misiewicz I, Skupinska K, Waclawek K, Fijalek Z, Kasprzycka-Guttman T. The activity of Selol in multidrug-resistant and sensitive human leukemia cells. Oncol Rep. 2007 Oct;18(4):893-9.

[84] Beck MA, Levander OA, Handy J (May 2003). "Selenium deficiency and viral infection". J. Nutr. 133 (5 Suppl 1): 1463S–7S. PMID 12730444.

[85] Ren LQ, Li XJ, Li GS, Zhao ZT, Sun B, Sun F (November 2004). "Coxsackievirus B3 infection and its mutation in Keshan disease". World J. Gastroenterol. 10 (22): 3299–302.

[86] Davis CD, Tsuji PA, Milner JA. Selenoproteins and cancer prevention. Annu Rev Nutr. 2012 Aug 21;32:73-95.

[87] Patterson BH, Levander OA. Naturally occurring selenium compounds in cancer chemoprevention trials: a workshop summary. Cancer Epidemiol Biomarkers Prev. 1997 Jan;6(1):63-9.

[88] Blot WJ, Li JY, Taylor PR, Guo W, Dawsey S, Wang GQ, Yang CS, Zheng SF, Gail M, Li GY, et al. Nutrition intervention trials in Linxian, China: supplementation with specific vitamin/mineral combinations, cancer incidence, and disease-specific mortality in the general population. J Natl Cancer Inst. 1993 Sep 15;85(18):1483-92.

[89] Young VR. Selenium: a case for its essentiality in man. N Engl J Med. 1981 May 14;304(20):1228-30.

[90] Hafeman DG, Sunde RA, Hoekstra WG. Effect of dietary selenium on erythrocyte and liver glutathione peroxidase in the rat. J Nutr. 1974 May;104(5):580-7.

[91] Batist G, Norton J, Katki AG, Wagman L, Ferrans VJ, Maher M, Myers CE. Cardiac and red blood cell glutathione peroxidase: results of a prospective randomized trial in patients on total parenteral nutrition. Cancer Res. 1985 Nov;45(11 Pt 2):5900-3.

[92] Schrauzer GN. Selenium and cancer: a review. Bioinorg Chem. 1976;5(3):275-81.

[93] Chakraborty P, Sk UH, Bhattacharya S. Chemoprotection and enhancement of cancer chemotherapeutic efficacy of cyclophosphamide in mice bearing Ehrlich ascites carcinoma by diphenylmethyl selenocyanate. Cancer Chemother Pharmacol. 2009 Oct; 64(5):971-80. doi: 10.1007/s00280-009-0950-8. Epub 2009 Feb 17.

[94] Poirier KA, Milner JA. Factors influencing the antitumorigenic properties of selenium in mice. J Nutr. 1983 Nov;113(11):2147-54.

[95] Greeder GA, Milner JA. Factors influencing the inhibitory effect of selenium on mice inoculated with Ehrlich ascites tumor cells. Science. 1980 Aug 15;209(4458):825-7.

[96] Weisberger, A. S.. and Suhrland, L. G. Studies on analogues of L-cysteine and L-cystine. The effect of selenium cystine on leukemia. Blood, / /: 19-30, 1956.

[97] Batist G, Katki AG, Klecker RW Jr, Myers CE. Selenium-induced cytotoxicity of human leukemia cells: interaction with reduced glutathione. Cancer Res. 1986 Nov; 46(11):5482-5.

[98] Weitberg AB, Weitzman SA, Clark EP, Stossel TP. Effects of antioxidants on oxidant-induced sister chromatid exchange formation. J Clin Invest. 1985 Jun;75(6):1835-41.

[99] Hendrickson W.A., Horton,J.R. and LeMaster,D.M. (1990) Selenomethionyl proteins produced for analysis by multiwavelength anomalous diffraction (MAD): a vehicle for direct determination of three-dimensional structure. EMBO J., 9, 1665–1672.

[100] Ching WM. Characterization of selenium-containing tRNAGlu from Clostridium sticklandii. Arch Biochem Biophys. 1986 Jan;244(1):137-46.

[101] Chung AS, Maines MD. Effect of selenium on glutathione metabolism. Induction of gamma-glutamylcysteine synthetase and glutathione reductase in the rat liver. Biochem Pharmacol. 1981 Dec 1;30(23):3217-23.

[102] Lagace A. Effect of selenium on white muscle disease in lambs.J Am Vet Med Assoc. 1961 Feb 15;138:188-90

[103] Schwarz S. Essentiality and metabolic functions of selenium. Med Clin North Am. 1976 Jul;60(4):745-58.

[104] Ferencík M, Ebringer L. Modulatory effects of selenium and zinc on the immune system. Folia Microbiol (Praha). 2003;48(3):417-26.

[105] Vogt TM, Ziegler RG, Graubard BI, Swanson CA, Greenberg RS, Schoenberg JB, Swanson GM, Hayes RB, Mayne ST. Serum selenium and risk of prostate cancer in U.S. blacks and whites. Int J Cancer. 2003 Feb 20;103(5):664-70.

[106] Hoekstra, W. G. Biochemicalfunction of seleniumand its relation to vitamin E. Fed. Proc., 34: 2083-2089,1975.

[107] Tappel AL. Biological antioxidant protection against lipid peroxidation damage. Am J Clin Nutr. 1970 Aug;23(8):1137-9.

[108] Ip C. Interaction of Vitamin C and Selenium Supplementation in the Modification of Mammary Carcinogenesis in Rats. JNCI J Natl Cancer Inst (1986) 77 (1): 299-303.

[109] Spallholz JE, Palace VP, Reid TW (2004) Methioninase and selenomethionine but not Se-ethylselenocysteine generate methylselenol and superoxide in an in vitro chemiluminescent assay: implications for the nutritional carcinostatic activity of selenoamino acids. Biochem Pharmacol 67:547–554.

[110] Stadtman TC. Selenium biochemistry. Mammalian selenoenzymes. Ann N Y Acad Sci. 2000;899:399–402.

[111] Badmaev V, Majeed M, Passwater RA. Selenium: a quest for better understanding. Altern Ther Health Med. 1996 Jul;2(4):59-62, 65-7.

[112] Hercberg S, Galan P, Preziosi P, Bertrais S, Mennen L, Malvy D, Roussel AM, Favier A, Briançon S. The SU.VI.MAX Study: a randomized, placebo-controlled trial of the health effects of antioxidant vitamins and minerals. Arch Intern Med. 2004 Nov 22;164(21):2335-42.

[113] Hercberg S, Kesse-Guyot E, Druesne-Pecollo N, Touvier M, Favier A, Latino-Martel P, Briançon S, Galan P. Incidence of cancers, ischemic cardiovascular diseases and mortality during 5-year follow-up after stopping antioxidant vitamins and minerals supplements: a postintervention follow-up in the SU.VI.MAX Study. Int J Cancer. 2010 Oct 15;127(8):1875-81.

[114] Sato S, Sueki H, and Nishijima A. "Two unusual cases of argyria: the application of an improved tissue processing method for X-ray microanalysis of selenium and sulphur in silver-laden granules," British Journal of Dermatology, vol. 140, no. 1, pp. 158–163, 1999.

Chapter 15

Adaptive Behaviour Change and Health in Adults with Down Syndrome: A Prospective Clinical Follow-Up Study

T. Määttä, T. Tervo-Määttä, A. Taanila, M. Kaski and M. Iivanainen

Additional information is available at the end of the chapter

http://dx.doi.org/10.5772/57461

1. Introduction

People with Down syndrome are prone to early ageing and Alzheimer's disease (Zigman & Lott 2007). The functional decline in adults with Down syndrome starts decades earlier, compared to the mainstream population and other people with intellectual disabilities (Zigman *et al.* 1996; Strydom *et al.* 2007). The coping skills necessary for daily life, social interactions and work are gradually lost during the progression of dementia (Margallo-Lana *et al.* 2007).

Typical neuropathology of Alzheimer's disease is seen in virtually all people with Down syndrome by the age of 40 (Wisniewski *et al.* 1985). Depending on diagnostic criteria, 17-55% of them develop clinical dementia after that age (Holland *et al.* 2000; Janicki & Dalton 2000; Coppus *et al.* 2006). Genetic factors modifying the risk of dementia in adults with Down syndrome have been identified (Zigman & Lott 2007; Prasher *et al.* 2008; Patel *et al.* 2010). The rates of dementia in adults with intellectual disability without Down syndrome aged 60 years and older are greater than expected (Strydom *et al.* 2007).

The cognitive impairment in adults with Down syndrome has similarities to early cognitive changes in Alzheimer's disease (Brugge *et al.*1994). Personality and behaviour changes (Ball *et al.* 2006), executive dysfunction (Ball *et al.* 2008) and selective attention deficits (Krinsky-McHale *et al.* 2008) are early signs of dementia in adults with Down syndrome. Frontal-like dementia can be diagnosed in 33% in their thirties (Holland *et al.* 2000). Maladaptive behaviour is often seen and includes aggression, fearfulness, sadness, sleep problems, social inadequacy, stealing and general regressive behaviour (Urv *et al.* 2008). Increasing age associates with decreasing cognitive and language abilities; the deterioration with the age is largely explained by the presence of Alzheimer's disease (Iacono *et al.* 2010).

Identification of persons with risk of early dementia remains a challenge (Shulz *et al.* 2004). Direct assessments of cognitive functions of people with intellectual disabilities may be difficult (Pyo *et al.* 2007). Informant-based assessments are useful as complementary or alternative methods in clinical work (Ball *et al.* 2004; Prasher *et al.* 2004; Niuwenhuis-Mark 2009).

The Adaptive Behavior Scale - Residential and Community (Nihira *et al.* 1993) and its earlier versions have been widely used in research. Cross-sectional studies have demonstrated lower scores on people with Down syndrome older than 40 years compared to younger participants with Down syndrome (Collacott 1992). The age-related decline of adaptive behaviour associates to dementia (Prasher & Chung 1996). Prospective studies have confirmed changes in adaptive behaviour (Rasmussen & Sobsey 1994; Prasher *et al.* 1998). Zigman *et al.* (2002) described the incidence and temporal patterns of adaptive behaviour changes in adults with intellectual disabilities. Rasmussen and Sobsey (1994) found stability of adaptive behaviour in adults with Down syndrome in the age groups younger than 40 years and a pattern of decline in self-help and communication skills in several individuals with Down syndrome older than 40, including declines in dressing, receptive language, vocational and domestic behaviour.

Relative preservation of cognitive and functional ability in persons with Down syndrome older than 45 associates with better survival whereas clinically, the most important disorders that are related to mortality are dementia, mobility restrictions, visual impairment, and epilepsy (Coppus *et al.* 2008).

Health co-morbidities in ageing persons with Down syndrome and Alzheimer's dementia are common (McCarron *et al.* 2005). Depression often precedes the onset of dementia in people with Down syndrome (Burt *et al.* 1992). Visual impairment and hearing loss are very common in elderly people with Down syndrome (van Splunder *et al.* 2006; Meuwese-Jongejeugd *et al.* 2006; Meuwese-Jongejeugd *et al.* 2008). Epilepsy is often seen at the same age with dementia (Collacott 1993). Hypothyroidism may also affect adaptive behaviour (Bhaumik *et al.* 1991). The absence of a medical illness predicts a higher level of adaptive behaviour, while dementia is a predictive factor for increased maladaptive behaviour (Prasher & Chung 1996) and psychiatric symptoms (Urv *et al.* 2010)

Medication for Alzheimer's disease might benefit many people with Down syndrome by slowing the progression of the disease (Prasher *et al.* 2002). Accurate measures are important for the follow-up and evaluation of treatments. It is necessary to find and use valid, reliable and sensitive methods for assessments of adults and ageing people with Down syndrome and Alzheimer's disease.

http://dx.doi.org/10.5772/57461

The aim of the present study was to explore the clinical usefulness of repeated assessments of adaptive behaviour in people with Down syndrome and suspected or confirmed dementia. Repeated assessments of adaptive behaviour in people at risk of functional decline might help to confirm the change and lead to necessary additional evaluations of the underlying reasons and help in follow-up.

2. Methods

Study population

The participating adults with Down syndrome were recruited to the study at a specialized service centre for people with intellectual disabilities serving a population of 79 690 (December 2008), among them 723 people with identified intellectual disability. These include 84 people with Down syndrome; 19 of them were 0-19 years old, 65 were 20 years old or older. Forty of the 65 adults belonged to the age group 40 years old or older.

Assessments of adaptive behaviour were conducted to 42 persons with Down syndrome (Table 1). Twenty five persons had repeated assessments. These persons' proxies had noticed a change of mood, behaviour or performance. At the time of the first evaluation, their age range was 24-61 years, with a mean of 45.8 and SD of +/- 8.4; at the time of the last evaluation, the corresponding figures were 25-65.5, 48.8, and +/- 8.4 years, respectively. The mean time of follow-up was, thus, 3.0 years (range 0-8 years). Five participants died during the follow up. Twenty participants (80%) of the 25 were 40 years or older at the time of the first evaluation. Most participants (17/25, 68%) resided at the beginning of the follow-up in small group homes, seven (28%) at home with parents or siblings and one in institution. Fourteen participants (56%) had organized weekly activities outside the home and two participants had part time supported work.

Methods

Repeated informant evaluations regarding observed changes in behaviour were recorded prospectively. Evaluations of adults with Down syndrome were performed over ten years, beginning in 2001. Adaptive behaviour assessments were performed by the closest relatives or carers who lived or worked with the participants and knew the persons and their daily skills for a long time.

The current coping skills for daily living were assessed using the Adaptive Behavior Scale - Residential and Community, ABS-RC: 2 1993, Part I (Nihira *et al.* 1993). The Adaptive Behavior Scale (ABS) was chosen because the reliability and validity of this method are well established. Earlier research supports its feasibility in the use of scientific studies of ageing and dementia in people with intellectual disabilities (Rasmussen & Sobsey 1994; Prasher *et al.* 1998; Zigman *et al.* 2002).

The first part of ABS is focused on personal independence and includes ten domains or subscales: Independent Functioning, Physical Development, Economic Activity, Language

Development, Numbers and Time, Domestic Activity, Prevocational/Vocational Activity, Self-Direction, Responsibility and Socialization. The ABS Manual reports that factor analysis has found three Part One factors: Personal Self-Sufficiency, Community Self-Sufficiency, and Personal–Social Responsibility.

Clinical evaluations were done by the principal investigator. These included interviews of the proxies, referrals for differential diagnostics and specialist consultations, and prescriptions and assessments of medications. Additional clinical data was drawn from the case records of the health centres, central hospital and service centre regarding all persons with Down syndrome in the region. The data of medical treatments for Alzheimer's disease, depression, behavioural problems, epilepsy, and other major health concerns possibly affecting adaptive behaviour were analyzed. The age at the time of the first observation of functional decline was calculated.

Informant ratings by ABS were scored and analysed. Total scores, scores for the ten subscales and three factors of ABS and changes of scores from the first to the last evaluation were counted. The ABS score changes as percentages per three years were calculated for subgroups of participants with and without Alzheimer's disease, depression, epilepsy, hypothyroidism, and antipsychotic medication use for challenging behaviour.

The ethical committee of the Kainuu Central Hospital approved the study and permission for combining data from medical and social records was given by the Ministry of Social and Health Affairs.

3. Results

The number of people with Down syndrome living in the area is well known and their morbidity data was available for comparison. The participants with repeated ABS assessments were older than participants with single assessments. Dementia, medication use for challenging behaviour, depression and epilepsy were more common among participants than among adults with Down syndrome living in the region.

Alzheimer's disease

Alzheimer's disease with dementia was diagnosed in 15 out of the 25 participants assessed repeatedly. Four of them died during the survey. The diagnosis was confirmed in ten participants by a neurologist and in five participants by the first author with competence in intellectual disability medicine. Other causes of dementia were excluded. Computerized tomographies of the brain were performed in ten of these participants. Eleven persons received medication for Alzheimer's disease (donepezile, galantamine or rivastigmine, in three participants combined with memantine). Early dementia was suspected in an additional four participants; they had increasing difficulties following instructions and performing their usual domestic work.

The number of living people with diagnosed and suspected dementia (fifteen persons among the participants and two not participating in this study) among adults with Down syndrome

http://dx.doi.org/10.5772/57461

in the region gives prevalence's of dementia 38% (15 of 40 persons) in the age group 40 years and more, and 13% (two of 15 persons) in the age group 30-39 years. The prevalence estimate of dementia for the age group 30 years and more is thus 31% (17 of 55 persons).

Medical problems

Of the 25 participants eleven (44%) had experienced long periods of depression. Thirteen (52%) had received antipsychotic medication mainly for behavioural problems, six of them already during early adulthood and eight for behavioural problems with dementia. Eleven persons were treated for hypothyroidism. Varying degrees of visual impairment were common, and three had cataracts. Recurrent faints were seen in eight, with falls causing fractures in three persons. Epilepsy was diagnosed in eight persons.

Among participants with Alzheimer's disease (n=15), antipsychotic medication had been used for eleven (73%), depression had been diagnosed in ten (67%), thyroid disease in ten (67%), and epilepsy in seven (47%) participants. Among participants without Alzheimer's disease (n=10), antipsychotic medication had been used for two (20%), depression had been diagnosed in one (10%), thyroid disease in four (40%), and epilepsy in one participant (10%). Among eleven participants with depression (N=11), antipsychotic medication had been used for seven (64%), Alzheimer's disease had been diagnosed in ten (91%), thyroid disease in 6 (55%), and epilepsy in five (45%) participants.

Informant observations

A decline of daily functioning was observed by informants in regards to 19 of 25 persons, starting at the ages of 37-51 years with a mean of 44.9 and SD +/- 4 years in persons with full trisomy of chromosome 21. In addition, there was one participant with mosaic trisomy of chromosome 21 whose decline started only at the age of 60 (Figure 3, participant 2).

Adaptive Behavior Scale (ABS) scores

The mean ages, ABS total scores at first and last assessments and the calculated percentages of score changes per three years in subgroups of participants are presented in Table 1. The mean ABS total scores for the 25 participants with multiple assessments declined from 161 to 126 (21.8%) during the mean 3.0 years between the first and last assessments. The decline of ABS total scores associated very strongly to Alzheimer's disease: there was no decline in the mean ABS total scores in the group of participants with no suspected or confirmed Alzheimer's disease. The mean rates of ABS score change were higher in participant groups with Alzheimer's disease (33.6% in three years), and depression (32.0%) compared to participants without these conditions (0.6% and 13.9% respectively). The participants treated with medication for Alzheimer's disease had lower mean rates of score declines compared to untreated patients, 31% and 40% declines in three years respectively. The mean rates of change were almost similar in groups of persons with and without epilepsy, antipsychotic medication, and hypothyroidism. (Table 1)

Participants (number of persons)	Age of participants at first (last) assessment	ABS total scores, means at first (last) assessment	ABS score change percentage per three years, %
Participants with single assessments (17)	36.5 (36.5)	174 (174)	
males (10)	32.3 (32.3)	188 (188)	
females (7)	42.4 (42.4)	155 (155)	
Participants with repeated assessments (25)	45.8 (48.8)	161 (126)	-21.8
males (11)	43.8 (47.0)	135 (117)	-12.4
females (14)	48.4 (51.5)	193 (137)	-28.4
Alzheimer`s disease (AD, 15)	49.7 (52.9)	165 (106)	-33.6
AD, no medication (4)	47.8 (50.8)	155 (93)	-40.0
AD, medication (11)	50.6 (53.9)	170 (112)	-31.0
No AD (10)	40.0 (43.1)	154 (155)	+0.6
Depression (11)	47.6 (50.5)	159 (112)	-32.0
No depression (14)	44.4 (47.8)	162 (136)	-13.9
Epilepsy (8)	50.6 (54.5)	193 (141)	-23.0
No epilepsy (17)	43.5 (46.5)	145 (118)	-18.7
Antipsychotic medication (13)	49.0 (52.0)	168 (132)	-21.7
No antipsychotic medication (12)	42.3 (45.7)	152 (119)	-19.3
Hypothyroidism (11)	45.8 (48.7)	152 (125)	-19.4
No hypothyroidism (14)	45.8 (49.1)	166 (126)	-21.5

Table 1. Ages, ABS-RC:2 total scores and score changes in subgroups of participants with Down syndrome.

ABS-RC:2 subscale	Scores, first assessment Mean (SD)	Scores, last assessment Mean (SD)	Score change, %
Domestic Activity	9.6 (6.1)	5.8 (6.1)	-64.8
Responsibility	5.0 (3.0)	3.3 (3.1)	-51.2
Self-Direction	12.1 (5.9)	8.0 (6.9)	-50.3
Prevocational/Vocational Activity	5.8 (3.1)	4.0 (3.6)	-44.0
Numbers and Time	5.4 (3.4)	3.8 (3.8)	-41.1
Independent Functioning	64.8 (24.3)	52.3 (32.0)	-23.8
Language Development	21.0 (9.4)	17.2 (8.9)	-22.0
Economic Activity	3.6 (3.3)	3.2 (3.5)	-12.5
Physical Development	18.4 (3.5)	16.0 (5.5)	-15.0
Economic Activity	3.6 (3.3)	3.2 (3.5)	-12.5

Table 2. ABS-RC:2 subscale mean scores and their change during the prospective follow-up of 25 participants with Down syndrome.

The biggest mean declines were seen in the subscales Domestic Activity, Responsibility and Self-Direction, to 35.2, 48.8 and 49.7%, respectively. The slightest changes were seen in the domains of Economic Activity, Physical Development and Language Development (Table 2). The mean changes of scores for the ABS factors Personal Self-Sufficiency, Community Self-Sufficiency and Personal–Social Responsibility were 22.2, 27.9 and 36.8%, respectively.

Individual changes in ABS scores

The ABS scores remained stable in nine and improved in three persons. A progressive decline of ABS scores was seen in 13 of 25 (52%) participants after their early forties. The direction, amount and rate of change of ABS scores varied from an increase of 27% within a year in the youngest participant recovering from deep depression to 90% decline during seven years in an ageing participant.

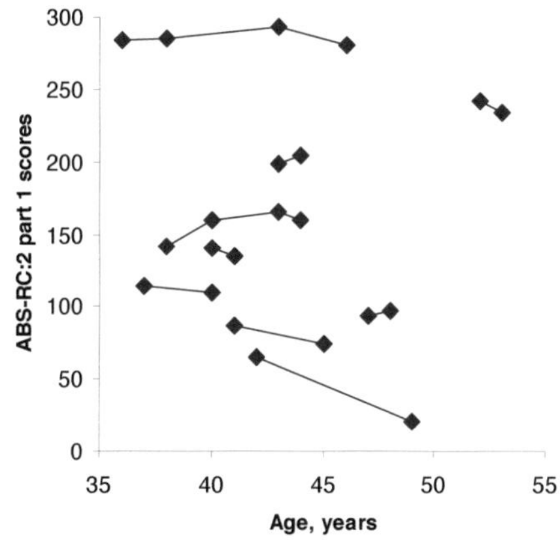

Figure 1. Adaptive behaviour in 9 participants without clinical Alzheimer's disease

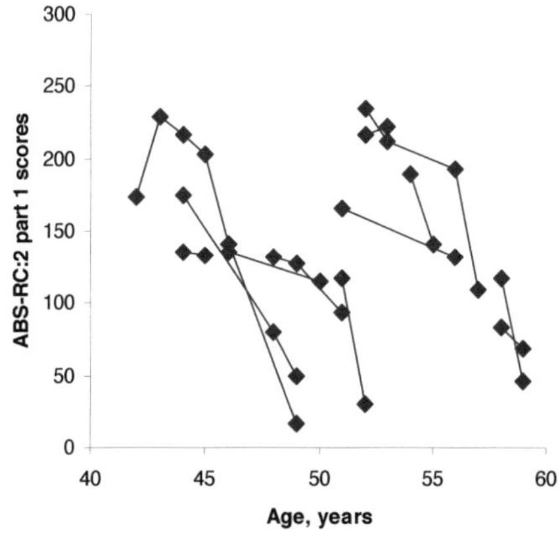

Figure 2. Adaptive behaviour in 12 participants with diagnosed Alzheimer's disease

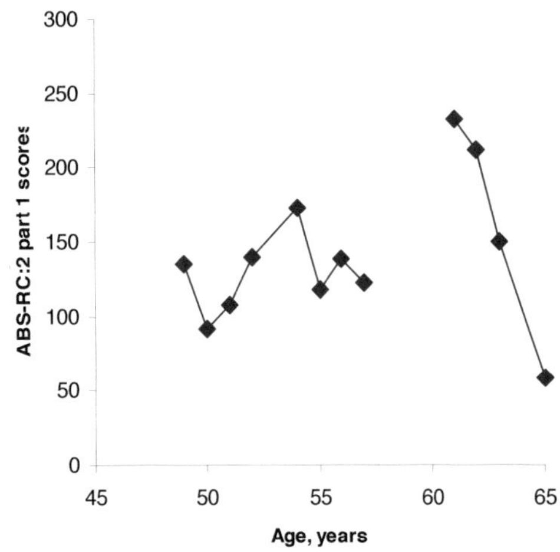

Figure 3. Adaptive behaviour in two participants with different clinical course of diagnosed Alzheimer's disease: participant 1 with slow progression of dementia (clinical case data given in text), participant 2 with mosaic trisomy of chromosome 21 and late onset of dementia

4. Late onset of dementia with mosaic trisomy of chromosome 21

For most of the younger and many of older participants too, changes in ABS scores were minimal (Figure 1). Slight improvement in scores at ages 38-40 was seen in an participant after a change of residence, coupled with increasing exercise, weight loss and improved fitness. The highest scores with slight improvement at ages 38-43 were seen in a participant in spite of many treated health problems, including a slight permanent visual impairment, hypothyroidism, fractures associated with osteoporosis and bronchial asthma.

The ABS scores declined in most participants with Alzheimer´s disease (Figure 2). Improvements in ABS scores were seen in two elderly participants. In the first participant (Figure 2), the improvement at age 42 to 43 associated to the change of residence and medical treatment of Alzheimer's disease with response for two years before advancing deterioration later. Epilepsy and loss of mobility after a fall resulting in a hip fracture, and poor visual acuity contributed to the loss of independent functioning.

The improvement of the other participant (Figure 3) during the treatment of confirmed Alzheimer's disease, after a decline at age 48 to 49 lasted five years before further deterioration. Contributing factors to the functional improvement were the removal of cataracts resulting in improved visual acuity, active participation in activities with support of the carers, and

http://dx.doi.org/10.5772/57461

stabilization of mood and behaviour. This participant had a long history of hypothyroidism, depression and challenging behaviour and he had long-term antidepressant and antipsychotic medication, and successful treatment of late onset epilepsy.

5. Discussion

We report experiences of a long term prospective clinical follow-up of adults with Down syndrome. The participants in this study were adults with Down syndrome and behavioural changes as perceived by carers. Adults without behavioural or mood changes observed by their proxies were not actively recruited and thus this group is not represented in this survey. The participants represent adults with Down syndrome with observed change of mood, behaviour or performance causing concern in their proxies.

Depression and, among participants in their forties and older, Alzheimer's dementia were the most common underlying reasons for the behavioural change. The number of participants with diagnosed and suspected dementia gave estimates of prevalence comparable to published epidemiological studies. Most people with Down syndrome and diagnosed Alzheimer's dementia in this population participated in this study. A change of behaviour or adjustment had been noticed by their proxies before the diagnosis of Alzheimer's dementia.

The current coping skills of the participants were assessed repeatedly using Adaptive Behaviour Scale - Residential and Community, Part I (Nihira *et al.* 1993). Earlier research supports its feasibility in scientific studies of ageing and dementia in people with intellectual disabilities. The clinical use of ABS to monitor ageing and dementia from the early non-symptomatic phase to the advanced stages at various levels of abilities proved to be possible and helpful for the clinician. A decline in ABS scores was seen in most participants after their early forties. This supported the suspicion of Alzheimer's disease, led to differential diagnostic assessments and also helped in monitoring the progression of the disease.

Adaptive behaviour can be assessed by ABS in adults with intellectual disability at all phases of ageing and dementia. This informant-based method overcame many of the problems of cognitive based measures. For example, no cooperation or communication skills of the person to be evaluated were needed for this assessment. Direct evaluations of cognitive functions were not possible in this study due to the limited neuropsychological resources available. Stable scores in clinically stable participants between repeated evaluations supported the reliability of ABS, when used by proxy informants. The informants with a close and long familiarity to their proxies observed and reported subtle changes in daily life and completed adaptive behaviour questionnaires without obvious difficulty.

A careful evaluation of the life situation and comprehensive assessment of physical and mental health is necessary when carers describe a decline in everyday functioning - that is a difficulty in accomplishing daily tasks which the individual would normally complete with ease (Ball et al. 2006). This is also needed in the elderly with established Alzheimer's disease because of common co-morbidities. In the case of a rapid deterioration of function, the underlying reasons should be assessed even when Alzheimer's disease has been diagnosed and treatment started. Visual acuity and hearing should be regularly monitored in all adults with Down syndrome because of high prevalence's of visual impairment and hearing loss. Alzheimer's disease does not protect from any other disease or disability. Other treatable conditions, including hypothyroidism, visual impairment and hearing loss, may be found.

The decline of the ABS total scores associated strongly to Alzheimer's disease; therefore the described declines in the ABS subscale scores probably reflect changes attributable to Alzheimer's disease. The relative rates of change among of the subscales of ABS differed. The scores of the domains Domestic Activity, Responsibility, Self-Direction and Vocational Activity declined more, as compared to other domains including Independent Functioning and Physical Activities. This may reflect the early impairment of frontal lobe functions among people with Down syndrome (Holland *et al.* 2000), including executive dysfunction in the development of Alzheimer's disease (Ball *et al.*2008).

Individual differences of the functional skills assessed by ABS scores were considerable. Decline of skills with ageing started at very different ages among participants in this study. The improvements of adaptive behaviour seen in several participants highlight the need for careful assessment of treatable medical conditions and possibilities for supporting the maintenance of functional independence. Stabilization of ABS scores was seen during medication for Alzheimer's disease in one participant for up to five years. Studies using population based representative larger samples would be needed to further analyse factors that represent potential confounders affecting adaptive behaviour more vigorously.

A considerable proportion of people with Down syndrome do not develop clinical dementia at all (Coppus et al. 2006). People with Down syndrome differ in their individual biological and genetic risk of dementia (Zigman & Lott 2007; Prasher et al. 2008; Patel et al. 2008). Better understanding of genetic and environmental influences and medical conditions contributing to these differences is needed.

Repeated prospective assessments overcome memory errors compared to retrospective evaluations. Short questionnaires of adaptive behaviour change may be sufficient for screening purposes (Prasher *et al.* 2004). However, repeated assessments are needed for the confirmation of dementia and evaluation of interventions. The possibility of performing an assessment in various settings without special professional expertise is a benefit of this approach.

The informant-based assessments of coping skills for daily living may prove practical and useful for the follow up of ageing and dementia from the early non-symptomatic phase to the advanced stages at various levels of abilities. The authors suggest repeated assessments of adaptive behaviour and careful clinical evaluations to detect treatable medical conditions in adults with Down syndrome.

http://dx.doi.org/10.5772/57461

Author details

T. Määttä[1*], T. Tervo-Määttä[2], A. Taanila[3,4], M. Kaski[5] and M. Iivanainen[5,6]

*Address all correspondence to: tuomo.maatta@kainuu.fi

1 Kainuu Social and Health Care Joint Authority, Finland

2 Department of Teacher Education, University of Oulu, Finland

3 Institute of Health Sciences, University of Oulu, Finland

4 Unit of General Practice, University Hospital of Oulu, Finland

5 The Rinnekoti Research Centre, Espoo, Finland

6 Department of Child Neurology, University of Helsinki, Finland

References

[1] Ball, S. L., Holland, A. J., Hon, J., Huppert, F. A., Treppner, P., & Watson, P. C. (2006). Personality and behaviour changes mark the early stages of Alzheimer's disease in adults with Down's syndrome: Findings from a prospective population-based study. *International Journal of Geriatric Psychiatry* 21, 661-673.

[2] Ball, S. L., Holland, A. J., Huppert, F. A., Treppner, P., Watson, P., & Hon, J. (2004). The modified CAMDEX informant interview is a valid and reliable tool for use in the diagnosis of dementia in adults with Down's syndrome. *Journal of Intellectual Disability Research* 48, 611-620.

[3] Ball, S. L., Holland, A. J., Treppner, P., Watson, P. C., & Huppert, F. A. (2008). Executive dysfunction and its association with personality and behaviour changes in the development of Alzheimer's disease in adults with Down syndrome and mild to moderate learning disabilities. *The British Journal of Clinical Psychology / the British Psychological Society* 47, 1-29.

[4] Bhaumik, S., Collacott, R. A., Garrick, P., & Mitchell, C. (1991). Effect of thyroid stimulating hormone on adaptive behaviour in Down's syndrome. *Journal of Mental Deficiency Research* 35, 512-520.

[5] Brugge, K. L., Nichols, S. L., Salmon, D. P., Hill, L. R., Delis, D. C., Aaron, L., et al. (1994). Cognitive impairment in adults with Down's syndrome: Similarities to early cognitive changes in Alzheimer's disease. *Neurology* 44, 232-238.

[6] Burt, D. B., Loveland, K. A., & Lewis, K. R. (1992). Depression and the onset of dementia in adults with mental retardation. *American Journal of Mental Retardation* 96, 502-511.

[7] Collacott, R. A. (1992). The effect of age and residential placement on adaptive behaviour of adults with Down's syndrome. *The British Journal of Psychiatry : The Journal of Mental Science* 161, 675-679.

[8] Collacott, R. A. (1993). Epilepsy, dementia and adaptive behaviour in Down's syndrome. *Journal of Intellectual Disability Research* 37, 153-160.

[9] Coppus, A., Evenhuis, H., Verberne, G. J., Visser, F., van Gool, P., Eikelenboom, P., et al. (2006). Dementia and mortality in persons with Down's syndrome. *Journal of Intellectual Disability Research* 50, 768-777.

[10] Coppus, A. M., Evenhuis, H. M., Verberne, G. J., Visser, F. E., Oostra, B. A., Eikelenboom, P., et al. (2008). Survival in elderly persons with Down syndrome. *Journal of the American Geriatrics Society* 56, 2311-2316.

[11] Holland, A. J., Hon, J., Huppert, F. A., & Stevens, F. (2000). Incidence and course of dementia in people with Down's syndrome: Findings from a population-based study. *Journal of Intellectual Disability Research* 44, 138-146.

[12] Iacono, T., Torr, J., & Wong, H. Y. (2010). Relationships amongst age, language and related skills in adults with Down syndrome. *Research in Developmental Disabilities* 31, 568-576.

[13] Janicki, M. P., & Dalton, A. J. (2000). Prevalence of dementia and impact on intellectual disability services. *Mental Retardation* 38, 276-288.

[14] Krinsky-McHale, S. J., Devenny, D. A., Kittler, P., & Silverman, W. (2008). Selective attention deficits associated with mild cognitive impairment and early stage Alzheimer's disease in adults with Down syndrome. *American Journal of Mental Retardation 113*, 369-386.

[15] Margallo-Lana, M. L., Moore, P. B., Kay, D. W., Perry, R. H., Reid, B. E., Berney, T. P., et al. (2007). Fifteen-year follow-up of 92 hospitalized adults with Down's syndrome: Incidence of cognitive decline, its relationship to age and neuropathology. *Journal of Intellectual Disability Research* 51, 463-477.

[16] McCarron, M., Gill, M., McCallion, P., & Begley, C. (2005). Health co-morbidities in ageing persons with Down syndrome and Alzheimer's dementia. *Journal of Intellectual Disability Research* 49, 560-566.

[17] Meuwese-Jongejeugd, A., van Splunder, J., Vink, M., Stilma, J. S., van Zanten, B., Verschuure, H., et al. (2008). Combined sensory impairment (deaf-blindness) in five percent of adults with intellectual disabilities. *American Journal of Mental Retardation* 113, 254-262.

http://dx.doi.org/10.5772/57461

[18] Meuwese-Jongejeugd, A., Vink, M., van Zanten, B., Verschuure, H., Eichhorn, E., Koopman, D., et al. (2006). Prevalence of hearing loss in 1598 adults with an intellectual disability: Cross-sectional population based study. *International Journal of Audiology* 45, 660-669.

[19] Nieuwenhuis-Mark, R. E. (2009). Diagnosing Alzheimer's dementia in Down syndrome: Problems and possible solutions. *Research in Developmental Disabilities* 30, 827-838.

[20] Nihira, K., Leland, H., & Lambert, N. (1993). *AAAMR adaptive behavior scales, residential and community edition (2nd ed), TX:Pro-ed.*

[21] Patel, A., Rees, S. D., Kelly, M. A., Bain, S. C., Barnett, A. H., Thalitaya, D., et al. (2010). Association of variants within APOE, SORL1, RUNX1, BACE1 and ALDH18A1 with dementia in Alzheimer's disease in subjects with Down syndrome. *Neuroscience Letters,*

[22] Prasher, V., Farooq, A., & Holder, R. (2004). The adaptive behaviour dementia questionnaire (ABDQ): Screening questionnaire for dementia in Alzheimer's disease in adults with Down syndrome. *Research in Developmental Disabilities* 25 385-397.

[23] Prasher, V. P., & Chung, M. C. (1996). Causes of age-related decline in adaptive behavior of adults with Down syndrome: Differential diagnoses of dementia. *American Journal of Mental Retardation* 101, 175-183.

[24] Prasher, V. P., Chung, M. C., & Haque, M. S. (1998). Longitudinal changes in adaptive behavior in adults with Down syndrome: Interim findings from a longitudinal study. *American Journal of Mental Retardation* 103, 40-46.

[25] Prasher, V. P., Huxley, A., Haque, M. S., & Down syndrome Ageing Study Group. (2002). A 24-week, double-blind, placebo-controlled trial of donepezil in patients with Down syndrome and Alzheimer's disease--pilot study. *International Journal of Geriatric Psychiatry* 17, 270-278.

[26] Prasher, V. P., Sajith, S. G., Rees, S. D., Patel, A., Tewari, S., Schupf, N., et al. (2008). Significant effect of APOE epsilon 4 genotype on the risk of dementia in Alzheimer's disease and mortality in persons with Down syndrome. *International Journal of Geriatric Psychiatry* 23, 1134-1140.

[27] Pyo, G., Kripakaran, K., Curtis, K., Curtis, R., & Markwell, S. (2007). A preliminary study of the validity of memory tests recommended by the working group for individuals with moderate to severe intellectual disability. *Journal of Intellectual Disability Research* 51, 377-386.

[28] Rasmussen, D. E., & Sobsey, D. (1994). Age, adaptive behavior, and Alzheimer disease in Down syndrome: Cross-sectional and longitudinal analyses. *American Journal of Mental Retardation* 99, 151-165.

[29] Shultz, J., Aman, M., Kelbley, T., LeClear Wallace, C., Burt, D. B., Primeaux-Hart, S., et al. (2004). Evaluation of screening tools for dementia in older adults with mental retardation. *American Journal of Mental Retardation* 109, 98-110.

[30] Strydom, A., Livingston, G., King, M., & Hassiotis, A. (2007). Prevalence of dementia in intellectual disability using different diagnostic criteria. *The British Journal of Psychiatry : The Journal of Mental Science* 191, 150-157.

[31] Urv, T. K., Zigman, W. B., & Silverman, W. (2008). Maladaptive behaviors related to dementia status in adults with Down syndrome. *American Journal of Mental Retardation* 113, 73-86.

[32] Urv, T. K., Zigman, W. B., & Silverman, W. (2010). Psychiatric symptoms in adults with Down syndrome and Alzheimer's disease. *American Journal on Intellectual and Developmental Disabilities, 115*(4), 265-276.

[33] van Splunder, J., Stilma, J. S., Bernsen, R. M., & Evenhuis, H. M. (2006). Prevalence of visual impairment in adults with intellectual disabilities in the netherlands: Cross-sectional study. *Eye (London, England), 20*(9), 1004-1010.

[34] Wisniewski, K. E., Wisniewski, H. M., & Wen, G. Y. (1985). Occurrence of neuropathological changes and dementia of Alzheimer's disease in Down's syndrome. *Annals of Neurology, 17*(3), 278-282.

[35] Zigman, W. B., & Lott, I. T. (2007). Alzheimer's disease in Down syndrome: Neurobiology and risk. *Mental Retardation and Developmental Disabilities Research Reviews, 13*(3), 237-246.

[36] Zigman, W. B., Schupf, N., Sersen, E., & Silverman, W. (1996). Prevalence of dementia in adults with and without Down syndrome. *American Journal of Mental Retardation : AJMR, 100*(4), 403-412.

[37] Zigman, W. B., Schupf, N., Urv, T., Zigman, A., & Silverman, W. (2002). Incidence and temporal patterns of adaptive behavior change in adults with mental retardation. American Journal of Mental Retardation : AJMR, 107(3), 161-174.

Chapter 16

The Nutritional Status of Children with Suspected Abuse

Eileen Harper, Shirley Ekvall, Valli Ekvall and
Wei Pan

Additional information is available at the end of the chapter

http://dx.doi.org/10.5772/57374

1. Introduction

Child abuse is the willful infliction of injury to a child. Estimated at 2.8 million children affected per year, over 2,000 die from maltreatment [1]. In 1998 alone, 900,000 cases were reported [2] and from 1986-1993 cases doubled in the United States. Up to 10% of children seen in the emergency room (ER) under the age of 6 had a non-accidental injury accounting for nearly 25% of all hospital admissions for head injury in infancy, producing significant morbidity [3, 4]. Abuse is not limited to poor or racial minorities [5]. Physical and sexual abuse during childhood/adolescence was reported by 22% on a questionnaire [6]. Abused children frequently have moderate to severe malnutrition [7] due to withholding of food which may lead to compromised nutritional state and failure to thrive (FTT) [8]. Twenty-nine percent of 42 children with severe trauma had under nutrition resulting in growth retardation [9].

Bonnier et al. reported that all 13 children with whiplash shaken infant syndrome had a weight <50th percentile and 9 had a weight <10th percentile. Average birth weight was at the 30th percentile, but body weight at admission for shaking was below the 10th percentile [10]. Poor physical growth/nutrition are seen in 25-35% of abused children [11]. The most common chronic illness of childhood is lead poisoning [11]. Siblings in foster care, physically abused or neglected children are at high risk of lead poisoning and incurring a developmental disability [12-14]. Lead poisoning is caused by ingesting contaminated paint from window sills, furniture, Mexican terra cotta pottery, imported tamarind candy, hot-running water through lead soldered pipes or anything covered in lead-based paint [12-14]. The interaction between nutrition and toxic hazards depends on the baseline nutritional status of the individual as well as total food intake, percent dietary fat, calcium, iron, zinc, vitamin D and phosphorus [15, 16]. Food restriction increased lead retention in animals fed lead containing diets [16, 17]. Yet, one study found a positive association between total caloric intake and blood lead levels [18]. Low calcium diets elevate lead tissue concentrations as calcium functions as a chelating agent reducing lead absorption [17, 19]. Lead competes with calcium in enzyme systems, alters calcium metabolism regulation, modifies the calcium second messenger system, impairs normal modulation of intracellular calcium homeostasis, modifies induction of calcium-regulating proteins and interferes with energy metabolism [19-22, 23]. Zinc status has been found to be approximately 20% lower in children with substantially elevated blood lead concentration. Children may have increased lead absorption following shorter fasting time than adults because of rapid gastric emptying [24]. As dietary zinc intake increases, tissue lead levels and toxicity decrease. Research suggests that higher dietary iron intake might be protective against high blood lead levels [24-26]. Another study found anemia in 13% of the 5,181 abused/neglected children screened; potentially due to lead interfering with heme synthetase.[27] When examining dietary iron intake and H/H levels, the degree of anemia from iron-deficient/lead-intoxicated rats was greater than either condition alone [16]. Lead ia a divalent cation which can deplete iron and zinc. In abused/neglected children, poor nutritional status and lead toxicity can result in severe neurological effects [16]. Increased lead levels, malnutrition and iron deficiency have negative effects on growth and development. Diets adequate in zinc, calcium, iron, vitamin D, phosphorus and protein can reduce high blood lead levels [22, 28]. Lead leakage from outdated non zinc-lined soldering seams in canned vegetables and fruits should be avoided (usually found in underdeveloped countries); accordingly, for homemade baby foods only fresh or frozen fruits and vegetables are recommended [29]. Calcium in evaporated or canned milk is rarely a problem as calcium chelates lead for excretion. Itoh and Suyama report another problem regarding calcium retention, high dietary sodium intake produces greater loss of calcium in urine as sodium and calcium compete for the same recovery mechanism in the kidney [30]. The purpose of this study was to determine the nutritional status of children with suspected abuse since it relates to health risk.

2. Methods

When the child was admitted to the ER with suspected abuse, a social worker was notified, who informed the investigator of the admission. The dietary department was contacted by nursing staff to record the child's dietary intake while a medical resident/staff was notified to perform laboratory levels as determined from the medical/social history. Medical records provided the following information: age, sex, race, type of injury, family size and family characteristics. Nutritional status was assessed using anthropometric measures, biochemical values and dietary intakes. Height and weight were plotted on the growth charts and head circumference, upper arm circumference and triceps skinfold measurements were performed according to the standard methods [31-34]. Biochemical values were obtained by established standard laboratory procedures. A calorie count one to three-day food record was obtained for each child and calculated by the dietitian for calories, protein, zinc, vitamin A, calcium, magnesium, phosphorus, iron, thiamin, riboflavin, niacin, vitamin C and vitamin D from standard data; below two-thirds of the standard being deficient [35]. Due to confidentiality and legal issues with these families, only hospital dietary intakes could be obtained A t-test was performed from anthropometric, biochemical, and dietary values against the standard and further compared PA against SA children. The research proposal was accepted by the Children's Hospital Medical Center's Institutional Review Board. Fingerprick lead screening was performed on 14 of the 28 children, as determined by medical staff from the medical/social history, and thus are listed as an outgrowth of the study.

3. Results/Discussions

Twenty-eight children suspected victims of child abuse, aged 1.5 months to 8.75 years [10 Caucasians, 17 African American, 1 bi-racial child; 14 male, 14 female) were admitted to ER. Type of injury, number of cases, and size of family are shown in Table 1. Many of the families received financial assistance, which is not atypical (Table 1). Anthropometric results showed the majority of subjects (61%) below the 50th percentile; 32% above the 75th percentile for height-for-age and 64% below the 50th percentile for weight-for-age (Table 2). The majority had TSF values of 8-9 mm; below the standard of 10.6 mm. Weight was significantly below the mean for PA children (p=0.05) and PA significantly below the mean of SA children (p=0.019). TSF for PA children were significantly below national government standards (p=0.01). All SA children were in upper percentiles of height-for-age and weight-for-age, while the majority of PA children were below the 50th percentile for weight-for-age. Biochemical results (Table 2) revealed the average hemoglobin was 11.6 gm%; significantly below the average of 12.7 gm% (p=0.0005) and. the average hematocrit was 35.5%; significantly below the standard of 37.1% (p=0.025) although dietary iron was adequate. Of 14 children, 36% had lead levels above normal and 28% were borderline indicating that lead levels may be high in some children with suspected abuse. SA children (p=0.005) and PA children (0.025) had significantly higher lead levels with PA children having more variability within the group. Hematocrits of SA children were slightly higher. PA subjects show that weight (p=0.05) and TSF (p=0.01) were significantly below standards (Table 2). Although diets offered to the hospitalized children were nutritionally adequate, diets consumed by children with suspected abuse were significantly lower than standard data in vitamin D and zinc (p=0.0005). When comparing PA and SA children, height (p=0.033) and weight (p=0.019) were significantly different and lower in PA children. A history of PA was more often found in males, with SA occurring more often in females [36, 37]. The incidence of abuse is not limited to racial minorities [38]; many children with suspected PA were Caucasian. The decreased weight of PA children found in this study is consistent with other findings that underweight and poor physical growth accompany child abuse [11, 39-42]. Low TSF values are consistent with findings and further indicate poor nutritional status. Leung et al. suggested FTT in child abuse may be due to withholding of food or the child not eating (appetite loss) associated with abuse/neglect. Twenty-five of 50 abused children had hemoglobin concentrations of less than 10gm% [38], while 25% fell below 10 gm% in this study. Bithoney et al. stated that every FTT child is malnourished [13]. Thirty-six percent [5 of 14 children) had elevated blood lead levels with 28% borderline, while Flaherty found 64.7% of abused and neglected children had elevated levels [14]. Behavioral manifestations of elevated lead may be more noticeable than effects on intelligence (elevated tempers and mental retardation) [43]. Zinc and vitamin D, which enhances calcium absorption, were low; thus, nutrient chelators were not available to reduce lead absorption [44]. Reduced weight and triceps values often accompany abuse, possibly indicating inadequate availability of food. Due to confidentiality of being classified with suspected abuse, home visits were not available as is typical in other reports on dysfunctional families. PA children have a higher rate of malnutrition, reduced growth, low iron status and elevated blood levels. Each is interrelated increasing the effects of the other. Leung et al [8] claim that if children are suffering from malnutrition, it is essential to begin early intervention because of unknown prognosis. Adequate energy needs should be addressed immediately, followed by treatment of iron deficiency anemia and elevated lead levels [13]. Furthermore, early intervention is essential as children may develop significant long-term cognitive and developmental delay.

Age Range:		1.5 months to 8.75 years	
Age		**Number of Subjects**	
0-3 years		10	
1-3 years		8	
4-6 years		8	
Over age 6		2	
Total:		28	
Type of Abuse		**Number of Subjects**	
1. Sexual		7	
2. Bruises/lacerations		8	
Subdural hematomas/facial trauma		6	
3. Dehydration/severe neglect		1	
4. Burns		3	
5. Fractures		3	
Total:		28	
Cross-Tabulation for Type of Abuse with Socioeconomic Variables:			
		Sexually Abused (SA)	**Physically Abused (PA)**
Race	Caucasian	1 (14.3%)	10 (47.6%)
	Non-Caucasian	6 (85.7%)	11 (53.4%)
Parents	One	4 (57.1%)	15 (71.4%)
	Two	3 (42.9%)	6 (28.6 %)
Receiving Government Aid	Yes	3 (42.9%)	13 (61.9%)
	No	4 (57.1%)	8 (38.1%)

Table 1. Summary of Characteristics of Children with Suspected Abuse

Factor	Mean	Standard Values	Standard Deviation	*p
All Subjects:				
Height (cm)	84.6	86.1	24.0	NS
Weight (kg)	12.4	16.6	8.4	NS
Head Circumference (cm)	46.6	46.6	5.3	NS

Triceps (mm)	9.2	10.6	4.7	0.10
Hemoglobin (g/dL)	11.6	12.7	1.0	0.0005*
Hematocrit (%)	35.5	37.1	4.0	0.025*
Vitamin D (I.U.)	247.7	400.0	69.7	0.0005*
Calcium (mg)	761.6	671.0	264.1	0.10+
Protein (g)	48.8	21.7	24.87	0.005*+
Magnesium (mg)	122.4	141.4	58.0	0.10+
Zinc (mg)	5.8	7.9	2.8	0.0005*
Physically Abused:				
Height (cm)	79.1	79.0	21.3	NS
Weight (kg)	10.3	12.2	5.9	0.05*
Head Circumference (cm)	45.7	45.5	5.9	ND
Triceps (mm)	8.5	10.4	2.9	0.01*
Hemoglobin (g/dL)	11.6	12.5	1.1	0.001*
Hematocrit (%)	35.4	36.8	4.3	0.05*
Vitamin D (I.U.)	254.7	400.0	76.8	0.0005*
Calcium (mg)	699.0	628.6	269.8	NS+
Protein (g)	42.0	18.6	25.1	0.0005*+
Magnesium (mg)	102.7	119.5	53.8	0.10+
Zinc (mg)	5.3	7.3	2.8	0.0005*

	Mean		
All Subjects	**Sexually Abused (SA)**	**Physically Abused (PA)**	***p**
Height (cm)	101.1	79.1	0.0033*
Weight (kg)	18.7	10.3	0.019*
Head Circumference (cm)	49.6	45.7	0.09
Triceps (mm)	11.4	8.5	0.10
Hemoglobin (g/dL)	11.6	11.6	NS
Hematocrit (%)	35.7	35.4	NS
Vitamin D (% DRI)	55.1	65.2	0.185
Calcium (% DRI)	112.8	112.5	NS+
Protein (%DRI)	299.4	230.0	NS+
Magnesium (% DRI)	79.9	85.0	NS+
Zinc (% DRI)	74.4	82.5	NS
Lead Screen (14 subjects) (% std) high 5(36%) borderline 4(28%) SA p=0.005* PAp=0.025*			

*Statistically significant p<0.05 by "t" test

+Nutrient intake and dietary iron adequate

Table 2. Nutritional Status Evaluation of Children with Suspected Abuse

4. Conclusion

Research indicates that abused children may be at nutritional risk upon hospital admission. PA children are especially vulnerable; therefore, awareness of the child's nutritional status by the health care team should be increased. Interdisciplinary cooperation involving physicians, social workers, nurses, and dietitians are needed to provide the best health care for these children. Dietitians should be responsible for employing various nutritional assessment techniques and teamwork with other disciplines. Further studies concerning dietary patterns in the home environment and nutritional knowledge of the caretaker/parent(s) should be conducted to prevent reoccurrence.

5. Applications

Dietitians/nutritionists should be included as members of a child abuse team. Child abuse/neglect training materials for medical/health professionals should incorporate nutritional status and provide nutrition education to caretakers/parents through Parents Anonymous Groups and similar therapeutic sessions. Nutritional as well as other environmental toxins, such as lead and mercury, also should be discussed with the families. Cooking sessions with culturally diverse nutrition education materials, nutrition counseling, and teamwork may need to be conducted by dietitians with families who have minimal cooking and/or nutritional skills using some of the available resources [45-51].

Author details

Eileen Harper[1], Shirley Ekvall[2,3*], Valli Ekvall[2,3] and Wei Pan[3]

*Address all correspondence to: shirley.ekvall@uc.edu

1 Providence Everett Medical Center, Seattle, Washington, USA

2 University Affiliated Cincinnati Center for Developmental Disabilities, Children's Hospital Medical Center, Cincinnati, Ohio, USA

3 University of Cincinnati, Cincinnati, Ohio, USA

References

[1] Child abuse doubles: investigation lags. *Public Health Reports*. 1997; 112:4.

http://dx.doi.org/10.5772/57374

[2] Department of Health and Human Services, Administration for Families Fact Sheet. Washington, D.C.; September 22, 2002.

[3] Famularo, R., Fenton, T., Kinscherff, R. Medical developmental histories of maltreated children. *Clin Pediatr.* 1992; 31:536-541.

[4] Duhaine, A.C., Christian, C., Moss, E., Seidl, T. Long-term outcome in infants with the shaking infant syndrome. *Pediatr Neurosurg.* 1996; 24:292-298.

[5] Depanfilis, D. Rates, patterns and frequency of child maltreatment recurrences among families known to CPS. *Child Maltreat.* 1998; 3:27-42.

[6] McCauley, J. Kern, D.E., Kolodner, K., Dill, L., Schroeder, A.F., DeChant, K. Clinical characteristics of women with a history of childhood abuse: unhealed wounds. *JAMA.* 1997; 277(17):1362-1368.

[7] Helfer, R. Pollock, C. The Battered Child Syndrome. *Adv Pediatr.* 1968; 15:9-27.

[8] Leung, A. Robson, W., Fagan, J. Assessment of the child with failure to thrive. *Am Fam Physician.* 1993; 48:1432-1438.

[9] Birrell, R., Birrell, J. The maltreatment syndrome in children. *Med J Aust.* 1968; 2:1023-1029.

[10] Bonnier, C., Nassaqne, M.C., Evard, P. Outcome and prognosis of whiplash shaken infant syndrome: late consequences after a symptom-free interval. *Dev Med Child Neurol.* 1995; 37:943-956.

[11] Martin, H.P., Beezley, P., Conway, E.F., Kempe, C.H. The development of abused children. *Adv Pediatr.* 1974;1074:21-25.

[12] Chung, E.K., Webb, D., Clampet-Lundquist, S., Campbell, C. A comparison of elevated blood lead levels among children living in foster care, their siblings, and the general population. *Pediatrics.* 2001; 107:E81-82.

[13] Bithoney, W., Vandeven, A., Ryan, A. Elevated lead levels in reportedly abused children. *J Pediatr.* 1993; 122:719-720.

[14] Flaherty, R. Risk of lead poisoning in abused and neglected children. *Clin Pediatr.* 1995; 34:128-132.

[15] Hu, H., Kotha, S., Brennan, T. The role of nutrition in mitigating environmental insults: policy and ethical issues. *Environmental Health Perspect.* 1995; 103(6):185-189.

[16] Mahaffey, K.R. Nutritional factors and lead poisoning. *Nutr Rev.* 1981; 39:353-365.

[17] Ahrens, F.A. Effects of lead on glucose metabolism, ion flux, and collagen synthesis in cerebral capillaries of calves. *Am J Vet Res.* 1993; 54:808-812.

[18] Lucas, S. Sexton, M., Langenburg, P. The relationship between blood lead levels and nutrition factors in preschool children: a cross-sectional study. *Pediatrics*. 1996; 97:74-78.

[19] Mahaffey, K.R., Garthside, P.S., Glueck, C.J. Blood lead and dietary calcium in 2926 1-through 11 year-old black and white children: The second national health and nutrition examination survey,. *Pediatrics*. 1986; 78:257-262.

[20] Schanne, F.A., Gupta, R.K., Rosen, J.F. lead inhibits 1, 25 dihydrovitamin D-3 regulation of calcium metabolis, in osteoblastic osteosarcoma cells (ROS 17/2.8). *Biochem Biophys Acta*. 1992; 1180:187-194.

[21] Long, G.J., Pounds, J.G., Rosen, J.F. Lead intoxication alters basal and parathyroid hormone-regulated cellular calcium homoeostasis in rat osteosarcoma (ROS 17/2.8) cells. *Calcif Tissue Int*. 1992; 50:451-458.

[22] Long, G.J., Rosen, J.F. Lead perturbs epidermal growth factor (EGF) modulation of intracellular calcium metabolism and collagen synthesis in clonal rat osteoblastic (ROS 17/2.8) cells. *Toxicol Appl Pharmacol*. 1992; 114:63-70.

[23] Bogden, J.D., Gertner, S.B., Christakos, S. Kemp, F.W., Yang, Z., Katz, S.R. Dietary calcium modified concentrations of lead and other metals and renal calbindin in rats. *J Nutr*. 1992; 122:1351-1360.

[24] Mahaffey, K.R. Nutrition and lead: Strategies for public health. *Environ Health Perspect*. 1995;103(S6):191-196.

[25] Lanphear, B.P., Hornung, R., Ho, M., Howard, C.R., Eberle, S., Knauf, B.S. Environmental lead exposure during early childhood. *J Pediatr*. 2002; 140:40-47.

[26] Hammand, T.A., Sexton, M., Langenberg, P. Relationship between blood lead and dietary iron intake in preschool children. *Ann Epidemiol*. 1996; 6(1):30-33.

[27] Flaherty, E., Weiss, H. Medical evaluation of abused and neglected children. *Am J Dis Child*. 1990; 144:330-334.

[28] Mushal, P. Cronenti, A.F. Lead and nutrition: biologic interactions of lead with nutrients. *Nutr Today*. 1996; 31:12-18.

[29] Ziegler, E.E., Edward, B.B., Jensen, R.I., Mahaffey, K.R., Fomon, S.J. Absorption and retention of lead by infants. *Pediatr Res*. 1978; 12:29-34.

[30] Itoh, R., Suyama, Y. Sodium excretion in relation to calcium and hydroxyproline excretion in a healthy Japanese population. *Am J Clin Nutr*. 1996; 63:735-740.

[31] Ekvall, S.W., Ekvall V.K., Nehring, W., Walberg-Wolfe, J.Nutritional Assessment, All Ages and Levels,In: Ekvall, S. W., Ekvall, V.K.eds. *Pediatric Nutrition in Chronic Diseases and Developmental Disabilities*. 2nd ed. New York: Oxford University Press; 2005:50-80.

[32] Owen, C. The assessment and recording of measurements of growth of children: report of a small conference. *Pediatrics*. 1973; 51:461-466.

[33] Lohman, T., Roche, A. Martorell, R. *Anthropmetry standardization reference manual*. Champaign, IL: Herman Kinetics Books; 1988.

[34] *National Center for Health Statistics: Growth Charts.* Rockville, MD: Health Resources Administration, Monthly Vital Statistics Report. 25(3), Suppl. (HRA), 76-1120.

[35] Bowes and Church. *Food Values of Portions Commonly Used*, 16th ed., Philadelphia, PA: JB Lippincott Co.; 1994 (incorporated into computer values).

[36] Sobsey, D., Randall, W. Parrilla, P.K. Gender differences in abused children with and without disabilities. *Child Abuse Negl.* 1997; 21:707-720.

[37] MacMillan, H.L., Fleming, J.E., Trocme, N, Boyle, M.H., Wong, M., Racine, Y.A., Beardslee, W.R., Offord, D.R. Prevalence of child physical and sexual abuse in the community. *JAMA*. 1997; 278:131-135.

[38] Ebbin, A.J., Gollub, M.H., Stein, A.M., Wilson, M.G. Battered child syndrome at Los Angeles County General Hospital. *Am J Dis Child*. 1969; 118:660-667.

[39] Elmer, E. *Children in Jeopardy*. Pittsburgh: University of Pittsburgh Press; 1974.

[40] Wehner, F. Schieffer, M.C., Wehner, H.D., Percentile charts to determine the duration of child abuse by chronic malnutrition. *Forensic Sci Int.* 1999; 105(3):191-194.

[41] Rao, N,K,, Begum, S., Benkataramana,V., Gangadharappa, N. Nutritional neglect and physical abuse in children of alcoholics. *Indian J Pediatr.* 2001; 68(9):843-845.

[42] Bonet Alcaina, M., Martinez Roig, A, Pujals Ferrer, J.M., Vall combelles, O. Kwashiorkor as a symptom of abuse and neglect in Barcelona. *An Esp Pediatr*. 2001; 54(4): 405-408.

[43] Glotzer, D.E., Weitzman, M. Commonly asked questions about childhood lead poisoning. *Pediatr Ann*. 1995;24(12):631-639.

[44] Hutchinson, J., Langlykke, K. *Adolescent Maltreatment: Youth as Victims of Abuse and Neglect* (Maternal and Child Health Technical Information Bulletin), Arlington, VA: National Center for Education in Maternal and Child Health; 1998.

[45] Huber, A., Ekvall,S. Lead Toxicity and Pica. In Ekvall, S.W., Ekvall, V.K.eds. *Pediatric Nutrition in Chronic Diseases and Developmental Disorders*. 2nd edition, New York, Oxford University Press, 2005; 168-170.

[46] Stevens, F., Ekvall, S. *Empowering Children with Good Nutrition and Early Intervention :Focusing on Culturally Diverse Children with Special Health Care Needs.* Maternal and Child Health Manual 4, Cincinnati, University of Cincinnati, 2002.

[47] Rokusek, C, Jarka, E., Hanley, B., Earle-Hahn, J. Community Based Services and Resources. In *Pediatric Nutrition in Chronic Diseases and Developmental Disorders.* 2nd edition, New York, Oxford University Press, 2005, 63-69.

[48] Graff. C., Murthy, L., Ekvall, S. Magnon, M. In home toxic chemical exposures and children with developmental disabilities. *Pediatr. Nursing.* November/December, 2006;32(6):597-602.

[49] American Dietetic Association (Diabetic Care and Education Practice Group), American Diabetes Association. *Ethnic and Regional Food Practices.* Chicago, American Dietetic Association, 1998.

[50] Ekvall S.,EkvallV. Nutrition Support for Children with Developmental Disabilities. In Baker,S, Baker,R, Davis,A. *Pediatric Nutrition Support*, Sudbury, Mass., Jones and Bartlett Publishers, 2007.

[51] Tyler,C,White-Scott,S, Ekvall, S, Abulafa, L. Environmental Health and Developmental Disabliltities: A Life Span Approach, *Family and Community Health.* 2008:31(4)28:287.

Chapter 17

Copper Deficiency a New Reason of Androgenetic Alopecia?

Margarita G. Skalnaya

Additional information is available at the end of the chapter

http://dx.doi.org/10.5772/58416

1. Introduction

Androgenetic alopecia is the common type of hair loss in men and women since puberty. Typically, AA is the complex result of an androgen-dependent process and this process is located to androgen receptor (AR) areas (frontal and vertex zone). Number of androgen receptors is genetic transmission. The polymorphism involving the CAG triple repeat expansion of the AR protein has been revealed in men with AA. This male pattern hair loss may represents from influence of minimal androgen excess basing on genetically sensitive hair papilla.

Dihydrotestosterone (DHT) is derived from circulating testosterone (T) inhibits cell proliferation in the dermal papilla and local production of vascular endothelial growth factor [1]. As a result, the DHT-dependent process leads to the miniaturization of sensitive hair follicles and progressive thinning the scalp hair. It is known that the follicular dermal papilla controls hair growth. Steroid hormones, including androgens, estrogens and glucocorticoids may influence on timing of hair cycle [2].

More recent studies have focused on androgen-regulated hair growth. But, studies of action of other steroids in the hair follicle have been relatively limited. There are two estrogen receptors (ERα and ERβ) which bind to 17β-estradiol. The effects of estrogens seem complex whereby estrogen prolongs the anagen phase of the hair follicle and stimulates hair shaft elongation [2]. ERβ expression was found in outer root shaft and epithelial matrix. In contrast, ERα and AR were expressed in dermal papilla [3].Therefore, the ratio of ERα to ERβ in dermal papilla cells is extremely important. Estrogen also modifies androgen metabolism. The local production of estrogens from androgen precursors has been converted by the aromatase cytochrome P 450 enzyme complex. It is now clear there is aromatase expression in the dermal papilla and the outer root sheath. The activity of aromatase is higher in women in occipital

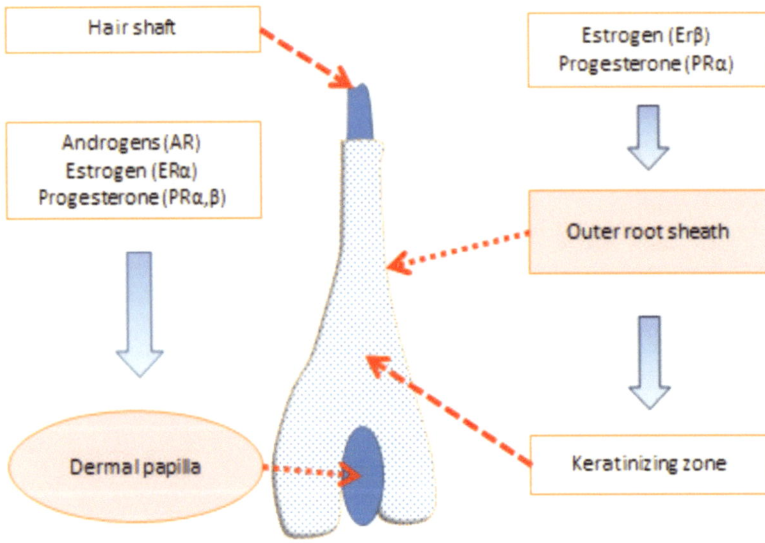

Figure 1. The hair shaft

scalp area compared to the frontal scalp and it has been diminished in AA [4]. Some researchers found that estradiol inhibited 5 alpha-reductase activities [5]. The effects on estrogens might be explained by an increased conversion of T to the weaker androgens such as androstendione and androstendiol. Progesterone is able to modulate activity of DHT in dermal papilla by 75% [4, 6]. Also, progesterone is widely recognized as a marker of estrogen action and has anti-inflammatory properties. Progesterone regulates the expression of matrix metalloproteinases (MMPs) by transforming growth factor-β [7].

However, in women hair loss is not limited to only this location and combined with diffuse alopecia. Except in some cases, treatment of 5 alpha reductase inhibitors is ineffective in women. The origin and mechanisms of AA in women are different and more complicated than in men and remain a challenge.

The aim of the work was to estimate a possible role of trace elements (TE) changes in AA in man and women.

2. Materials and methods

In this study, 97 women and 40 men, ages 20-55 y., with AA were selected for the determination of TE content and CP in serum, hormonal status. Diagnosis of AA was based on clinical findings, pattern of increased hair thinning on frontal/vertex scalp with greater hair density on occipital scalp zone; retention of frontal hairline; and the presence of miniaturized hairs (vellus hair, diameter less 30 μkm). Detailed study of the consumption of drugs, iron intake and thyroid metabolism ruled out other types of alopecia. The degree of AA was determined

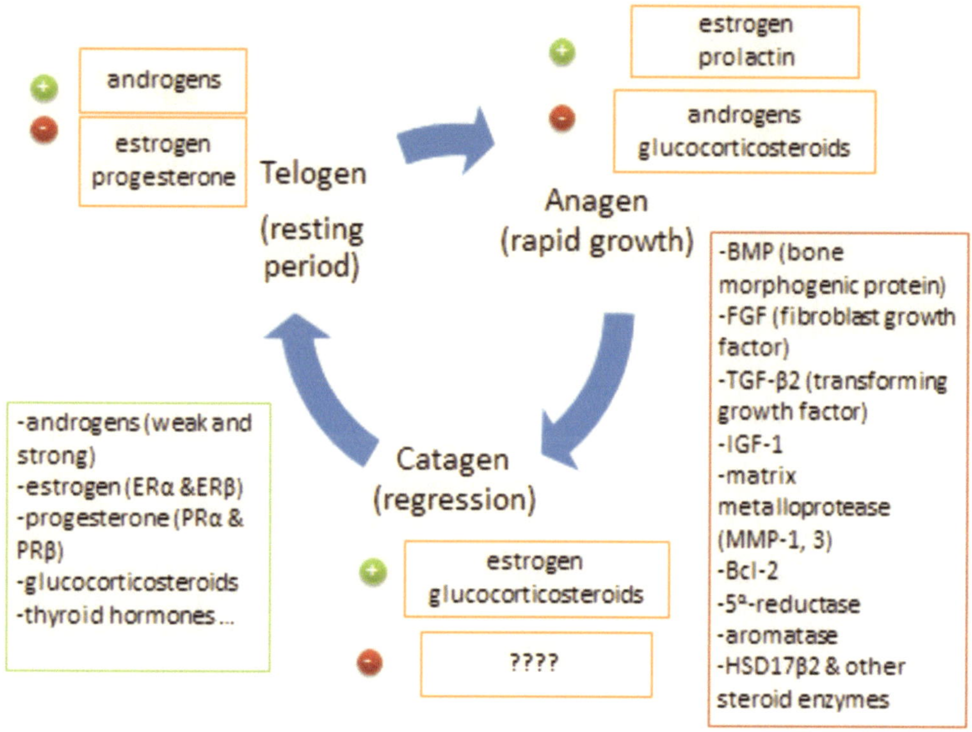

Figure 2. The timing of the hair cycle

by application of Ludwig scales (II–III). Exclusion criteria were: replacement hormone therapy (RHT) with estrogens, progesterone, testosterone, L-thyroxin or corticoids during last 6 months. Women's group was divided by 5 subgroups: women with excess of androgens, ages before 40 and after 40 y.o. (22 and 19 correspondently), women with excess of estrogens before and after 40 y.o. (24 and 17) and women with obesity at age of 20-40 year (16 patients). Women had both AA and the other sings of elevated androgens level (hirsutism and acne) were included in group with excess of androgens (HA 1 and 2). Women in group with excess of estrogens had endometriosis, uterine leiomyoma or combining both of these (HE 1 and 2). Childbearing aged women with abdominal obesity (waist >88 cm.) and excess of ALT concentration in blood were enrolled in group with obesity (O1). Control group included in age-matched men and women (76 and 32 patients correspondently) who presented no diseases at the time of examine. The concentration of TE has been analyzed by ICP mass-spectrometer Nexion-300D and Elan-9000 (Perkin Elmer Corp., USA). Reference materials of serum and hair samples were used. The level of FSH (follicle-stimulated hormone), LT (leuteotpophic), 17β-estradiol (E2), progesterone (PR), prolactin, androstendione (A), dihydrotestosterone (DHT) and sex hormone bound globulin (SHPG) was tested by routine laboratory methods.

Statistical analyses were performed with the ANOVA software (Statistics version 7). We applied non parametrical statistics: median, 25 and 75 percentiles. Student's t-test was used to compare the values of quantitative variables. Correlations among variables were studied using the Pearson's coefficient. P ≤ 0.05 was considered significant in all analyses.

3. Results

No significant differences of TE serum content in men and women were found between AA patients and control group. The exception was the concentration of copper (Cu) which was statistically significant differences between men and women suffering from AA and matched control (Table 1). In present work in women with hyperandrogenism there are the some trends in TE content in serum than in men. The key disorder was decreased Cu level in frontal zones of scalp hair and serum.

Element	Men				Women			
	AA group, n=40		Control, n=32		AA group, n=97		Control, n=76	
	Median	Persencile (25-75)	Median	Persencile (25-75)	Median	Persencile (25-75)	Median	Persencile (25-75)
As	0,019	0,015-0,025	0,015	0,008-0,028	0,018	0,007-0,028	0,02	0,01-0,032
Ca	92,3	88,2- 98,5	96,1	91,0-101,0	95,8	90,6-102,4	95,3	89,6-103,3
Co	0,0005	0,0004-0,0006	0,0006	0,0004-0,0007	0,006	0,0005-0,0008	0,0006	0,0005-0,0008
Cu	***0,80***	***0,70-0,85***	***0,88****	***0,75-1,06***	***0,85***	***0,77-0,94***	***0,99****	***0,90-1,11***
Fe	1,3	1,0-1,5	1,4	1,3-1,5	1,3	1,0-1,6	1,2	0,78-1,46
K	183	169-196	187	178-199	170	158-193	178	157-204
Mg	20,7	19,9-21,2	20,7	19,3-22,4	20,3	19,1-21,5	20,8	19,4-22,4
Mn	0,0034	0,0030-0,0038	0,0037	0,0031-0,0048	0,0032	0,0027-0,0039	0,0032	0,0026-0,0043
Mo	0,0008	0,0007-0,0012	0,0009	0,0007-0,0012	0,0009	0,0007-0,0012	0,001	0,0008-0,0014
Ni	0,006	0,005-0,007	0,006	0,005-0,008	0,006	0,005-0,007	0,006	0,005-0,008
Se	0,14	0,13-0,16	0,16	0,13-0,17	0,14	0,13-0,17	0,14	0,13-0,16
Zn	0,89	0,83-1,04	0,91	0,82-1,10	0,81	0,72-0,95	0,83	0,69-1,06

*-P<0, 01 (differences between control group and AA's group)

Table 1. Trace elements content (mkg/ml) in serum in men and women with AA

In spite of sex decreased Cu concentration in serum were obtained in patients with AA. However, Cu level in women was higher in comparison to men.

Median, 25-th and 75-th percentiles values in women with AA and accompanying other diseases are summarized in Table 2.

Element	HA1 n=22	HA2 n=19	O1 n=24	HE1 n=17	HE2 n=16	Control n=76
As	0,017 (0,007-0,031)	0,020 (0,008-0,031)	0,016 (0,006-0,038)	0,014 (0,006-0,023)	0,012 (0,007-0,031)	0,020 (0,010-0,032)
Ca	95,8 (91,5-98,0)	101,1 (89,3-104,0)	91,3 (87,2-97,5)	97,8 (87,1-100,5)	93,5 (91,7-97,1)	95,3 (89,6-103,3)
Co	0,0006 (0,0005-0,0007)	0,0005 (0,0004-0,0007)	0,0006 (0,0004-0,0008)	0,0007 (0,0005-0,0008)	0,0007 (0,0005-0,0010)	0,0006 (0,0005-0,0008)
Cu	0,81* (0,72-0,89)	0,85* (0,80-0,91)	0,94 (0,81-1,08)	0,97** (0,86-1,19)	0,99** (0,89-1,21)	0,99 (0,90-1,11)
Fe	1,3 (1,1-1,7)	1,2 (1,1-1,4)	1,2 (0,8-1,6)	1,3 (0,4-1,5)	1,1 (0,6-1,4)	1,2 (0,8-1,5)
K	183 (164-204)	193 (169-291)	183 (165-194)	195 (175-234)	170 (153-190)	178 (157-204)
Mg	20,4 (19,1-21,8)	20,9 (20,1-22,1)	19,6 (18,4-21,4)	20,5 (18,7-22,3)	19,6 (18,1-20,5)	20,8 (19,4-22,4)
Mn	0,0033 (0,0027-0,0040)	0,0035 (0,0030-0,0039)	0,0031 (0,0026-0,0034)	0,0030 (0,0027-0,0035)	0,0033 (0,0027-0,0036)	0,0032 (0,0026-0,0043)
Mo	0,0009 (0,0007-0,0013)	0,0007 (0,0005-0,0010)	0,0009 (0,0006-0,0011)	0,0008 (0,0006-0,0009)	0,0007 (0,0007-0,0008)	0,0010 (0,0008-0,0014)
Ni	0,006 (0,005-0,007)	0,006 (0,005-0,007)	0,006 (0,004-0,007)	0,005 (0,005-0,006)	0,005 (0,004-0,006)	0,006 (0,005-0,008)
Se	0,15 (0,13-0,16)	0,14 (0,14-0,16)	0,15 (0,13-0,16)	0,14 (0,12-0,16)	0,14 (0,13-0,15)	0,14 (0,13-0,16)
Zn	0,93 (0,82-1,05)	0,85 (0,75-1,07)	0,70* (0,66-0,76)	0,89 (0,80-0,95)	0,79 (0,69-1,19)	0,83 (0,69-1,06)
Cu/Mn	239 (187-306)	245 (213-277)	319 (278-369)	336** (300-438)	349** (282-420)	288 (253-370)
Cu/Zn	0,82* (0,73-1,06)	1,01 (0,76-1,14)	1,31* (1,22-1,40)	1,12 (1,04-1,25)	1,12 (0,82-1,50)	1,22 (0,94-1,42)

*-P<0,005 (differences between control group and others)

**-P<0, 05 (differences between groups with excess of androgens (HA1) and estrogens (HE 1 or 2)).

Table 2. TE content and ratio Cu/Mn and Cu/Zn (Median, 25-75th percentiles) in women with AA and associated with different diseases.

When we separated women with AA into subgroups there have obtained differences between control and investigated groups. No significant differences were found between AA patients and control in the majority of TE content in serum. Although the lowest Cu content was observed in group combining AA with other sing of excess of androgens such as hirsutism and acne.

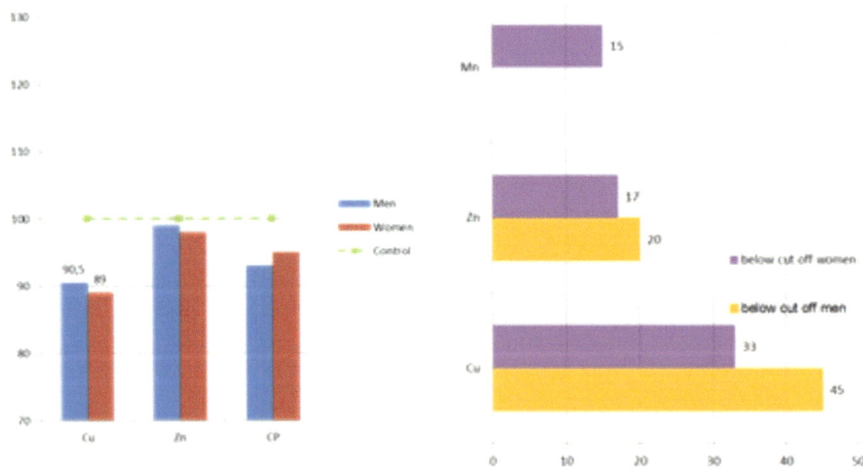

Figure 3. Content of Cu, Zn and ceruloplasmin (CP) in men and women with AA

Cu concentration in groups with elevated androgens level and with appearance of several marks of androgens abundance was lower than in the whole women group with AA. There were statistically significant differences between Cu level in groups with plenty of androgens and estrogen. In case of being endometriosis or uterine leiomyoma (HE1 and 2) in women Cu concentration in serum have maintained the same than in control, although not decreased in patients with AA. The overflowed androgens in women were conducted the reduction Cu content in serum considerably. The zinc (Zn) level was the lowest in women who combined AA and abdominal obesity. There was variety Zn content in serum in women at ages. In women under 40 year of age either elevated androgens or excess of estrogen the Zn level was getting low as compared to women before 40 year. The ratio Cu/Mn in women HE1 and 2 groups has been elevated significantly in comparison with groups with excess of androgens.

There was a tendency to raise the ratio Cu/Mn in women with elevated estrogen level as compared to control. The ratio Cu/Zn was significant lower in women any ages with abundant of androgens than in control. But, in case of abdominal obesity the values of this ratio were higher in comparison with control group.

4. Discussion

The hair follicle represents a unique, highly regenerative neuroectodermal – mesodermal interaction system. These transformations are controlled by changes in the expression/ activity

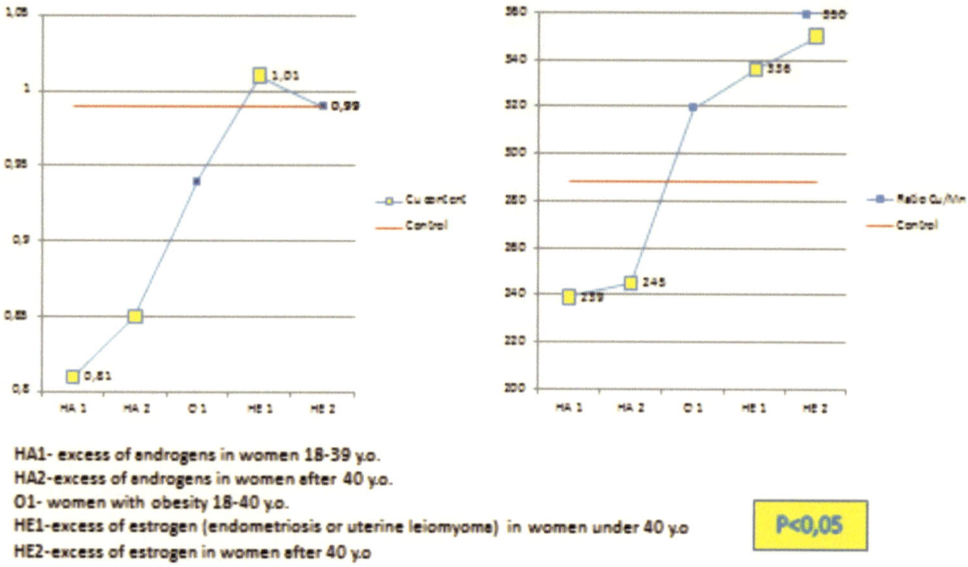

Figure 4. Cu content and ratio Cu/Mn in women with AA

of a numerous growing factors, cytokines, hormones, neurotransmitters, as well as transcription factors and enzymes.

Alopecia areata (AA) is the most common type of alopecia that the onset after puberty in both sexes. AA may affect up to 70 of men and 40% of women [8]. Male and female pattern hair loss are clinically distinct entities but pathogenically indistinguishable. The main role in the onset of AA in men is local disturbances in androgens metabolism which based on genetic predisposes to converse of terminal hair in vellus-like hair. AA is a polygenetic hereditary disease. A low number of CAG repeats in the androgen receptor gene implies increased risk factor for AA; prostate hyperplasia, coronary heart disease. But the role of sex hormones in females is less understood. Same of women suffering from AA are revealed androgens excess with other signs of elevated androgens such as hirsutism, acne, polycystic ovary syndrome. In women there is the appearance of AA combining with diffuse hair loss [9].

AA in men is due to implicate DNT production by 5 alpha-reductase type 2. The primary precursor of DHT in men is testosterone. The androgen receptor (AR) binding leads to increase production of cytokines such as TGFβ-1 and 2, which promote telogen, thinning and shortening hair. There is a low number of AR in occipital hair follicles that hair loss is mostly restricted to the scalp vertex and frontal and temporal areas. The using of a type 2 – selective inhibitor demonstrated the improvements in scalp hair growth in men. On stopping finasteride treatment, the balding process resumed. However, finasteride has been associated with depressive symptoms, persistent sexual side effects (loss of libido and erectile function). In contract to its beneficial effects of finasteride (5 alpha–reductase's inhibitor) in men; it didn't improve hair growth in women with AA. These findings suggested that the molecular mechanisms involved in the different metabolic ways in regulations hair growth in women.

Women with some markers of insulin resistant have increased risk of AA [9]. Several studies have analyzed the relationship between androgenetic alopecia and cardiovascular disease. Women with AGA showed higher significant mean values than non-alopecic women for all the parameters (triglyceridaemia, LDL-C, total cholesterol, total cholesterol/HDL-C and LDL-C/HDL-C) and lower significant HDL-C than controls.

Estrogens are indirect anti-androgens which increase SHMG production by binding to androgens and reducing their bioavailability. The production of estrogens from androgens via aromatase is of the importance in hair follicles. The comparison of scalp biopsies from men and women with AA revealed aromatase levels to be higher in hair follicles from occipital area in comparison to the frontal hair follicles. Furthermore, aromatase levels has found in six times higher in women when compared to men. Recent study has demonstrated that both dermal papilla and outer root sheath expressed aromatase activity. The levels of ER expression and aromatase activity may be modulated by steroid hormones in other tissues it would be important in the hair follicle. Likewise androgens have been reported to alter the ration of ERα to ERβ [2]. The alteration in the ratio of ERα to ERβ in dermal papilla cells could promote E2 signaling via ERβ in preference to ERα.

Since the hair follicles has been shown to express AR, glucocorticoid receptor, ERα, ERβ and progesterone receptors (PRα and PRβ). Both the dermal papilla cells and surrounding epithelial cells express ER. Additional local productions of E2 via conversion from A by aromatase may act in either an autocrine or paracrine manner to control lair growth and differentiation. In experimental studies PR inhibited the synthesis of DHT in dermal papilla by 75%. E2 was less able inhibit its production [6].

However, no direct effects of prolactin on hair growth have been reported [11]. Progesterone acts via PR receptors on cells to induce secretion of paracrine factor that in turn stimulate the expression 17β –hydroxysteroid dehydrogenase type 2 (HSD17β2). HSD17β2 metabolizes E2 to weak estrogenic estrone. The control of hair growth by E2 is much more complex than previously appreciated.

The E2 may modulate hair growth by interfering with androgen metabolism [12]. The estrogenic effects on dermal papilla cells are mediated via ERα.The role of ERβ may be to protect tissues from oxidative stress by inducing battery of antioxidative enzymes. Under hyperestrogenic conditions, the ratio PRβ to PRα is decreased but ratio ERβ to ERα is elevated in endometriosis and uterine leiomyoma. Serum Cu level is known to control by estrogens. Under excess of androgens Cu content in serum was decreased and associated with elevated DHT level which results of 5alpha-reductase type 2 activities. The pathogenic mechanism of AA is case of abundant of androgens doesn't differ in men and women with high androgens level. The development of AA shows up other clinical marks of androgens excess (hirsutism and acne) and reflect the interaction androgens and estrogen metabolism. Both AR and ERα are located into dermal papilla and influenced on hair growth [4]. In some studies have shown there was depressed ratio E2 to androgens [13].

http://dx.doi.org/10.5772/58416

We demonstrated the development of AA in women with endometriosis or /and uterine leiomyoma. These diseases have usually revealed of estrogens excess, high activity of aromatase and decreased level of progesterone. There was a high level of ratio ERβ to ERα against the background of changed ratio progesterone receptor (PRα/PRβ). The onset and development of AA in this group didn't link to abundant androgens level.

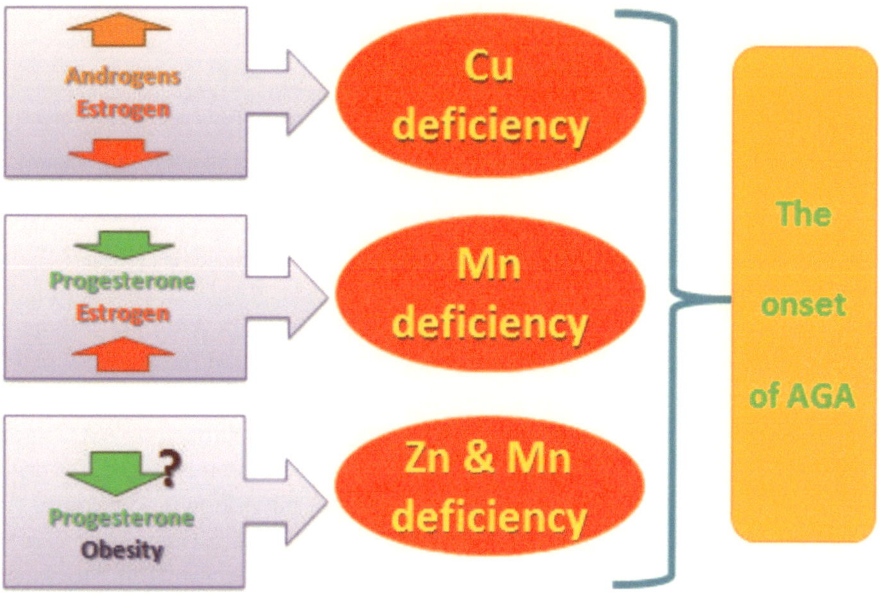

Figure 5. Proposed schema of TE dependent androgenetic alopecia

Normal or excess estrogens concentration and deficiency or resistant to progesterone were typical in these women. Cu content in serum and ratio Cu/Mn determined higher than in control. But, Mn level in these groups remains lower to compare with control. These data suggest that the important value in appearance of AA belongs to the relationship between E2 and PR and ratio of their receptors in peripheral tissues. About 15% from all examined women with AA have been detected the cut-off Mn level. Mn is known to impede the female and male reproductive function. In experimental studies the relationship Mn concentration and progesterone level have been shown. There is the high level of Mn-COD in lutein phase of menstrual cycle [14]. Manganese superoxide dismutase (Mn–COD), an antioxidant enzyme in the mitochondria, protects cells by scavenging superoxide radicals. Mn–COD increases by inducing progesterone. Experimental data suggests that Mn down-regulated steroidogenesis in Leydig cells [15]. Mn influences the receptor signaling pathways and contractile machinery of vascular smooth muscle cells [16]. The expression of Mn-COD was significantly increased by 17β–estrogen and testosterone in neutrophil granulocytes in healthy volunteers [17]. In our work we hypothesize that the assignment of low Mn content may reflect depressed value of PR, changed ratio PR receptors or cell's resistance to PR.

In women serum ferritin levels may also be assessed to determine hair loss. Appreciating the importance of iron as a factor in hair loss may be important in the therapy in a variety of etiologically distinct forms of hair loss. According to obtained findings there was no statistical difference in iron content between control and experimental groups [18].

Condition	**excess of A**	**excess of estrogen**
Hormonal status	↑ A→DHT	↑E, ↓Progesterone, ± A
Receptors	AR→ alteration ratio ERα/ERß	alteration ratio ERα/ERß and PRβ/PRα
Age	after puberty	middle age and premenopausal
Treatment	decrease level of A and modulation of ratio ER's	increase level of progesterone and modulation of ratio ER's

Table 3. The difference of the onset and development of AA under excess of androgen or estrogen.

In this hypothetic scenario, there were two groups' women with AA. One of them has been registered excess of A in serum (Table 3). The other demonstrated normal level of A but had the alteration of estrogen and progesterone contents in blood. A lot of hormones, growth's factors take part in development of AA. Many diseases have followed by AA. Typically, the excess of A in blood in both men and women with AA have been revealed. Surprisingly, in women with hyperestrogenic condition the onset of AA have shown. The comparable with control level of A has been demonstrated in this group. Therefore, the ratio of ERα to ERß in follicular dermal papilla cells may be important. The alteration of estrogen, progesterone and androgen receptors has the key of metabolic disturbances in dermal papilla cells and outer root sheath. That is why the typical approaches for treatment of AA which include in using hormonal replacement therapy, inhibitors of DHT production and others were not fruitful.

Author details

Margarita G. Skalnaya*

Address all correspondence to: skalnaya@yandex.ru

Center for Biotic Medicine, Moscow, Russia

References

[1] Jamin C. Androgenetic alopecia. //Ann. Dermato.l Venereol.-2002.-Vol. 129.-N.5 (Pt 2).-P.801-803.

[2] Thornton M.J. et al. The modulation of aromatase and estrogen receptor alpha in cultured human dermal papilla cells by dexamethasone: a novel mechanism for selective action of estrogen via estrogen receptor beta? //J. Investigative Dermatology.-2006.-Vol. 126.-P. 2010-2018.

[3] Ohnemus U. et al. The Hair Follicle as an Estrogen Target and Source. // Endocrine Reviews.-2006.-Vol. 27.-N. 6.-P. 677-706.

[4] Hoffmann R. Enzymology of the hair follicle. //European J. Dermatology.-2001.-Vol. 11.-N. 4.-P. 296-300.

[5] Hoffmann R. et al. 17alpha-estradiol induces aromatase activity in intact human anagen hair follicles ex vivo. //Exp. Dermatol. – 2002.-Vol.11.-N.4.-P. 376-380.

[6] Niiyama S, Happle R, Hoffmann R. //Influence of estrogens on the androgen metabolism in different subunits of human hair follicles. //Eur. J. Dermatol. – 2001.-Vol.11.-N.3.-P. 195-198.

[7] Chevronnay G.H.P. et al. Regulation of matrix metalloproteinases activity studied in human endometrium as a paradigm of cyclic tissue breakdown and regeneration. // Biochim. Biophys. Acta.-2012.-Vol. 1824.-N. 1.-P. 146-156.

[8] Kevin J. et al. Promising therapies for treating and /or preventing androgenic alopecia. //Skin Therapy Lett.-2012.-Vol. 17.-N. 6.-P.1-4.

[9] Arias-Santiago S. et al. A comparative study of dyslipidaemia in men and women with androgenic alopecia. //Acta Derm. Venereol.-2010.-Vol. 90.-P. 485-487.

[10] Niiyama R., Happle R. and Hoffmann R. Influence of estrogens on the androgen metabolism in different subunits of human hair follicles. //Eur. J. Dermatol.-2001.-Vol. 11.-N.3.-P. 195-198.

[11] Craven A.J. et al. Prolactin signaling influences the timing mechanism of the hair follicle: analysis of hair growth cycles in prolactin receptor knockout mice. //Endocrinology.-2001.-Vol. 142.-N. 6.-P. 2533-2539.

[12] Ohnemus U. et al. Hair cycle control by estrogens: catagen induction via estrogen receptor (ER)-α is checked by ER-β signaling. //Endocrinology.-2005.-Vol. 146.-N. 3.-P. 1214-1225.

[13] Matthew D. et al. Extra-adrenal glucocorticoids and mineralocorticoids: evidence for local synthesis, regulation and function. //Am. J. Physiol. Endocrinol. Metab.-2011.-Vol. 301.-P. 11-24.

[14] Sugino N. et al. Superoxide dismutase expression in the human corpus luteum during the menstrual cycle and in early pregnancy. //Mol. Hum. Reprod. – 2000. – Vol. 6. – N. 1. – P. 19-25.

[15] Cheng J., Fu J.L. and Zhou Z.C. The inhibitory effects of manganese on steroidogenesis in rat primary Leydig cells by disrupting steroidogenic acute regulatory (StAR) protein expression. // Toxicology.-2003.-Vol. 187.-N. 2-3.-P. 139-148.

[16] Kalea A.Z., Harris P.D. and Klimis-Zacas D.J. Dietary manganese suppresses alpha 1 adrenergic receptor-mediated vascular contraction. //J. Nutr. Biochem. – 2005.-Vol. 16.-N. 1.-P. 44-49.

[17] Adler I. et al. The effect of certain steroid hormones on the expression on genes involved in the metabolism of free radicals. //Gynecol. Endocrinol.-2012.-Vol.

[18] Kantor J.et al. Decreased serum ferritin is associated with alopecia in women. // J. Investigative Dermatology.-2003.-Vol.121.-P. 985–988.

Chapter 18

Pharmacological Interventions of Selenium in Duchene Muscular Dystrophy: The Role of Reactive Oxygen Species in Mediating Lipid Peroxide Formation

Tuomas Westermarck, Shirly Ekvall and
Kaski Markus

Additional information is available at the end of the chapter

http://dx.doi.org/10.5772/57370

1. Introduction

The muscular dystrophies are a group of muscle diseases which have three features in common: they are hereditary; they are progressive; and each causes a characteristic, selective pattern of weakness. Duchenne muscular dystrophy (DMD) is the most common inherited muscular disease, affecting one in 3,500 male births. DMD is characterized by rapid, progressive muscle wasting that typically kills patients in their twenties. Complete muscle dystrophin deficiency is a common mechanism for DMD.

Duchenne muscular dystrophy (DMD) is a severe X-linked recessive, progressive muscle-wasting disease affecting one in 3500 boys (Emery AEH, 1993). Patients are usually confined to a wheelchair before the age of 12 and die in their late teens or early twenties usually of respiratory failure. A milder form of the disease, Becker muscular dystrophy (BMD), has a later onset and a much longer survival.

The most widely studied dystrophies are those due to mutations in the dystrophin gene. In humans, dystrophin deficiency leads to the severe disease, Duchenne muscular dystrophy, whereas reductions or truncations of dystrophin lead to a milder disease, Becker muscular dystrophy. Numerous animal models of dystrophin deficiency are actively studied, but none more so than the *mdx* mouse. Despite over a decade of study of dystrophin and its associated proteins, some of which themselves cause muscular dystrophies when deficient or defective, the mechanisms by which the primary biochemical defects lead to muscle cell death remain to be determined.

Both disorders are caused by mutations in the DMS gene that encodes a 427-kDa cytoskeletal protein called dystrophin. The vast majority of DMD mutations result in the complete absence of dystrophin, whereas the presence of low levels of a truncated protein is seen in BMD patients. The defected gene causes a shortage or absence of the structural protein dystrophin, which is near the sites of Ca^{2+} release from sarcoplasmic reticulum and uptake of intracellular Ca^{2+}. The genetic alteration produces an abnormality in the membrane of muscular fibers that consists of a disturbance in the calcium transport (Ca^{++}), inside the muscular fibers, which is the base mechanism of cellular degeneration, necrosis, and apoptosis (Simonian and Coyle 1996). A nucleotide degeneration and decreased muscle AP and ADP content has been reported. Of the total body selenium reserves consists of muscle selenium supply. Selenium is gradually wasted out by the kidneys during the proceeding of the dystrophy of the legs (Westermarck et al 1982). Open follow-up trials with antioxidants are indicating positive clinical response (Gebre-Medhin et al 1985; Timberg 1989; Westermarck et al 1997).

2. Description and clinical features of Duchenne

Typically, DMD patients are clinically normal at birth, although serum levels of muscle isoform of creatine kinase are elevated. The onset of pseudohypertrophy of the calf muscles, proximal limb muscle weakness suggests DMD. Weakness of the arms occurs later along with progressive kyphoscoliosis (Dubowitz. Major Probl Clin Pediatr 1978).

Most patients die in their early twenties as a result of respiratory complications due to intercostal muscle weakness and respiratory infection. Death can also be the result of cardiac dysfunction with cardiomyopathy. BMD and DMD patients also present with mild cognitive impairment, indicating that brain function is also abnormal in these disorders (Blak and Martin-Rendon, 2002).

Fetal DMD is histologically normal except for occasional eosinophilic hypercontracted fibers (Bertorini et al. 1984). Necrotic or degenerating muscle fibers are seen in all postnatal DMD muscle biopsies even before muscle weakness is clinically seen. The necrotic fibers are phagocytized, and muscle biopsies from DMD patients reveal the presence of inflammatory cells at perimysial and endomysiel sites (Arahata and Engel 1984). The regenerative capacity of the muscle is lost and muscle fibers are gradually replaced by adipose and fibrous connective tissue, giving rise to the clinical appearance of pseudohypertrophy followed by atrophy (Emery 1993), resulting in muscle wasting and ultimately muscle weakness (Blake et al 2002). Most patients die in their early twenties as a result of respiratory complications due to intercostal muscle weakness and respiratory infection. Death can also be the result of cardiac dysfunction with cardiomyopathy. BMD and DMD patients also present with mild cognitive impairment, indicating that brain function is also abnormal in these disorders (Blake and Kroger 2000).

DMD muscle shows signs of oxidative damage (Murphy and Kehrer 1989). Muscle diseases in which oxidative damage may play a primary role show features in common with DMD (Mendell Et al 1971). Moreover, muscle cells from mdx mice have an increased susceptibility to oxidative stress (Rando et al 1998). The lack of neuronal-type nitric oxide synthase (nNOS) seen in DMD causes disregulation of vascular tone, and ischemia (Crosbie 2001, Blake et al 2002). This henomenon may increase the generation of free radicals. Open follow-up trials with antioxidants are indicating positive clinical response (Gebre-Medhin et al 1985; Timber 1989; Westermarck et al 1997).

A low blood selenium level has previously been observed in healthy inhabitants of Finland (WESTERMARCK, 1977). In this study even lower blood selenium values were observed in patients with acrodermatitis enteropathica, dystrophia musculorum progressiva (Duchenne), infantile and juvenile type of neuronal ceroid lipofuscinosis (NCL), severe mental retardation caused by various factors, and myocardial infarction. The selenium content of the brain, heart, kidney and liver in patients of different ages was also determined. The highest selenium level was found in the kidney. The mean liver selenium concentrations in stillborn, premature and full-term neonates were 1.11 +/- 0.23 (8), 1.21 +/- 0.17 (12) and 0.93 +/- 0.16 microgram/g dry weight (12) respectively (the number of subjects in parentheses). The selenium values are considerably higher than those in infants of from one to nine months of age and adults, whose liver selenium values were 0.58 +/- 0.21 (8) and 0.67 +/- 0.08 microgram/g dry weight (8) respectively. The vitamin E levels of serum in patients with NCL, as well as in subjects with severe mental retardation (controls), were low compared with values in healthy normal subjects. Sodium selenite supplementation in patients with NCL produced at least a transitory improvement without causing any toxic effects during one year of administration. In Duchenne muscular dystrophy we found that ^{75}Se-selenite was not absorbed in the lower extremities in the equal level compared to healthy ones.

3. Oxidative stress

Oxidative stress is often defined as an imbalance between the generation of reactive oxygen species and the removal of such species by enzymatic and nonenzymatic cellular defense systems (Figure 1). This imbalance could arise from overproduction of reactive species, as occurs under certain pathologic conditions and in association with inflammation, or from an impairment of the defense mechanisms, as occurs in certain genetic loss-of-function disorders and deficiency states. Implicit in this definition is the notion that such an imbalance is sufficient to lead to the oxidation of various cellular constituents and to cause cellular dysfunction and injury. As such, oxidative stress may also be viewed as a condition in which the production of oxidative products exceeds their removal by cellular repair mechanisms. Such conditions may lead to acute cellular dysfunction or cell death, and chronic tissue degeneration, if such changes accumulate.

During normal cellular metabolism, the primary generation of reactive oxygen species comes from the leakage of superoxide anions from the electron transport chain. A series of linked enzymatic reactions are responsible for the detoxification of superoxide. Superoxide is converted to hydrogen peroxide by the action of superoxide dismutase (SOD). Most animal cells contain two forms of SOD, a cytoplasmic Cu,Zn-SOD and a mitochondrial Mn-SOD. In addition, there is an extracellular form of the enzyme. Hydrogen peroxide is subsequently metabolized to oxygen and water by the selenium-containing enzyme glutathione peroxidase, which uses glutathione (GSH) as a cofactor in the reaction. Glutathione peroxidase converts most of the hydrogen peroxide in the cytoplasm. At sites of relatively high concentrations of hydrogen peroxide, such as peroxisomes, catalase is an important antioxidant enzyme that also converts hydrogen peroxide to water. Hydrogen peroxide can react with metal ions in the cell to produce the highly reactive hydroxyl radical, and superoxide can react with nitric oxide (NO•) to produce peroxynitrite. Hydroxyl radical and peroxynitrite are among the most reactive species present in biological systems and are capable of oxidizing nucleic acids, proteins, lipids, and carbohydrate moieties in the cell.

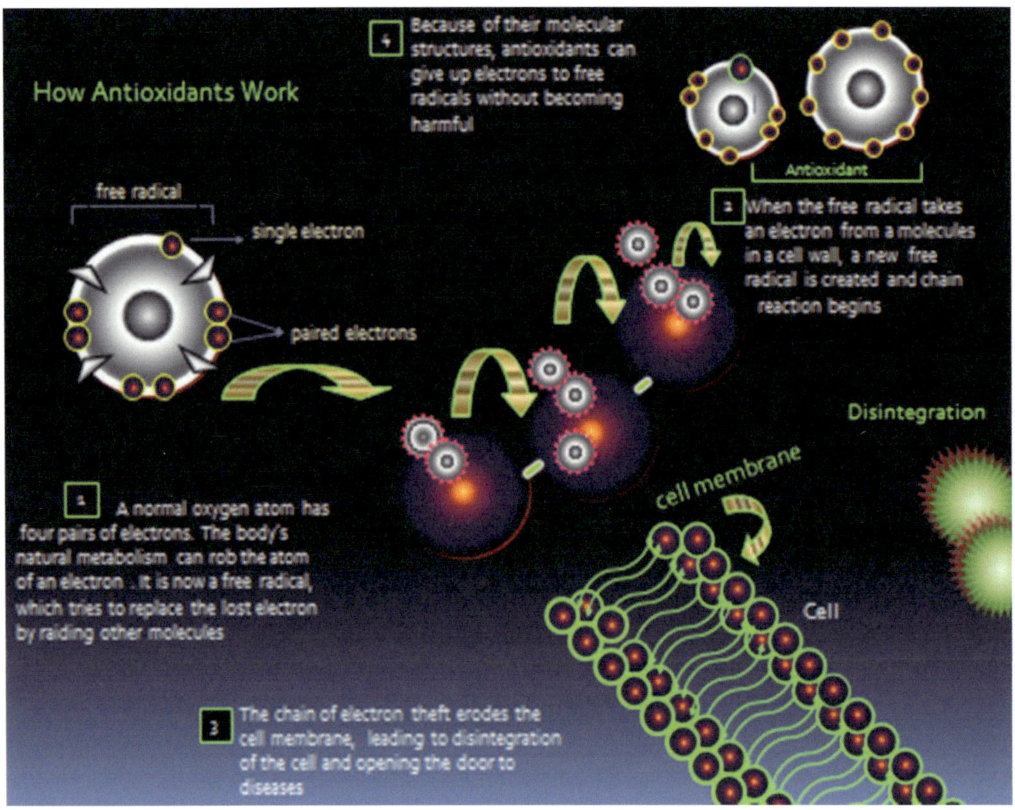

Figure 1. The role of free radical in inflammation

4. Oxidative stress cause dystrophic changes

One of the first observations that led to the oxidative stress hypothesis was the finding that vitamin E deficiency in animals leads to muscle degeneration with pathologic characteristics very similar to those of the muscular dystrophies. The similarities are most striking in avian species in which vitamin E deficiency myopathies closely mimic the hereditary dystrophies both anatomically and biochemically. In humans, vitamin E deficiency is associated with myopathic changes, and in these disorders, there is selective involvement of type IIB fibers as in the inherited muscular dystrophies. Vitamin E refers to a group of compounds of which [alpha]-tocopherol is the most potent and most prevalent in animal tissues as the major lipid-soluble antioxidant in the cell. Deficiencies of vitamin E are associated with increases in lipid peroxidation and decreases in polyunsaturated fatty acids in muscle and compensatory increases in muscle antioxidant enzymes and GSH levels. Although it is clear that inherited muscular dystrophies are not due to primary deficiencies in vitamin E, as was once proposed, the cumulative data strongly support the proposition that the mechanism of muscle injury is the same in both conditions.

5. Can antioxidant treatment ameliorate muscular dystrophy

In addition to evidence of oxidative damage preceding pathologic changes, amelioration of the pathology of a muscular dystrophy by antioxidant treatment would be strong support for the hypothesis that oxidative stress is a primary pathogenetic process. Various antioxidant treatments have been tried in humans and animals with muscular dystrophy. However, the benefit from any individual antioxidant treatment would depend on the actual nature of the oxidative stress that is occurring in the muscle tissue. For example, supplementation of vitamin E–deficient animals with the most prevalent cellular soluble antioxidant, ascorbic acid (vitamin C), does not significantly improve the myopathy. Different susceptibilities to oxidative stress are not identical. Even if oxidative stress is indeed the primary pathophysiologic process leading to muscle cell death in the dystrophies, effective treatment will need to be targeted to the specific deficit in antioxidant defense in the dystrophic muscle and thus will depend on a detailed understanding of the nature of that susceptibility.

Antioxidant treatments in animals with hereditary muscular dystrophies have provided modest benefits. Penicillamine, a sulfhydryl compound with antioxidant properties, and vitamin E slowed the degenerative process in avian dystrophy. Research showed that iron deprivation resulted in a significant reduction of necrosis in the mdx mouse, presumably by a decrease in the production of hydroxyl radical. Dietary supplementation rich in antioxidants significantly reduced an index of muscle weakness in mdx mice.

Clinical trials of antioxidant therapy in humans with Duchenne muscular dystrophy have included treatments with tocopherols, ascorbate, penicillamine, and SOD. No clear benefit has been found from any of these treatments. However, these trials have been very limited in duration and size. Furthermore, in no human study has antioxidant treatment begun early in the course of the disease. In fact, all of these studies involved boys with advanced disease (average age, >=10 yr). Based on the notion that oxidative injury is critical to the pathogenesis of muscle cell death and that antioxidant treatment might be effective to prevent such death, trials in humans would need to be initiated early in the course of the disease, and efficacy would need to be assessed primarily as the slowing, not a reversal, of muscle loss. The difficulties and pitfalls of clinical trials for new treatments of muscular dystrophies are well known. Thus, based on both statistical power and theoretical benefit, none of these human trials would even be predicted to demonstrate any benefit, and the negative results do not in any way refute the oxidative stress hypothesis.

6. Selenium in the brain and brain diseases

Oxidative stress and generation of reactive oxygen species (ROS) are strongly implicated in a number of neuronal and neuromuscular disorders, including stroke and cerebrovascular disease, Alzheimer's disease, Parkinson's disease, familial amyotrophic lateral sclerosis, and Duchenne muscular dystrophy (Dexter et al. 1989a,b; Smith et al. 1991; Ragusa et al. 1997; Cornett et al. 1998b; Facchinetti et al. 1998; Sagara et al. 1998; Tan et al. 1998). Selenium is known to provide protection from ROS-induced cell damage, and the proposed mechanisms mainly invoke the functions of glutathione peroxidases (GPxs) and selenoprotein P (SelP).

Considerable evidence exists linking heavy metals to neurodegenerative diseases (Thompson et al. 1988; Deibel et al. 1996; Cuajungco and Lees 1997; Schionning et al. 1997; Cornett et al. 1998b; Ely 2001). Heavy metals trigger the conversion of hydrogen peroxide to hydroxyl radical through Fenton reaction. Selenium has long been known to function as an antidote to toxicity of heavy metals. Co-administration of selenium was reported to play a role in reducing the toxic effects of mercury as early as the 1970s (Koelman et al. 1973; Kosta et al. 1975). Among the selenoproteins, SelP has been reported in several studies to possess metal-binding function (see below). The GPxs might also detoxify heavy metals through their well-known function of eliminating peroxides (Figure 2).

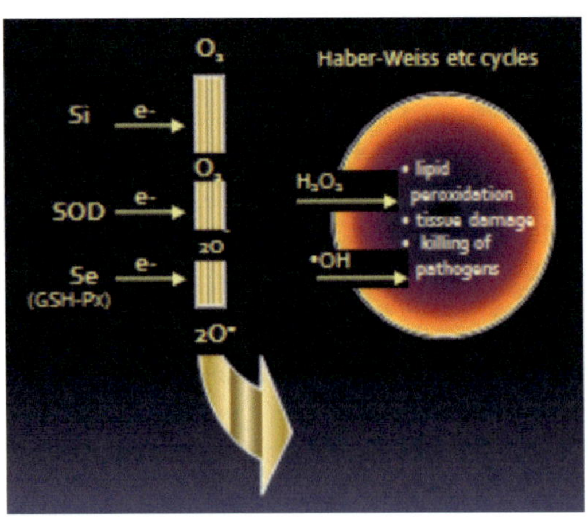

Figure 2. Complementary actions of selenium (GSH-Px) in free radical formation and lipid peroxidation (from Parantainen et al., 1987)

http://dx.doi.org/10.5772/57370

7. Treatment of brain diseases with selenium

Two children with severe neurodevelopmental retardation and elevated liver function tests developed intractable seizures during the first years of life. They were found systemically selenium deficient. Oral substitution with selenium supplements in both children (3–5 μg/kg body weight) resulted in reduction of seizures, improvement of the electroencephalogram (EEG) recordings, and return of normal liver function after 2 weeks (Ramaekers et al. 1994). It is unknown if selenium deficiency is a direct factor for the neurodevelopmental retardation or it affected the brain via abnormal liver function.

Methamphetamine (MA) exposure of animals results in enhanced formation of superoxide radical ($O2^-$) and nitric oxide (NO), which interact to produce peroxynitrite ($OONO^-$). Peroxynitrite is a potent oxidant, leading to dopaminergic damage (Imam and Ali 2000). Thus, multiple dose administration of MA to mice results in long-lasting toxic effects in the nigrostriatal dopaminergic system, which is a relevant model of PD. In selenium-replete mice, this dopaminergic toxicity was significantly attenuated, compared with selenium-deficient mice (Kim et al. 1999; Kim et al. 2000). Pre-treatment of animals with selenium and melatonin can completely protect against the depletion of striatal dopamine induced by MA exposure (Imam et al. 2001). The reason for the protective effects of selenium against MA was reported to be the efficient scavenging of peroxynitrite by selenoproteins (Sies and Arteel 2000).

6-hydroxydopamine (6-OHDA) is a neurotoxin specific for catecholamine neurons in both the central and peripheral nervous system. PD induced by this compound in rats was prevented by selenium in a dose-dependent manner, through up-regulating the antioxidant status and lowering the dopamine loss. This study revealed that selenium may be helpful in slowing down the progression of neurodegeneration in Parkinsonism (Zafar et al. 2003).

8. Hypotesis and intervention

It is possible to improve the life quality of Duchenne patients by biological active substances (antioxidants), and psychotherapeutic intervention. Therapy of DMD has been an elusive goal. Studies with isolated myocytes have shown that lipid peroxidation with an enhanced free radical production can be activated by increasing Ca concentration. No wonder that several kinds of antioxidants have been proposed as a treatment since increased levels of thiobarbituric acid (TBA) reactive material has been found in the muscles and blood of patients with DMD.

Vitamin E has been observed to decrease the amount of TBA reactive material in dystrophic muscle. Previously we have reported that the biological half-life of selenium -75 (75Se) in DMD patients is significantly shorter than in healthy controls (Westermarck et al 1982). On the basis of these facts we started to treat some DMD patients with selenium and other antioxidants. Selenium is activating a well-known antioxidative enzyme glutathione peroxidase (GSH-Px, iodothyronine desiodinase, selenoprotein P, thioredoxin reductase and the selenoprotein W, that all contain selenocystein. Beside iodothyronine desiodinase that facilitates the activation of thyroid hormones; all other selenoproteins have a role in the metabolisation and detoxification of reactive oxygen species and in the maintenance of the antioxidant defense of cells.

For example, in 1981 the antioxidant treatment of two siblings with DMD, aged six and ten years, was started. At that time the older brother was wheel-chair bound and was not able to walk since eight years of age, the younger one was still able to walk almost normally. The condition of the older brother, who practically had not got carnitine or coenzyme Q^{10} supplementation, was gradually deteriorated, and he deceased at 17 years of age. However, at the age of 15 years the younger brother was still able to walk without any assistance. Six months later he became wheel-chair bound. The younger brother was one of the most talented graduated students in his high-school. The mean IQ of DMD patients is without treatment 15-20 points lower than that of normal populations. Anyway for some years he was able to study at the University of Joensuu. Now he is 31 years old and still able to swim some meters, and to produce computer art. Actually he had his first art-show in 2003 in Helsinki. Moreover, only during the nights it is necessary to give him non-invasive breathing assistance.

The present daily megadoses of nutrients supplements (vitamin E 1200mg; sodium selenite 8mg; riboflavin 3mg; pyridoxine 75mg; carnitine 600mg; and coenzyme Q10 180mg) have been well tolerated and no side effects have observed in our opcn controlled trial (Westermarck et al 1997). The long-term pilot study speaks in favor for a larger study. Dr. Anders Erikson from Sweden (personal communication) has made the same observations with two Swedish siblings suffering from DMD, as we have also made with two 13- and 14-year old cousins 2with DMD.

Author details

Tuomas Westermarck[1], Shirly Ekvall[2,3] and Kaski Markus[1]

1 Rinnekoti Foundation, Espoo, Finland

2 University Affiliated Cincinnati Center for Developmental Disabilities, Children's Hospital Medical Center, Cincinnati, Ohio, USA

3 University of Cincinnati, Cincinnati, Ohio, USA

References

[1] Arahata K, Engel AG: Monoclonal antibody analysis of mononuclear cells in myopathies. I. Quantitation of subsets according to diagnosis and sites of accumulation and demonstration And counts of muscle fibers invaded by T cells. Ann Neurol 16: 193-208, 1984

[2] Blake DJ, Kroger S: The neurobiology of Duchenne muscular ystrophy: learning lessons From muscle? Trends Neurosci 23: 92-99, 2000

[3] Blake DJ, Weir A, Newey SE, Davies KE: Function and genetics of Dystrophin and Dystrophin-Related Proteins in Muscle: Physiol. Rev 82: 291-329, 2002.

[4] Blake DJ, Martin-Rendon E. Intermediate filaments and the function of the dystrophin-protein complex. Trends Cardiovasc Med 2002; 12:224-228.

[5] Dubowitz V: Muscle disorders in childhood. Major Probl Clin Pediatr 16: 1-282, 1978

[6] Emery AEH: Duchenne Muscular Dystrophy. Oxford Monographs on Medical Genetics (2nd ed. Oxford, UK: Oxford Univ Press, 1993, vol XV, p 392, 1993

[7] Gebre-Medhin M, Gustavson KH,Gamstorp I, Plantin LO: selenium supplementation in X-linked muscular Dystrophy. Effects on erythrocyte glutathione peroxidase activity. Acta Pediatr Scand 7:886-890, 1985

[8] Jackson MJ, Edwards RHT: Free radicals and trials of antioxidant therapy in muscle diseases. Adv Exp Med Biol 264:485-491, 1990

[9] Simonian NA, Coyle JT: Oxidative stress in neurodegenerative diseases. Annu Rev Pharmacol Toxical 36:83-106, 1996

[10] Timberg H: Progradu- studies. University of Helsinki 1989

[11] Westermarck T, Rahola T, Kallio A-K, Suomela M: Long turnover of selenite Se in children With motor disorders. Klin Pädiat 194:301-02, 1981

[12] Westermarck T, Antila E, Kaksonen S, Laakso J, Härkönen M, Atroshi F: Long-term follow-up Of two Duchenne muscle dystrophy patients treated with antioxidants. Publ.: Food and free radicals, Eds M. Hiramatsu, T. Yosikawa, M. Inoue. Plenum Press, New York 1997, pp 161-163.

[13] Basun H., Forssell L. G., Wetterberg L. and Winblad B. (1991) Metals and trace elements in plasma and cerebrospinal fluid in normal aging and Alzheimer's disease. *J. Neural. Transm. Park. Dis. Dement. Sect.* 3, 231–258.

[14] Behne D. and Kyriakopoulos A. (2001) Mammalian selenium-containing proteins. *Annu. Rev. Nutr.* 21, 453–473.

[15] Berr C., Nicole A., Godin J., Ceballos-Picot I., Thevenin M., Dartigues J. F. and Alperovitch A. (1993) Selenium and oxygen-metabolizing enzymes in elderly community residents: a pilot epidemiological study. *J. Am. Geriatr. Soc.* 41, 143–148.

[16] Burk R. F. (1991) Molecular biology of selenium with implications for its metabolism. *FASEB J.* 5, 2274–2299.

[17] Ceballos-Picot I., Merad-Boudia M., Nicole A., Thevenin M., Hellier G., Legrain S. and Berr C. (1996) Peripheral antioxidant enzyme activities and selenium in elderly

subjects and in dementia of Alzheimer's type – pace of the extracellular glutathione peroxidase. *Free Rad. Biol. Med.* 20, 579–587.

[18] Chanoine J. P., Braverman L. E., Farwell A. P., Safran M., Alex S., Dubord S. and Leonard J. L. (1993) The thyroid gland is a major source of circulating T3 in the rat. *J. Clin. Invest.* 91, 2709–2713.

[19] Clausen J., Jensen G. E. and Nielsen S. A. (1988) Selenium in chronic neurological diseases, multiple sclerosis and Batten's disease. *Biol. Trace Elem. Res.* 15, 179–203.

[20] Cornett C. R., Ehmann W. D., Wekstein D. R. and Markesbery W. R. (1998a) Trace elements in Alzheimer's disease pituitary glands. *Biol. Trace Elem. Res.* 62, 107–114.

[21] Covas M. I., Elosua R., Fito M., Alcantara M., Coca L. and Marrugat J. (2002) Relationship between physical activity and oxidative stress biomarkers in women. *Med. Sci. Sports Exerc.* 34, 814–819.

[22] Cuajungco M. P. and Lees G. J. (1997) Zinc metabolism in the brain: relevance to human neurodegenerative disorders. *Neurobiol. Dis.* 4, 137–169.

[23] Damier P., Hirsch E. C., Zhang P., Agid Y. and Javoy-Agid F. (1993) Glutathione peroxidase, glial cells and Parkinson's disease. *Neuroscience* 52, 1–6.

[24] Deibel M. A., Ehmann W. D. and Markesbury W. R. (1996) Copper, iron, and zinc imbalances in severely degenerated brain regions in Alzheimer's disease: possible relation to oxidative stress. *J. Neurol. Sci.* 143, 137–142.

[25] Dexter D. T., Carter C. J., Wells F. R., Javoy-Agid F., Agid Y., Lees A., Jenner P. and Marsden C. D. (1989a) Basal lipid peroxidation in substantia nigra is increased in Parkinson's disease. *J. Neurochem.* 52, 381–389.

[26] Dexter D. T., Wells F. R. and Lees A. (1989b) Increased nigra iron content and alterations in other metal ions occurring in brain in Parkinson's disease. *J. Neurochem.* 52, 1830–1836.

[27] Ely J. T. A. (2001) Mercury induced Alzheimer's disease: accelerating incidence? *Bull. Environ. Contam. Toxicol.* 67, 800–806.

[28] El-Yazigi A. A. L.,-Saleh I. and Al-Mefty O. (1984) Concentrations of Ag, Al, Au, Bi, Cd, Cu, Pb, Sb, and Se in cerebrospinal fluid of patients with cerebral neoplasms. *Clin. Chem.* 30, 1358–1360.

[29] Facchinetti F., Dawson V. L. and Dawson T. M. (1998) Free radicals as mediators of neuronal injury. *Cell Mol. Neurobiol.* 18, 667–682.

[30] Flentjar N. J., Crack P. J., Boyd R., Malin M., de Haan J. B., Hertzog P., Kola I. and Iannello R. (2002) Mice lacking glutathione peroxidase-1 activity show increased TUNEL staining and an accelerated inflammatory response in brain following a cold-induced injury. *Exp. Neurol.* 177, 9–20.

[31] Glauser T. A., Titanic-Schefft M. and Pippenger C. E. (1999) Racial differences in free radical scavenging enzyme activity in children. *J. Child Neurol.* 14, 382–387.

[32] Ho Y. S., Magnenat J. L., Bronson R. T., Cao J., Gargano M., Sugawara M. and Funk C. D. (1997) Mice deficient in celular glutathione peroxidases develop normally and show no increased sensitivity to hyperoxia. *J. Biol. Chem.* 272, 16644–16651. l

[33] Hock A., Demmel U., Schicha H., Kasperek K. and Feinendegen L. E. (1975) Trace element concentration in human brain. *Brain* 98, 49–64.

[34] Ip C. (1998) Lessons learned from basic research in selenium and cancer prevention. *J. Nutr.* 128, 1845–1854.

[35] Jeong D., Kim T. S., Chung Y. W., Lee B. J. and Kim I. Y. (2002) Selenoprotein W is a glutathione-dependent antioxidant *in vivo*. *FEBS Lett.* 517, 225–228.

[36] Johannsen P., Velander G., Mai J., Thorling E. B. and Dupont E. (1991) Glutathione peroxidase in early and advanced Parkinson's disease. *J. Neurol. Neurosurg. Psychiatry* 54, 679–682.

[37] Kalra J., Rajput A. H., Mantha S. V. and Prasad K. (1992) Serum antioxidant enzyme activity in Parkinson's disease. *Mol. Cell Biochem.* 110, 165–168.

[38] Kim H. C., Jhoo W. K., Choi D. Y., Im D. H., Shin E. J., Suh J. H., Floyd R. A. and Bing G. (1999) Protection of methamphetamine nigrostriatal toxicity by dietary selenium. *Brain Res.* 851, 76–86.

[39] Kim H. C., Jhoo W. K., Shin E. and Bing G. (2000) Selenium deficiency potentates methamphetamine-induced nigral neuronal loss; comparison with MPTP model. *Brain Res.* 862, 247–252.

[40] Kish S. J., Morito C. and Hornykiewicz O. (1985) Glutathione peroxidase activity in Parkinson's disease brain. *Neurosci. Lett.* 58, 343–346.

[41] Kosta L., Byrne A. R. and Zelenko V. (1975) Correlations between selenium and mercury in man following exposure to inorganic mercury. *Nature* 254, 238–239.

[42] Marttila R. J., Lorentz H. and Rinne U.K. (1988) Oxygen toxicity protecting enzymes in Parkinson's disease. *J. Neurol. Sci.* 86, 321–331.

[43] Meseguer I., Molina J. A., Jimenez-Jimenez F. J., Aguilar M. V., Mateos-Vega C. J., Gonzalez-Munoz M. J., de Bustos F., Orti-Pareja M., Zurdo M., Berbel A., Barrios E. and Martinez-Para M. C. (1999) Cerebrospinal fluid levels of selenium in patients with Alzheimer's disease. *J. Neural. Transm.* 106, 309–315.

[44] Oster O., Schmiedel G. and Prellwitz W. (1988) The organ distribution of selenium in German adults. *Biol. Trace Elem. Res.* 15, 23–45.

[45] Poirier J. and Barbeau A. (1987) Erythrocyte antioxidant activity in human patients with Parkinson's disease. *Neurosci. Lett.* 75, 345–348.

[46] Prohaska J. R. and Ganther H. E. (1976) Selenium and glutathione peroxidase in developing rat brain. *J. Neurochem.* 27, 1379–1387.

[47] Ramaekers V. T., Calomme M., Vanden Berghe D. and Makropoulos W. (1994) Selenium deficiency triggering intractable seizures. *Neuropediatrics* 25, 217–223.

[48] Rayman M. P. (2000) The importance of selenium to human health. *Lancet* 356, 233–241.

[49] Rotruck J. T., Pope A. L., Ganther H. E., Swanson A. B., Hafeman D. G. and Hoekstra W. G. (1973) Selenium: biological role as a component of glutathione peroxidase. *Science* 179, 588–590.

[50] Sagara Y., Tan S., Maher P. and Schubert D. (1998) Mechanisms of resistance to oxidative stress in Alzheimer's disease brain. *Neurotoxicology* 19, 339–345.

[51] Saito Y. and Takahashi K. (2002) Characterization of selenoprotein P as a selenium supply protein. *Eur. J. Biochem.* 269, 5746–5751.

[52] Saito Y., Hayashi T., Tanaka A., Watanabe Y., Suzuki M., Saito E. and Takahashi K. (1999) Selenoprotein P in human plasma as an extracellular phospholipids hydroperoxide glutathione peroxidase. *J. Biol. Chem.* 274, 2866–2871.

[53] Schomburg L., Schweizer U., Holtmann B., Flohe L., Sendtner M. and Kohrle J. (2003) Gene disruption discloses role of Selenoprotein P in selenium delivery to target tissues. *Biochem. J.* 370, 397–402.

[54] Sies H. and Arteel G. E. (2000) Interaction of peroxynitrite with selenoproteins and glutathione peroxidase mimics. *Free Rad. Biol. Med.* 28, 1451–1455.

[55] Smith C. D., Carney J. M., Starke-Reed P. E., Oliver C. N., Stadtman E. R., Floyd R. A. and Markesbery W. R. (1991) Excess brain protein oxidation and enzyme dysfunction in normal aging and in Alzheimer disease. *Proc. Natl Acad. Sci. USA* 88, 10540–10543.

[56] Stadtman T. C. (1996) Selenocysteine. *Ann. Rev. Biochem.* 65, 83–100.

[57] Syburra C. and Passi S. (1999) Oxidative stress in patients with multiple sclerosis. *Ukr. Biokhim. Zh.* 71, 112–115.

[58] Takizawa S., Matsushima K., Shinohara Y., Ogawa S., Komatsu N., Utsunomiya H. and Watanabe K. (1994) Immunohistochemical localization of glutathione peroxidase in infracted human brain. *J. Neurol. Sci.* 122, 66–73.

[59] Tan S., Wood M. and Maher P. (1998) Oxidative stress induces a form of programmed cell death with characteristics of both apoptosis and necrosis in neuronal cells. *J. Neurochem.* 71, 95–105.

[60] Thompson C. M., Markesbery W. R., Ehmann W. D., Mao X. Y. and Vance D. E. (1988) Regional brain trace-element studies in Alzheimer's disease. *Neurotoxicology* 9, 1–7.

http://dx.doi.org/10.5772/57370

[61] Torreilles F., Salman-Tabcheh S., Guerin M. C. and Torreilles J. (1999) Neurodegenerative disorders: the role of peroxynitrite. *Brain Res. Rev.* 30, 153–163.

[62] Turan B., Acan N. L., Ulusu N. N. and Tezcan E. F. (2001) A comparative study on effect of dietary selenium and vitamin E on some antioxidant enzyme activities of liver and brain tissues. *Biol. Trace Elem. Res.* 81, 141–152.

[63] Vahter M., Lutz E., Lind B., Herin P., Bui T. H. and Krakau I. (1997) Concentrations of copper, zinc and selenium in brain and kidney of second trimester fetus and infants. *J. Trace Elem. Med. Biol.* 11, 215–222.

[64] Vitorica J., Machado A. and Satrustegui J. (1984) Age-dependent variations in peroxide-utilizing enzymes from rat brain mitochondria and cytoplasm. *J. Neurochem.* 42, 351–356.

[65] Westermarck T. Selenium content of tissues in Finnish infants and adults with various diseases, and studies on the effects of selenium supplementation in neuronal ceroid lipofuscinosis patients. Acta Pharmacol Toxicol. 1977;41(2):121-8.

[66] Westermarck, T; Antila, E; Kaksonen, S; Laakso, J; Härkönen, M ; Atroshi, F. Long-term follow-up of two Duchenne muscle dystrophy patients treated with antioxidants. Food and free radicals (1997): 161-163.

[67] Whanger P. D. (2001) Selenium and the brain: a review. *Nutr. Neurosci.* 4, 81–97.

[68] Wilson D. S. and Tappel A. L. (1993) Binding of plasma selenoprotein P to cell membranes. *J. Inorg. Biochem.* 51, 707–714.

[69] Zachara B. A., Pawluk H., Bloch-Boguslawska E., Sliwka K. M., Korenkiewicz J., Skok Z. and Ryc K. (2001) Tissue level, distribution, and total body selenium content in healthy and diseased humans in Poland. *Arch. Environ. Health* 56, 461–466.

[70] Zafar K. S., Siddiqui A., Sayeed I., Ahmad M., Salim S. and Islam F. (2003) Dose-dependent protective effect of selenium in rat model of Parkinson's disease: neurobehavioral and neurochemical evidences. *J. Neurochem.* 84, 438–446.

[71] Zhang L., Maiorino M., Roveri A. and Ursini F. (1989) Phospholipid hydroperoxide glutathione peroxidase: specific activity in tissues of rats of different age and comparison with other glutathione peroxidase. *Biochim. Biophys. Acta* 1006, 140–143.

Chapter 19

Green Tea: Just a Drink or Nutraceutical

Sakaewan Ounjaijean, Suthat Fucharoen and
Somdet Srichairatanakool

Additional information is available at the end of the chapter

http://dx.doi.org/10.5772/57519

1. Introduction

Brewed tea has been the most widely consumed beverage throughout history. Attractively, this is attributed to its present taste, aromatic odor and healthful effects to the human body. Tea (*Camellia sinensis*) is used for the production of green tea, oolong tea and black tea, depending on the fermentation process. Without fermentation, green tea can be made from fresh tea shoots at a high temperature, thereby inactivating the oxidizing enzymes such as polyphenol oxidase (PPO) and leaving the intact polyphenols. Many ingredients persisting in green tea products are flavonols, flavanols, chlorogenic acid, coumarylquinic acid, theogallin (3-galloylquinic acid), vitamin P (flavonoids), alkaloids, caffeine, theophylline, theobromine, theanine, volatile compounds, fluoride, minerals (e.g. aluminium and magnesium), trace elements and other unidentified compounds. During fermentation, these polyphenolic compounds undergo PPO-catalyzed oxidative polymerization giving rise to the formation of theaflavins and thearubigins which are the major antioxidants in black tea [1]. Besides being a world-wide, well-known beverage, green tea has many benefits for health, including anti-oxidative, free radical scavenging, iron-chelating, anti-hyperglycemic and anti-diabetic, weight-lowering, anti-aging, neuro-protective and rescue, thrombosis-inhibitory, anti-inflammatory, exercise-endurating, hepatoprotective, hepatic phase II enzyme activity-inducing, cardioprotective, neoangioprotective, anti-mutagenic, anti-carcinogenic and cancer-preventive, anti-microbial, as well as immunomodulatory activities. Tea products generally provide refreshment and diuretic benefits, as well as contributing to feelings of alertness; however; green tea extraordinarily exhibits such biological and pharmacological properties depending on several specific active phytochemical constituents; particularly catechins. Nowadays, crude extracts, purified catechin fractions and synthetic catechin derivatives of green tea are applicable in alternative and complementary medicines for the prevention, treatment and co-treatment of many diseases and disorders.

2. Sources and compositions of green tea

Tea has traditionally been cultivated across four continents in the manufacturing of a refreshing drink. The tea products that are available are directly related to the process used at the origin, and can be classified as black tea, green tea, yellow tea, red tea, green pressed tea, as well as instant tea and tea dyes [1]. Green tea is manufactured by using conventional and modified methods. One of these methods involves a 2-3-day process of to drying fresh tea leaves and then rolling the dry leaves with a commercial machine. Alternatively, another method involves the very rapid process of baking the tea leaves in a house-hold microwave oven (800 watt, 3 minutes) at a working temperature of 115 °C. This process will shock the persisting PPO enzyme and result in higher catechins content [2]. A typical green tea beverage is normally prepared at a proportion of 1 g dry weight of tea leaves in 100 ml of hot water in a 3-minute brew (an approximate temperature of 80 °C). This brew usually contains 250 – 350 mg tea solids, 30 – 42% catechins (74 mg) and 3–6% caffeine [3]. HPLC analysis shows the green tea extract (GTE) is comprised of at least six major catechins, including (-)-epicatechin (EC), (-)-epicatechin 3-gallate (ECG), (-)-epigallocatechin (EGC), (-)-epigallocatechin 3-gallate (EGCG), (+)-catechin (C) and (-)-gallocatechin (GC), of which EGCG is the major isomer followed by ECG, EGC and EC (Figure 1) [4]. Gallic acid (GA) is derivatized to one of the hydroxyl groups of the catechins, which has been directly attributed to the biological activities of the catechin species.

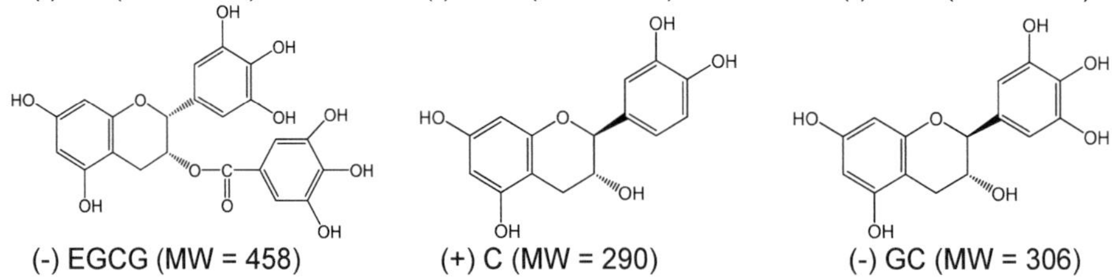

Figure 1. Chemical structures of catechins in green tea (Redrawn from [4])

Moreover, tea products have different amounts and compositions of catechins, which is possibly due to biodiversity, different processing methods, different planting areas and different varieties of tea strains. For instance, Khokhar and colleagues reported that 1 g dry weight of tea product contained 48.4 mg total catechins (9.1 mg EGC, 7.9 mg EC, 22.9 mg EGCG, and 8.5 mg ECG) for Ceylon (NL) black tea; 5.6 mg total catechins (<0.5 mg EGC, 3.1 mg EC,

1.8 mg EGCG, and 0.8 mg ECG) for Yule (India) black tea; 7.5 mg total catechins (<0.5 mg EGC, 4.0 mg EC, 2.6 mg EGCG, and 1.0 mg ECG) for PG tips (UK) black tea;5.15 mg total catechins (16.3 mg EGC, 4.7 mg EC, 26.3 mg EGCG, and 4.4 mg ECG) for Chinese green tea; 84.9 mg total catechins (28.7 mg EGC, 9.4 mg EC, 40.8 mg EGCG, and 5.9 mg ECG) for Japanese green tea; and 21.1 mg total catechins (7.7 mg EGC, 1.7 mg EC, 11.5 mg EGCG, and 0.5 mg ECG) for Chinese oolong tea [5]. EGCG has so far received the most attention because it represents approximately 59% catechin content, EGC at approximately 19%, ECG at approximately 13.6%, and EC at approximately 6.4% of the total catechin content [6]. Green tea also contains other phenolic acids, such as chlorogenic acid and caffeic acid, as well as other flavonols, such as kaempferol, myricetin and quercetin [7].

Green tea catechins have proven to be quite stable in water that is room temperature; however, they can be destroyed at a rate of 20% under brewing at 98 °C for 7 hours and epimerized to other derivatives (e.g. EGCG → GCG) under autoclaving at 120 °C for 20 minutes [8]. Fresh tea leaves are unusually rich in polyphenolic catechins that may constitute up to 30% of the dry leaf weight [9]. As a result of the immediate inactivation of PPO enzyme, the compositions of catechins in green tea are very similar to those of the fresh tea leaves. Various quinines, which are subsequently produced by the enzymatic oxidations, undergo condensation reactions to produce *bis*-flavanols, theaflavins, epitheaflavic acids and thearubigens. These compounds impart the characteristic taste and color properties of black and oolong tea [10].

In our Thai green tea, EGCG was found to be the most abundant catechin (at about 60% of the total catechin content), followed by EGG, ECG, and EC, respectively and the assay yield of the total green tea catechin content was found to be 26-29 g/100 g dry tea leaves (Table 1) [2]. In comparison, Taiwan green tea (1 g dry weight) contained 93.3 mg total catechin content, followed by 43.2 mg EGCG, 33.6 mg ECG, 0.7 mg C, 3.3 mg EC and 2.7 mg ECG [11].

Amounts	EGCG	EGC	ECG	EC	Total catechins
mg/g dry weight	169.4±7.2	60.1±6.2	19.3±2.6	16.3±5.6	279.8±15.2
% (*w/w*)	60.6±2.2	21.5±1.4	6.9±1.0	5.9±2.1	100

Table 1. HPLC analysis of catechin compositions in six green tea extract solutions (2 g%, *w/v*).

3. Nutritional value of green tea

In general, an antioxidant refers to any substance capable of preventing the oxidation catalyzed by reactive oxygen species (ROS)/reactive nitrogen species (RNS). Thus, an antioxidant that protects against iron toxicity is a substance that can: i) chelate iron and prevent the reaction with oxygen or peroxides; ii) chelate iron and maintain it in a redox state that makes iron unable to reduce molecular oxygen; iii) trap already formed radicals, which is a putative action of any substance that can scavenge free radicals in biological systems, regardless of whether they have originated from iron-dependent reactions or not. Not only can natural products chelate iron, but also synthetic compounds are capable of chelating iron *in vivo*, thereby limiting its participation in free radical reactions. Thus, iron chelators also serve as antioxidants by suppressing iron-mediated oxidation in biological systems. Surprisingly, thiol compounds (e.g. glutathione) that are synthesised by mammals can afford significant antioxidant protection. This protection is related to the ability of glutathione to trap radicals, reduce peroxides, as well asits ability to work to maintain the redox state of the cells [12].

The potential of green tea to prevent or ameliorate chronic diseases is currently the subject of considerable scientific investigations. Although a number of mechanisms have been proposed for their beneficial effects, the radical scavenging and antioxidant properties of green tea catechins are frequently cited as important contributors. Emerging evidence has also shown that catechins and their metabolites possessmany additional mechanisms of action [13] by affecting numerous sites, potentiating endogenous antioxidants and eliciting dual actions during oxidative stress. Much of the evidence supporting an antioxidant function for green tea catechins is derived from assays of their antioxidant activity *in vitro*. However, the evidence that green tea catechins are acting either directly or indirectly as antioxidants *in vivo* is limited [14]

4. Anti-oxidative and iron-chelating properties

Green tea catechins stoichiometrically bind ferric ion to form a redox-inactive iron-phenolic complex [15, 16] and potentially protect vital biomolecules from oxidative damage. Incredibly, the catechins could be capable of chelating excessive redox iron in iron overloaded diseases, such as thalassemia, and play important preventive or/and protective roles in this unpleasant condition [2, 17-19]. The phytochemical compounds therefore play a double role in reducing the rate of oxidation because they can participate in: i) iron chelation [19], and ii) trapping radicals [2, 20]. Catechins can protect culture cells from iron-mediated damage [21, 22], ameliorate iron accumulation [17] and inhibit hepatic iron-induced lipid oxidation [23], and also play a dual effect in decreasing labile plasma iron (LPI) in iron-loaded rats [18]. Animal studies offer a unique opportunity to assess the contribution of green tea administration to the physiological effects on different models of oxidative-related diseases. In a combination of free-radical scavenging activity with iron-chelating properties, green tea may have a capacity of chelating excess iron in iron-overloaded conditions and play important preventive and/or protective roles in this unpleasant condition.

Like the deferiprone (DFP) treatment, oral administrations of GTE and EGCG significantly lowered levels of plasma non-transferrin bound iron (NTBI) and LPI in wild-type (WT), heterozygous β-globin gene knockout (BKO) thalassemic and double heterozygous β-globin gene knockout carrying human β^E gene (DH) mice (strain C57BL/6J) with iron overload, when compared to the DW group (Table 2) (Sakaewan Ounjaijean and Somdet Srichairatanakool, unpublished data). Elimination of these two toxic irons by green tea extract and EGCG fraction would relieve redox iron-induced oxidative stress and tissue damage in the body. GTE treatment efficiently depleted plasma malondialdehyde (MDA) concentrations in the iron-loaded mice (approximately 50% in WT, 30% in BKO and 40% in DH mice), whereas EGCG treatment caused significantly lower plasma MDA levels (approximately 30% in all the mice), suggesting that GTE and EGCG are strong antioxidants and exert potent anti-plasma lipid peroxidation. Consistently, the GTE and EGCG increased levels of reduced glutathione (GSH) in the plasma of all the mice despite under iron overload. Thus, it can be said that green tea catechins, particularly EGCG, chelate the redox irons and consequently inhibit the iron-catalyzed lipid peroxidation reactions in plasma lipids, as well as membrane phospholipids, resulting in an improvement of a powerful antioxidants as reduced glutathione is reduced in the plasma compartment.

Mice	N diet +DW	Fe diet (0.2% ferrocene, w/w) +DW	+GTE (90 mg/kg/day)	+EGCG (50 mg/kg/day)	+DFP (50 mg/kg/day)
			Plasma NTBI concentrations (μM)		
WT (n = 24)	-0.27±0.23	11.17±0.26*	6.83±1.49†	6.80±1.75†	6.81±2.23†
BKO (n = 16)	0.34±0.26	19.78±1.36*	10.20±1.92†	10.66±1.60†	11.75±1.21†
DH (n = 10)	-0.07±0.11	13.41±1.84*	7.74±1.38†	7.81±0.71†	7.83±1.41†
			LPI concentrations (μM)		
WT (n = 24)	-2.49±1.00	1.19±0.42*	-2.26±1.98†	-2.47±1.25†	-2.01±2.76†
BKO (n = 16)	0.87±0.22	2.30±1.08*	0.30±2.57†	-0.21±1.37†	0.35±1.05†
DH (n = 10)	-0.15±0.52	0.81±0.26*	0.26±0.61†	0.47±0.63	0.34±0.70
			Plasma MDA concentrations (μM)		
WT (n = 24)	13.39±5.10	39.97±8.67*	23.26±8.30†	28.39±6.66†	32.58±8.73†
BKO (n = 16)	26.80±3.59	54.34±9.88*	37.62±9.23†	41.85±11.8†	52.29±7.51†
DH (n = 10)	18.79±2.31	46.89±4.56*	26.62±5.14†	32.72±2.46†	38.13±5.09†
			Plasma GSH concentrations (μM)		
WT (n = 24)	11.53±2.50	7.73±4.70*	15.15±7.72†	16.04±6.61†	15.89±8.43†
BKO (n = 16)	7.73±4.25	6.24±3.89	15.12±9.76*,†	15.63±7.74*,†	16.50±8.75*,†
DH (n = 10)	10.97±5.00	5.81±1.44*	14.78±5.16†	17.03±7.27†	14.19±4.89†

*p <0.05 compared to N diet; †p <0.05 compared to DW.

Table 2. NTBI, LPI, MDA and GSH concentrations (mean+SD) in the WT, BKO and DH mice fed with a normal (N) diet (iron content 180 mg/kg) and an iron (Fe) diet (iron content 780 mg/kg) and treated with deionized water (DW), 90 mg/kg/day GTE, 50 mg/kg EGCG and 50 mg/kg DFP for 6 months.

5. Fate of green tea catechins in the body

5.1. Gastrointestinal absorption

Among these polyphenolic compounds, the hierarchy of antioxidant activity is ECG > EGCG > EGC > GA > EC ≈ C [24]. With the chelating activity of such prooxidant metals as iron (Fe^{2+}), green tea is able to reduce dietary nonheme iron absorption [25]. The ratio of EGC, EGCG, ECG or EC to the iron was 3:2, 2:1, 2:1 and 3:1, respectively [26]. Unlike most flavonoids, tea catechins existing as aglycone are found in the blood following oral ingestion and subsequently metabolized in the liver by methylation, sulfation and glucoronidation reactions [27]. Structure-activity studies have shown that the presence of the galloyl ring in the 3-position and trihydroxyphenyl B ring are of significant importance in terms of the antioxidant properties of the catechins [26].

After green tea (25 mg/kg) and pure EGCG fractions (10 mg/kg) were intravenously administered into rats, a study of the pharmacokinetic (concentration-time curves) properties of the catechins in the plasma was conducted. Beta-elimination half-lives ($T_{1/2}\beta$) were found to be 212, 45, and 41 minutes; clearances were 2.0, 7.0, and 13.9 ml•minute/kg; and apparent distribution volumes (V_d) were 1.5, 2.1, and 3.6 dl/kg for EGCG, EGC, and EC, respectively. In comparison, EGCG had a shorter $T_{1/2}\beta$ (135 minute), a larger clearance (72.5 ml•minute/kg), and a larger volume (V_d) (22.5 dl/kg) than the other two. When the green tea was intragastrically given (200 mg/kg), around 0.1, 13.7 and 31.2% of EGCG, EGC and EC were detected in the plasma compartment. The EGCG level was found to be the highest in the intestine samples and declined with a $T_{1/2}$ of 173 minute. EGC and EC levels were found to be the highest in the kidneys and declined rapidly with $T_{1/2}$ of 29 and 28 minute, respectively. EGCG, EGC, and EC levels in the liver and lungs were lower than those recorded in the intestine and the kidney [28]. This implies that EGCG is mainly excreted through bile, while EGC and EC are excreted through urine and bile. Inter-individual variations in the bioavailability of green tea catechins can be substantial and may be due, in part, to differences in colonic microflora and genetic polymorphisms among the enzymes involved in polyphenol metabolism [29]. The effect of green tea drinking may also differ by genotype [30].

Following oral administration of green tea catechin solutions (0.6%, *w/v*) to the rats, plasma levels of the catechins measured at 6:00 AM., 9:00 AM., 0:00 PM and 6:00 PM on the same day were found to be 983.9±114.2, 372.89±56.7, 186.89±34.5 and 548.1±221.6 ng/ml EGC; 1,527.3±163.7, 449.2±82.7, 224.6±58.0 and 845.6±374.0 ng/ml ECG; and 105.0±12.6, 85.5±15.8, 95.7±18.3 and 114.8±45.6 ng/ml EGCG, respectively, for which the plasma EGCG concentrations were found to be even lower than those of EGC and EC. There wasa gradual increase in plasma concentrations of EGC, EC and EGCG during Days 1-4. Levels of EGC and EC in the plasma on Day 14 were approximately three times higher than those on Day 1. Plasma levels of these three catechins decreased after Day 14, and by Day 28, plasma levels of the EGC and EC returned to the levels recorded on Day 1. On Days 4, 14 and 28, the catechins were mostly present in glucuronic acid (MW=194)/sulfuric acid (MW=98) conjugated-EGC (91.4, 95.6 and 86.4 ng/ml, respectively) and-EC (92.4, 95.5 and 89.4 ng/ml, respectively), while a much lower proportion of EGCG was found in the conjugated form (21.2, 60.7 and 39.3 ng/ml, respectively). The highest EGC concentration was found in the bladder; the highest EGCG concentration was found in the large intestine; very high concentrations of EGC and EGCG were found in the kidneys, prostate gland and lungs; and low levels of these three catechins were present in the liver, spleen, heart, and thyroid glands [31].

5.2. Organ metabolism

EC was not glucuronidated by uridine diphosphate-glucuronosyltransferases (UGT) and sulfotransferases (SULT) in human liver and small intestinal microsomes. However, the compound was efficiently glucuronidated in rat liver microsomes with the formation of two different glucuronides, and was also sulfated in human liver cytosol, mainly through the SULT1A1 isoform, as well as in the intestine through the SULT1A1 and SULT1A3 isoforms. In comparison, the EC was much less sulfated in the rat liver than in the human liver [32]. EGCG and ECG constituents in green tea drinks (10%, *w/v*) almost completely, competitively inhibited the activities of the SULT1A1 and SULT1A3 enzymes that play an important role in the presystemic inactivation of β_2 agonists in the liver and intestine, respectively [33]. When EGCG was glucuronidated by the liver microsomal UGT enzymes; four EGCG-glucuronides were identified as EGCG-3-glucuronide, EGCG-3′-glucuronide, EGCG-4′-glucuronide and EGCG-7-glucuronide. Under the same conditions, EGC was metabolized into two EGC-glucuronides as EGC-7-glucuronide and EGC-3′-glucuronide [34]. Since rate of the glucuronidation of EGCG and ECG in liver microsomes is rather low (12.2±0.2 and 7.5±0.2%, respectively for 3 hours) due to the galloyl ring, the two potent catechins are therefore recognized to be circulating in the plasma in unconjugated forms [35]. One study claimed that catechins were toxic to rat liver cells in the order of EGCG (LD_{50} 200±19 μM) > ECG (LD_{50} 2,000±214 μM) > GA (LD_{50} 3,000±298 μM), EGC (LD_{50} 3,000±304 μM) > EC (LD_{50} >10,000 μM), and this was likely due to the mitochondrial membrane potential ($\Delta\psi_m$) collapse, and the depletion of GSH and ROS formation. The EGCG and GA dose dependently affected GSH conjugation, methylation, metabolism by NAD(P)H:quinoneoxidoreductase 1 (NQO1) in the hepatic detoxification step (Figure 2), as monitored by a significant increase of plasma alanine aminotransferase (ALT) activity in mice [36].

5.3. Excretion

Most polyphenolic catechins in green tea may not be absorbed in the small intestine. The nonabsorbed catechins will be converted by large bow bacterial flora into simpler phenolic compounds, such as hippuric acid, then absorbed into the blood and excreted in the urine (4.22±0.28 mmol/24 hours), when compared to non-consumption (1.89+0.28 mmol/24 hours) [37].

6. Health benefits

6.1. Health promotion

The potential health effects of green tea catechins depend not only on the amount consumed, but also on their bioavailability, which appears to be substantially varied. Following the oral administration of tea catechins to rats [38] and mice [39], the four principal catechins have been identified in the portal vein, indicating that tea catechins are absorbed intestinally. There appear to be species-related differences in the bioavailability of EGCG compared to other tea

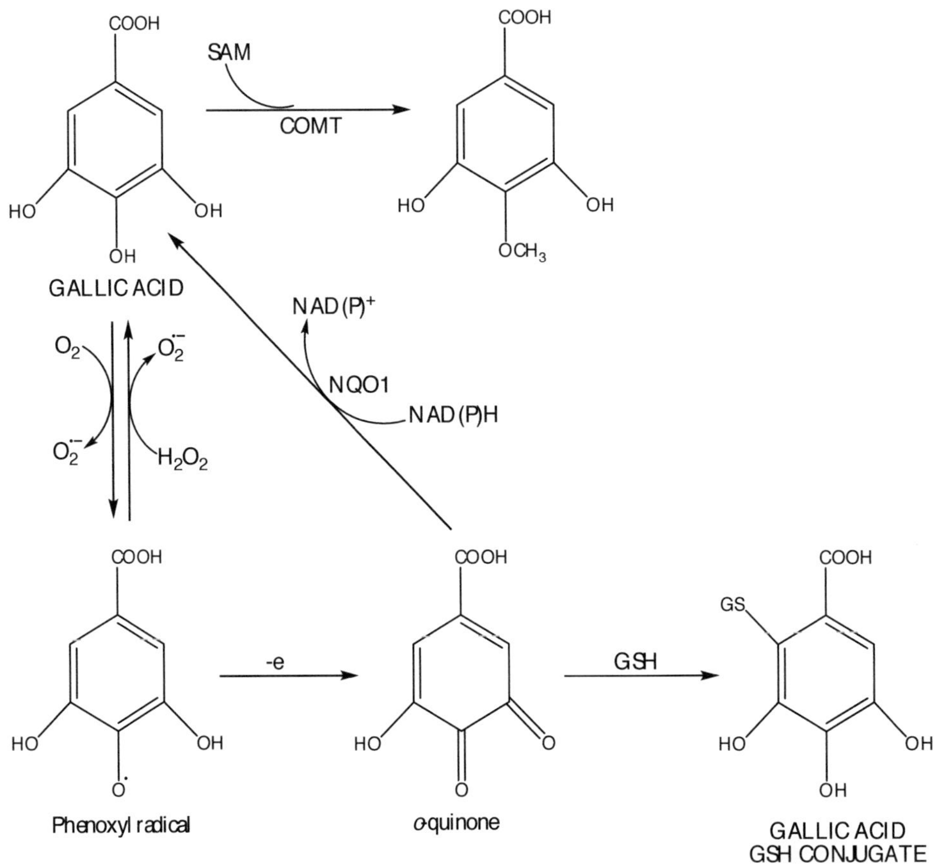

Figure 2. Possible mechanism for the hepaticgalloyl ring metabolism (Redrawn from [36]). Abbreviations: COMT=catechol-*O*-methyltransferase; GSH=reduced glutathione;NAD(P)$^+$=nicotinamide adenine dinucleotide phosphate; NAD(P)H=reduced nicotinamide adenine dinucleotide phosphate; NQO1=NAD(P)H:quinone oxidoreductase-1; SAM=*S*-adenosyl methionine

catechins [7]. The epicatechin isomers purified from green tea were effective agents in protecting human low-density lipoproteins (LDL) and red blood cell (RBC) membranes from oxidative modification [40]. These effects are partly due to their free-radical scavenging abilities [20] and their iron-chelating properties, which are capable of binding any available iron, thus greatly reducing their bioavailability. They also have many pharmacological properties, including anti-hypertensive [41], anti-atheroslcerotic [42], anti-carcinogenic [43-45] and hypocholesterolemic effects [46, 47]. Health benefits of green tea consumption were achieved in the rodents within relatively short periods: three weeks [48], four weeks [49, 50], five weeks [51, 52] and eight weeks [53, 54].

Surprisingly, catechins inhibited xanthine oxidase (XO) activity *in vitro* [55– 58] and the XO inhibition constant (K_i) of EGCG was comparable to that of the common XO inhibitor allopurinol (0.76 versus 0.30 μmol) [56]. GTE consumption was found to decrease levels of serum uric acid concentrations observed in human subjects [59-61]; for instance, by decreasing serum uric acid levels from 4.54 to 4.22 mg/dl ($p<0.05$) within 7 days [59]. Our group has currently found that the consumption of GTE (2, 4 and 6 g/day), of which the 2 g/day dose was found to be the most effective, lowered levels of serum uric acid (3.53%) and also increased serum trolox-equivalent antioxidant capacity (TEAC) values in healthy volunteers (n=11) (unpublished data), suggesting an hypouricemic effect by XO inhibition or an increase of urinary uric acid excretion.

6.2. Hematologic disorders

In consideration of the evidence for its iron chelating properties, strong antioxidant capacity, low toxicity, and orally available administration, green tea has potential to be used as a pharmacological agent in the management of diseasesrelated to iron overload. Hypothetically, the removal of iron could reduce oxidative damage to the cellular biomolecules, including lipids, proteins, carbohydrates and nucleic acids, and this can consequently prevent, as well as improve the vital organ dysfunctions. DFP, known to readily permeate and mobilize nonheme iron from β-thalassemic patient erythrocytes, serves as a benchmark against which orally effective agents; catechins in GTE and purified EGCG products have been compared. Our studies have paid particular attention to the efficacy of GTE and EGCG in terms of the aspects of anti-oxidation and the potential for iron chelation in order to alleviate oxidative stress and iron overload in β-thalassemic mice in the past experiments, and in Thai β-thalassemia patients with regard to the near future.

Though the pathological role of redox iron in the hemosiderosis (such as hereditary hemochromatosis and thalassemia) is well characterized, excessive accumulation of the iron can result in significant organ dysfunction and abnormality. Recognition of the role of iron in conditions beyond transfusion-dependent iron overload may bring significant implications for the management of metabolic, infectious, and degenerative diseases. New findings obtained during the past years, especially in terms of the discovery of mutations in the genes associated with brain iron metabolism, have provided key insights into the mechanisms of brain iron homeostasis and the pathological mechanisms responsible for neurodegenerative diseases. Increased iron in the brain, which is rich in oxygen and fatty acids, provides an ideal environment for oxidative stress and possible irreparable tissue damage. Oxidative stress, resulting from increased brain iron levels, and possibly also from defects in antioxidant defense mechanisms, is widely believed to be associated with neuronal death in brain disorders.

The interaction between iron overload and dietary antioxidants has been well characterized; especially, with respect to vitamins E and C. Vitamin E has been extensively studied with respect to its capacity to protect molecules from the *in vitro* and *in vivo* effects of iron toxicity [62, 63]. Elevated levels of ROS tended to normalize in response to oral therapy with vitamin E, with patients exhibiting improvement in the antioxidant–oxidant balance in plasma and decreased lipid peroxidation in erythrocytes [64]. However, prolonged administration of vitamin E did not result in any significant changes in Hb levels in patients with β-thalassemia intermedia [65]. Therefore, vitamin E by itself is probably insufficient in inducing major changes in the rate of RBC hemolysis and in prolonging their survival, resulting in increased Hb levels.

The interaction of another dietary antioxidant, vitamin C (ascorbic acid) and iron is less clear. Ascorbic acid can reduce 'free iron' (ferric) to a ferrous form, promoting the initiation and propagation of free radical reactions [66, 67]. In people under a risk of iron overload, in which the elevated levels of iron could lead to higher 'free iron' concentrations, an excess of vitamin C could have deleterious effects. Plant flavonoids (including rutin and curcumin) are another group of antioxidants, which may have therapeutic potential in thalassemia. However, despite their apparent salutary effects on erythrocytes, antioxidants have not yet been shown to ameliorate the anemia of the patients [68]. Antioxidants may be more effective if used in combination with an iron chelator. This approach, if successful, could be particularly useful in countries with limited financial resources.

The potential of green tea to prevent or ameliorate chronic disease is currently the subject of considerable scientific investigation. Although a number of mechanisms have been proposed as being responsible for green tea's beneficial effects, the radical scavenging and antioxidant properties of green tea catechins are frequently cited as important contributors. Emerging evidence has shown that catechins and their metabolites have many additional mechanisms of action [69] by affecting numerous sites, potentiating endogenous antioxidants and eliciting dual actions during oxidative stress. Much of the evidence supporting the antioxidant function for green tea catechins has been derived from assays of their antioxidant activity *in vitro*. However, evidence that green tea catechins are acting directly or indirectly as antioxidants *in vivo* is more limited [14]. Interestingly, green tea catechins can play a double role in reducing the rate of oxidation, as they can participate in: i) iron chelation [19]; and ii) trapping radicals [2, 20]. The catechins have been shown to protect culture cells from iron-mediated damage [21, 22]. In animal models of iron overload, they have been reported to ameliorate iron accumulation [17] and inhibit iron-induced lipid oxidation in the liver [23]. They also play a dual effect in decreased labile iron in the plasma and consequently depleting oxidative stress in iron-loaded rats [18]. Animal studies offer a unique opportunity to assess the contribution of the antioxidant properties of the catechins in terms of the physiological effects of tea administration in different models of oxidative-related diseases. Combining free-radical scavenging with iron-chelating properties, green tea catechins may have a capacity of chelating an excess of iron under iron-overloaded conditions and play the important preventive and/or protective roles in this unpleasant condition. None of the treatments over 2 months affected the levels of blood hemoglobin (Hb) in the WT, BKO and DH mice challenged by iron overload, there were fed a high iron-diet. Nonetheless, iron-induced oxidative stress as well as GSH content in the RBC cytoplasm, and lipid-peroxidation in the RBC plasma membrane were reversed by the GTE that was used in the testing, as well as the EGCG, when compared to the DW treatment (Table 3). We also found that these two green tea products increased the survival rate or half-life of the RBC of the WT and BKO mice significantly (Sakaewan Ounjaijen and Somdet Srichairatanakool, unpublished data). Our results suggest that GTE and EGCG treatment might directly increase the erythropoietic rate, either in normal mice or in thalassemic mice, but probably do protect red cells from ROS-induced hemolysis.

Mice	Fe diet (0.2% ferrocene, w/w)								
	+DW			+GTE (90 mg/kg/day)			+EGCG (50 mg/kg/day)		
	Month 0	Month 1	Month 2	Month 0	Month 1	Month 2	Month 0	Month 1	Month 2
	Blood Hb concentration (g/dl)								
WT (n = 24)	14.80±1.14	15.19 ±1.11	15.15±1.06	15.22±1.23	15.37±1.23	15.32±1.14	15.29±1.25	15.40±1.13	15.41±1.00
BKO (n = 16)	9.45 ±0.56	9.35 ±0.40	9.28 ±0.31	9.55 ±0.59	9.60 ±0.45	9.54 ±0.48	9.45 ±0.56	9.53 ±0.36	9.56 ±0.39
DH (n = 10)	15.97±1.09	15.80±1.01	15.85±0.88	16.11±0.84	16.25±0.85	16.17±0.77	16.33±0.76	16.41±0.72	16.29±0.71
	Erythrocyte ROS (Fluorescent intensity unit)								
WT (n = 10)	38.46±9.17	38.29 ±10.93	42.62±9.63	31.74±9.14	23.29±3.99†	22.45±3.39†	33.07±8.08	26.87±3.72†	23.26±3.02†
BKO (n = 10)	48.29±8.01	53.92 ±9.69	59.81±8.96	35.07±7.68	33.69±7.83†	38.50±6.90†	33.88±7.08	31.47±8.93†	36.67±5.16†
DH (n = 10)	43.08±4.38	44.38 ±3.78	49.60±4.25	31.97±4.23	31.57±4.31	27.88±3.65†	31.51±5.38	31.50±4.38	28.17±4.64†
	Erythrocyte MDA (pmol/g Hb)								
WT (n = 8)	ND	ND	48.23±6.15	ND	ND	36.80±3.23†	ND	ND	36.82±2.71†
BKO (n = 8)	ND	ND	60.63±3.28	ND	ND	44.26±2.87†	ND	ND	44.74±2.79†
DH (n = 8)	ND	ND	50.86±1.90	ND	ND	42.00±2.85†	ND	ND	40.36±2.83†
	Erythrocyte GSH (μmol/g Hb)								
WT (n = 8)	ND	ND	2.80 ±0.52	ND	ND	3.61 ±0.32†	ND	ND	3.73 ±0.29†
BKO (n = 8)	ND	ND	2.56 ±0.22	ND	ND	3.31 ±0.40†	ND	ND	3.24 ±0.36†
DH (n = 8)	ND	ND	2.76 ±0.18	ND	ND	3.49 ±0.22†	ND	ND	3.46 ±0.19†

†$p < 0.05$ compared to DW.

Table 3. Levels of blood Hb, erythrocyte ROS, GSH and MDA (mean±SD) in WT, BKO and DH mice fed with an Fe diet (iron content 780 mg/kg) and treated with DW, GTE and EGCG for 2 months.†$p < 0.05$ compared to DW treatment. ND=not done.

The inhibition of the growth of blast cells from patients with acute myelocytic leukemic (AML) by EGCG affected hematopoietic growth factors (HGF), granulocyte colony stimulating factor (G-CSF), granulocyte macrophage colony stimulating factor (GM-CSF) or interleukin-3 (IL-3), was useful in terms of the stimulation of leukemic cell proliferation. EGCG dosage and time dependently reduced the survival of NSF60 leukemic cell lines [69, 70]. These factors can lead to an induction of cell apoptosis, including endonuclease activation, p53 induction, caspase 3 protease activation *via* a Bcl-2-insensitive pathway, free-radical production and sphinganine accumulation. Chemopreventive effects in multi-step carcinogenesis by EGCG have also been mentioned [71]. From in vitro studies, green tea and EGCG (dose 9-27 μg/ml) displayed a significant level of inhibition of the peripheral blood T-lymphocytes of adult T-lymphocytes patients, along with a moderate level of inhibition of human T-cell lymphotropic virus type I (HTLV-I)-infected T-cell line, but not of T-lymphocytes in the healthy controls. This was possibly due to a suppression of HTLV-I pX gene expression and induction of cell apoptosis [72].Consistently, Japanese HTLV-1 carriers who had taken green tea extract powder (9 capsules/day equivalent to 10 cups of regular green tea drinking) for 5 months showed a significant decrease in the HTLV-1 provirus load, suggesting that green tea drinking could inhibit the proliferation of HTLV-1-infected lymphocytes [73].

Surprisingly, EGCG diminished the phosphorylation of vascular endothelial growth factor (VEGF) receptors, potent angiogenic cytokines that are essential for the survival of tumor cells in the autocrine pathway, in chronic lymphocytic leukemia B cells that have been isolated from leukemic patients, leading to cell apoptosis [74]. EGCG decreased human telomerase reverse transcriptase (hTERT) promoter methylation and histone H_3 Lys9 acetylation, but increased hTERT repressor E_2F-1 binding at the promoter of MCF-7 breast cancers and HL60 promyelocytic leukemia cell cultures [75]. EGCG treatment induced death-associated protein kinase 2 (DAPK2) in multiple myeloma cells and dose dependently increased levels of the DAPK2 in HL60 and NB4 AML cells, while a combined treatment of EGCG (0 – 40 μM) with all-*trans* retinoic acid (ATRA) (1 μM) cooperatively induced and potentially differentiated the DAPK2 enzyme [76]. After ten patients with stage-0 chronic lymphocytic leukemia (CLL) had been orally given GTE for 6 months; eight patients showed decreases in lymphocytosis and circulating regulatory T cells (T_{reg}) numbers, while one patient revealed stable lymphocytosis with decreased T_{reg} numbers, and one patient showed increased lymphocytosis and T_{reg} numbers [77].

The results of the phase 2 clinical study demonstrated that patients with early stage CLL consumed GTE (Polyphenon E preparation, dose of 2000 mg/day, twice daily) for 6 months showed decreases in the absolute lymphocyte counts and lymphadenopathy [78].

6.3. Cardiovascular diseases

Epigenetics, hypercholesterolemia, diabetes, hypertension, heavy smoking, physical inactivity, stress and obesity are all risk factors for atherosclerosis and cardiovascular diseases (CVD). Green tea catechins have been reported to exert anti-obesity effects, including a reduction of adipocyte differentiation and proliferation; decreases in lipogenesis, fat mass, body weight,

http://dx.doi.org/10.5772/57519

fat absorption, plasma levels of triglycerides, free fatty acids, cholesterol, glucose, insulin and leptin; and increases in β-oxidation and thermogenesis.

Yang and Koo reported that the ECG and EGCG that are present in Chinese green tea reduced lipid deposition-caused weight, as well as the cholesterol content of the liver, importantly lowered levels of serum cholesterol levels and the atherogenic index in the rats fed with a cholesterol-enriched diet [54]. Rats fed with the green tea powder (20 g/kg)-enriched diet showed a significant increase in the lag-phase oxidation of plasma with very low density in lipoproteins (VLDL) and LDL by 33% when compared to the control diet [48]. EGCG was proposed to be a competitive inhibitor of β-ketoacyl reductase of the FAS enzyme complex in the liver [79]. EGCG and ECG lowered FAS and malate enzymes in rat liver cytosol, resulting in a significant decrease in visceral fat deposition and hepatic triglyceride content [80]. Nonetheless, experiments showed that GTE lowered serum cholesterol and triglyceride concentrations in the hamsters fed with high fat diet (200 g lard and 1 g cholesterol/kg) in a concentration-dependent manner, for which the mechanism was most likely due to its influence on the absorption of dietary fat and cholesterol, but not on the inhibition of the synthesis of cholesterol or fatty acid [49]. Another study supports the evidence that Chinese green tea lowered plasma cholesterol levels by increasing fecal bile acids and cholesterol excretion, but not by inhibiting activities of three major lipid metabolizing enzymes, including 3-hydroxy-3-methylglutaryl-coenzyme A (HMG-Co A) reductase, cholesterol 7α-hydroxylase and FAS [53]. More importantly, high plasma cholesterol levels, fatty liver, renal dysfunctions and severe atherosclerotic aorta were observed in the LDL knockout mice fed with a normal diet, but not in those fed with a 4% green tea catechins-enriched diet for 35 weeks [81].

GTE, which had greater effects than oolong tea and black tea, decreased high serum triglyceride (195 vs. 119 mg/dl) and cholesterol (104 vs. 73 mg/dl) levels to normal levels, and also decreased hepatic triglyceride content in sucrose-induced hyperlipidemic rats (8.4±1.5 vs. 27.7±7.9 mg/g wet weight ($p<0.05$); possibly by limiting the intestinal absorption of dietary fat and storage of fat in the liver [52]. EGCG (dose of 0.5 g/kg for 4 weeks) can interfere with the micellar solubilization of dietary cholesterol in the gastrointestinal tract and subsequently reduce cholesterol absorption in the rats fed with a high cholesterol diet [50].

Green tea catechins functioned against membrane phospholipid peroxidation [82], showed a strong synergistic anti-oxidative activity with α-tocopherol in micelles [83],as well as in human LDL levels [84], and had a protective effect of high-density lipoprotein (HDL) on endothelial cell-dependent vasodilatation [85]. They have many pharmacological activities, including anti-hypertensive [41] and anti-atherosclerotic [86, 87] effects. Clearly, green tea catechins; especially EGCG, has a potential hypolipidemic effect, possibly by interfering with the emulsification, digestion, and micellar solubilization of lipids in the critical steps of intestinal absorption of dietary lipids [88]. Bursill and coworkers found that GTE (2% catechins, *w/w*) decreased the levels of total cholesterol (-60%), VLDL-and intermediate density lipoprotein (IDL)-cholesterol (-70%), LDL-cholesterol (-80%) in plasma, total cholesterol (622 versus 800 μmol/g,-10%) and unesterified cholesterol (323 versus 399 μmol/g,-15%) in the liver, and cholesterol (-25%) in the thoracic aorta (0.73 versus 0.98 μmol/g,-25%) and aortic arch fatty streak (1.93 versus 2.35 μmol/g) of the rabbits fed with a high cholesterol (0.25%, *w/w*) diet compared with the placebo group, possibly due to a decrease in cholesterol synthesis and an upregulation of hepatic LDL receptor gene expression [89, 90]. Controversial data has indicated that the consumption of high doses of green tea polyphenols (714 mg/day) for 3 weeks resulted in decreases in the total cholesterol:HDL-cholesterol ratio, but had no effects on the risk biomarkers of CVD [91].

6.4. Neurological diseases

The errors in brain iron metabolism found in neurological disorders are found to be multifactorial, however treatment conditions seem to be particularly important. Epilepsy, an oxidative related disorder of the brain, has served as a model for the investigation in the role of iron, especially NTBI in neurological disorders. The effect of antiepileptic drug treatment on changes of iron status and oxidative stress parameters were determined [92]. Recent genetic and biochemical manipulations of iron overload have placed iron at the centre of research into neurodegenerative diseases. This is supported by the discovery of genetic and non-genetic misregulations of the iron metabolism in these disorders. In many neurodegenerative disorders, abnormally high levels of iron in specific regions of the brain have been reported [93]. Evidence for iron contribution to diseases by augmentation of oxidative stress have led to an examination of the contribution of iron to other diseases, in which oxidative stress may be involved, including epilepsy [94]. It has not been possible to determine whether the accumulated iron is in the labile iron pool (LIP), which can participate in the Fenton reaction to generate the reactive hydroxyl radical. The reduction in GSH during disease progression and in response to neurotoxins, together with increased iron accumulation and ROS generation, might be taken as evidence for the presence of free iron [95].

Oxidative stress, resulting from increased brain iron levels, and possibly also from defects in antioxidant defensive mechanisms, is widely believed to be associated with neuronal death in these disorders [96, 97], along with a reduced availability of GSH and other antioxidant substances in the brain. Changes in the integrity of the blood brain barrier (BBB) due to altered vascularization of the tissue or inflammatory events could be another initial cause. However, neuronal death by any initial cause could lead to large amounts of iron release and increased ROS formation [98]. Therefore, iron and iron-induced oxidative stress could possibly be a common mechanism involved in the development of neurodegeneration [99] (Figure 3). Available data strongly support this hypothesis [100, 101]

Based on this hypothesis, therefore, therapeutic efforts should be devoted to reducing brain iron levels and inhibiting the generation of ROS. A few recent studies have shown that the iron chelator, deferrioxamine, may be a significant factor in an effective therapy for the prevention and treatment of brain disorders [102]. One possible non-toxic approach with natural metal chelators could make use of green tea catechins, especially EGCG. This compound comprising antioxidant, iron chelating and anti-inflammatory activities; has been shown to be neuroprotective in animal models of Parkinson's disease (PD) and Alzheimer's disease (AD), and also regulates the processing of amyloid precursor protein (APP) through a non-amyloidogenic pathway [103, 104]. Understanding the timing of iron mismanagement in relation to the progression of neuronal losses would provide important information on pathogenesis, and

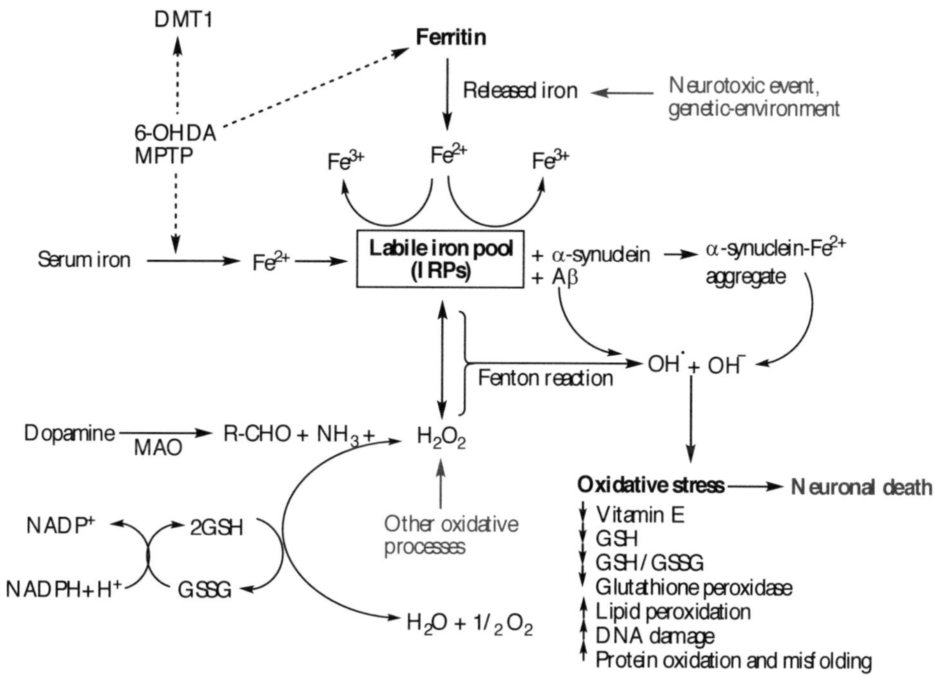

Figure 3. Mechanism of iron-induced neurodegeneration and its prevention [95]. Abbreviations: DMT1=divalent metal ion transporter-1; GSH=reduced glutathione; GSSG=oxidized glutathione; IRPs=iron regulatory proteins; MAO=monoamine oxidase; MPTP=1-methyl-4-phenyl-1,2,3,6-tetrahydropyridine;NADP+=nicotinamide adenine dinucleotide phosphate; NADPH=reduced nicotinamide adenine dinucleotide phosphate; 6-OHDA=6-hydroxydopamine

would raise the possibility of monitoring iron changes as a marker of disease progression, and perhaps even in a pre-clinical diagnosis in conditions where iron misregulation is an early event.

More *in vitro* and *in vivo* studies should be done to investigate how iron misregulation/accumulation synergizes with common endogenous and environmental toxins. Iron misregulation/accumulation alone can kill neurons only in genetic disorders where iron imbalance occurs rapidly and is extensive. However, in most cases, the amount of iron build-up is relatively low and the neurotoxic mechanism might involve a combination of iron and other toxins. Future investigations of iron in the brain, including how to best monitor iron deposition *in vivo*, the clinical relevance of excessive iron deposition, and the mechanistic relationship between iron deposition and disease pathophysiology, hold the promise of advancements in the field of neurotherapeutics.

6.5. Mutagenicity and cancinogenesis

Topical applications of green tea polyphenol fractions (such as EGCG, EGC and ECG) inhibitedbenz[a]-pyrene (BP)-and 7,12-dimethylbenz[a]-anthracene (DMBA)-initiated and 12-*O*-tetradecanoylphorbol-13-acetate (TPA)-promoted tumorigenesis of mouse skin, possibly by inhibiting ROS production, inflammation and hyperplasia [105]. Green tea catechins can counteract against tumorigenesis and DNA damage [106]. Mu and colleagues have identified an association between tea consumption and decreased cancer risk [107]. Surprisingly, EGCG in green tea exerted inhibitory effects on skin cancer, hepatocellular carcinoma and duodenal cancer, on metastasis of the melanoma cell line in lung cancer in mice, possibly by blocking the interaction of their tumor promoters with their own membrane receptors called sealing effects. Green tea significantly prevented growth of Namalwa, RAP1-EIO and HS-Sultan tumors transplanted intraperitoneally in the NOD/SCID mice; possibly by impairment of tumor invasion, anti-angiogenesis and by cell apoptosis induction [108]. EGCG decreased ornithine decarboxylase (ODC) and Ras and Jun oncogene levels, and also inhibited tyrosine kinase (TK) as well as mitogen-activated protein kinase (MAPK) activities in the transformed NIH-pATMras fibroblasts [109].

7. Conclusions

Green tea has long been considered a refreshing beverage that is prepared from tea (*Camellia sinensis*) shoots. It exerts many beneficial health effects, including anti-oxidant, anti-diabetic, hypolipidemic, anti-aging, anti-gout, neuroprotective, cardioprotective, hepatoprotective, anti-inflammatory, anti-carcinogenesis properties, among others. Variations of strain, source, geographic area, altitude, climate, cultivation, duration of fermentation and the preparation process can give rise to differences in the amounts of catechins derivatives, nutritional values, biological activities and the pharmacological properties of green tea products. EGCG is the most abundant type of catechin found in green tea and also the most relevant phytochemical displaying an influencing in several diseases and disorders. Some green tea catechins are not absorbed, while some catechins are absorbed from the intestine into the blood, and then are biologically transformed in liver microsomes by glucuronidation, sulfation and methylation reactions and ultimately excreted through the bile and urine. In this article, we have focused on the efficacy of green tea crude extract and catechins fractions, particularly EGCG in 1) depleting free radicals in normal cells, 2) removing chelatable iron from vital organs with iron overload, 3) lowering the levels of the risk factors of cardiovascular diseases, 4) inhibiting growth and proliferation of leukemic cells and solid malignant tumors, and 5) scavenging ROS and a repletion in the reducing power in neuronal tissues. The recognized benefits of green tea are that it is 1) potent in antioxidation, 2) effective in iron chelation, 3) beneficial in the inhibition of fat digestion, absorption and synthesis, 4) apoptotic induction, and 5) neuroprotection, respectively. Green tea has played a prominent role in the lives of many over time as a beverage, as a component of the diet, and now a substance that can be applied in drugs. The benefits of which have now been evidently documented.

Abbreviations

AD=Alzheimer's disease

ALT=alanine aminotransferase

http://dx.doi.org/10.5772/57519

AML=acute myelocytic leukemia

APP=amyloid precursor protein

ATRA=all-*trans* retinoic acid

BBB=blood brain barrier

BKO=β-globin gene knockout

BP=benz[a]-pyrene

C=catechin

CLL=chronic lymphocytic leukemia

COMT=catechol-*O*-methyltransferase

CVD=cardiovascular diseases

DAPK2=death-associated protein kinase 2

DFP=deferiprone

DH=double heterozygous β-globin gene knockout carrying human β^E gene

DMBA=7,12-dimethylbenz[a]-anthracene

DMT1=divalent metal ion transporter-1

DW=deionized water

EC=epicatechin

ECG=epicatechin 3-gallate

EGC=epigallocatechin

EGCG=epigallocatechin 3-gallate

FAS=fatty acid synthase

GA=gallic acid

GC=gallocatechin

G-CSF=granulocyte colony stimulating factor

GM-CSF=granulocyte macrophage colony stimulating factor

GSH=reduced glutathione

GSSG=oxidized glutathione

GTE=green tea extract

Hb=hemoglobin

HDL=high-density lipoprotein

HGF=hematopoietic growth factors

HMG-Co A=3-hydroxy-3-methylglutaryl-coenzyme A

hTERT=human telomerase reverse transcriptase

HTLV-I=human T-cell lymphotropic virus type I

IDL=intermediate density lipoprotein

IL-3=interleukin-3

IRPs=iron regulatory proteins

K_i=inhibition constant

LD_{50}=lethal dose at 50%

LDL=low-density lipoprotein

LIP=labile iron pool

LPI=labile plasma iron

MAO=monoamine oxidase

MAPK=mitogen-activated protein kinase

MDA=malondialdehyde

MPTP=1-methyl-4-phenyl-1,2,3,6-tetrahydropyridine

MW=molecular weight

$NAD(P)^+$=nicotinamide adenine dinucleotide phosphate

NAD(P)H=reduced nicotinamide adenine dinucleotide phosphate

ND=not determined

NQO1=NAD(P)H:quinoneoxidoreductase 1

NTBI=non-transferrin bound iron

ODC=ornithine decarboxylase

6-OHDA=6-hydroxydopamine

PD=Parkinson's disease

PPO=polyphenol oxidase

RBC=red blood cell

RNS=reactive nitrogen species

ROS=reactive oxygen species

SAM=*S*-adenosyl methionine

SULT=sulfotransferases

$T_{1/2}\beta$=beta-elimination half-lives

TEAC=trolox-equivalent antioxidant capacity

TK=tyrosine kinase

TPA=12-*O*-tetradecanoylphorbol-13-acetate

T_{reg}=regulatory T cells

UGT=uridine diphosphate-glucuronosyltransferase

V_d=distribution volume

VEGF=vascular endothelial growth factor

WT=wild-type

XO=xanthine oxidase

Acknowledgements

This work was partially supported by the Office of Higher Education Commission and Mahidol University under the National Research University Initiative, Thailand Research Fund through Professor Suthat Fucharoen, MD. and by a Research Chair Grant from the National Science and Technology Development Agency (NSTDA) and Mahidol University through Professor Suthat Fucharoen, MD.

Author details

Sakaewan Ounjaijean[1], Suthat Fucharoen[2] and Somdet Srichairatanakool[3*]

*Address all correspondence to: ssrichai@med.cmu.ac.th

1 Research Institute for Health Sciences, Chiang Mai University, Chiang Mai, Thailand

2 Thalassemia Research Center, Institute of Bioscience, Mahidol University, NakornPathom, Thailand

3 Department of Biochemistry, Faculty of Medicine, Chiang Mai University, Chiang Mai, Thailand

References

[1] Bokuchava MA, Skobeleva NI. The Biochemistry and Technology of Tea Manufacture. Critical Reviews in Food Science and Nutrition 1980;12(4) 303-70.

[2] Srichairatanakool S, Ounjaijean S, Thephinlap C, Khansuwan U, Phisalpong C, Fucharoen S. Iron-chelating and Free-radical Scavenging Activities of Microwave-processed Green Tea in Iron Overload. Hemoglobin 2006;30(2) 311-27.

[3] Balentine DA, Wiseman SA, Bouwens LC. The Chemistry of Tea Flavonoids. Critical Reviews in Food Science and Nutrition 1997;37(8) 693-704.

[4] Zuo Y, Chen H, Deng Y. Simultaneous Determination of Catechins, Caffeine and Gallic Acids in Green, Oolong, Black and Pu-erh Teas Using HPLC With a Photodiode Array Detector. Talanta 2002;57(4) 307-16.

[5] Khokhar S, Venema D, Hollman PC, Dekker M, Jongen W. A RP-HPLC Method for the Determination of Tea Catechins. Cancer Letters 1997;114(1-2) 171-2.

[6] McKay DL, Blumberg JB. The Role of Tea in Human Health: an Update. Journal of the American College of Nutrition 2002;21(1) 1-13.

[7] Cabrera C, Artacho R, Gimenez R. Beneficial Effects of Green Tea--a Review. Journal of the American College of Nutrition 2006;25(2) 79-99.

[8] Chen Z, Zhu QY, Tsang D, Huang Y. Degradation of Green Tea Catechins in Tea Drinks. Journal of Agricultural and Food Chemistry 2001;49(1) 477-82.

[9] Rababah TM, Hettiarachchy NS, Horax R. Total Phenolics and Antioxidant Activities of Fenugreek, Green Tea, Black Tea, Grape Seed, Ginger, Rosemary, Gotu Kola, and Ginkgo Extracts, Vitamin E, and Tert-butylhydroquinone. Journal of Agricultural and Food Chemistry 2004;52(16) 5183-6.

[10] Graham HN. Green Tea Composition, Consumption, and Polyphenol Chemistry. Preventive Medicine 1992;21(3) 334-50.

[11] Kuo YC, Yu CL, Liu CY, Wang SF, Pan PC, Wu MT, et al. A Population-based, Case control Study of Green Tea Consumption and Leukemia Risk in Southwestern Taiwan. Cancer Causes and Control 2009;20(1) 57-65.

[12] Milchak LM, Douglas Bricker J. The Effects of Glutathione and Vitamin E on Iron Toxicity in Isolated Rat Hepatocytes. Toxicology Letters 2002;126(3) 169-77.

[13] Sutherland BA, Rahman RM, Appleton I. Mechanisms of Action of Green Tea Catechins, With a Focus on Ischemia-induced Neurodegeneration. Journal of Nutritional Biochemistry 2006;17(5) 291-306.

[14] Frei B, Higdon JV. Antioxidant Activity of Tea Polyphenols in Vivo: Evidence From Animal Studies. Journal of Nutrition 2003;133(10) 3275S-84S.

[15] Grinberg LN, Newmark H, Kitrossky N, Rahamim E, Chevion M, Rachmilewitz EA. Protective Effects of Tea Polyphenols Against Oxidative Damage to Red Blood Cells. Biochemical Pharmacology 1997;54(9) 973-8.

[16] Morel I, Lescoat G, Cillard P, Cillard J. Role of Flavonoids and Iron Chelation in Antioxidant Action. Methods in Enzymology 1994;234 437-43.

[17] Saewong T, Ounjaijean S, Mundee Y, Pattanapanyasat K, Fucharoen S, Porter JB, et al. Effects of Green Tea on Iron Accumulation and Oxidative Stress in Livers of Iron challenged Thalassemic Mice. Medicinal Chemistry 2010;6(2) 57-64.

[18] Ounjaijean S, Thephinlap C, Khansuwan U, Phisalapong C, Fucharoen S, Porter JB, et al. Effect of Green Tea on Iron Status and Oxidative Stress in Iron-loaded Rats. Medicinal Chemistry 2008;4(4) 365-70.

[19] Thephinlap C, Ounjaijean S, Khansuwan U, Fucharoen S, Porter JB, Srichairatanakool S. Epigallocatechin-3-gallate and Epicatechin-3-gallate From Green Tea Decrease Plasma Non-transferrin Bound Iron and Erythrocyte Oxidative Stress. Medicinal Chemistry 2007;3(3) 289-96.

[20] van Acker SA, van Balen GP, van den Berg DJ, Bast A, van der Vijgh WJ. Influence of Iron Chelation on the Antioxidant Activity of Flavonoids. Biochemical Pharmacology 1998;56(8) 935-43.

[21] Kostyuk VA, Potapovich AI, Vladykovskaya EN, Korkina LG, Afanas'ev IB. Influence of Metal Ions on Flavonoid Protection Against Asbestos-induced Cell Injury. Archives of Biochemistry and Biophysics 2001;385(1) 129-37.

[22] Raza H, John A. In Vitro Protection of Reactive Oxygen Species-induced Degradation of Lipids, Proteins and 2-Deoxyribose by Tea Catechins. Food and Chemical Toxicology 2007;45(10) 1814-20.

[23] Higuchi A, Yonemitsu K, Koreeda A, Tsunenari S. Inhibitory Activity of Epigallocatechin Gallate (EGCg) in Paraquat-induced Microsomal Lipid Peroxidation--a Mechanism of Protective Effects of EGCg against Paraquat Toxicity. Toxicology 2003;183(1-3) 143-9.

[24] Salah N, Miller NJ, Paganga G, Tijburg L, Bolwell GP, Rice-Evans C. Polyphenolic flavanols as Scavengers of Aqueous Phase Radicals and As Chain-breaking Antioxidants. Archives of Biochemistry and Biophysics 1995;322(2) 339-46.

[25] Samman S, Sandstrom B, Toft MB, Bukhave K, Jensen M, Sorensen SS, et al. Green Tea or Rosemary Extract Added to Foods Reduces Nonheme-iron Absorption. American Journal of Clinical Nutrition 2001;73(3) 607-12.

[26] Guo Q, Zhao B, Li M, Shen S, Xin W. Studies on Protective Mechanisms of Four Components of Green Tea Polyphenols Against Lipid Peroxidation in Synaptosomes. Biochimica et Biophysica Acta 1996;1304(3) 210-22.

[27] Valcic S, Burr JA, Timmermann BN, Liebler DC. Antioxidant Chemistry of Green Tea Catechins. New Oxidation Products of (-)-Epigallocatechin Gallate and (-)-Epigallocatechin From Their Reactions With Peroxyl Radicals. Chemical Research in Toxicology 2000;13(9) 801-10.

[28] Chen L, Lee MJ, Li H, Yang CS. Absorption, Distribution, Elimination of Tea Polyphenols in Rats. Drug Metabolism and Disposition 1997 Sep;25(9) 1045-50.

[29] Scalbert A, Williamson G. Dietary Intake and Bioavailability of Polyphenols. Journal of Nutrition 2000;130(8S Suppl) 2073S-85S.

[30] Loktionov A, Bingham SA, Vorster H, Jerling JC, Runswick SA, Cummings JH. Apolipoprotein E Genotype Modulates the Effect of Black Tea Drinking on Blood Lipids and Blood Coagulation Factors: a Pilot Study. British Journal of Nutrition 1998;79(2) 133-9.

[31] Kim S, Lee MJ, Hong J, Li C, Smith TJ, Yang GY, et al. Plasma and Tissue Levels of Tea Catechins in Rats and Mice During Chronic Consumption of Green Tea Polyphenols. Nutrition and Cancer 2000;37(1) 41-8.

[32] Vaidyanathan JB, Walle T. Glucuronidation and Sulfation of the Tea Flavonoid (-)-Epicatechin by the Human and Rat Enzymes. Drug Metabolism and Disposition 2002;30(8) 897-903.

[33] Nishimuta H, Ohtani H, Tsujimoto M, Ogura K, Hiratsuka A, Sawada Y. Inhibitory Effects of Various Beverages on Human Recombinant Sulfotransferase Isoforms SULT1A1 and SULT1A3. Biopharmaceutics & Drug Disposition 2007;28(9) 491-500.

[34] Lu H, Meng X, Li C, Sang S, Patten C, Sheng S, et al. Glucuronides of Tea Catechins: Enzymology of Biosynthesis and Biological Activities. Drug Metabolism and Disposition 2003;31(4) 452-61.

[35] Crespy V, Nancoz N, Oliveira M, Hau J, Courtet-Compondu MC, Williamson G. Glucuronidation of the Green Tea Catechins, (-)-Epigallocatechin-3-gallate and (-)-Epicatechin-3-gallate, by Rat Hepatic and Intestinal Microsomes. Free Radical Research 2004;38(9) 1025-31.

[36] Galati G, Lin A, Sultan AM, O'Brien PJ. Cellular and in Vivo Hepatotoxicity Caused by Green Tea Phenolic Acids and Catechins. Free Radical Biology and Medicine 2006;40(4) 570-80.

[37] Mulder TP, Rietveld AG, van Amelsvoort JM. Consumption of Both Black Tea and Green Tea Results in an Increase in the Excretion of Hippuric Acid into Urine. American Journal of Clinical Nutrition 2005;81(1 Suppl) 256S-60S.

[38] Okushio K, Matsumoto N, Kohri T, Suzuki M, Nanjo F, Hara Y. Absorption of Tea Catechins into Rat Portal Vein. Biological and Pharmaceutical Bulletin 1996;19(2) 326-9.

[39] Lambert JD, Lee MJ, Lu H, Meng X, Hong JJ, Seril DN, et al. Epigallocatechin-3-gallate is Absorbed but Extensively Glucuronidated Following Oral Administration to Mice. Journal of Nutrition 2003;133(12) 4172-7.

[40] Zhang A, Zhu QY, Luk YS, Ho KY, Fung KP, Chen ZY. Inhibitory Effects of Jasmine Green Tea Epicatechin Isomers on Free Radical-induced Lysis of Red Blood Cells. Life Sciences 1997;61(4) 383-94.

[41] Henry JP, Stephens-Larson P. Reduction of Chronic Psychosocial Hypertension in Mice by Decaffeinated Tea. Hypertension. 1984;6(3) 437-44.

[42] Hertog MG, Feskens EJ, Hollman PC, Katan MB, Kromhout D. Dietary Antioxidant Flavonoids and Risk of Coronary Heart Disease: the Zutphen Elderly Study. Lancet 1993;342(8878) 1007-11.

[43] Cutter H, Wu LY, Kim C, Morre DJ, Morre DM. Is The Cancer Protective Effect Correlated with Growth Inhibitions by Green tea (-)-Epigallocatechin Gallate Mediated Through an Antioxidant Mechanism? Cancer Letters 2001;162(2) 149-54.

[44] Shi ST, Wang ZY, Smith TJ, Hong JY, Chen WF, Ho CT, et al. Effects of Green Tea and Black Tea on 4-(Methylnitrosamino)-1-(3-pyridyl)-1-butanone Bioactivation, DNA Methylation, and Lung Tumorigenesis in A/J mice. Cancer Research 1994;54(17) 4641-7.

[45] Wang ZY, Huang MT, Lou YR, Xie JG, Reuhl KR, Newmark HL, et al. Inhibitory Effects of Black Tea, Green Tea, Decaffeinated Black Tea, and Decaffeinated Green Tea on Ultraviolet B Light-induced Skin Carcinogenesis in 7,12-Dimethylbenz[a]anthracene-initiated SKH-1 Mice. Cancer Research 1994;54(13) 3428-35.

[46] Imai K, Nakachi K. Cross Sectional Study of Effects of Drinking Green Tea on Cardiovascular and Liver Diseases. British Medical Journal 1995;310(6981) 693-6.

[47] Kono S, Shinchi K, Ikeda N, Yanai F, Imanishi K. Green Tea Consumption and Serum Lipid Profiles: a Cross-sectional Study in Northern Kyushu, Japan. Preventive Medicine 1992;21(4) 526-31.

[48] Anderson JW, Diwadkar VA, Bridges SR. Selective Effects of Different Antioxidants on Oxidation of Lipoproteins from Rats. Proceedings of the Society for Experimental Biology and Medicine 1998;218(4) 376-81.

[49] Chan PT, Fong WP, Cheung YL, Huang Y, Ho WK, Chen ZY. Jasmine Green Tea Epicatechins are Hypolipidemic in Hamsters (Mesocricetus auratus) Fed a High Fat Diet. Journal of Nutrition 1999;129(6) 1094-101.

[50] Raederstorff DG, Schlachter MF, Elste V, Weber P. Effect of EGCG on Lipid Absorption and Plasma Lipid Levels in Rats. Journal of Nutritional Biochemistry 2003;14(6) 326-32.

[51] Skrzydlewska E, Ostrowska J, Farbiszewski R, Michalak K. Protective Effect of Green Tea Against Lipid Peroxidation in the Rat Liver, Blood Serum and the Brain. Phytomedicine 2002;9(3) 232-8.

[52] Yang M, Wang C, Chen H. Green, Oolong and Black Tea Extracts Modulate Lipid Metabolism in Hyperlipidemia Rats Fed High-sucrose Diet. Journal of Nutritional Biochemistry 2001;12(1) 14-20.

[53] Yang TT, Koo MW. Chinese Green Tea Lowers Cholesterol Level Through an Increase in Fecal Lipid Excretion. Life Science 2000;66(5) 411-23.

[54] Yang TT, Koo MW. Hypocholesterolemic Effects of Chinese Tea. Pharmacological Research 1997;35(6) 505-12.

[55] Lam le H, Sakaguchi K, Ukeda H, Sawamura M. Flow Injection Determination of Xanthine Oxidase Inhibitory Activity and Its Application to Food Samples. Analytical Sciences 2006;22(1) 105-9.

[56] Aucamp J, Gaspar A, Hara Y, Apostolides Z. Inhibition of Xanthine Oxidase by Catechins From Tea (Camellia sinensis). Anticancer Research 1997;17(6D) 4381-5.

[57] Ozyurek M, Bektasoglu B, Guclu K, Apak R. Measurement of Xanthine Oxidase Inhibition Activity of Phenolics and Flavonoids With a Modified Cupric Reducing Antioxidant Capacity (CUPRAC) Method. Analytica Chimica Acta 2009;636(1) 42-50.

[58] Lin JK, Chen PC, Ho CT, Lin-Shiau SY. Inhibition of Xanthine Oxidase and Suppression of Intracellular Reactive Oxygen Species in HL-60 Cells by Theaflavin-3,3'-digallate, (-)-Epigallocatechin-3-gallate, and Propyl Gallate. Journal of Agricultural and Food Chemistry 2000;48(7) 2736-43.

[59] Kimura M, Umegaki K, Kasuya Y, Sugisawa A, Higuchi M. The Relation Between Single/double or Repeated Tea Catechin Ingestions and Plasma Antioxidant Activity in Humans. European Journal of Clinical Nutrition 2002;56(12) 1186-93.

[60] Gomikawa S, Ishikawa Y, Hayase W, Haratake Y, Hirano N, Matuura H, et al. Effect of Ground Green Tea Drinking for 2 Weeks on the Susceptibility of Plasma and LDL to the Oxidation ex Vivo in Healthy Volunteers. Kobe journal of medical sciences 2008;54(1) E62-72.

[61] Sone T, Kuriyama S, Nakaya N, Hozawa A, Shimazu T, Nomura K, et al. Randomized Controlled Trial For an Fffect of Catechin-enriched Green Tea Consumption on Adiponectin and Cardiovascular Disease Risk Factors. Food and Nutrition Research 2011;55. doi: 10.3402/fnr.v55i0.8326.

[62] Fraga CG, Oteiza PI. Iron Toxicity and Antioxidant Nutrients. Toxicology 2002;180(1)23-32.

[63] Galleano M, Puntarulo S. Dietary Alpha-tocopherol Supplementation on Antioxidant Defenses After in Vivo Iron Overload in Rats. Toxicology 1997;124(1) 73-81.

[64] Tesoriere L, D'Arpa D, Butera D, Allegra M, Renda D, Maggio A, et al. Oral Supplements of Vitamin E Improve Measures of Oxidative Stress in Plasma and Reduce Oxidative Damage to LDL and Erythrocytes in Beta-thalassemia Intermedia Patients. Free Radical Research 2001;34(5) 529-40.

[65] Rachmilewitz EA, Weizer-Stern O, Adamsky K, Amariglio N, Rechavi G, Breda L, et al. Role of Iron in Inducing Oxidative Stress in Thalassemia: Can It Be Prevented by Inhibition of Absorption and by Antioxidants? Annals of the New York Academy of Sciences 2005;1054 118-23.

[66] Buettner GR, Jurkiewicz BA. Catalytic Metals, Ascorbate and Free Radicals: Combinations to Avoid. Radiation Research 1996;145(5) 532-41.

[67] Herbert V, Shaw S, Jayatilleke E. Vitamin C-driven Free Radical Generation from Iron. Journal of Nutrition 1996;126(4 Suppl) 1213S-20S.

[68] Rund D, Rachmilewitz E. Beta-thalassemia. The New England Journal of Medicine 2005;353(11) 1135-46.

[69] Otsuka T, Ogo T, Eto T, Asano Y, Suganuma M, Niho Y. Growth Inhibition of Leukemic Cells by (-)-Epigallocatechin Gallate, the Main Constituent of Green Tea. Life Sciences 1998;63(16) 1397-403.

[70] Asano Y, Okamura S, Ogo T, Eto T, Otsuka T, Niho Y. Effect of (-)-Epigallocatechin Gallate on Leukemic Blast Cells from Patients With Acute Myeloblastic Leukemia. Life Sciences 1997;60(2) 135-42.

[71] Surh Y. Molecular Mechanisms of Chemopreventive Effects of Selected Dietary and Medicinal Phenolic Substances. Mutation Research 1999;428(1-2) 305-27.

[72] Li HC, Yashiki S, Sonoda J, Lou H, Ghosh SK, Byrnes JJ, et al. Green Tea Polyphenols Induce Apoptosis in Vitro in Peripheral Blood T Lymphocytes of Adult T-Cell Leukemia Patients. Japanese Journal of Cancer Research 2000;91(1) 34-40.

[73] Sonoda J, Koriyama C, Yamamoto S, Kozako T, Li HC, Lema C, et al. HTLV-1 Provirus Load in Peripheral Blood Lymphocytes of HTLV-1 Carriers is Diminished by Green Tea Drinking. Cancer Science 2004;95(7) 596-601.

[74] Beliveau R, Gingras D. Green tea: Prevention and Treatment of Cancer by Nutraceuticals. Lancet 2004;364(9439) 1021-2.

[75] Berletch JB, Liu C, Love WK, Andrews LG, Katiyar SK, Tollefsbol TO. Epigenetic and Genetic Mechanisms Contribute to Telomerase Inhibition by EGCG. Journal of Cellular Biochemistry 2008;103(2) 509-19.

[76] Britschgi A, Simon HU, Tobler A, Fey MF, Tschan MP. Epigallocatechin-3-gallate Induces Cell Death in Acute Myeloid Leukaemia Cells and Supports All-trans Retinoic Acid-induced Neutrophil Differentiation via Death-associated Protein Kinase 2. British Journal of Haematology 2010;149(1) 55-64.

[77] D'Arena G, Simeon V, De Martino L, Statuto T, D'Auria F, Volpe S, et al. Regulatory T-cell Modulation by Green Tea in Chronic Lymphocytic Leukemia. International Journal of Immunopathology and Pharmacology 2013;26(1) 117-25.

[78] Shanafelt TD, Call TG, Zent CS, Leis JF, LaPlant B, Bowen DA, et al. Phase 2 Trial of Daily, Oral Polyphenon E in Patients With Asymptomatic, Rai Stage 0 to II Chronic Lymphocytic Leukemia. Cancer 2012;119(2) 363-70.

[79] Wang X, Tian W. Green Tea Epigallocatechin Gallate: a Natural Inhibitor of Fatty acid Synthase. Biochemical and Biophysical Research Communications 2001;288(5) 1200-6.

[80] Ikeda I, Hamamoto R, Uzu K, Imaizumi K, Nagao K, Yanagita T, et al. Dietary Gallate Esters of Tea Catechins Reduce Deposition of Visceral Fat, Hepatic Triacylglycerol, and Activities of Hepatic Enzymes Related to Fatty Acid Synthesis in Rats. Bioscience, Biotechnology, and Biochemistry 2005;69(5) 1049-53.

[81] Suzuki J, Ogawa M, Izawa A, Sagesaka YM, Isobe M. Dietary Consumption of Green Tea Catechins Attenuate Hyperlipidaemia-induced Atherosclerosis and Systemic Organ Damage in Mice. Acta Cardiologica 2005;60(3) 271-6.

[82] Kondo K, Kurihara M, Miyata N, Suzuki T, Toyoda M. Scavenging Mechanisms of (-)-Epigallocatechin Gallate and (-)-Epicatechin Gallate on Peroxyl Radicals and Formation of Superoxide During the Inhibitory Action. Free Radical Biology and Medicine 1999;27(7-8) 855-63.

[83] Zhou B, Wu LM, Yang L, Liu ZL. Evidence for Alpha-tocopherol Regeneration Reaction of Green Tea Polyphenols in SDS Micelles. Free Radical Biology and Medicine 2005;38(1) 78-84.

[84] Liu Z, Ma LP, Zhou B, Yang L, Liu ZL. Antioxidative Effects of Green Tea Polyphenols on Free Radical Initiated and Photosensitized Peroxidation of Human Low Density Lipoprotein. Chemistry and Physics of Lipids;106(1) 53-63.

[85] Li XP, Zhao SP, Zhang XY, Liu L, Gao M, Zhou QC. Protective Effect of High Density Lipoprotein on Endothelium-dependent Vasodilatation. International Journal of Cardiology 2000;73(3) 231-6.

[86] Geleijnse JM, Launer LJ, Hofman A, Pols HA, Witteman JC. Tea Flavonoids May Protect Against Atherosclerosis: the Rotterdam Study. Archives of Internal Medicine 1999;159(18) 2170-4.

[87] Vinson JA, Teufel K, Wu N. Green and Black Teas Inhibit Atherosclerosis by Lipid, Antioxidant, and Fibrinolytic Mechanisms. Journal of Agricultural and Food Chemistry 2004;52(11) 3661-5.

[88] Koo SI, Noh SK. Green Tea as Inhibitor of the Intestinal Absorption of Lipids: Potential Mechanism for Its Lipid-lowering Effect. Journal of Nutritional Biochemistry 2007;18(3) 179-83.

[89] Bursill CA, Abbey M, Roach PD. A Green Tea Extract Lowers Plasma Cholesterol by Inhibiting Cholesterol Synthesis and Upregulating the LDL Receptor in the Cholesterol-fed Rabbit. Atherosclerosis 2007;193(1) 86-93.

[90] Bursill CA, Roach PD. A Green Tea Catechin Extract Upregulates the Hepatic Low-Density Lipoprotein Receptor in Rats. Lipids 2007;42(7) 621-7.

[91] Frank J, George TW, Lodge JK, Rodriguez-Mateos AM, Spencer JP, Minihane AM, et al. Daily Consumption of an Aqueous Green Tea Extract Supplement Does Not Impair Liver Function or Alter Cardiovascular Disease Risk Biomarkers in Healthy Men. Journal of Nutrition 2009;139(1) 58-62.

[92] Ounjaijean S, Westermarck T, Partinen M, Plonka-Poltorak E, Kaipainen P, Kaski M, et al. Increase in Non-transferrin Bound Iron and the Oxidative Stress Status in Epilepsy Patients Treated Using Valproic Acid Monotherapy. International Journal of Clinical Pharmacology and Therapeutics 2011;49(4) 268-76.

[93] Snyder AM, Connor JR. Iron, the Substantia Nigra and Related Neurological Disorders. Biochimica et Biophysica Acta. 2009;1790(7) 606-14.

[94] Thompson KJ, Shoham S, Connor JR. Iron and Neurodegenerative Disorders. Brain Research Bulletin 2001;55(2) 155-64.

[95] Zecca L, Youdim MB, Riederer P, Connor JR, Crichton RR. Iron, Brain Ageing and Neurodegenerative Disorders. Nature Reviews Neuroscience 2004;5(11) 863-73.

[96] Andrews NC. Iron Homeostasis: Insights from Genetics and Animal Models. Nature Reviews Genetics 2000;1(3) 208-17.

[97] Halliwell B. Role of Free Radicals in the Neurodegenerative Diseases: Therapeutic Implications for Antioxidant Treatment. Drugs and Aging 2001;18(9) 685-716.

[98] Andersen JK. Oxidative Stress in Neurodegeneration: Cause or Consequence? Nature Medicine 2004;10 Suppl S18-25.

[99] Ke Y, Qian ZM. Brain Iron Metabolism: Neurobiology and Neurochemistry. Progress in Neurobiology 2007;83(3) 149-73.

[100] Youdim MB, Stephenson G, Ben Shachar D. Ironing Iron Out in Parkinson's Disease and Other Neurodegenerative Diseases With Iron Chelators: a Lesson From 6-Hydroxydopamine and Iron Chelators, Desferal and VK-28. Annals of the New York Academy of Sciences 2004;1012 306-25.

[101] Richardson DR. Novel Chelators for Central Nervous System Disorders That Involve Alterations in the Metabolism of Iron and Other Metal Ions. Annals of the New York Academy of Sciences 2004;1012 326-41.

[102] Liu G, Men P, Perry G, Smith MA. Nanoparticle and Iron Chelators As a Potential Novel Alzheimer Therapy. Methods in Molecular Biology 2010;610 123-44.

[103] Mandel SA, Amit T, Weinreb O, Reznichenko L, Youdim MB. Simultaneous Manipulation of Multiple Brain Targets by Green Tea Catechins: a Potential Neuroprotective Strategy for Alzheimer and Parkinson Diseases. CNS Neuroscience and Therapeutics 2008;14(4) 352-65.

[104] Mandel S, Amit T, Reznichenko L, Weinreb O, Youdim MB. Green Tea Catechins as Brain-permeable, Natural Iron Chelators-antioxidants For the Treatment of Neurodegenerative Disorders. Molecular Nutrtion and Food Research 2006;50(2) 229-34.

[105] Huang MT, Ho CT, Wang ZY, Ferraro T, Finnegan-Olive T, Lou YR, et al. Inhibitory Effect of Topical Application of a Green Tea Polyphenol Fraction on Tumor Initiation and Promotion in Mouse Skin. Carcinogenesis 1992;13(6) 947-54.

[106] Anderson RF, Fisher LJ, Hara Y, Harris T, Mak WB, Melton LD, et al. Green Tea Catechins Partially Protect DNA From (.)OH Radical-induced Strand Breaks and Base Damage Through Fast Chemical Repair of DNA Radicals. Carcinogenesis 2001;22(8) 1189-93.

[107] Mu LN, Zhou XF, Ding BG, Wang RH, Zhang ZF, Chen CW, et al. [A Case-control Study on Drinking Green Tea and Decreasing Risk of Cancers in the Alimentary Canal Among Cigarette Smokers and Alcohol Drinkers]. Zhonghua Liu Xing Bing Xue Za Zhi 2003;24(3) 192-5.

[108] Bertolini F, Fusetti L, Rabascio C, Cinieri S, Martinelli G, Pruneri G. Inhibition of Angiogenesis and Induction of Endothelial and Tumor Cell Apoptosis by Green Tea in Animal Models of Human High-grade Non-Hodgkin's Lymphoma. Leukemia 2000;14(8) 1477-82.

[109] Wang YC, Bachrach U. The Specific Anti-cancer Activity of Green Tea (-)-Epigallocatechin-3-gallate (EGCG). Amino Acids 2002;22(2) 131-43.

Chapter 20

Possible Relation Between Trace Element Status and Clinical Outcomes in Parkinson Syndrome

Erland Johansson, Tuomas Westermarck and
Faik Atroshi

Additional information is available at the end of the chapter

http://dx.doi.org/10.5772/57612

1. Introduction

Parkinson disease (PD) is a degenerative disorder of the central nervous system and one of the most common neurologic disorders, affecting approximately 1% of individuals older than 60 years and causing progressive disability that can be slowed, but not halted, by treatment (Poewe, 2006; DeLong & Juncos, 2008). The epidemiology of Parkinson disease is not genetically predetermined, but influenced by environmental factors which may be geographically heterogeneousn (Tanner & Langston, 1990). Major gene mutations cause only a small proportion of all cases and that in most cases; non-genetic factors play a part, probably in interaction with susceptibility genes (de Lau & Breteler, 2006). A number of environmental factors have been associated with an increased risk of Parkinson's including: pesticide exposure, head injuries, and living in the country or farming (Noyce et al. 2012; Van Maele-Fabry et al. 2012). Parkinson disease is characterised by focal loss of melanin –containing neurons of the central and caudal parts of the zona compacta of the substantia nigra (Jellinger 1987). Dopamine deficiency of the nigrostrial system is the hallmark of PD disorder. The cause of the degeneration of the dopamine containing neurons in the substantia nigra of patients with PD is nknown. Excessive free radical production has been suggested as a consequence of the catabolism of the monoamines (Dexter et al 1989). It has been shown those catalase and glutathione peroxidases are reduced in the substantia nigra of PD patients (Sofic et al. 1992). It has therefore been suggested that additional antioxidant therapy ncluding vitamins-E and C may be helpful to slowing the progression of PD. Increasing evidence indicates that PD is primarly a Mitochondrial disorder and thus the use of compounds With good mitochondrial penetrance, (CoQ10), could Potentially be of benefit in this disease (Matthews et al 1998).

2. Current treatment pathways

Parkinson's disease is a degenerative disease of the nervous system. The exact cause for Parkinson's disease is not well understood. There is no definitive test for PD – diagnosis is often based on medical history and the presence of the classic symptoms and signs of PD (Samii et al. 2004; Tolosa & Katzenschlager, 2007). Sometimes people are given anti-PD drugs to see if they respond, or other tests may be performed, such as MRI and CAT scans, to rule out other disorders with similar symptoms (Gelb et al. 1999; Hughes et al. 2002). The presence of other diseases, such as dementia and general ageing can obscure PD symptoms and reduce the chance of an accurate diagnosis. Certain drugs, when taken for long periods of time or in amounts greater than recommended, can cause Parkinsonism (Di Fabio et al. 2013) and have side effects. These medications do not result in Parkinson's disease, however, and symptoms resolve when the medications are no longer used.

3. Environmental and nutritional factors in Parkinson disease

Environmental factors and nutrients may play an important role in early life. In people who are genetically predisposed to Parkinson's disease, many experts believe that environmental exposures, such as unusual exposure to herbicides and pesticides, increase a person's risk of developing Parkinson's disease (Tanner & Langston, 1990; Van Maele-Fabry et al. 2012).

Numerous epidemiological studies and interventional trials have suggested a link, in aging, between an adequate nutritional status and health (de Lau & Breteler, 2006; Barichella et al. 2009). Nutrient deficiencies and constipation may also play a role (Dan Beth, 1992; Schelosky et al, 1995). Parkinson's patients are often deficient in vitamins, minerals and trace elements (Ames, 2011). Micronutrient sufficiency and quality of the lipid supply may play key roles in brain development. It is because of their diverse and vital roles that nutrient element imbalances are frequently found to be factors in degenerative diseases. Since the body cannot manufacture the elements-and daily losses are unavoidable-the nutrient elements are all "essential" and must regularly be taken in through the diet. Erythrocyte element levels are good indicators of body pools of essential elements such as selenium, zinc, magnesium, potassium, and calcium. Often referred to as minerals, the chemical elements are fundamental to every function in the body. It is because of their diverse and vital roles that nutrient element imbalances are frequently found to be factors in degenerative diseases. Since the body cannot manufacture the elements-and daily losses are unavoidable-the nutrient elements are all "essential" and must regularly be taken in through the diet. But they are easily lost in food processing, so it's easy to see how deficiencies can occur. It has been reported that moderate selenium and vitamin K deficiency show damage accumulates over time as a result of vitamin and mineral loss, leading to age-related diseases (Ames, 2006; McCann & Ames, 2011). Therefore, understanding how best to define and measure optimum nutrition will make the application of new technologies to allow each person to optimize their own nutrition a much more realistic possibility than it is today McCann & Ames, 2011).

http://dx.doi.org/10.5772/57612

4. Oxidative stress and Parkinson's disease

Oxidative stress could play an important role in the degenerative process leading to Parkinson's disease. These considerations provide a rationale for therapeutic strategies to diminish oxidative stress in dopaminergic regions of brain. If oxidative stress is a major factor, the agents that selectively and safely chelate iron may be of value. It was reported that the mitochondrial deficiency (Shoffner et al. 1991; Jenner, 1991; Saggu et al. 1989; Perry & Yong, 1986) in electron transport, enhanced lipid peroxidation, elevated superoxide dismutase, diminished capacity to remove excess hydrogen peroxide (suggested by low glutathione and glutathione peroxidase levels) and the presence of increased iron, which catalyses formation of highly reactive hydroxyl ions from hydrogen peroxide, make attractive the suggestion that oxidative stress could play an important role in the degenerative process leading to Parkinson's disease (Ambani et al. 1975).

5. Selenium and other antioxidants in Parkinson

Deficiency of the minerals and other antioxidants required for life are relatively uncommon, however, modest deficiency is very common and often not taken seriously. Selenium is an essential trace element which is necessary for growth and protein synthesis. Selenium protects cellular elements from oxidative damage and may participate in redox type reactions. Low plasma selenium concentrations are associated with subtle neurological impairments reflected in soft neurological signs (Shahar et al. 2010). A statistically significant increase in plasma Se was identified for PD patients (McIntosh et al. 2012). This has been evidenced by an increased lipid peroxidation and reduced glutathione levels (Delanty and Dichter, 2000) and high concentration of iron and free radical generation via autocatalytic mechanisms within neuromelanin-containing catecholaminergic neurons in the substantia nigra. In addition, the observation that exogenous administration of cysteine, N-acetyl cysteine or glutathione decreased the neurotoxic effects of 6-hydroxydopamine in vitro and in vivo reinforces this hypothesis (Soto-Otero et al. 2000). McCann et al. (2011), tested whether selenium-dependent proteins that are essential from an evolutionary perspective are more resistant to selenium deficiency than those that are less essential. The authors demonstrated a highly sophisticated array of mechanisms at cellular and tissue levels that, when selenium is limited, protect essential selenium-dependent proteins at the expense of those that are nonessential. It was also found that mutations in selenium-dependent proteins that are lost on modest selenium deficiency result in characteristics shared by age-related diseases including cancer, heart disease, and loss of immune or brain function (McCann et al., 2011). It was concluded that taking a multivitamin that contains selenium is a good way to prevent deficiencies that, over time, can cause harm in ways that we are just beginning to understand.

6. Zinc in Parkinson

Zinc is essential as a cofactor for a variety of enzymes and transcription factors and plays a role in various biological processes ranging from gene expression to the immune response. There are two distinct gene families of zinc transporters, 10 ZnT (Slc30a) and 14 Zip (Slc39a) transporter genes (Ohno et al., 1985; Liuzzi & Cousins, 2004). The zinc concentration is ~15 times greater in mature RBC than in plasma (Eide, 2006). More than 90% of RBC zinc functions as a component essential for the activity of zinc metalloenzymes, particularly carbonic anhydrase and Cu2+/Zn2+-superoxide dismutase (Ryu et al. 2008). Abnormal levels of Zn2+plays a role in many diseases, including Alzheimer's and type-2 diabetes. Zn is an essential element for plants and other organisms and is involved in many cellular processes, including activation of enzymes, protein synthesis, and membrane stability (Welch et al., 1982). Zinc is involved in numerous aspects of cellular metabolism (Jiménez-Jiménez et al. 1992; Forsleff et al. 1998; Brewer et al. 2010). Zinc deficiency is characterized by growth retardation. The global extent of zinc deficiency is debated, but diets that are high in whole grains and low in meat could lead to deficiency (Qureshi et al. 2006; MacDiarmid et al. 2013). Low zinc supply has the same effect on human cells as on yeast, zinc deficiency might contribute to human diseases that are associated with a build-up of "junked" proteins, such as Parkinson's and Alzheimer's. A similar protective system to Tsa1 also exists in animals, and the research group plans to move ahead by studying that system in human cell culture (MacDiarmid et al. 2013). The authors demonstrated that cells that are low in zinc also produce proteins that counter the resulting stress, including one called Tsa1. Tsa1 could reduce the level of harmful oxidants in cells that are short of zinc (MacDiarmid et al. 2013).

It has been reported that zinc deficiency may be linked to increased inflammation. Liu et al (2013) studied the activity of zinc to control sepsis, the severe systemic response to infection that can lead to death. Using cell models, the team focused on the role of zinc to prevent the inflammation that leads to sepsis; they found that when a pathogen is recognized, the gene that produces the zinc transporter SLC39A8 (ZIP8) is expressed. This transporter then rapidly moves to cell's walls, where it shuttles zinc from the bloodstream into the cell; after cell entry, zinc is then directed to and bonds to a protein that halts further activity (Liu et al., 2013).

7. Is there a role for trace element in human diseases?

Trace elements are metal ions and non-metal ions (e.g. selenium, arsenic) in human body in low concentrations, less than about 0.05 %. Calcium in the body, about 1.4 % is usually considered a macro element but it should be kept in mind that inside cells calcium is present in low concentration as a trace element and needs carefully control as it is a powerful second messenger. Trace elements like vitamins must be added through food as the body can't synthesize trace elements. Some of them are essential e.g. lack may disturb metabolism, sometime causative a disease, Keshan disease. Some examples of essential trace elements: Si, Fe, F, Zn, Cu, Mn, Se, Mo, Co. Knowledge of trace elements has increased a lot since accurate, sensitive, selective analytical technique was developed around 1980, ICP-MS (inductively coupled plasma mass spectrometry).

Trace elements were originally viewed as nutrients and they excerpt pharmacological actions. Some of these possibly essential elements also are receiving attention because of their toxicological or pharmacological properties that can affect health and wellbeing. However possible relation between trace element status and clinical outcomes are insufficient. Extrapyramidal symptoms reflecting nigrostrial dopaminergic hypofunction are common in patients with neuronal ceroid lipofuscinosis and Parkinson's disease. Inadequacy or imbalance of trace elements supply consequently affects a number of physiological functions. Zinc as an elements that may play a protective anti-atherosclerotic role, decreases. Zn is considered an efficient antioxidant (Prasad, 2008). Zn controls metallothionein expression and is involved in, cellular redox regulation (Maret, 2000). Oxidative stress can be corrected by dietary Zn as demonstrated of hepatic antioxidant enzymes (Tupe et. al. 2010). Zn metabolism may be influenced by low intake, lack of protective factors, e.g. Se. Another possibility may be Cd competition with Zn. Cd has higher binding capacity than Zn, e.g. in metallothionein and may displace Zn from its carrier sites. In a study of Parkinson's disease Mn was implicated (Normandie and Hazell, 2002) and another study demonstrated elevated concentrations of Cd in the erythrocytes (Johansson et.al. 2007). Lack of protective elements e.g. selenium in the metabolism makes it easier for heavy metal ions to enter and interfere the metabolism. As trace elements are active in many parts of the cell metabolism the discussion will be focused on possible effects of imbalance due to heavy metal ions in Parkinson's disease.

8. Elemental profiles as an indicator of metal ion and ligand homeostasis

The cell metabolism is a complex balance of proteins, fatty acids, carbohydrates, metal ions and trace elements regulated by DNA and RNA in nucleus and mitochondria. As the metabolism involve many molecular reactions and species not practical to be monitored a simplified indication of metal ion-ligand status, elemental profile, may be a substitute to monitor effects of important cell reactions. The elemental profile may be looked upon as the integrated results of reactions at the moment the sample was taken. It is important to underline that deviations in the elemental profile may also include effects of compounds with strong association to the examined elements. These deviations may give biochemical and physiological insights to observe early changes in the metabolism. Changes of metabolism of metal ions in e.g. erythrocytes may help to understand early reactions, if it is normal or an indication of an early pathophysiological process.

9. Membrane trafficking and dynamics in presence of heavy metal ions

In a study of 12 patients (9 men and 3 women) with Parkinson's disease (Johansson et.al. 2013) erythrocytes showed significant increased concentration of Pb and Ag. The concentration of Cd (9/12) was also higher than that of controls. The observed increased of concentrations of Pb, Ag and Cd may have effects at different levels, e.g. 1. ATP-metabolism and heavy metal ion metabolism 2. Pb, Ag, Cd interactions with dopamine metabolism 3. Axonal transport and membrane trafficking 4. ROS formation by increased activity of hemeoxidases and displaced iron 5. Preapoptosis signals and possible activation of second messengers 6. Pb and porphyrine synthesis

10. Possible sources of metal ion supply

10.1. ATP-metabolism and heavy metal ion interactions

Pb, Cd and Ag has higher association to binding sites than Mg, Ca. Possible effect is displacement of Mg from enolase enzyme which introduces a double bond in the phosphate group. Mg may also be blocked in the phospho-mutase reaction when phosphoglycerate is transferred from position 3 to position 2. Another effect of cadmium ions is inhibition of Na/K ATPase enzyme by 50% in ABC-transporters (Lijnen et. al. 1991). Examples above indicate possible effects of heavy metal ions in the ATP-metabolism.

10.2. Pb, Ag, Cd interactions with dopamine metabolism

In patients with Parkinon's disease the micoenvironment is full of misfolded alfa-Synuclein (George et.al. 2013) in brain (striatum) which may promote aggregation of cells and cause losses in dopamine synthesis. The synthesis in substantia nigria may be blocked by the increased concentrations of Pb, Ag and Ag. Transport of compounds (dopamine, acetylcholine) by vesicles (Kornberg and McConnell, 1971) in axons may be blocked by reactions with heavy metal ions.

10.3. Axonal transport and membrane trafficking

The axonal transport of mitochondria (Hollenbeck and Saxton, 2006, Gunter et.al 2000) may be disturbed by Pb, Cd and Ag by carry over effects. Mitochondria were transported by kinosin, dynein and myosin motors (Zhang and Zhao, 2007). Interactions with the motor transport in axons may be expected to slow down or stop movements when exposed to Pb, Ag and Cd. The transport of Ca (Perin et.al.1990) may be blocked by Pb, Cd and due to stronger association to binding sites in the mitochondria and ER (endoplasmatic reticulum) resulting in poor nerve signals in the axons.

10.4. ROS formation by increased activity of hemeoxidases and displaced iron

The accumulated heavy metal ions in the erythrocytes may disturb oxygen transport and interact with important brain cells. Cd may be used in heme metabolism, reducing heme concentration when sufficient. In a previous study significantly increased concentration of Cd was observed in the erythrocytes (Johansson et.al. 2007). The gene for hemeoxygenases HO-1, HO-2 is Cd dependent (Koizumi et.al.2007, Alami et.al.2000). HO-1, HO-2 hemeoxygenases are important for cleaning up residues of senescent erythrocytes. Low concentrations of Cd may be involved in cleaning up heme residues, too high concentration of Cd may support formation of reactive oxygen species (ROS), superoxide anion, hydroxy free radicals, and singlet oxygen. In the porphyrine synthesis it is important that introduction of iron (ferrochelatase, frataxin) is not blocked by excess Cd, Pb, Ag (Johansson et.al. 2007). Uncontrolled iron may react with oxygen and produce free radicals, Haber-Weiss reactions.

10.5. Preapoptosis signals and possible activation of second messengers

Cd may enter Ca channels (e.g. Gardos channels) in the erythrocyte membrane and introduce interactions in cells (Verbost et.al.1989). Cd, Pb, Ag may release Ca from calmodulin (superfamily of Ca-carriers) due to weaker binding. Ca Is an important secondary messengers in cells activating e.g. flippases. Liberated Ca may activate translocators, flippases, within the cell (Devaux et.al. 2006). Phosphatidylserine in the inner leaflet may be transferred by trans locators to outer membrane giving an apoptosis marker for the macrophages. Phosphatidylserine is normally situated below leflet (Martin et.al. 1995). Increased Pb, Cd, Ag may start too early apoptosis of important cells e.g. neurons (Sopjani et.al.2009).

10.6. Pb and porphyrine synthesis

Pb is not known to be essential to man. Pb has redox capacity (Pb2+or Pb4+) and usually associated in reduced form to other molecules. As about 99% of Pb is associated to erythrocytes in blood one target will be the metabolism of erythrocytes. Pb is known to interfere with aminolevulinic acid dehydratase in the heme synthesis (Flindt et.al. 1976, Kelada et.al.2001). Pb is also known to interact with Ca channels by allowing increased input of calcium starting too early senescence (Lang et.al. 2010).

10.7. Possible sources of metal ion supply

In the study of 12 Parkinson patients (Johansson et.al.2013) there was no information of food habits for individual patients. In Finland cadmium uptake from food is about 5-10 μg/day, lead 20-66 μg /day, silver was not mentioned. In Sweden cadmium uptake from wheat, rice, potatoes, root-crops is about 10-20 μg /day, lead 15-30 μg /day, silver was not reported. In view of contribution from nutrition of heavy metal ions it is interesting to note that cadmium rich diet in Nigeria decreased Hb and erythrocyte counts in mice (Asagba & Eriyamremu 2007). It cannot be excluded that cadmium, lead in food after long time may accumulate in human erythrocytes and likely decrease erythrocyte counts and hemoglobin synthesis. Smoker may have higher cadmium values in blood but there was no information about smoking habits. Implanters may be a source of metal ion supply. Amalgam is an alloy which is not stable but will release mercury, silver (Johansson E1991, Johansson E et.al.1994, Johansson E and Liljefors T, 1991). Studies indicate that released mercury from amalgam will be found in liver, kidney and brain only minor amounts of mercury will be found in the blood indicating need for looking after other indicators. The effects of silver are often missing but should be included due to effects of silver on important antioxidant compounds containing selenium, sulphur. Some amalgam fillings may have small sticks of guttapercha in the cavity. Some trademarks of Gutta-percha contain cadmium but the released amount is not known for the examined patients (Johansson E and Liljefors T 1991).The observations of problems possibly attributed to implanters should be considered in the early diagnosis.

10.8. The discoid shape of erythrocytes and heavy metal ions

Erythrocytes must be able to shrink and expand during transport (Huang et.al. 2010). If Cd, Pb, Ag, are associated to stabilizing proteins, erythrocytes possess a spectrin-based cytoskeleton they may lose their capacity to shrink and expand (Zhang and Zhao, 2007, Bosman et.al. 2008) in the capillaries.

Author details

Erland Johansson[1], Tuomas Westermarck[2] and Faik Atroshi[3]

1 Selenium consultant Ltd, Sweden

2 Rinnekoti Research Centre, Espoo, Finland

3 Pharmacology & Toxicology, University of Helsinki, Finland

References

[1] Liu MJ, Bao S, Galvez-Peralta M, Pyle CJ, Rudawsky AC, Pavlovicz RE, Killilea DW, Li C, Nebert DW, Wewers MD, Knoell DL. “ZIP8 Regulates Host Defense through Zinc-Mediated Inhibition of NF-[kappa]B.” Cell Rep. 2013;3(2):386-400.

[2] Gellein K, Syversen T, Steinnes E, Nilsen TI, Dahl OP, Mitrovic S, Duraj D, Flaten TP Trace elements in serum from patients with Parkinson's disease--a prospective case-control study: the Nord-Trøndelag Health Study (HUNT).Brain research 1219: 2008 Jul 11: 111-5.

[3] Schelosky L, Raffauf C, Jendroska K, Kava and dopamine antagonism (letter). J Neurol Neurosurg Psychiatry 58: 639-40. 1995.

[4] Dan Beth-El. Magic beans? Natural sources of L-Dopa in the treatment of Parkinson's Disease. International J of Comp Med: 11-13. September 1992.

[5] Samii A, Nutt JG, Ransom BR (May 2004). "Parkinson's disease". Lancet 363 (9423): 1783–93.

[6] Poewe W (December 2006). "The natural history of Parkinson's disease". J. Neurol. 253 (Suppl 7): VII2–6.

[7] Davie CA (2008). "A review of Parkinson's disease". Br. Med. Bull. 86 (1): 109–27.

[8] de Lau LM, Breteler MM (June 2006). "Epidemiology of Parkinson's disease". Lancet Neurol. 5 (6): 525–35.

[9] Castagnoli K, Murugesan T (2004 Jan). "Tobacco leaf, smoke and smoking, MAO inhibitors, Parkinson's disease and neuroprotection; are there links?". Neurotoxicology 25 (1–2): 279–91.

[10] Tolosa E, Katzenschlager R (2007). "Pharmacological management of Parkinson's disease". In Tolosa E, Jankovic JJ. Parkinson's disease and movement disorders. Hagerstwon, MD: Lippincott Williams & Wilkins. pp. 110–45.

[11] Hughes AJ, Daniel SE, Ben-Shlomo Y, Lees AJ. The accuracy of diagnosis of parkinsonian syndromes in a specialist movement disorder service. Brain 2002;125:861–870.

[12] Gelb DJ, Oliver E, Gilman S. Diagnostic criteria for Parkinson disease. Arch Neurol 1999;56:33–39.

[13] Sofic E, Lange KW, Jellinger K, Riederer P. Reduced and oxidized glutathione in the substantia nigra of patients with Parkinson's disease. Neurosci Lett. 1992 Aug 17;142(2):128-30

[14] Barichella M, Cereda E, Pezzoli G (October 2009). "Major nutritional issues in the management of Parkinson's disease". Mov. Disord. 24 (13): 1881–92.

[15] Tanner, C. M., Langston, J. F. 1990. Do environmental toxins cause Parkinson's disease? A critical review.Neurology 40(3): 17-31.

[16] de Lau LM, Breteler MM. Epidemiology of Parkinson's disease. Lancet Neurol. 2006 Jun;5(6):525-35.

[17] Noyce AJ, Bestwick JP, Silveira-Moriyama L, Hawkes CH, Giovannoni G, Lees AJ, Schrag A. "Meta-analysis of early nonmotor features and risk factors for Parkinson disease". Annals of Neurology, 2012, 72 (6): 893–901.

[18] Van Maele-Fabry G, Hoet P, Vilain F, Lison D. "Occupational exposure to pesticides and Parkinson's disease: a systematic review and meta-analysis of cohort studies". 2012, Environ Int 46: 30–43.

[19] DeLong MR, Juncos JL. Parkinson's Disease and Other Movement Disorders. In: Kasper DL, Fauci AS, Longo DL, Braunwald E, Hauser SL, Jameson JL, editors. Harrison's Principles of Internal Medicine. 17th ed. New York: McGraw-Hill Medical Publishers; 2008. pp. 2406–17

[20] Di Fabio R, De Filippis S, Cafariello C, Penna L, Marianetti M, Serrao M, Pierelli F. Low doses of rotigotine in patients with antipsychotic-induced parkinsonism. Clin Neuropharmacol. 2013 Sep-Oct;36(5):162-5.

[21] Samii A, Nutt JG, Ransom BR (May 2004). "Parkinson's disease". Lancet 363 (9423): 1783–93.

[22] Poewe W (December 2006). "The natural history of Parkinson's disease". J. Neurol. 253 (Suppl 7): VII2–6.

[23] Davie CA (2008). "A review of Parkinson's disease". Br. Med. Bull. 86 (1): 109–27.

[24] de Lau LM, Breteler MM (June 2006). "Epidemiology of Parkinson's disease". Lancet Neurol. 5 (6): 525–35.

[25] Castagnoli K, Murugesan T (2004 Jan). "Tobacco leaf, smoke and smoking, MAO inhibitors, Parkinson's disease and neuroprotection; are there links?". Neurotoxicology 25 (1–2): 279–91.

[26] Tolosa E, Katzenschlager R (2007). "Pharmacological management of Parkinson's disease". In Tolosa E, Jankovic JJ. Parkinson's disease and movement disorders. Hagerstwon, MD: Lippincott Williams & Wilkins. pp. 110–45.

[27] McCann JC, Ames BN. Adaptive dysfunction of selenoproteins from the perspective of the triage theory: why modest selenium deficiency may increase risk of diseases of aging. The FASEB Journal, 2011; DOI: 10.1096/fj.11-180885

[28] Ames BN. Proc. Low micronutrient intake may accelerate the degenerative diseases of aging through allocation of scarce micronutrients by triage. Natl. Acad. Sci. USA,Vol. 103, pp. 17589-17594, November 2006

[29] Shoffner, J. M . , Watts, R. L. , Juncos,J. L . , Torroni, A . , Wallace, D. C .1991 . Mitochondrial oxidative phosphorylation defects in Parkinson's disease.Ann. Neurol. 30:332-39.

[30] Jenner, P. 1991 . Oxidative stress as a cause of Parkinson's disease. Acta N eurol. Scand. 1 36:6-15 (Supp\.)

[31] Saggu, H., Cooksey, J . , Dexter, D., Wells, F. R . , Lees, A . , et a1. 1989. A selective increase in particulate superoxide dismutase activity in parkinsonian substantia nigra. J. Neurochem.1 53:692-97

[32] Perry, T. L . , Yong, V. W. 1986. Idiopathic Parkinson's disease, progressive supranuclear palsy and glutathione metabolism in the substantia nigra of patients. Neurosci. Lett. 67:269-74.

[33] Ambani, L. M . , Van Woert, M. H . ,Murphy, S . 1975 . Brain peroxidase and catalase in Parkinson's disease.Arch. Neurol. 32: 1 14-1 8.

[34] Shahar A, Patel KV, Semba RD, Bandinelli S, Shahar DR, Ferrucci L, Guralnik JM. Plasma selenium is positively related to performance in neurological tasks assessing coordination and motor speed. Mov Disord. 2010 Sep 15;25(12):1909-15.

[35] McIntosh KG, Cusack MJ, Vershinin A, Chen ZW, Zimmerman EA, Molho ES, Celmins D, Parsons PJ. Evaluation of a prototype point-of-care instrument based on

monochromatic x-ray fluorescence spectrometry: potential for monitoring trace element status of subjects with neurodegenerative disease. J Toxicol Environ Health A. 2012;75(21):1253-68.

[36] Delanty N.; Dichter M. Antioxidant Therapy in Neurologic Disease. Archives of Neurology. 57(9):1265-1270, 2000.

[37] Dworkin RH. Linoleic acid and multiple sclerosis. Lancet 1981; 1153-4.

[38] Soto-Otero R, Mendez-Alvarez E, Hermida-Ameijeiras A, et al. Autoxidation and neurotoxicity of 6-hydroxydopamine in the presence of some antioxidants: potential implication in relation to the pathogenesis of Parkinson's disease. J Neurochem 2000; 74:1605-1612.

[39] McCann JC, Ames BN. Adaptive dysfunction of selenoproteins from the perspective of the triage theory: why modest selenium deficiency may increase risk of diseases of aging. The FASEB Journal, 2011; DOI: 10.1096/fj.11-180885.

[40] Jiménez-Jiménez FJ,; Fernández-Calle, P.; Martínez-Vanaclocha, M.; Herrero, E.; Molina, J.A.; Vázquez, A. and Codoceo, R. Serum levels of zinc and copper in patients with Parkinson's disease. J. Neurol. Sci. 1992, 112(1-2) 30-33.

[41] Forsleff, L.; Schauss, A.G.; Bier, I.D. and Stuart, S. J. Evidence of functional zinc deficiency in Parkinson's disease. Altern. Complement. Med. 1998, 5(1):57-64.

[42] Brewer G.J.; Kanzer, S.H.; Zimmerman, E.A.; Molho, E.S.; Celmins, D.F.; Heckman, S.M. and Dick, R. Subclinical zinc deficiency in Alzheimer's disease and Parkinson's disease. Am. J. Alzheimers Di.s Other Demen. 2010, 25(7):572-575.

[43] MacDiarmid CW, J. Taggart, K. Kerdsomboon, M. Kubisiak, S. Panascharoen, K. Schelble, D. J. Eide. Peroxiredoxin chaperone activity is critical for protein homeostasis in zinc-deficient yeast. Journal of Biological Chemistry, 2013; DOI: 10.1074/jbc.M113.512384.

[44] Qureshi GA, Qureshi AA, Memon SA, Parvez SH.Impact of selenium, iron, copper and zinc in on/off Parkinson's patients on L-dopa therapy. J Neural Transm Suppl. 2006;(71):229-36.

[45] Liuzzi JP, Cousins RJ. Mammalian zinc transporters. Annu Rev Nutr. 2004;24:151–72.

[46] Eide DJ. Zinc transporters and the cellular trafficking of zinc. Biochim Biophys Acta. 2006;1763:711–22.

[47] Ohno H, Doi R, Yamamura K, Yamashita K, Iizuka S, Taniguchi N. A study of zinc distribution in erythrocytes of normal humans. Blut. 1985;50:113–6

[48] Ryu MS, Lichten LA, Liuzzi JP, Cousins RJ. Zinc Transporters ZnT1 (Slc30a1), Zip8 (Slc39a8), and Zip10 (Slc39a10) in Mouse Red Blood Cells Are Differentially Regulated during Erythroid Development and by Dietary Zinc Deficiency.J. Nutr. November 2008 vol. 138 no. 11 2076-2083.

[49] Welch RW, Webb MJ, Loneragan JF (1982) Zinc in membrane function and its role in phosphorus toxicity. In A Scaife, ed, Plant Nutrition 1982, Proceedings of the Ninth International Plant Nutrition Colloquium, Warwick University, UK, August 22–27, 1982. Commonwealth Agricultural Bureaux, Farnham House, Farnham Royal, UK, pp 710–715

[50] Liu MJ, Bao S, Galvez-Peralta M, Pyle CJ, Rudawsky AC, Pavlovicz RE, Killilea DW, Li C, Nebert DW, Wewers MD, Knoell DL. "ZIP8 Regulates Host Defense through Zinc-Mediated Inhibition of NF-[kappa]B." Cell Rep. 2013 Feb 8.

[51] Prasad AS: Clinical, immunological, and antioxidant roles of zinc. Exp.gerontol. 2008.

[52] Maret W: The function of zinc metallothionein, a link between cellular zinc and redox state. J.Nutr.2000,130 (5S Suppl):1455S-8S.

[53] Tupe RS, Tupe SG,Tarwadi KV, Agte VV: Effect of different dietary zinc levels on hepatic antioxidant and micronutrients indices under oxidative stress conditions . Metabolism. 2010. 59(11): 1603-1611.

[54] Normandie I and Hazell AS: Manganese, neurotoxicity: an update of pathophysiological mechanisms. Metab.BrainDis. 2002,17(4), 375-387.

[55] Johansson E, Westermarck T, Hasan MY, Nilsson B, Stephen S, Adem A: Alteration in nickel and cadmium concentrations in erythrocytes and plasma of patients with Parkinson's disease, 2007. Trends in Biomedicine in Finland XXI, vol.2(4), 17-32.

[56] Johansson E, Holmkvist M, Ek P, Westermarck T, Atroshi F: Erythrocytes as biomarkers of changed metal ion homeostais in patients Parkinson's disease. Abstract ISTERH, 2013, Tokyo.

[57] Lijnen P, Staessen J, Fagard R, Amery A :Effect of cadmium on transmembrane Na+ and K+ transport systems in human erythrocytes. 1991. Br.J.Ind.Med.48, 392-398.

[58] George S, Rey NL, Reichenbach N, Steiner JA, Brundin P. ▪ -Synuclein:The long distance runner. 2013. Brain Pathol. 23(3), 350-357.

[59] Kornberg RD and McConnell HM: Inside-outside translocation of phospholipids in vesicle membranes. 1971. Biochemistry 10, 1111-1120.

[60] Hollenbeck PJ and Saxton WM: The axonal transport of mitochondria. 2006. CellScience 118, 5411-5419.

[61] Gunter TE, Buntinas L, Sparagna G, Eliseev R and Gunter K: Mitochondrial calcium transport: mechanisms and functions. 2000. Cell calcium, 288, 285-296.

[62] Zhang Q and Zhao Y: The diverse biofunctions of LIM domain proteins determined by subcellular localization and protein-protein interaction. 2007. Biol.Cell 99, 489-502.

[63] Perin MS, Fried VA, Mignery GA, Jahn R, Südhof TC: Phospholipid binding by a synaptic vesicle protein homologous to the regulatory region of protein kinase C. 1990. Nature 345,260-263.

[64] Koizumi S, Gong PG, Suzuki K and Murata M: Cadmium responsive element of the human heme oxygenase-1 gene mediates heat shock factor 1-17. 2007. J.Biol.Chem. 282, 8715-8723.

[65] Alami J, Wickel C, Syewart D, Gongi P, Touchardi C, Otterbein S, Choi AMK, Burow ME, Ton Jen-sie: Mechanism of heme oxygenase-1, gene activation by cadmium on MCF-7 epithelial cells. 2000, J.Biol.Chem. 275(36), 27694-27702.

[66] Verbost PM, Flik G. Pang PK, Lock RAC and Bonga: SEW: Cadmium inhibition of the erythrocyte Ca2+ pump. 1989. J.Biol.Chem. 264(10), 5613-5616.

[67] Devaux PF, Lopez-Montero I, Bryde S: Proteins involved in lipid translocation in eucaryotic cells. 2006. Chemistry and physics of lipids, 141, 119-132.

[68] Martin SJ, Reutelingsperger CP, McGahon AJ, Rader JA, van Schie RC, LaFace DM, Green DR: Early redistribution of plasma membrane phosphatidylserine is a general feature of apoptosis regardless of the initiating stimulus: inhibition by overexpression of Bcl-2 and Abl. 1995. J.Exp.Med.182(5), 1545-1556.

[69] Sopjani M, Föller M, Haendeler J, Götz F, Lang F: Silver ion-induced suicidal erythrocyte death. 2009. J.Appl.Toxicol.29(6), 531-536.

[70] Flindt ML, King E, Walsh DB: Blood level and erythrocyte delta-aminolevulinic acid dehydratase levels in Manchester taxi drivers. 1976. Br.J.Ind.Med. 33(2), 79-84.

[71] Kelada SN, Shelton E, Kaufmann RB, Khory MJ: δ-Aminolevulinic acid dehydratase genotype and lead toxicity: a HuGe review. 2001. Am.J.Epidemiol.154(1), 1-13.

[72] Lang F, Gulbins E, Lang FA, Zappulla D and Föller M: Ceramide in suicidal death of erythrocytes Cell Physiol. Biochem. 2010. 26(1), 21-28..

[73] Asagba SO & Eriyamremu GE: Oral cadmium exposure alters haematological and liver function parameters of rats fed a Nigerian-like diet. 2007. J.Nutr.Environ.Med. 16(3-4), 267-274.

[74] Johansson E: Selenium and its protection against the effects of mercury and silver. 1991. J.TraceElem.ElectrolytesHealthDis., 5(4), 273-274.

[75] Johansson E, Liljefors T and Plantin L-O: Comparison ICP-MS estimation of elements using quantitative mode and conditional factors, In Trace Element Analytical Chemistry in Medicine and Biology, Madrid 1994, pp.141-146.

[76] Johansson E and Liljefors T: Heavy elements in root tips from teeth with amalgam fillings, In TEMA-7, Zagreb 1991, pp. 11-18-11-20.

[77] Hollenbeck PJ and Saxton WM: The axonal tranport of mitochondria. 2006. J. Cell Science, 118(23), 5411-5419.

[78] Huang Y-X, Wu Z-J, Mehrishi J, Huang B-T, Chen X-Y, Zheng X-Y, Liu W-J, Liu M: Human red cell aging:correlative changes in surface charge and cell properties. 2010. J.Cell Mol. Med., 15(12), 2634-2642.

[79] Bosman GJ, Werre JM, Willekens FL, Novotny VM: Erythrocyte ageing in vivo and in vitro: structural aspects and implications for transfusion. 2008. Transfus.Med.18(6), 335-347.

Chapter 21

Metabolism Changes as Indicated by the Erythrocytes of Patients with Alzheimer's Disease

Erland Johansson, Tuomas Westermarck,
Paul Ek and Faik Atroshi

Additional information is available at the end of the chapter

http://dx.doi.org/10.5772/57511

1. Introduction

The aging processes proceed in small steps making it difficult to separate aging symptoms from early pathological processes. Cell metabolism involves metal ions and trace elements together with compounds necessary for optimal function. In case of imbalance in cells both compounds and distribution of metal ions may be changed but the change of metal ions and trace elements may probably be easier to identify than the large quantity of metabolized compounds. In cells there are distributions of elements, an elemental profile, indicating normal metabolism. Brain has a high demand of oxygen supply and need optimal supply of protection of reactive products. The erythrocytes pass brain many times and other organs accumulating information of elements during their way. We have chosen erythrocytes because oxygen dependent cells need regular supply of oxygen for a stable metabolism. Erythrocytes collect information for about 120 days and then will be replaced by new cells. Elemental profiles of erythrocytes reflect information in their own metabolism (limited metabolism) but may also give important information from other cells by deviations in the homeostasis, the element profile. For monitoring elemental profiles of the erythrocytes we have used inductively coupled plasma mass spectrometry (ICP-MS) which is selective, sensitive and allow analysis of elements in low concentration in a short time.

2. Material and methods

2.1. Patients

Thirteen diagnosed Alzheimer patients, 9 men and 4 women (mean age 61 y) and age matched controls (mean age 58 y) were selected for the study living in the same area. All patients participated voluntarily according to Helsinki declaration.

2.2. Samples

Whole blood (2x7 ml) was drawn into Vacutainer tubes for trace element analysis (BDH, with sodium heparin as anticoagulant). Centrifugation was started half an hour after venopuncture. The erythrocytes were separated by centrifugation at 120xg at 4 C for 15 minutes. After removing the buffy coat the erythrocytes were washed twice with 0.9 % NaCl at 1000xg for 5 minutes. The erythrocytes were transferred to cryo vials (Nunc) weighed and freezed at-18 C. The samples (0.6-0.8g, wet weight) were digested with nitric acid and hydrogen peroxide (both ultra pure) in microwave oven. The samples were diluted with Milli-Q water in 25 ml polypropylene bottles.

2.3. ICP-MS instrumentation

For the elemental analysis of the erythrocytes ICP-MS, Elan 6100 DRC was used in peak hopping mode. The isotopes monitored: ^{107}Ag, ^{114}Cd, ^{208}Pb and ^{238}U. Integration time: 5 sweep, 100 msek. Internal standard 10 ppb Rh was supplied by externally feeding. ^{114}Cd was corrected for ^{114}Sn. The analytical technique used is described in more details [1, 2, 3].

2.4. Reagents and standards

Ultra pure nitric acid and hydrogen peroxide was obtained from Merck. ICP-MS standards were obtained from Johnson & Matthey, SRM 1566a and 1577a from NIST. The different isotopes were validated against Oyster tissue 1566a, Bovine liver 1577a.

The estimated accumulated mean error in the analysis of samples was ± 10 % or less generated in the sampling procedure, preparation, digestion, volumetric and weighing errors and error in the ICP-MS analysis. For statistical calculations of ICP-MS results Wilcoxon's nonparametric test was used.

3. Results

3.1. Elemental profiles of erythrocytes

The main transport of erythrocytes is oxygen from the lungs to cells and carbon dioxide back to lungs serving different organs including brain. The elemental profile of the erythrocytes reflect metabolism of oxygen supplied cells but also the metabolism of the erythrocyte itself.

As erythrocytes carry ferro ions in hemoglobin and other divalent elements e.g. zinc, magnesium, calcium they will also reflect external influence of metabolism. The elemental profile of erythrocytes will be a status report of cell metabolism translated in terms of metal ions and trace elements. In this study we report accumulated ions: silver, cadmium, lead and uranium in the erythrocytes of patients with Alzheimer's disease. The concentration of lead (wet weight) in the erythrocytes of patients with Alzheimer's disease is demonstrated in Figure 1. The result of cadmium analysis (wet weight) of the erythrocytes is shown in Figure 2. The concentration of silver in the erythrocytes is indicated in Figure 3. The concentration of uranium in the erythrocytes was significant higher that of controls Figure 4. In summary the concentrations of Pb, Cd, Ag and U were significant higher than those of controls.

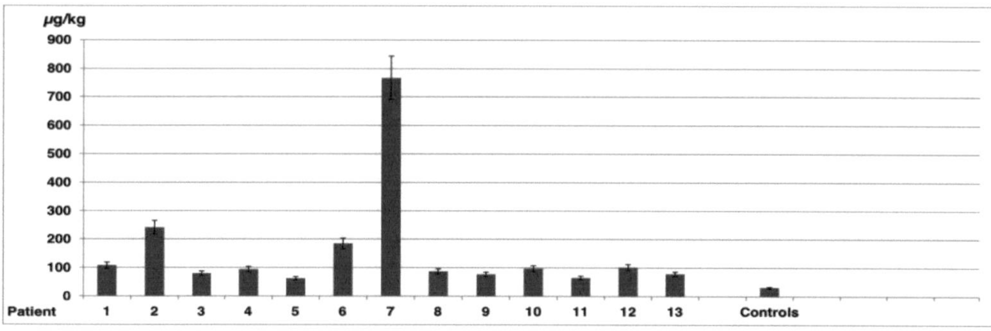

Figure 1. Lead concentration in erythrocytes of 13 patients with Alzheimer's disease. Patient 1-9 men, 10-13 women. Error bar 10%. The mean value of Pb in Alzheimer's patients was 157 μg/kg, mean of controls 31 μg/kg, standard error 52.8 μg/kg. Pb increases normally with age but the Alzheimer group indicate significant (Wilcoxon, $p < 0.005$) higher accumulation.

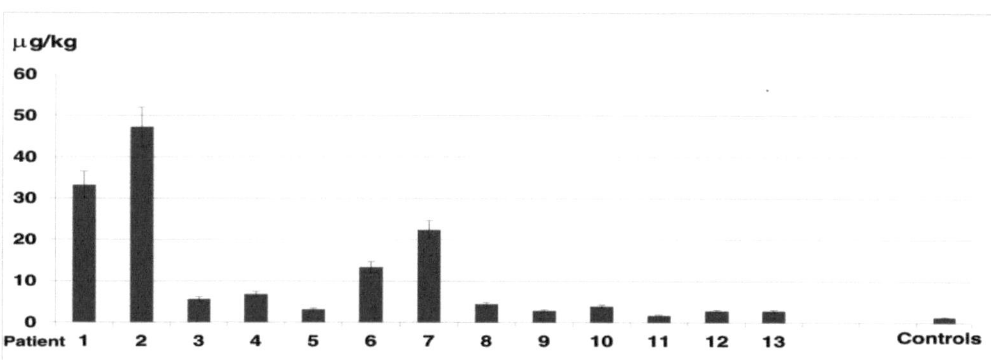

Figure 2. Distribution of cadmium in erythrocytes of 13 patients with Alzheimer's disease. Patient 1-9 men, 10-13 women. Error bar 10%. The mean value of Cd in Alzheimer's patients was 11.5 μg/kg, standard error 3.9 μg/kg, mean of controls 1.3 μg/kg, The concentration of Cd in the erythrocytes of patients with Alzheimer's disease was significant higher (Wilcoxon, $p < 0.05$) than that of controls.

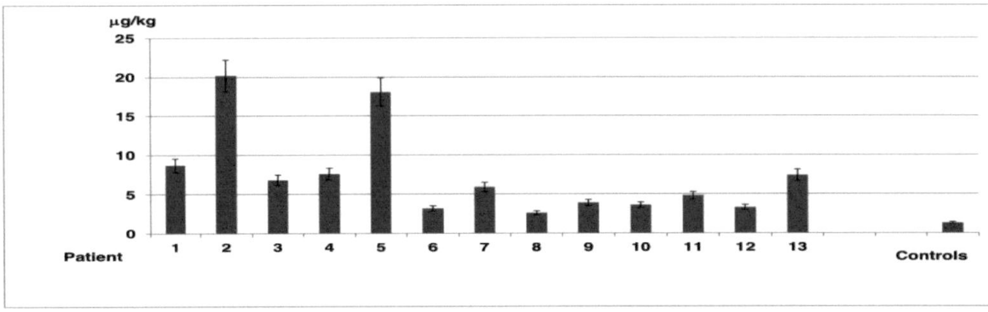

Figure 3. Distribution of silver in erythrocytes of 13 patients with Alzheimer's disease. Patient 1-9 men, 10-13 women. Error bar 10%. The mean value of Ag in Alzheimer's patients was 7.4 µg/kg, standard error 1.5 µg/kg, mean of controls 1.3 µg/kg, The concentration of silver in the erythrocytes of patients was significant higher (Wilcoxon, $p < 0.005$) than that of controls.

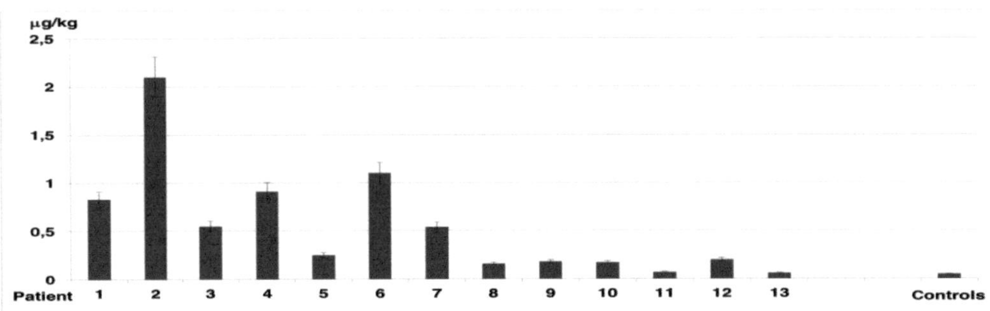

Figure 4. Concentration of uranium in erythrocytes of 13 patients with Alzheimers disease. Patient 1-9 men, 10-13 women. Error bar 10 %. The mean value of U in Alzheimer's patients was 0.55 µg/kg, standard error 0.16 µg/kg, mean of controls 0.11 µg/kg, The concentration of uranium in the erythrocytes of patients with Alzheimer's disease was significant higher (Wilcoxon, $p<0.01$) than that of controls

4. Discussion

Brain has low storing capacity of oxygen though it is a demanding consumer: brain uses about 20 % of oxygen total supply. In degenerative diseases like Alzheimer's, Parkinson's disease the etiology often are not fully known. In Alzheimer's disease pathophysiological theories have been proposed e.g. heat shock protein interactions [4], Tau-protein abnormality [5] neuroinflamation and neuronal loss [6, 7], β-amyloid interactions [8], mitochondrial misfunction [9]. An overlooked possibility may be using ICP-MS for analysis of elemental profiles of erythrocytes as biomarker for Alzheimer 's disease. Small changes in metabolism of oxygen dependent cells may give symptoms difficult to identify due to lack of suitable biomarkers [10, 11, 12. 13, 14]. Erythrocytes carrying excess lead, cadmium, silver and uranium ions may induce damages

http://dx.doi.org/10.5772/57511

in cells including brain cells. Accumulation of elements in the human erythrocytes are a result of low exposure and not of a sudden insult which calls for sensitive biomarkers.

4.1. Effects of accumulated lead, cadmium, silver and uranium in the erythrocytes

At present there is lack of methods to describe the accumulated effects of metal ions in erythrocytes in terms of stability constants or conditional constants. There is lacking information of e.g. solvent properties, pH, temperature, redox properties, lack of knowledge of interacting compounds. Elemental profiles of erythrocytes may be an alternative to estimate changes of trace elements and metal ions at the cellular level. The discussion below will be focused on some effects on membrane integrity by lead, cadmium, silver and uranium because it is not fully known how these ions are associated to other compounds.

4.2. Initiation of eryptosis by accumulated lead, cadmium silver and uranium in erythrocytes

It has been suggested that mature erythrocytes may enter programmed death without the aid of caspase systems [15,16]. Heavy metal ions and organic compounds may be involved in early senescence [17, 18, 19]. When erythrocytes are growing old they will change gradually, fragments will be cleaned up [20, 21], mainly in spleen, liver, bone marrow by the macrophages. Most material of captured senescent erythrocytes e.g. iron and metabolized organic material will be reused [22, 23].

Silver, cadmium ions induce suicidal erythrocyte death [24, 25] and it is likely that erythrocytes and cells dependent on erythrocytes of patients with Alzheimer's disease with accumulated silver and also lead, cadmium and uranium may show early eryptosis. Eryptosis may also be initiated via formation of phosphatidylserine by lead, cadmium, hemin as stimulator [26, 27, 28].

4.3. Erythrocyte channels exposed to accumulated ions of lead, cadmium, silver and uranium

The accumulated lead, cadmium, silver and uranium may interfere the activity in the erythrocyte channels for cations, anions and water. Cadmium, lead, silver may interfere with potassium, calcium [29, 30] and other ions in erythrocyte membranes [31, 32]. Binding in vitro of cadmium to β-amyloid channels was reported by [33]. Exposure to accumulated lead, cadmium, silver, uranium ions to β-amyloid or other compounds is likely to support the pathophysiological process by association to available binding sites.

Anions e.g. chlorides, carbonates ions are transported in anion channels [34, 35, 36] may react with silver, lead, cadmium and uranium disturbing channel transport and oxygen handling.

Aquaporin channels in the erythrocyte membrane are important for flow of water and shape [37, 38, 39]. Accumulated cadmium, lead, silver, uranium ions associated to erythrocyte aquaporin channels may decrease the capacity to shrink and expand. Water exchange may also be important for osmotic regulation when the erythrocytes enter capillaries. It cannot be excluded that lead, cadmium, silver, uranium may release important elements. e.g. calcium from their association sites. Released calcium may form non-selective channels in membranes [40].

4.4. Accumulated cadmium, lead, silver and uranium ions may compete with essential elements in carrier systems

Cadmium is known to compete with zinc in e.g. metallothionein (MT), carrier of zinc. Metal ions having higher affinity than zinc may interact with the binding sites in MT or other carrier. Lead and uranium ions is known to compete with calcium metabolism. Magnesium and calcium ions in calmodulin (calcium carrier) may be displaced by accumulated lead, cadmium, silver, uranium ions and release essential elements e.g. Mg, Ca, Zn. Release of secondary messenger e.g. Mg may disturb ATP metabolism, Ca may activate translocases flippases, floppases, scramblases and start apoptosis signals. Ca may also activate platelets and make them sticky, ready for clot. Sticky platelets may associate to proteins and form placks.

4.5. Sources of cadmium, lead, silver and uranium — Food and implants

The food intake is not known for individual patients. In Finland cadmium uptake from food is about 5-10 μg/day, lead 20-66 μg /day, uranium and, silver was not mentioned [41]. In Sweden is reported cadmium uptake from wheat, rice, potatoes, root-crops 10-20 μg /day, lead 15-30 μg /day, uranium 1-4 μg /day, silver not indicated [42]. Cd uptake from nutrition may disturb the heme synthesis. Cadmium rich diet in Nigeria decreased Hb and erythrocyte counts in mice [43]. It cannot be excluded that cadmium, lead, silver, uranium contaminated food may accumulate in human erythrocytes and in similar manner decrease erythrocyte counts and hemoglobin synthesis. Smoker may have higher cadmium values in blood but there was no information about smoking habits. Elevated uranium in drinking water may damage the kidneys and increase protein loss in urine [44, 45].

In Finland some districts have drinking water with high uranium concentrations (> 100 μg/L) which together with cadmium, lead and silver may increase kidney damage and disturb erythrocyte metabolism. Uranium in the drinking water may explain the significant elevated uranium concentrations of erythrocytes of Alzheimer patients.

Implants may be a source of metal ion supply. Amalgam is an alloy which is not stable [2, 3, 46, 47, 48] (release mercury, silver). Guttapercha may sometime contain cadmium [2] but the released amount is not known for the examined patients. Mercury was not analyzed as mercury will associate strong to liver, kidney also to pituary, low mercury will be found in blood. Mercury has also capacity to displace secondary messenger e.g. Mg, Ca, Zn, Fe when not properly associated.

4.6. Elemental profiles of erythrocytes as biomarkers of Alzheimer's disease by ICP-MS

The early diagnosis of a neurological disease like Alzheimer's and Parkinson's disease is difficult. In Parkinson's disease about 25 % of the patients may get wrong diagnosis [49]. The present study indicate that the elemental profile of erythrocytes may be used as a support in the diagnosis and pathophysiology of Alzheimer's disease. Changes in the elemental profile should be possible to identify earlier due to high sensitivity of ICP-MS. Monitoring elements in the erythrocytes may also be used to observe effects of applied pharmacy and effects on

http://dx.doi.org/10.5772/57511

secondary messengers. More research is needed to interpret early symptoms of Alzheimer disease and pathophysiological processes.

5. Conclusions

Monitoring changes of elements in the erythrocytes by ICP-MS may be used as an early biomarker of Alzheimer's disease and may support the pharmaceutical treatment. The accumulated lead, cadmium, silver and uranium may interfere with channel activities, have effects on apoptosis, react with secondary messenger and support pathophysiological processes.

Acknowledgements

We thank Crafoord foundation for economic support and Åbo Academy for putting instrumental facilities to our disposal. We also thank dr Sture Brishammar, Evert Karlsson for discussions.

Author details

Erland Johansson[1*], Tuomas Westermarck[2], Paul Ek[3] and Faik Atroshi[4]

*Address all correspondence to: erland.johansson@uppsala.mail.telia.com

1 EJSelenium Consultant Ltd, Uppsala, Sweden

2 Rinnekoti Research Center, Helsinki, Finland

3 Laboratory of Analytical Chemistry, Åbo Academy, Finland

4 Department of Pharmacology and Toxicology, University of Helsinki, Finland

References

[1] Johansson E, Westermarck T, Hasan MY, Nilsson B et.al. Alterations in nickel and cadmium concentrations in erythrocytes and plasma of patients with Parkinson's disease. Trends in Biomedicine in Finland 2007; XXI 2(4),17-32.

[2] Johansson E and Liljefors T. Heavy elements in root tips from teeth with amalgam fillings: in TEMA 7 (ed. Momcilovic B), pp 11-18-11-20. Zagreb 1991.

[3] Johansson E, Liljefors T, Plantin L-O. Comparative ICP-MS estimation of elements using quantitative and conditional Saha factors: in Trace Element Analytical Chemistry in Medicine and Biology, vol.7. (eds. Brätter P, Ribas B, Schramel P) pp 141-146. Madrid 1995.

[4] Ji-Sook H. The Hsp90 chaperone machinery from structure to drug development BMB reports 2009;342(10), 623-630.

[5] Lee VM, Goedert M and Trojanowski JQ Neurodegenerative Taupathies Annu Rev Neurosci 2001; 24,1121-1159.

[6] Eikelenboom P, Verhuis R, Scheper W, Roozemuller AJ, van Gool WA et.al. The significance of neuroinflammation in understanding Alzheimer's disease J Neurol Transm 2006; 113(11), 1685-1695.

[7] Eikelenboom PR, van Exel E, Hoozemans JJM, Verhuis R, Roozemuller AJM et.al. Neuroinflammation, an early event in both the history and pathogenesis of Alzheimer's disease. Neurodegenerative disease 2010; 7(1-3), 38-41.

[8] Gharibyan A. Amyloids here, amyloids there.....whats wrong with them? PhD thesis. University of Umeå, Sweden, 2012.

[9] Hedskog L. Mitochondria in Alzheimer disease:regulatory mechanisms and cell-death. PhD thesis, Karolinska Institute, Stockholm, Sweden, 2012.

[10] Bosman GJ, Van der Linden PA, Bartholomeus IG. De Man A.J, De Grip WJ, Van Kalmthout PJ. Erythrocyte aging in the demented elderly: a fluctuating process? Mech Ageing Dev 1998;100(1), 53-58.

[11] Franco RS. The measurement and importance of red cell survival. Am J Haematol 2009;84, 109-114.

[12] Bosman GJ, Willekens FL, Werre JM. Erythrocyte aging: a more than superficial resemblance to apoptosis? Cell Physiol Biochem 2005; 16(1-3), 1-8.

[13] Huang Y-X, Wu Z-J, Marishi J, Huang B-T, Chen X-Y et.al. Human red blood cell aging: correlative changes in surface charge and cell properties J Cell Mol Med 2010; 15(12), 2634-2642.

[14] Daniels G. Structure and function of red cell surface antigens Science Series 2006;1, 3-8.

[15] Bratosin D, Estaquier J, Petit F, Arnoult D, Quatannens B et.al. Programmed cell death in mature erythrocytes: a model for investigating death effector pathways operating in the absence of mitochondria Cell Death Differ 2001; 8(12), 1143-1156.

[16] Lang F, Lang KS, Lang PA, Huber SM, Wieder T. Mechanisms and significance of eryptosis Antioxid Redox Signal 2006; 8(7-8), 1183-1192.

[17] Lang F, Gulbins E, Lang FA, Zappulla D, Föller M. Ceramide in suicidal death of erythrocytes Cell Physiol Biochem 2010;26(1), 21-28.

[18] Föller F, Bobbala D, Koka S, Huber SM, Lang F. Suicide for survival-death of infected erythrocytes as a host mechanisms to survive malaria Cell Physiol Biochem 2009; 24,133-140.

[19] Gatidis S, Fšller M, Lang F. Hemin-induced suicidal erythrocyte death Ann Hematol 2009; 88, 721-725.

[20] Ryter ST, Alami J, Choi AMK. Heme oxygenase-1/Carbon monoxide: from basic science to therapeutic applications Physiol Rev 2006; 86, 583-656.

[21] Koizumi S, Gong P, Suzuki K, Murata M. Cadmium responsive element of the human heme oxygenase-1 mediates heat shock dependent transcriptional activation J Biol Chem 2007:282(12), 8715-8723.

[22] Kay MMB. Mechanism of removal senescent cells by human macrophages in situ Proc Natl Acad Sci USA 1973;72(9), 3521-3525.

[23] Tenhunen R, Marver HS, Schmidt R The enzymatic conversion of heme to bilirubin by microsomal heme oxygenase Proc Natl Acad Sci USA 1968; 61(2), 748-755.

[24] Sopjani M, Föller M, Haendeler J, Gštz F, Lang F. Silver ion-induced suicidal erythrocyte death J Appl Toxicol 2009;29(6), 531-536.

[25] Sopjani M, Fšller M, Dreischer P, Lang F. Stimulation of eryptosis by cadmium ions Cell Physiol Biochem 2008; 22(1-4), 245-252.

[26] Kempe SD, Lang PA, Eisele K., Klart BA., Wieder T., Huber SM. Stimulation of erythrocyte phosphatidylserine exposure by lead ions. Am.J.Physiol Cell Physiol 2005;288(2), C396-C402.

[27] Nguyen DB. Phosphatidylserine exposure in red cells: a suggestion for the active role of red blood cells in blood clot formation PhD thesis. University of Saarland, Saarbrücken, Germany. 2010.

[28] Boas FL, Forman L, Beutler E. Phosphatidylserine exposure and red cell viability in red cell aging and in hemolytic anemia ProcNatl Acad Sci USA. 1998; 95, 3077-3081.

[29] Gardos G. The function of calcium in the permeability of human erythrocytes Biochem Biophys Acta 1958; 30, 653-654.

[30] Lijnen P, Staessen J, Fagard R. Amery A. Effect of cadmium on transmembrane Na+ and K+-transport systems in human erythrocytes Br J Ind Med 1991; 48, 392-398.

[31] Leinders T., van Kleef RGDM,Vijberberg HPM. Distinct metal ion binding sites on Ca2+activated K+channels in inside-out patches of human erythrocytes Biochem BiophysActa 1992; 11-12,75-82.

[32] Lang PA, Kaiser S, Mysaina S, Wieder T, Lang F, Huber SM. Ca2+ -activated K+-channels in human erythrocyte apoptosis. Am J Physiol.Cell Physiol 2003;285(6), C1553-C1560.

[33] Gabriella N, Enrico G, Silvia M, Daniela M. Effect of cadmium ions on amyloid beta peptide 1-42 channels activity J Environ Chem Ecotoxicol. 2011;. 3(12), 309-319.

[34] Akkaya C, Shumulina E, Bobballa D, Brand VB, Mahmud H et.al. The Plasmodium falciparum-induced anion channel of human erythrocytes is an ATP-release pathway Eur J Physiol 2009; 457,1035-1047.

[35] Yamaguchi T, Ikeda Y, Abe Y, Kuma H, Kang DM, Hamasaki N, Hirai T. Structure of the membrane domain of human erythrocyte anion exchanger-1 revealed by electron crystallography J Mol Biol 2010; 397(1), 179-189.

[36] Obaid AL and Crandall ED. $HCO\text{-}_3$ and Cl^-. Exchange across the human erythrocyte membrane: effects of pH and temperature J Membrane Biol 1979; 50, 23-41.

[37] Roudier N, Verhavatz J-M, Maurel C, Ripoche P, Tacnet F. Evidence for the presence of Aquaporin-3 in human red cells J Biol Chem 1998;273, 8407-8412.

[38] Murata K, Mitsuoka K, Walz T, Agre P, Heymann JB, Engel A, Fujiyoshi Y. Structural determinants of water permeation through aquaporin-1 Nature 2000; 407, 599-605.

[39] Bietz S, Montila I, Przyborski JM, Lingelbach K. Recruitment of human aquaporin 3 to internal membranes in the Plasmodium falciparum infectant erythrocyte Mol Biochem Parasitol 2009;167(19), 48-53.

[40] Mironova GD, Gateau-Rosch O, Levrat C, Gritsenko E, Pavlov E, Lazareva AV, Linarenko E, Rey C, Louisot P, Saris N-E. Palmitic and stearic acids bind Ca^{2+} with high affinity and form nonspecific channels in black-lipid membranes, possible relation to Ca^{2+} -activated mitochondrial pores. J Bioenergetics and Biomembranes; 2000; 33(4), 319-330.

[41] Varo P and Koivistonen P Mineral element composition of Finnish Foods in Acta Agr Scand. Suppl.22 (ed. Koivistonen P) pp165-171, Stockholm 1980.

[42] Bielak AT, Holmes J, SavgŒrd J, Schaefer KA Comparison of European and North American approaches to the management and communication of environmental research. Swedish Environmental Protection Agency Report 2009; 5958.

[43] Asagba SO and Eriyamremu GE. Oral cadmium exposure alters haematological and liver function parameters of rats fed a Nigerian-like diet J Nutr Environ Med 2007;16(3-4), 267-274.

[44] Kurttio P, Auvinen A, Salonen L, Saha H, Pekkanen J et.al. Renal effects of uranium in drinking water Environ Health Perspective 2002;110(4), 337-342.